Fat-Soluble Vitamins			Water-Soluble Vitamins						
Vitamin A (µg RE)‡	Vitamin D (µg)§	Vitamin E (mg α-TE) ‖	Vitamin C (mg)	Thiamin (mg)	Riboflavin (mg)	Niacin (mg NE)¶	Vitamin B_6 (mg)	Folacin** (µg)	Vitamin B_{12} (µg)
420	10	3	35	0.3	0.4	6	0.3	30	0.5††
400	10	4	35	0.5	0.6	8	0.6	45	1.5
400	10	5	45	0.7	0.8	9	0.9	100	2.0
500	10	6	45	0.9	1.0	11	1.3	200	2.5
700	10	7	45	1.2	1.4	16	1.6	300	3.0
1000	10	8	50	1.4	1.6	18	1.8	400	3.0
1000	10	10	60	1.4	1.7	18	2.0	400	3.0
1000	7.5	10	60	1.5	1.7	19	2.2	400	3.0
1000	5	10	60	1.4	1.6	18	2.2	400	3.0
1000	5	10	60	1.2	1.4	16	2.2	400	3.0
800	10	8	50	1.1	1.3	15	1.8	400	3.0
800	10	8	60	1.1	1.3	14	2.0	400	3.0
800	7.5	8	60	1.1	1.3	14	2.0	400	3.0
800	5	8	60	1.0	1.2	13	2.0	400	3.0
800	5	8	60	1.0	1.2	13	2.0	400	3.0
+200	+5	+2	+20	+0.4	+0.3	+2	+0.6	+400	+1.0
+400	+5	+3	+40	+0.5	+0.5	+5	+0.5	+100	+1.0

stresses. Diets should be based on a variety of common foods in order to provide other nutrients for which human requirements have been less well

women; therefore the use of 30-60 mg of supplemental iron is recommended. Iron needs during lactation are not substantially different from those of pregnancy.

polyglutamyl forms of the vitamin available to the test organism.
intake (as recommended by the American Academy of Pediatrics) and consideration of other factors such as intestinal absorption.

Estimated Safe and Adequate Daily Dietary Intakes of Additional Selected Vitamins and Minerals*

		Vitamins			Trace Elements†						Electrolytes		
	Age (years)	Vitamin K (µg)	Biotin (µg)	Panto-thenic Acid (mg)	Copper (mg)	Man-ganese (mg)	Fluoride (mg)	Chromium (mg)	Selenium (mg)	Molyb-denum (mg)	Sodium (mg)	Potas-sium (mg)	Chloride (mg)
Infants	0-0.5	12	35	2	0.5-0.7	0.5-0.7	0.1-0.5	0.01-0.04	0.01-0.04	0.03-0.06	115-350	350-925	275-700
	0.5-1	10-20	50	3	0.7-1.0	0.7-1.0	0.2-1.0	0.02-0.06	0.02-0.06	0.04-0.08	250-750	425-1275	400-1200
Children and	1-3	15-30	65	3	1.0-1.5	1.0-1.5	0.5-1.5	0.02-0.08	0.02-0.08	0.05-0.1	325-975	550-1650	500-1500
adolescents	4-6	20-40	85	3-4	1.5-2.0	1.5-2.0	1.0-2.5	0.03-0.12	0.03-0.12	0.06-0.15	450-1350	775-2325	700-2100
	7-10	30-60	120	4-5	2.0-2.5	2.0-3.0	1.5-2.5	0.05-0.2	0.05-0.2	0.1-0.3	600-1800	1000-3000	925-2775
	11 +	50-100	100-200	4-7	2.0-3.0	2.5-5.0	1.5-2.5	0.05-0.2	0.05-0.2	0.15-0.5	900-2700	1525-4575	1400-4200
Adults		70-140	100-200	4-7	2.0-3.0	2.5-5.0	1.5-4.0	0.05-0.2	0.05-0.2	0.15-0.5	1100-3300	1875-5625	1700-5100

From Recommended Dietary Allowances. Revised 1979. Food and Nutrition Board National Academy of Sciences–National Research Council. Washington, D.C.

*Because there is less information on which to base allowances, these figures are not given in the main table of the RDA and are provided here in the form of ranges of recommended intakes.

†Since the toxic levels for many trace elements may be only several times usual intakes, the upper levels for the trace elements given in this table should not be habitually exceeded.

Cont'd on inside back cover

Times Mirror/Mosby
Series In Nutrition

Essentials of Nutrition and Diet Therapy

Sue Rodwell Williams, Ph.D., M.P.H., R.D.

Director, The Berkeley Nutrition Group, and
President, SRW Productions, Inc., Berkeley,
California; Nutrition Consultant, Kaiser-
Permanente Northern California Regional
Metabolic Program, Kaiser Medical Center,
Oakland, California; Field Faculty, M.P.H.-Dietetic
Internship Program and Coordinated
Undergraduate Program in Dietetics, University of
California, Berkeley, California

Fourth Edition
with 94 illustrations

Times Mirror/Mosby College Publishing

St. Louis • Toronto • Santa Clara   1986

A000002319575

Editor: Nancy K. Roberson
Developmental Editor: Rebecca A. Reece
Manuscript Editor: Helen C. Hudlin
Design: Diane Beasley
Cover Design: Christine Leonard Raqnepaw
Production: Barbara Merritt, Florence Fansher

Cover/Photomicrograph of PM crystallizations of citric acid. Institut für Wissenschaftliche Fotografie und Kinematografie.
Photo credits: p. 3 NASA; pp. 19, 181, 243, 269, 295, and 331 H. Armstrong Roberts; pp. 41, 57, 87, 105, 353, 371, 389, and 477 Dan Sindelar; pp. 73, 139, 215, 313, 415, 453, 507, and 559 G. Robert Bishop; and p. 533 Mallinckrodt Institute of Radiology.

Fourth Edition
Copyright © 1986 by Times Mirror/Mosby College Publishing
A division of The C. V. Mosby Company
11830 Westline Industrial Drive, St. Louis, Missouri 63146

Previous editions copyrighted 1974, 1978, 1982

Printed in the United States of America

Library of Congress Cataloging-in-Publication Data

Williams, Sue Rodwell.
    Essentials of nutrition and diet therapy.

    Includes bibliographies and index.
    1. Diet therapy.   2. Nutrition.   I. Title.
[DNLM: 1. Diet Therapy.   2. Nutrition.   QU 145 W727e]
RM216.W683   1986   613.2   85-28355
ISBN 0-8016-5539-0

C/VH/VH   9 8 7 6 5 4 3 2 1   03/B/318

To **My Students**
whose "whys" and "hows" and "so whats"
keep my feet to the fire of knowledge
and make the learning process exciting
and ever new to me

Preface

Through three previous editions, this compact "little" book has served the needs of students and teachers in the health sciences in many colleges, as well as providing a sound but simple reference for busy practitioners. In truth, in all its editions as its title indicates, it has captured and distilled the essence of my larger more comprehensive college and university text-book, *Nutrition and Diet Therapy,* to lay a faithful foundation for further study and practice.

In this new fourth edition I have adhered to these same fundamental goals. But in reality this is a new book. Here I have largely rewritten and greatly expanded the material and its organization to meet the more comprehensive needs of beginning students in the health professions today. It displays a completely new design and format, yet retains its sound, simple, substantive content, thoroughly updated and realistically applied to meet human health needs in our rapidly changing modern world.

Major Changes in This Edition

As indicated, this book is in essence an abridgement of my larger text. It follows a similar new look and style to facilitate learning and lay an initial foundation for sound clinical practice. To achieve these expanded goals in this new edition, I have made a number of major changes.

1. New Chapters
   Several new chapters apply the expanding science of nutrition to changing health care needs and provide in our developing technology tools for its clinical practice and management. These chapters include Chapter 14, "Nutrition and Physical Fitness"; Chapter 17, "Drug-Nutrient Interaction"; and Chapter 24, "Computers in Nutrition Practice."

2. New Book Format and Design
   To enhance its appeal and draw students into its content, this edition uses an entirely new format and design. Its one-column, two-color text is easier to read, and its greater visual impact heightens interest and learning.

3. New Learning Aids
   The new format involves a number of new learning aids, described later, that stimulate the dynamic teaching-learning process. These aids provide numerous clinical reference tools, apply the science of nutrition to current practice, and address current nutrition-related issues and controversies.

4. New Illustrations
   To help create an enhanced design and enriched learning support, new illustrations have been used. Many anatomic illustrations, graphic flow charts, and photographs portray concepts discussed and help students grasp the clinical problems encountered in patient care.

5. Enhanced Readability and Student Interest
   At least 90% of the text has been rewritten to draw students into the material, with a writing style designed to capture interest and present a comprehensive substance that is both simple and sound. Many issues of student interest and public-professional controversy are introduced. The many examples open up meaning and understanding. Topics of current relevance clarify questions and concerns.

Additional Changes New to This Edition

In addition to these major changes, I have made substantive changes in the development and organization of material in this new edition:

1. Chapter 1 has been rewritten to provide a much broader updated focus needed by all health professionals in our rapidly changing world. This introductory focus centers on four basic areas: (1) an interdependent world view of problems in nutrition and human health; (2) a concern with our major U.S. health problems, which require a team approach to providing care and finding solutions; (3) a new outlook on changing health care systems and practices; and (4) a consideration of the expanded role of nutrition in health care and clinical practice to help meet these changing needs.

2. Part One, "Introduction to Human Nutrition," includes much updating and new material based on current research in the nutritional sciences and its application in clinical practice. For example, new content is included on dietary fiber, apolipoproteins, vitamins, and the trace minerals to help students distinguish faddish claims from sound ideas and practice in their study and patient care.

3. Part Two, "Community Nutrition: The Life Cycle," includes new organization of material on community nutrition that focuses on family and individual nutritional needs through the life cycle with emphasis on *health maintenance*. A newly integrated chapter on the food environment and food habits, a new chapter on nutrition and *physical fitness*, and a completely rewritten chapter on *weight management* reflect new research and practice based on a "health model."

4. Part Three, "Introduction to Diet Therapy," presents an expanded clinical nutrition section, all areas updated and rewritten to reflect current research and practice. The section's new introductory chapter bases sound nutritional therapy squarely on sound *assessment* of need and the unfolding patient care process. A new chapter relates *drug-nutrient interactions* to more comprehensive nutritional assessment and therapy. All clinical care topics then correlate nutritional care with these modern approaches to overall patient care and education. For example, the chapter on diabetes mellitus relates new trends in all phases of therapy, including diet, insulins, glucose monitoring, exer-

cise; the renal disease chapter includes new sections on dialysis; the surgery chapter has expanded material on current parenteral feeding (TPN, PPN); the cancer chapter reviews nutritional support approaches and current enteral modes. Finally, a new chapter on *computers in nutritional care* concludes the section, describing applications of this new technology in practice management.

Learning Aids Within the Text

Throughout the text, many learning aids help to unify and teach the comprehensive material:

1. *Chapter openers* focus immediate attention on the key chapter topic, giving a brief summary statement and related photograph.

2. *Chapter headings and subheadings* of special type and color make for easy reading, organization of content, and relationship of key concepts.

3. *Marginal material* highlights definitions, data, comments, charts, line drawings, and includes photos to expand understanding of text discussion.

4. *Boxed clinical application material* displays various principles and concepts explained in the text.

5. *Definitions of terms* are clarified in three tiers—running text, accompanying marginal expansion, and a summary glossary complete with pronounciation guide at end of the book to give ready alphabetized reference to all key terms used. This three-level approach to vocabulary development greatly improves overall study and use of the text.

6. *Illustrations and color emphasis* integrate page design and content with clarifying artwork.

7. *Chapter summaries* review chapter highlights and help students place details in the "big picture."

8. *Review questions* help test comprehension of chapter material and lead students to analyze key concepts.

9. *Further readings* provide brief annotated guides to expanded background sources relevant to chapter topics.

10. *Issues and Answers* present short articles on current issues and controversies related to chapter material to stimulate thinking, practical application, and questions.

11. *Diet guides* in clinical chapters provide sample food lists for patient care and education.

12. *Appendixes* include many new reference tables and tools to enhance study projects and practice. The Food Value Tables include major nutrient references and material on fiber, sodium, and fast foods. Current American Dietary Association food lists are given for diet calculations and meal patterns.

13. *The Index* extends the basic text cross-referencing and alphabetizes the book's content topics.

Supplementary Materials

As a companion to this new edition of the basic text, an expanded and updated student guide is also provided—*Self-Study Guide for Nutrition and Diet Therapy, edition 4*. This concise little companion includes many items to support learning of each chapter's content: (1) chapter focus; (2) summary-review quiz; (3) discussion questions to stimulate thinking; (4) true-false and multiple choice test items to test comprehension; (5) numerous guides for individual and group projects that involve experiments, case studies, and situational problems that apply learning; and (6) inquiry questions that relate an "Issues and Answers" article to current health care problems.

Personal Approach

My person-centered approach in past editions remains in this new text. It is further enhanced here by (1) a writing style that reflects my own personal convictions about patient care; (2) extensive use of personal files and materials gathered from my own clinical practice, teaching, and biochemical work; and (4) practical applications of scientific knowledge in realistic *human* terms to find personal solutions to individual problems.

Acknowledgements

Many persons have helped me in this book project and I am grateful for their contributions. To these persons I give my thanks: to my publisher and editorial staff, especially my fine developmental editor, Rebecca Reece, for her constant skill and support and to the reviewers for their valuable time and suggestions. A first group of reviewers examined the third edition to help lay valuable ground work for manuscript development: Marcia Floyd, Guilford Technical Community College; David Holder, Wallace State College; Susan A. Schongalla, Southern Conneticut State University; and Darlene Stewart, William Rainey Harper College. A second group reviewed the initial manuscript for the fourth edition and gave valuable suggestions for developing the final draft: Barbara Bloom, Cypress College; Nancy Burminski, University of Evansville; Marcia Floyd, Guilford Technical Community College; Elizabeth Parrela, Mattatuck Community College; and Elizabeth Pinar, Front Range Community College.

I also thank my own staff, especially my production manager, Ruth Williams, for her skillful manuscript production and personal help; my many students, interns, colleagues, clients, and patients, all of whom have taught me much; and my family who never cease to support all my efforts and who always share in whatever I am able to achieve.

Sue Rodwell Williams
Berkeley, California

Contents

Part One

Introduction to Human Nutrition

Chapter 1
Nutrition and Health

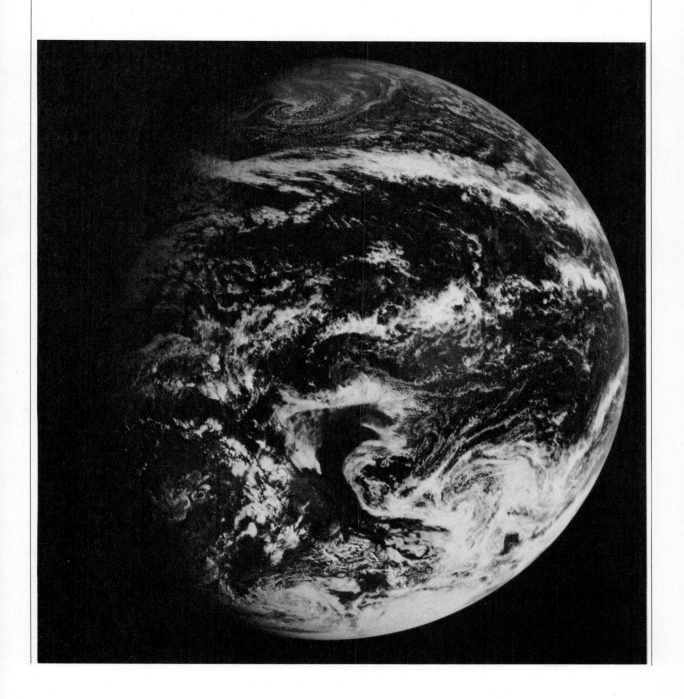

Preview

Why should persons working in health care be concerned about nutrition? What is health? How is nutrition related? What is nutrition? What does it *do?*

To answer such basic questions and meet realistic and practical needs in today's world, a study of nutrition and health care must focus first on *change.* Our physical bodies and personalities, our scientific knowledge and society are all constantly changing. For health maintenance, these constant changes must be in some kind of *positive balance* to produce an integrated whole. Thus in our study the learning concepts of *change* and *balance* will provide a fundamental framework.

In this first chapter we introduce three interdependent issues: a broad world nutrition view, an understanding of our own major U.S. health problems, and a person-centered health team approach for meeting these problems, promoting health, and preventing disease. We will consider the far-reaching effects of change in today's world on nutrition and health, the ways persons view and define health and disease, and the role of nutrition in health care.

Chapter Objectives

After study of this chapter the student should be able to:

1. Identify today's main world health problems and describe their root causes in terms of food security.

2. Define the major U.S. health problems and relate them to social and nutritional factors.

3. Identify four major social influences on our changing concepts of health and disease.

4. Identify four basic changes in the current U.S. health care system and their effects on our health care practices, especially team care.

5. Describe the expanding role of nutrition in health care and define human nutrition in terms of health needs and personal/social needs.

Nutrition and World Health

Main World Health Problems
Food Security

Perhaps in no other area does the realization of the necessity of mutual interaction and dependency among the countries of our world become more evident than in the issue of food security and, hence, survival. This new concept of food security is of great concern in international discussions today. The 1983 World Food Report of the Food and Agriculture Organization of the United Nations (FAO) focused on food security and the three basic sets of issues on which it depends: *food production, stability of food supplies,* and *economic access to food.*[1] We have long since learned, often through sad experience, that in our small world events in one place cause disrupting effects in other parts of the world. We know increasingly that in a very real sense we are all bound together for survival.

Population Expansion and Food Supply

With our expanding world population, the ultimate objective of world food security is to ensure that all people are able to buy or grow the basic food they need. But this is not a simple problem with simple solutions. Although the world has made some progress in coping with its food problems over the past decade, the tasks that still lie ahead are monumental. As the FAO report[1] indicates, the surplus food stocks of exporting countries do not fill the bellies of the undernourished in a major part of the world. A major determinant of food security in the world is the agricultural production possible in developing countries of south and east Asia, since these countries contain about half of the world's population. Food security in these populous regions is still fragile. The most devastated area is the African sub-Sahara region where countries face staggering problems, as evidenced by the appalling famine in Ethiopia.[2] Although the multifaceted nature of malnutrition has many roots, several interrelated problems lie at its heart: (1) poverty, (2) population growth, (3) soil deterioration as a result of poor farming methods, (4) political turmoil, and (5) maldistribution of the world's food supply.

Malnutrition Diseases

By far the greatest world health problem is that of **protein-energy malnutrition** with its attendant infectious diseases, followed by *nutritional anemias* principally caused by iron deficiency, and *vitamin A deficiency,* which causes widespread blindness. Other continuing problems include classic nutritional deficiency diseases such as endemic goiter, pellagra, beriberi, scurvy, and rickets. In 1982 the FAO began a long-term program to help raise nutritional standards in the poorest countries by applying nutritional guidelines to all its development projects and providing assistance in community education and training.[1] It also began regional workshops in 1983 to improve national skills in nutrition assessment and planning.

Major U.S. Health Problems

In the past, our killer diseases were infections such as smallpox, diphtheria, pneumonia, and tuberculosis. For these, we found "magic bullets" in specific antibodies and vaccines. Today, however, our problems are more

Protein-energy malnutrition Malnutrition caused by a deficiency of both protein and kilocalories as compared with protein deficiency in the presence of adequate kilocalories.

Approximately 15 to 20 million people in the world, principally in the poorer countries, die each year of hunger-related causes. It is estimated that some 450 million persons throughout the world suffer from severe malnutrition, consuming less than 1.2 times the kilocalories required to maintain even the basal metabolic rate.

complex and there are no simple solutions. Our major health problems center on the so-called "diseases of civilization"—heart disease and cancer. Additional problems include those stemming from complications of diabetes mellitus, which are related to heart disease and renal disease.

Heart Disease

Every day, about 3400 Americans, more than two each minute, suffer a heart attack. In addition, every day approximately 1600 people suffer strokes. Coronary heart disease alone is responsible for some 650,000 deaths per year, with more than 150,000 of these occurring in people less than 65 years old.

The major cause of death in the United States and other Western societies for the past half century has been and continues to be diseases of the heart and blood vessels. The magnitude of this health care problem is enormous. In addition to the human toll, diseases of the heart and blood vessels extract a severe social and economic cost on the families affected. Major nutrition-related problems center on (1) the body's handling of fats and cholesterol and (2) the large amount of dietary sodium found in an individual's diet in relation to a major risk factor for heart disease—hypertension. Look for a broader discussion of this major U.S. health problem in Chapter 20.

Cancer

About 440,000 Americans die each year of cancer. A majority of these persons, about 25%, die of lung cancer.

In its many forms, cancer has become one of our major public health problems, accounting for about 20% of the total deaths in the United States, close on the heels of our number one killer, heart disease, which accounts for about 50% of the total. Although published research results are conflicting, important relationships between nutrition and cancer seem to exist in two basic areas: (1) prevention of cancer by improvement of the environment and the body's defense system and (2) therapeutic nutritional support for medical treatment and rehabilitation. Look for more detail about these nutritional relationships in Chapter 23.

Diabetes Mellitus Complications

Atherosclerosis Condition in which yellowish plaques (atheromas) are deposited within the medium-sized and large arteries.

Glomerulosclerosis Scarring and aging of renal glomeruli.

In the United States diabetes has become the fifth ranking cause of death from disease. Among older persons with diabetes the cause of death from diabetic complications is mainly myocardial infarction, or heart attack. The underlying pathology of coronary heart disease, or **atherosclerosis,** is two to three times more common in persons with diabetes than in the general population. The major complicating cause of death among younger persons with diabetes is renal failure as a result of **glomerulosclerosis**. Kidney disease is a leading cause of lost work time and income and is the fourth leading health problem in America today. Good dietary control supported by insulin and exercise often helps prevent these diabetic complications. A broader discussion of these related problems—diabetes and renal disease—occurs in Chapters 18 and 21.

General Malnutrition and Poverty

Although small in scope in comparison to the difficulties affecting underdeveloped countries as described previously, the encroaching problem of malnutrition occurs in low income American families caught in the grip of unemployment and poverty. General economic problems involving regional and racial poverty have caused more and more middle income families to slip below the national identified poverty income level. For the families involved, this problem has enormous repercussions in their standard of living and food intake. Look for more details about this food economics problem in Chapter 10.

The Team Approach to Health Care

Health care Term used to refer to the preventive philosophy of helping persons maintain optimum wellness, productivity, and enjoyment of life—a broader, more positive term as compared with the traditional term "medical care," which has been used to denote a curative or illness (crisis) intervention approach.

How do we handle these **health care** problems? What kind of care is needed? Born of necessity, a two-fold approach is emerging: *person-centered care* provided through the coordinated efforts of a strong **health care team**.

Person-Centered Care

Each person is a unique individual and brings to the practitioner-patient encounter that which no professional can supply— the individual's personal experience with the health problem. Despite the attitudes of some practitioners, the ultimate decisions concerning management of a person's health care problem will be made not by the practitioners but by the persons in the family involved. Thus, throughout this text, you will find constant applications of this basic premise—that effective health care must focus on the identified needs of the individual and involve that individual directly in the care provided.

Health care team Interrelated network of components by which health care is made available to persons. May include such components as group or team of health care providers (physicians, nurses, nutritionists, etc.), prepaid health insurance plans, places of care (hospitals, health centers, community projects), health screening, education, therapies, etc.

Health Care Providers

The strong team efforts of a group of health care providers can effectively meet a broad range of health care needs. A rapidly increasing number of people needing care has brought tremendous pressure on community health resources. Most physicians realize that the time is long past when they can be all things to all people. The modern physician is usually interested in the joint effort of building an effective health care team.

Changing Concepts of Health and Disease

Reasons for Changes in Health Views
View of Health

In the past, health has usually been defined simply as the absence of disease. Thus the basic approach to care was curative. The education and training of hospital and community workers centered primarily on learning certain skills for treatment of illness or for crisis intervention. In more primitive societies, disease was associated with evil spirits, or mysterious supernatural powers to be driven out of the body. Treatment of disease, therefore, was in the hands of a religious leader of the group, the shaman, who acted as both priest and physician. In underdeveloped countries this approach still exists and is being blended with more modern medical knowledge. Gradually, as scientific knowledge has increased, the biologic basis for disease has become well established. Consequently, in developed countries public and personal hygiene has improved, treatment for specific diseases has become more scientific and skilled, and many of the most lethal childhood diseases have been eliminated.

Human Values

Faced now with the so-called gift of longer life, we view health increasingly in more qualitative human terms. *Health concepts* have moved from the wholly negative view of health as the absence of disease—the *curative approach*—to a more positive view of optimal human fulfillment and productivity—the *preventive approach* of health promotion.[3] But health is a relative concept in any culture. Health competes with other values and is relative to a culture's way of life. This recognition of differences in needs extends the concept of health to include moral, philosophical, and religious dimensions. Perhaps, then, a realistic goal would be to achieve a level of physical and mental health that would make for social well-being within the individual's social system. Such a goal must provide opportunity for personal self-fulfillment and productivity. To meet it, today's education for students in the health care fields requires an integrated study of the whole person, the community, and personal health needs.

Social Influences

A number of factors in our rapidly developing society have contributed to changes in attitudes toward health values and practices:

Expansion of scientific knowledge The rate of expansion of present scientific knowledge is almost incomprehensible. Knowledge of nutrition—the body's intricate chemistry—and its interaction with the environment is constantly increasing. Also, technology for applying this basic knowledge is rapidly advancing. Using this knowledge challenges and taxes health care facilities. Cures for specific diseases and a wide variety of treatment techniques, drugs, and electronic instruments have all become a regular part of medical care, and, although life saving and extending in many ways, such rapidly expanding scientific knowledge has created problems. Increased specialization brings fragmentation of care and removal of patients still farther from their physicians and other allied practitioners, sometimes creating feelings of being lost within the system. Also, with this increasing complexity of care have come increasing costs and ethical questions about the use of our costly new medical technology.

1980 census indicates a percentage increase of Asian immigration during the past decade of 127.6%. Most of these people have settled in the West helping to give California the largest population (23.7 million) among the states and making it the most urban of the states.

Population increase The population is increasing in many nations of the world, especially those that can least afford to feed such growing numbers. According to the 1980 census, the U.S. population has grown to 232.6 million.[4] The "baby-boom" generation of the 1940s continues to create a demographic bulge affecting everything from the housing market to Social Security payments. This generation is not conforming to historical patterns of American life: they are marrying later, divorcing more frequently, postponing childbirth, and setting up smaller households. Also, recent immigration has affected the nature of our population. During 1977-1979, the number of persons admitted to the United States surpassed figures for any year since the early 1920s. In particular, the Asian population increased because of the influx of thousands of refugees and immigrants. Attendant health care needs have grown.

At any given point in time, about 20% of our total population is moving to a different place.

In general, the recent American population increase is reflected not only in total numbers but also in percentage shifts in age and location. There is an increasing percentage of older people and there is greater overall mobility. Urban-suburban trends have created changes in individual psychologic patterns, in family patterns, and in community and national social patterns. All these changes affect health needs and social values.

Social changes Radical changes in family and community patterns have developed in our highly industrialized society. Crowded, low-income housing in the cities contrasts with sprawling, affluent suburbs that consume, at an alarming rate, open land that was once used for agriculture. Economic affluence, the higher cost of living, and more emphasis on post-secondary education—all in the face of increasing poverty in urban and rural areas—have changed human goals, health values, and medical care programs.

Development of the social sciences The behavioral sciences—psychology, sociology, and anthropology—are contributing insights concerning human behavior in response to illness and food habits. There is a new effort within the health professions to understand and help the total patient. More time is devoted to analysis of the impact of social and cultural factors on the concept of good health.

Functional illness is recognized as a very real phenomenon. An individual's life situation and reaction to stress must be considered if total health needs are to be met.

Effects of Change on Health Care Practices

Basic Changes in the Health Care System
Focus of Care

The change in focus of care includes attention to the social issues that lie at the roots of disease and are involved in health status. This goal places value and emphasis on preventive health maintenance and promotion rather than on the exclusive traditional medical approach of crisis intervention and curative practice. In the future, health workers at all levels will be more involved in dealing with the "whole self" and in working more in the areas of community and legislative action, family and community health projects, and primary family care and health education.

Systems of Providing Care

Changes in our health care delivery systems are increasingly based on the work of *health care teams* providing primary care in a *variety of settings*. Primary care practitioners, assisted by support personnel, work in a number of various satellite clinics or health centers, as well as in central-core medical centers. There are extended-care facilities based on degree of care needed; community health centers and special clinics such as those for nutrition, home-management counseling, and maternity and child care; and outreach clinics in more remote rural areas.

Role of Patients and Clients

Changing relationships with patients and clients is evident in their increasingly active role in their own care. They must be involved in planning and decision-making. They must be given more opportunity for better education in nutrition and general health to help them toward more positive health behavior, wiser use of health care facilities, and self-care. (See Issues and Answers on pp. 17-18)

Payment for Services

The traditional fee-for-service practice of American medicine and the rapidly rising costs of medical care often place such care beyond the reach of many persons who need it most. Changes in payment mechanisms are therefore moving toward a variety of plans such as prepaid group medical practice, health maintenance organizations (HMOs), various forms of individual and group health insurance, including some form of national health insurance.

Changing Health Care Values and Attitudes
The Science and Art of Clinical Care

Science is a body of systematic knowledge, facts, and principles born of controlled research that shows the operation of natural law. The rapid advances in scientific knowledge have provided all clinicians with a stronger base on which to build professional practice. *Art* is the exceptional ability to conduct any human activity. All practitioners must base their practice on sound scientific knowledge *and* they must know and care about people and their needs.

Unique Team Position of Nutritionist and Nurse

RD—Registered Dietitian.

Whether functioning in the hospital, the clinic, or the community, the clinical dietitian, or clinical nutrition specialist,[5,6] and the nurse hold positions on the health team that are in a unique relation to the patient. Their roles are changing as their team responsibilities expand. The clinical dietitian (RD), holding both professional certification and graduate degrees in nutritional science, determines nutritional care needs in relation to medical diagnosis and care as well as individual patient needs. The nurse assists the dietitian with this nutritional care, applying it in her general nursing care. In many respects these two health professionals are closest to the patient and the family and have the opportunity to determine many of the patient's needs. They must coordinate services and help the patient understand and participate in personal care. Such sensitive practitioners realize that their most therapeutic contribution is their genuine involvement and concern.

In personalized patient care, remember that often your most therapeutic tool is *yourself.*

Nutrition in Health Care

In the midst of such significant changes in society and in approaches to health care, nutrition can no longer be viewed in the narrow, isolated sense that may have been common in the past (see box, p. 11). It is intimately involved in these broader changes in total health care.[7]

Changing Concepts of Nutrition

Several interrelated areas of social and scientific change are reflected in changing nutritional needs, problems, and priorities.

Rapidly Changing Food Environment

From 1970 to 1980, fast-food sales rose 300%, from $6.5 billion to $23 billion per year. About 90% of all Americans eat periodically in a fast-food restaurant; 10% eat fast foods more than five times a week.

No longer do we always have "regular food" and home meals as in past generations. The number of "fast food" outlets has been increasing rapidly (see p. 209). Also, the growing food industry is producing an increasing number of new processed food products. These include a wide variety of combination, "convenience," synthetic, and textured foods. Two basic problem areas result: (1) primary single foods of known nutrient composition tend to be used less often so more practical guides related to nutrient contribution of a variety of foods and food products need to be developed, and (2) the need for nutrition education in schools, homes, clinics, hospitals, and the marketplace has increased. Confusing claims and

Clinical Application

Practical Applied Nutrition

Since sound nutrition is fundamental to health maintenance and a significant support in any medical care, it is imperative that all practitioners incorporate it in everyday practice. You will help to strengthen the nutritional base of your patient care by doing three basic things:

- **Develop a sound basic working knowledge of nutrition** This includes a knowledge of nutrients and their functions and the ability to distinguish between sound and unreliable references and resources.
- **Use the human approach** In dealing with individuals, personal lifestyle and living situation must be considered. Practical problems related to meeting nutritional needs are always important considerations.
- **Apply principles of nutrition education to every patient situation** Nutrition education is necessary to: (1) improve individual nutritional status, (2) combat malnutrition and misinformation, (3) provide tools for expanded, sound self-care, and (4) motivate persons toward desired food behavior changes. All of this has to be accomplished through a recharged and sensitized *person-centered* approach.

counter claims and misleading advertising increase the difficulty of buying wisely.

Increased Consumer Awareness and Action

The development of broad communications media, especially television, and the national attention given to nutritional problems of the poor and the aged and to questionable food additives have increased public awareness of the role of nutrition in health. Questions are being raised, and consumers are seeking information on nutrition.

Changing Socioeconomic and Population Trends

Shifts in population patterns and an increase in the number of older persons have focused attention on nutrition problems in two basic areas:

Malnutrition in poverty areas An increasing number of persons in large cities especially among minority groups, in migrant working populations, and in rural areas face the pressure of unemployment and reduced income.

Malnutrition and chronic health problems in the aging population Attitudes of our youth-and-action-oriented society toward the aged, compounded by problems of health and economic security, often isolate and bring despair to elderly persons (see Chapter 16). Realistic programs are needed to promote nutrition education, food assistance related to better nutrition, and the care of chronic conditions such as heart disease and diabetes.

Definition of Human Nutrition

At its fundamental level, *human nutrition* may be defined as the process of meeting human health needs in the context of basic human personal needs by nutritional means.

Human Health Needs

Four basic frames of reference help us identify human health needs in our patients and clients:

Age group needs Human beings progress through normal growth and development from the prenatal period, birth, infancy, and childhood through adulthood in the continuing aging process leading to death. In each of these stages specific physical growth patterns and psychosocial development occur. Each age group has its special needs and nutritional requirements (see Chapters 11, 12, and 13). Food habits are specifically related to the growth and development process.

Stress factors Stresses in individual life situations are caused by physical, mental, or emotional problems. Depending on personal strength, reserves, and resources available, the stress may be handled well or it may become unmanageable. The effect of stress on the body and the degree of adjustment or method of coping will have to be considered in determining needs.

Health status A person's degree of health or disease, not only the actual situation but the situation as each person perceives it, influences nutritional or food modification needs.

Basic human needs Such physiologic survival needs as food and water and safety and comfort, respectively, must be met before the higher needs for love, self-esteem, and creative growth can be met. Basic nutrition and health needs are related to each of these general human needs in achieving the overall goal of personal integrity.

Relation of Nutrition to Health

It is evident, therefore, that nutrition is specifically related to both physical and emotional health:

Physical health Life in its most fundamental sense—survival—depends on air, water, and food. These basic life-support materials supply the body with certain essential chemicals that enable it to do its work. Oxygen from the air combines with chemical materials—nutrients—in food and water to enable the body to carry on all its functions. We must have energy for work and physical activities, and we must build body cells and tissues. The essential nutrients supply the fuel and building blocks for carrying on these activities. In a biologic sense, we are what we eat. Some general signs of good nutrition are a well-developed body, average weight for body size, and good muscles. The skin is smooth and clear, the hair is glossy, the eyes are clear and bright; and the posture is good and facial expression alert. Appetite, digestion, and elimination are good. Compare evidence of good and poor states of nutrition given in Table 1-1.

Table 1-1
Clinical Signs of Nutritional Status

	Good	Poor
General appearance	Alert, responsive	Listless, apathetic; cachexia
Hair	Shiny, lustrous; healthy scalp	Stringy, dull, brittle, dry, depigmented
Neck glands	No enlargement	Thyroid enlarged
Skin, face, and neck	Smooth, slightly moist; good color, reddish pink mucous membranes	Greasy, discolored, scaly
Eyes	Bright, clear; no fatigue circles	Dryness, signs of infection, increased vascularity, glassiness, thickened conjunctiva
Lips	Good color, moist	Dry, scaly, swollen; angular lesions (stomatitis)
Tongue	Good pink color, surface papillae present, no lesions	Papillary atrophy, smooth appearance; swollen, red, beefy (glossitis)
Gums	Good pink color; no swelling or bleeding; firm	Marginal redness or swelling; receding, spongy
Teeth	Straight, no crowding; well-shaped jaw; clean, no discoloration	Unfilled cavities, absent teeth, worn surfaces, mottled, malpositioned
Skin, general	Smooth, slightly moist, good color	Rough, dry, scaly, pale, pigmented, irritated; petechiae, bruises
Abdomen	Flat	Swollen
Legs, feet	No tenderness, weakness, or swelling; good color	Edema, tender calf; tingling, weakness
Skeleton	No malformations	Bowlegs, knock-knees, chest deformity at diaphragm, beaded ribs, prominent scapulae
Weight	Normal for height, age, body build	Overweight or underweight
Posture	Erect, arms and legs straight, abdomen in, chest out	Sagging shoulders, sunken chest, humpback
Muscles	Well developed, firm	Flaccid, poor tone; undeveloped, tender
Nervous control	Good attention span for age; does not cry easily; not irritable or restless	Inattentive, irritable
Gastrointestinal function	Good appetite and digestion; normal, regular elimination	Anorexia, indigestion, constipation, diarrhea
General vitality	Good endurance; energetic, vigorous; sleeps well at night	Easily fatigued, no energy, falls asleep in school, looks tired, apathetic

Human personal needs Although food and water are essential for survival, we do not eat to sustain our physical body alone. Food has many meanings and helps us to meet a number of personal, social, and cultural needs. Unmet personal needs may contribute to actual physical illness. Nutrition and food, therefore, are related to both physical and emotional health.

Plan of Study

To meet the basic objectives of stressing nutrition in health care as outlined, our plan of study concentrates on two basic areas: (1) organization of content material, including basic science principles, community resources, and patient care, and (2) providing a variety of learning tools to aid your study.

Organization of Material
Part One—Introduction to Human Nutrition

In this section of the text, we introduce the basic elements of nutrition and discuss the essential nutrients and their functions in the body. These functions are developed around three fundamental problems of human nutrition: energy, tissue building, and regulation and control.

Part Two—Community Nutrition: The Life Cycle

Here we consider the food environment and the web of factors that controls it—factors that influence individual choices from available foods, cultural food patterns and nutrition education, various age group needs in the life cycle, and health maintenance through physical fitness and weight management.

Part Three—Introduction to Diet Therapy

Here we discuss the hospitalized patient, nutrition assessment, drug-nutrient interactions, and the principles of diet therapy in various disease situations. Finally, we look at the use of computers in the management of nutritional practice.

Learning Tools for Study

To aid your study of human nutrition and its multiple applications in our lives both in health and disease, a number of learning tools are used.

Concepts

Concept Combined ideas forming a whole.

Each idea is considered first in terms of basic principles or **concepts** which are then applied to specific situations to help clarify meaning. Diagrams and line drawings further illustrate basic concepts.

Terms

Words are important vehicles for communicating ideas in any body of knowledge. You will find many key words analyzed along with their derivations and meanings in practice.

Clinical Application

Abstract theory is of little practical value. It finds meaning only as it is applied to key needs or problems. Numerous Clinical Application boxes are inserted to guide your learning. Look for nuggets of nutritional science applied to specific situations and needs.

Summaries

At the end of each chapter you will find a brief summary of the material presented. Using these summaries and the following Questions for Review, you may review what you have read and organize your understanding of the principal concepts presented.

References and Further Readings

Many specific current references from research, clinical work, conferences, and reviews are used to indicate source materials. These may stimulate your interest to seek an even broader base of background knowledge. The Further Readings section provides an annotated listing of a few selected materials for additional reading.

Issues and Answers

Nutritional science is often controversial because it is constantly growing and developing. A section included at the end of each chapter, Issues and Answers, addresses questions or controversies, with current practice applications that may help you seek related answers.

Reference Tools

Additional tools for reference are included in the appendixes. Finally, an index is provided for quick location or cross-referencing of desired topics for study.

Results of this Approach to the Study of Nutrition

Growing evidence of linkages between diet and disease is bringing increased awareness of the importance of nutrition in health care. Nutrition is playing an increasing role in the management of health problems and in the control of rising health care costs.[5] Recognizing the importance of food and nutrition in health care will deepen and facilitate your own patient care.

To Sum Up

Basic issues in nutrition and health center on world nutrition needs, major U.S. health problems and their relation to nutrition, and methods of organizing effective health care systems to meet these problems.

World nutrition needs are inevitably linked to our own in the United States since food security in the underdeveloped countries is interrelated with world food markets and our own food production and storage systems. The Food and Agriculture Organization (FAO) of the United Nations has a major responsibility in helping to coordinate work in many nations toward meeting world food security problems.

Our own major U.S. health problems include heart disease, cancer, and complications of diabetes and renal disease. All of these problems have a close relationship to nutrition. Wise approaches to health care must be person-centered and seek to meet the needs of the whole person, both physical and psychosocial. This can best be done with a team approach that pursues the goal of health promotion and personal well-being.

Questions for Review

1. Name some major causes of food problems in undeveloped countries. What is the work of the FAO in helping to solve some of the food security problems of the poorer nations? How effective do you think this work is?
2. What are some world health problems resulting from lack of food? How do you think these problems can be solved? What role do you think we have, on both a national and personal level, in dealing with these problems?
3. What are the major U.S. health problems? What do you know about the possible relationships of nutrition to these health problems?
4. What values do you see in the health team approach to patient care?

References

1. FAO Report: World Food Report, Rome, 1983, Publications Division, Food and Agriculture Organization (FAO) of the United Nations.
2. Watson, R.: An African nightmare, Newsweek, Nov. 26, 1984, p. 50.
3. DuVal, M.K.: Health education, health promotion, and the allied health professions, J. Allied Health **11**:13, 1982.
4. Sheilds, M.: A portrait of America, Newsweek, Jan. 17, 1983, p. 20.
5. ADA reports: Role delineation for the field of clinical dietetics, J. Am. Diet. Assoc. **78**(4):370, 1981.
6. Groziak, P., and Kaud, F.: Dietitians play growing role, Hospitals **57**(2):46, 1983.
7. Nestle, M.: Nutrition instruction for health professions students and practitioners: strategies for the 1980s, J. Parent. Enteral Nutr. **6**(3):191, 1982.

Further readings

American Dietetic Association: Position paper on clinical dietetics, J. Am. Diet. Assoc. **80**(3):256, March, 1982.

This professional organization paper helps to define the group's position concerning the role of the registered dietitian in clinical care and stimulates extended discussion of the health team approach.

Cousins, N.: Human options: an autobiographical notebook, London, 1982, W.W. Norton & Co.

This excellent background material by a well-known writer, publisher, and editor about his own odyssey through serious illness will help sensitize you to the human aspects of dealing with patient care.

Issues and Answers

If You're Not Healthy, It's Your Own Fault!

Some critics of the current health promotion/self-care movement, concerned with maintaining the traditional medical model of patient care, are once again blaming the victim for health problems. This is a misplaced accusation. It apparently started in the 1970s, when the public and practitioners alike became increasingly alarmed at the soaring costs of health care and sought ways in which individuals could cut their chances of being ill. The result was the now-growing field of preventive health care.

Many preventive health care practitioners are sensitive, skilled professionals who have used different methods of sharing their knowledge and skills with the public:

- Identification of risks
- Patient education regarding special illnesses
- Medical self-care
- Alternatives to traditional medical care (e.g., holistic health)
- Promotion of "wellness" as a state of mind or an attitude

Their task has not been easy because (1) their recommendations are often taken over and redefined by business opportunists, (2) there are no guarantees that every recommendation will achieve the same results (e.g., everyone who jogs 10 miles a day does not escape heart disease), (3) our culture stresses "antihealth" habits (e.g., availability of high-sodium convenience foods, high alcohol use, and overeating promoted by the media), and (4) health activists are viewed as attempting to impose their personal value system on others.

However, recommendations of some of these practitioners are not based on solid research and tend to yield inconsistent results. Because these "opinions" almost always involve the personal habits of the client, the "wellness" promoter *is* in effect telling persons that it's their fault if they're sick—they don't eat the "right" foods, they aren't keeping their weight down, they smoke/drink too much, they even *think* too much. In doing so they may be confusing the issue:

- Is it really the 16-year-old's fault that he eats too much when, in his lifetime, he's seen over 300,000 television commercials, most of which advertise readily available food?
- Is it the fault of the working woman that she relies on high sodium/high-fat convenience foods to feed her family?
- Is the low-income patient with no recreation available other than meal preparation totally at fault for obesity?

Health professionals who have improved their own health because of wellness practices can contribute to the wellness of their patients. They can teach those same health-promoting ideas nonjudgmentally, rather than concentrating *only* on the "challenge" of illness. Otherwise, if the "victim" role is reinforced, circumstances that created vulnerability to poor health are perpetuated and legitimized,

Continued.

Issues and Answers—cont'd

and further attempts to "help" are often turned down. To avoid this type of situation:

Examine personal value systems Is my own work designed to point a finger at the victim or to truly help the client help himself?

Consider every aspect of the client Is it really within my client's power to control food intake at home? What social, financial, or other factors may be limiting choice of foods or activities other than eating?

Be realistic If current research is not conclusive, do I avoid presenting recommendations as being "failure-proof"?

References
Dismuke, S.E., and Miller, S.T.: Why not share the secrets of good health? JAMA **249**(23):3181, 1983.
DuVal, M.K.: Health education, health promotion, and the allied health professions, J. Allied Health **11**:13, 1982.

Chapter 2
Digestion, Absorption, and Metabolism

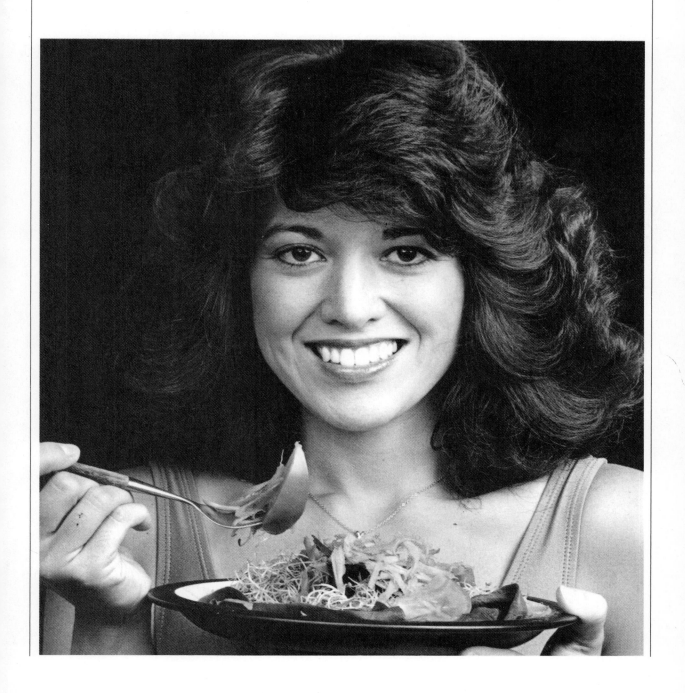

Preview

A health worker's knowledge of the process of digestion can be a vital tool for conveying scientifically sound information about nutrition. Thus, as a basic framework for introducing the individual nutrients, we will look first at the overall integrated body system that handles them.

This unique system of organ structures and functions energizes our bodies. This marvelous physiologic process consists of three integrated events: digestion, absorption, and metabolism. But as you view these three processes separately, remember that they are not functioning singly but as one continuum—a *dynamic whole* to give us life.

Chapter Objectives

After study of this chapter, the student should be able to:

1. Identify the processes by which the food we eat is prepared for our body's use and determine why this preparation is necessary.

2. Describe the integrated work of specific muscles and secretions in achieving this preparation work.

3. Relate the roles played by the nervous and endocrine systems in this preparation work.

4. Relate specific intestinal structures to the extensive task of nutrient absorption.

5. Identify processes by which the cells complete the task of making specific fuel and building nutrients available to sustain and nourish the whole body.

The Human Body as a Dynamic Whole

The Concepts of Change and Balance

Through a sucessive interrelated system of balanced change, the foods we eat must be transformed into simpler substances and then into other, still simpler, substances that our cells can use to sustain life. All these many changes whereby food is prepared for use by the body constitute the over-all digestion-absorption-metabolism process.

The Concept of Wholeness
Body Integrity

The parts of this overall process of change do not exist separately. Rather they comprise one continuous *whole*. Look carefully at the respective components of the gastrointestinal tract and their relative position in the over-all body system (Figure 2-1). In your study, follow the fate of food components as they travel *together* through the successive parts of the gastrointestinal tract and into the body cells.

Figure 2-1
The gastrointestinal system. Through the successive parts of the system, multiple activities of digestion liberate and re-form food nutrients to our use.

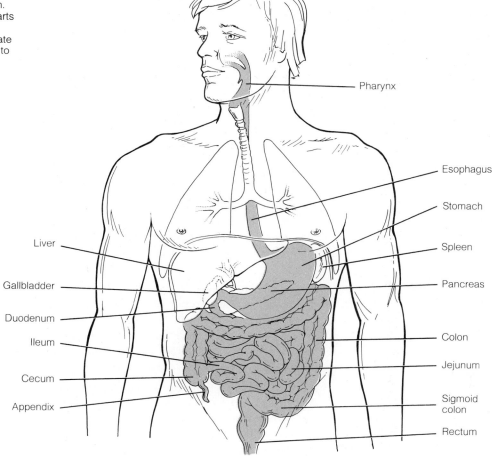

Pharynx

Esophagus

Stomach

Spleen

Pancreas

Colon

Jejunum

Sigmoid colon

Rectum

Liver

Gallbladder

Duodenum

Ileum

Cecum

Appendix

Reasons for Human Life Systems

Why is this intricate complex of biochemical and physiologic activities so necessary to human life? Two reasons are apparent: (1) *Food* as it naturally occurs and as we eat it is not a single component but a mixture of substances. If these substances are to release their energy for use, they must be separated into their respective components so that each one may be handled by the body as a separate unit. (2) *Nutrients* released from food may still remain unavailable to the body, and some additional means of changing their form must follow. The intermediate units must be broken down, simplified, regrouped, and rerouted. This exceeding complex chemical work must take place because the human being, whose life is developed and sustained in a fantastic internal chemical environment, is the most highly organized and intricately balanced of all organisms. This view of the human body as an integrated physiochemical organism is basic to an understanding of human nutrition.

Digestion

Digestion Process by which food is broken down chemically in the gastrointestinal tract through the action of secretions containing specific enzymes. Digestion separates complex food structures into their simpler parts, which are the chemicals needed by the body to sustain life.

Basic Principles of Digestion

Digestion initially prepares the food for use by the body. Two basic types of action are involved: (1) *mechanical* or muscular activity and (2) *chemical* or enzymatic activity.

Gastrointestinal Motility

Mechanical digestion takes place through a number of neuromuscular, self-regulatory processes. These actions work together to move the food components along the alimentary tract at the best rate for digestion and absorption of the nutrients to take place.

Types of muscles Four types of muscle in the stomach and intestine contribute to this motility:
1. **Contractile rings** A layer of circular contractile muscle rings that break up, mix, and churn the food particles.
2. **Longitudinal muscles** Long, smooth muscles that help to propel the food mass along.
3. **Sphincter muscles** Muscle rings at strategic points that act as valves—pyloric, ileocecal, and anal—to control passage of material to the next segment of the intestine.
4. **Mucosal muscles** A thin layer of smooth muscle that raises intestinal folds to increase the absorbing surface.

Types of muscle action The interaction of these four types of muscles produces two basic types of movement: (1) a general muscle tone or tonic contraction that ensures continuous passage and valve control and (2) periodic, rhythmic contractions that mix and propel the food mass. These alternating muscular contractions and relaxations that force the contents forward are known by the term *peristalsis*.

Intramural nerve plexus Network of interwoven nerve structures within a particular organ. The action of smooth muscle layers comprising the gastrointestinal wall is controlled by such a network of nerve fibers.

Nervous system control Specific nerves regulate these muscular actions. A complex, interrelated network of nerves within the gastrointestinal wall, the **intramural nerve plexus** (Figure 2-2), extends from the esophagus to the anus. This network controls muscle tone of the gastrointestinal wall, regulates the rate and intensity of muscle contractions, and coordinates the various movements.

Gastrointestinal Secretions

Food is digested chemically by the combined action of a number of secretions. Generally these secretions are of four types:

1. **Enzymes** Specific kind and quantity for the breakdown of a given nutrient.
2. **Hydrochloric acid and buffer ions** Essential agents to produce the pH necessary for the activity of given enzymes.
3. **Mucus** Necessary for lubrication and protection of the gastrointestinal tract.
4. **Water and electrolytes** In quantities sufficient to carry or circulate the organic substances.

All these secretions are produced by special cells in the mucosal tissue of the gastrointestinal tract or in accessory organs adjacent to it. The secretory action of these cells or glands is stimulated by the presence of food, by the sensory nerve network, or by hormones specific for certain foods.

Digestion in the Mouth and Esophagus
Mechanical Digestion

Mastication Initial biting and chewing begins the breaking up of food into smaller particles. The teeth and other oral structures are particularly suited for this function. The incisors cut; the molars grind. Tremendous force is supplied by the jaw muscles. Mastication makes possible an enlarged surface area of food for constant enzyme action. Also, the fineness of the food particles eases the continued passage of material through the gastrointestinal tract.

Swallowing The mixed mass of food particles is swallowed and passes down the esophagus largely by peristaltic waves controlled by nerve reflexes. Muscles at the base of the tongue aid the process of swallowing and, in the usual upright position, gravity aids the movement of food down the esophagus.

Entry into the stomach At the point of entry into the stomach, the *gastroesophageal constrictor muscle* relaxes to allow food to enter, then constricts again to prevent regurgitation of stomach contents up into the esophagus. When regurgitation does occur, through failure of this mechanism, the person feels it as "heartburn." Two clinical problems may hinder normal food passage at this point: (1) *cardiospasm,* caused by failure of the constrictor muscle to relax properly, or (2) *hiatal hernia,* caused by protrusion of the stomach into the thorax through an abnormal opening of the diaphragm (see p. 419).

Chemical or Secretory Digestion

Salivary secretions: 1000 to 1500 ml/day; pH range around neutral or 6.0 to 7.0.

Three pairs of salivary glands—*parotid, submaxilary,* and *sublingual*—secrete serous material containing *salivary amylase (ptyalin).* This is an enzyme specific for starches. A mucus material is also secreted that lubricates and binds the food particles. Stimuli such as sight, smell, taste, and touch—and even the thought of likes and dislikes in food—greatly influence these secretions. Food remains in the mouth only a short time, so starch digestion by ptyalin is brief and is terminated by the more acid medium of the stomach.

Digestion in the Stomach
Mechanical Digestion

Gastric secretions: 2000 ml/day; acid pH around 2.0.

The major parts of the stomach are shown in Figure 2-3. Muscles in the stomach wall provide three basic motor functions: storage, mixing, and controlled emptying. As the food mass enters the stomach, it lies against the stomach walls, which can stretch outward to store as much as 1 L. Gradually local tonic muscle waves increase their kneading and mixing action as the mass of food and secretions move on toward the pyloric valve at the distal end of the stomach. Here waves of peristaltic contractions reduce the mass to a semifluid *chyme*. Finally, with each peristaltic wave, small amounts of chyme are forced through the pyloric valve. This sphincter muscle controls the emptying of the stomach contents into the duodenum by constrictive action. This control releases the acid chyme slowly enough so it can be buffered by the alkaline intestinal secretions. Recent studies indicate that the caloric density of a meal, not just its particular composition or volume, influences the rate of stomach emptying.[1]

Chemical or Secretory Digestion

Types of secretions These contain three basic types of materials:
1. **Acid** Hydrochloric acid is produced to prepare certain enzymes and materials for digestion and absorption by creating the necessary degree of acidity for given enzymes to work.

Figure 2-3
Stomach.

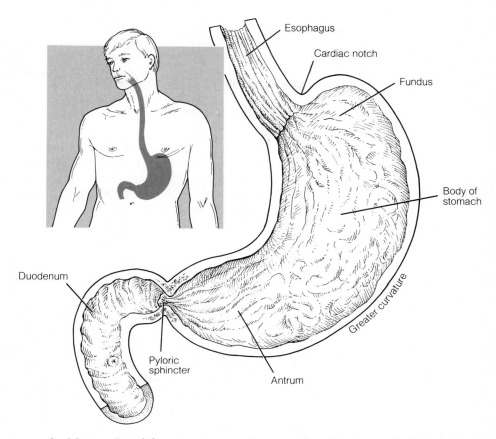

Mucus Viscid fluid secreted by mucous membranes and glands, consisting mainly of mucin (a glycoprotein), inorganic salts, and water.

2. **Mucus** Special mucous secretions protect the stomach lining from the eroding effect of the acid. This **mucus** also binds and mixes the food mass and helps move it along.

3. **Enzymes** The main enzyme in the stomach is *pepsin,* which begins the breakdown of protein. It is first secreted in the inactive form *pepsinogen,* which is then activated by the hydrochloric acid present. A small amount of *gastric lipase (tributyrinase)* is present and works on emulsified fats such as butterfat. This is a relatively minor activity, however. In childhood an enzyme called *rennin* (not to be confused with the vital lifelong renal enzyme *renin* [see p. 173]) is also present in gastric secretions, aiding in the coagulation of milk. However, in adults this enzyme is absent.

Control of secretions Stimuli for these gastric secretions come from two sources:

1. **Nerve stimulus** is produced in response to the senses, ingested food, and emotions. For example, chemical secretions increase in response to anger and hostility. Fear and depression decrease secretions and inhibit blood flow and motility as well.

2. **Hormonal stimulus** is produced in response to the entrance of food into the stomach. Certain stimulants, especially coffee, alcohol, and meat extractives, cause the release of a local hormone **gastrin** from mucosal cells in the antrum, which in turn stimulates the secretion

Gastrin Hormone secreted by mucosal cells in the antrum of the stomach that stimulates the parietal cells to produce hydrochloric acid.

of more hydrochloric acid. When the pH reaches 2.0, a feedback mechanism stops secretion of the hormone to prevent excess acid formation. Another local hormone, **enterogastrone,** produced by glands in the duodenal mucosal, counteracts excessive gastric activity by inhibiting acid and pepsin secretion and gastric motility.

Enterogastrone Hormone produced by glands in the duodenal mucosa that counteracts excessive gastric activity by inhibiting acid and pepsin secretion and gastric motility.

Digestion in the Small Intestine

Up to this point, the digestion of food has been mainly mechanical, with limited chemical activity. It is now delivered to the small intestine as a semifluid chyme made up of find food particles mixed with watery secretions. The major task of digestion, and of absorption that follows, occurs in the small intestine. Its structural parts, synchronized movements, and array of enzymes are highly developed for this all-important final task of mechanical and chemical digestion.

Mechanical Digestion

Note the exquisite structural arrangement of the intestinal wall shown in Figure 2-4. Finely coordinated intestinal motility is achieved by the three basic layers of muscle: (1) the thin layer of smooth muscle, the mucosa or *muscularis mucosa* with fibers extending up into the villi, (2) the circular muscle layer, and (3) the longitudinal muscle next to the outer *serosa*. Under the control of the nerve plexus, the wall-stretch pressure from food, and/or the hormonal stimuli, these muscles produce several types of movement that aid mechanical digestion:

Bolus Rounded mass of food ready to swallow or a mass passing through the gastrointestinal tract.

1. **Segmentation contractions** of circular muscle rings progressively chop the food mass into successive **boluses**, mixing food and secretions.

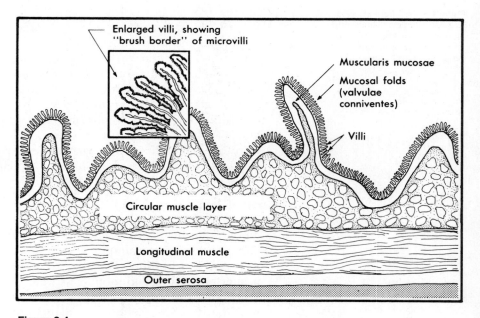

Figure 2-4
Intestinal wall. Note arrangement of muscle layers and structures of mucosa that increase surface area for absorption—mucosal folds, villi, and microvilli.

2. **Longitudinal rotation** of the long muscle running the length of the intestine rolls the slowly moving food mass in a spiral motion, mixing it and exposing new surfaces for absorption.
3. **Pendular movements** of small local muscle contractions sweep back and forth and stir chyme at the mucosal surface.
4. **Peristalsis** produces waves by the contraction of deep circular muscle, propelling the food mass slowly forward. The intensity of the wave may be increased by food intake or by the presence of irritants. In some cases this causes long, sweeping waves over the entire length of the intestine.
5. **Villi motions** constantly sweep the intestinal surface with alternating contractions and extentions of mucosal muscle fibers, agitating the mucosal surface, stirring and mixing chyme that is in contact with intestinal wall, and exposing additional nutrient material for absorption.

Chemical Digestion

The major burden of chemical digestion falls upon the small intestine. Thus this area secretes a large number of enzymes, each of which is specific for one of the fundamental types of nutrients. These important specific enzymes are secreted from the intestinal glands and from the pancreas. They are summarized in Table 2-1. Four basic types of digestive secretions in the small intestine aid in this final process:

1. **Enzymes** As indicated, specific enzymes act on specific nutrients to bring about the final breakdown of the nutrient materials in food to a form that the body can absorb and use.

Combined secretions of the mucous glands of the intestine and pancreas total about 2400 ml daily.

2. **Mucus** Large quantities of mucus are secreted by intestinal glands located immediately inside the duodenum. This secretion protects the mucosa from irritation and digestion by the highly acid gastric juices that enter the intestine at this point. Emotions inhibit these mucous secretions and are an important factor in the production of duodenal ulcers. Additional mucous cells on the intestinal surface continue to secret mucus when touched by the moving food mass. This secretion provides lubrication and protection of tissues.

Secretin Hormone produced in the mucous membrane of the duodenum in response to the entrance of the acid contents of the stomach into the duodenum.

3. **Hormone** A hormone called **secretin** is produced by the mucosa in the upper part of the small intestine. The presence of acid in the entering food mass causes this secretion. Its purpose in turn is to cause the pancreas to send pancreatic juices into the duodenum and buffer the acid chyme. The unprotected intestinal mucosa alone at this point could not withstand this high degree of acidity.
4. **Bile** Another important aid to digestion and absorption in the small intestine is bile, since it is an emulsifying agent for fats. A large volume of bile is produced in the liver as a dilute watery secretion. It is then concentrated and stored by the gallbladder. When fat enters the duodenum, the hormone *cholecystokinin*, secreted by the glands of the intestinal mucosa, stimulates the gallbladder to contract and release the needed bile.

Many factors influence the various secretions of the gastrointestinal tract; controls by hormone, nerve, and physical contact are summarized in Figure 2-5.

Table 2-1
Summary of Digestive Processes

Nutrient	Mouth	Stomach	Small Intestine

Carbohydrate	Starch $\xrightarrow{\text{Ptyalin}}$ Dextrins		**Pancreas**
			
			Starch $\xrightarrow{\text{Amylase}}$ (Disaccharides)
			          Maltose and sucrose
			
			Intestine
			
			Lactose $\xrightarrow{\text{Lactase}}$ (Monosaccharides)
			            Glucose and galactose
			
			Sucrose $\xrightarrow{\text{Sucrase}}$ Glucose and fructose
			
			Maltose $\xrightarrow{\text{Maltase}}$ Glucose and glucose

Protein		Protein $\xrightarrow[\text{Hydrochloric acid}]{\text{Pepsin}}$ Polypeptides	**Pancreas**
			
			Proteins, Polypeptides $\xrightarrow{\text{Trypsin}}$ Dipeptides
			
			Proteins, Polypeptides $\xrightarrow{\text{Chrymotrypsin}}$
			                          Dipeptides
			
			Polypeptides, Dipeptides $\xrightarrow{\text{Carboxypeptidase}}$
			                          Amino acids
			
			Intestine
			
			Polypeptides, Dipeptides $\xrightarrow{\text{Aminopeptidase}}$
			                          Amino acids
			
			Dipeptides $\xrightarrow{\text{Dipeptidase}}$ Amino acids

Fat		Tributyrin $\xrightarrow{\text{Tributyrinase}}$ Glycerol
		 (butterfat) Fatty acids
			Pancreas
			
			Fats $\xrightarrow{\text{Lipase}}$ Glycerol
			          Glycerides (di-, mono-)
			          Fatty acids
			
			Intestine
			
			Fats $\xrightarrow{\text{Lipase}}$ Glycerol
			          Glycerides (di-, mono-)
			          Fatty acids
			
			Liver and Gallbladder
			
			Fats $\xrightarrow{\text{Bile}}$ Emulsified fat

Absorption

Absorption Process by which digested food materials pass through epithelial cells of the alimentary canal (mainly of the small intestine) into the blood or lymph.

After digestion of the food nutrients is complete, the simplified end products are ready for **absorption**, aided by a number of transport mechanisms. These end products include *monosaccharides* such as glucose, fructose, and glactose from carbohydrates; *fatty acids* and *glycerides* from fats; and *amino acids* from protein. In some cases, incompletely digested nutrients, such as lactose in the absence of lactase, remain in the intestine and cause absorptive problems. (See Issues and Answers on pp. 39-40.) Some small peptides may be absorbed intact and hydrolyzed to amino acids within the mucosal absorptive cells. Vitamins and minerals are also liberated. Finally, with a water base for solution and transport plus necessary electrolytes, the total fluid food mass is now prepared for absorption as part of the large gastrointestinal circulation (Table 2-2).

Figure 2-5
Summary of factors
influencing secretions of the
gastrointestinal tract.

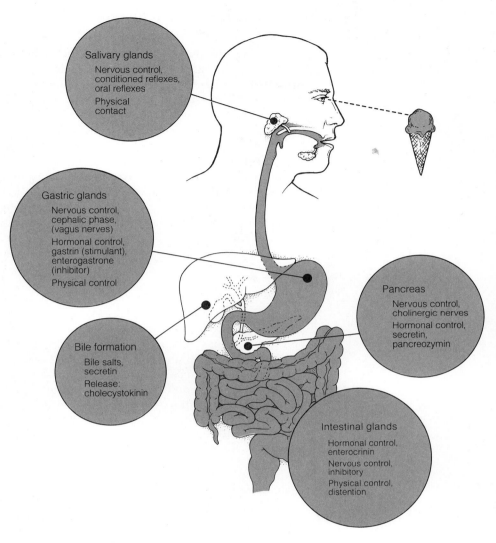

Salivary glands
Nervous control,
conditioned reflexes,
oral reflexes
Physical
contact

Gastric glands
Nervous control,
cephalic phase,
(vagus nerves)
Hormonal control,
gastrin (stimulant),
enterogastrone
(inhibitor)
Physical control

Pancreas
Nervous control,
cholinergic nerves
Hormonal control,
secretin,
pancreozymin

Bile formation
Bile salts,
secretin:
Release:
cholecystokinin

Intestinal glands
Hormonal control,
enterocrinin
Nervous control,
inhibitory
Physical control,
distention

Table 2-2
Daily Absorption Volume in
Human Gastrointestinal
System

	Intake (L)	Intestinal Absorption (L)	Elimination (L)
Food ingested	1.5		
Gastrointestinal secretions	8.5		
TOTAL	10.0		
Fluid absorbed in small intestine		9.5	
Fluid absorbed in large intestine		0.4	
TOTAL		9.9	
Feces			0.1

Absorption in the Small Intestine
Surface Structures

Viewed from the outside, the intestine appears smooth, but the inner mucosal surface lining is quite different. Refer again to Fig. 2-4 and note the three types of convolutions and projections that greatly enhance the absorbing surface area: (1) *Mucosal folds* similar to hills and valleys in a mountain range, which are easily seen by the naked eye, (2) *villi* or finger-like projections on these folds, which can be seen by a simple microscope, and (3) *microvilli* or extremely small projections on each villus, which can be seen only with an electron microscope.

Microvilli Minute surface projections that cover the edge of each intestinal villus, visible only through the electron microscope. This vast array of microvilli on each villus is called the "brush border." The microvilli add a tremendous surface area for absorption.

The array of **microvilli** covering the edge of each villus is called the *brush border* because it looks like bristles on a brush. Each villus has an ample network of blood capillaries as well as a central lymph vessel called the *lacteal* vessel. This name was given to these lymphatic vessels in the small intestine because the material that fills them during absorption consists mainly of fat substances, giving it a creamy, milk-like appearance.

Absorbing Surface Area

The three structural elements of the intestine—mucosal folds, villi, and microvilli—increase the inner surface area some 600 times over that of the outside serosa. These special structures, plus the contracted length of the live organ—630 to 660 cm (21 to 22 ft)—produce a tremendously large absorbing surface. The inner surface of the small intestine, if stretched out flat, would be as large or larger than half a basketball court! All three of these mucosal surface structures function as a unit for the absorption of nutrients. Although the small intestine is popularly thought of as the lowly "gut," it is actually one of the most highly developed, exquisitely fashioned, specialized tissues in the human body.

Mechanism of Absorption

Absorption is accomplished through the wall of the small intestine by means of a number of processes. These include passive diffusion and osmosis, active "ferrying" or a carrier-mediated diffusion, energy-driven active transport, and penetration by engulfment or pinocytosis.

Routes of Absorption

Cisterna chyli Dilated sac at the origin of the thoracic duct, which is the common trunk that receives all the lymphatic vessels.

After their absorption by these processes, the nutrient components from carbohydrates and proteins enter the portal blood system directly and travel by way of the liver to the body tissues. Only fat is unique in its route. After enzyme processing in the cells of the intestinal lumen, fat is largely converted to a complex with protein as a carrier, packaged as lipoproteins (p. 458). These packages flow into the lymph vessels, empty into the **cisterna chyli**, then travel upward into the chest through the thoracic duct, and empty into the venous blood at the left subclavian vein. Exceptions are the medium-chain and short-chain fatty acids, which are absorbed directly into blood circulation.[2] However, most of the fats consumed are long-chain fatty acids, which travel the lacteal lymphatic route.

Absorption in the Large Intestine (Colon)

Water absorption is the main task remaining for the large intestine. Related nutrient factors are involved, such as minerals, vitamins, amino acids, intestinal bacteria, and nondigestible residue.

Water Absorption

Within a 24-hour period about 500 ml of the remaining food mass leaves the *ileum,* the last portion of the small intestine, and enters the *cecum,* the pouch at the start of the large intestine. Here the *ileocecal valve* controls passage of the semiliquid chyme. Normally the valve remains closed, but each peristaltic wave relaxes the valve and squirts a small amount of chyme into the cecum. This mechanism holds the food mass in the small intestine long enough to ensure digestion and absorption of vital nutrients.

The chyme continues to move slowly through the large intestine, aided by mucous secretion from glands in the colon and muscle contractions. The major portion of the water in the chyme, 350 to 400 ml, is absorbed in the proximal half of the colon. Only about 100 to 150 ml remains to form the feces.

This food-residue mass now begins to slow its passage. Usually a meal, having traveled the 630 to 660 cm (21 to 22 ft) of the small intestine, starts to enter the cecum about 4 hours after it is consumed. About 8 hours later it reaches the sigmoid colon, having traveled about 90 cm (3 ft) through the large intestine. In the sigmoid colon the food mass descends still more slowly toward the anus. Even 72 hours after a meal has been eaten, as much as 25% of it may still remain in the rectum.

Mineral Absorption

Electrolytes, mainly sodium, are transported into the blood stream from the colon. Intestinal absorption is a major balance control point for many of the minerals, and much of the dietary intake remains unabsorbed for elimination in the feces. For example, 20% to 70% of the ingested calcium is eliminated here and 80% to 85% of the iron.

Iron from meat sources is absorbed more readily than iron from plant foods.

Bacterial Action

Vitamin absorption Bacteria in the colon are closely associated with a number of vitamins. At birth the colon is sterile, but very shortly intestinal bacterial flora become well established. The adult colon contains large numbers of bacteria, and great masses of bacteria are passed in the stool. The colon bacteria synthesize vitamin K and some vitamins of the B complex, which are absorbed from the colon to help meet daily requirements.

Other bacterial action Intestinal bacteria also affect the color and odor of the stool. The brown color represents bile pigments that are formed by the colon bacteria from *bilirubin.* In conditions where bile flow is hindered, the stools may become clay colored or white. The characteristic odor results from amines, especially *indole* and *skatole,* which are formed by bacterial enzymes from amino acids. Intestinal gas, or flatus, contains hydrogen sulfide or methane produced by the bacteria. Gas formation, however, is often caused not so much by specific foods as by the state of the body

---

Clinical Application

When Digestion Becomes Embarrassing

After eating a meal or certain foods, many persons experience the common discomfort of "gas."

Gas is a normal byproduct of digestion. The gastrointestinal tract normally holds about 3 ounces worth, an amount that is silently absorbed into the bloodstream. Sometimes extra gas collects in the stomach or intestine, creating an embarrassing, though usually harmless, situation.

Stomach gas results from uncomfortable air bubbles trapped in the stomach. It occurs when you eat too fast, drink through a straw, or otherwise take in extra air while eating. Burping relieves it. However, there are a few tips you can follow to avoid this social slip:
- Avoid carbonated beverages.
- Don't gulp.
- Chew with your mouth closed.
- Don't drink out of a can or through a straw or chew gum.
- Don't eat when you're nervous.

Intestinal gas is embarrassing in any culture. It is formed in the colon, where bacteria attack nondigested items, causing them to decompose and produce gas. Carbohydrates release hydrogen, carbon dioxide, and in people with certain types of bacteria in the gut, *methane*—three odorless (though noisy) gases. Protein produces *hydrogen sulfide* and such volatile amines as *indole* and *skatole*, which add a distinctive aroma to expelled air.

Follow this step-by-step approach for treatment:
- Cut down on simple carbohydrates. Observe milk's effect—lactose intolerance may be the real culprit.
- Eliminate all known offenders. These vary among individuals, although beans, onions, cabbage, and wheat are among the most common.

Once relief is achieved, you may add more complex carbohydrates and high-fiber foods back to the diet—slowly. Once small amounts are tolerated, slightly greater amounts can be tried.

References
Ribakove, B.M.: Private enemies: gas, Health **15**(5):44, 1983.

---

that receives them (see box above). Many foods have been labeled "gas formers" but in reality these effects are highly variable from one person to another and such classifications have little or no scientific basis.

Dietary Fiber

Since we have no microorganisms or enzymes to breakdown fiber, this plant product remains after digestion and absorption as residue. Pectin, however, is degraded in the large intestine.[3] Undigested fiber contributes

Table 2-3
Intestinal Absorption of Some Major Nutrients

Nutrient	Form	Means of Absorption	Control Agent or Required Cofactor	Route
Carbohydrate	Monosaccharides (glucose and galactose)	Competitive	—	Blood
		Selective	—	
		Active transport via sodium pump	Sodium	
Protein	Amino acids	Selective	—	Blood
	Some dipeptides	Carrier transport systems	Pyridoxine (pyridoxal phosphate)	Blood
	Whole protein (rare)	Pinocytosis	—	Blood
Fat	Fatty acids	Fatty acid-bile complex (micelles)	Bile	Lymph
	Glycerides (mono-, di-)		—	Lymph
	Few triglycerides (neutral fat)	Pinocytosis	—	Lymph
Vitamins	B_{12}	Carrier transport	Intrinsic factor (IF)	Blood
	A	Bile complex	Bile	Blood
	K	Bile complex	Bile	From large intestine to blood
Minerals	Sodium	Active transport via sodium pump	—	Blood
	Calcium	Active transport	Vitamin D	Blood
	Iron	Active transport	Ferritin mechanism	Blood (as transferritin)
Water	Water	Osmosis	—	Blood, lymph, interstitial fluid

important bulk to the diet and helps form the feces. Fully formed and ready for elimination, the feces contain about 75% water and 25% solids. The solids include fiber, bacteria, inorganic matter such as minerals, a small amount of fat and its derivatives, some mucus, and sloughed-off mucosal cells.

Some major features of nutrient absorption are summarized in Table 2-3.

Metabolism

Metabolism Sum of all physical and chemical changes that take place within an organism, by which it maintains itself and produces energy for its functioning.

The various absorbed nutrient components, including water and electrolytes, are carried to the cells to produce a large number of substances needed by the body to sustain life. Cell **metabolism** encompasses the total, continuous complex of chemical changes that determine the final use of the individual nutrients.

Carbohydrate Metabolism
Sources of Blood Glucose

Both carbohydrate and noncarbohydrate substances provide sources of blood glucose.

Glycogenolysis Specific term for conversion of glycogen into glucose in the liver; the chemical process of enzymatic hydrolysis or breakdown by which this conversion is accomplished.

Glycolysis Catabolism of carbohydrate (glucose and glycogen) by enzymes with release of energy and production of pyruvic acid or lactic acid.

Gluconeogenesis Formation of glucose from noncarbohydrate sources (protein or fat).

Carbohydrate sources Three carbohydrate sources provide blood glucose: (1) dietary starches and sugars, (2) glycogen stored in liver and muscle tissue (the hydrolysis of glycogen to form glucose is called **glycogenolysis** or **glycolysis**), and (3) products of intermediary carbohydrate metabolism, such as lactic acid and pyruvic acid.

Noncarbohydrate sources Both protein and fat provide additional sources of glucose. Certain amino acids are called *glucogenic amino acids* because they form glucose after they are metabolically broken down. About 58% of the protein in a mixed diet is composed of such glucogenic amino acids. Therefore more than half of dietary protein may ultimately be used for energy if sufficient carbohydrates and fat are not available for fuel. After the breakdown of fat into fatty acids and *glycerol*, the glycerol portion (about 10% of the fat) can be converted to glycogen in the liver and made available for glucose formation. The production of glucose from protein, fat, and intermediate carbohydrate metabolites is called **gluconeogenesis**.

Uses of Blood Glucose

Three uses of glucose serve to regulate the blood sugar within a normal range of the 70 to 120 mg/dl:

Energy production The primary function of glucose is to supply energy to meet the body's constant demand. A vast array of interacting metabolic pathways employing many specific successive cell enzymes accomplish this task in a highly efficient manner.

Energy storage Two storage forms may be used for glucose: (1) *Glycogen*—glucose may be converted to glycogen and stored in limited amounts in the liver and muscle tissue. Only a small supply of glycogen is present at any one time, and it turns over rapidly. (2) *Fat*—after energy demands have been fulfilled, any excess glucose is converted to fat and stored as adipose tissue.

Glucose products Small amounts of glucose are used in the production of various carbohydrate compounds, which have significant roles in overall body metabolism. Examples include DNA and RNA, galactose, and certain amino acids.

These sources and uses of glucose act as checks and balances to maintain the blood sugar within its normal range by adding sugar to the blood or removing it as needed.

Hormonal Controls

A number of hormones directly and indirectly influence the metabolism of glucose and regulate the blood sugar level according to need:

Blood sugar–lowering hormone Only one hormone, *insulin,* acts to lower the blood sugar. It is produced by specialized beta cells in the pancreas. These beta cells, which are scattered cell clusters, form "islands" in the pancreatic tissue and are called *islets of Langerhans* (see p. 394), named for the scientist Paul Langerhans, who, as a young German medical student, first discovered them and studied them. Insulin regulates blood sugar through several actions:

1. **Glycogenesis** Stimulates conversion of glucose to glycogen in the liver for constant energy reserve.
2. **Lipogenesis** Stimulates conversion of glucose to fat for storage in adipose tissue.
3. **Cell permeability** Increases cell permeability to glucose, allowing it to pass from the extracellular fluids into the cells for oxidation to supply needed energy.

Blood sugar–raising hormones A number of hormones effectively raise blood sugar:
1. **Glucagon** Produced by pancreatic islet alpha cells, it acts opposite to insulin, increasing breakdown of liver glycogen to glucose and maintaining blood glucose during fasting sleep hours.
2. **Somatostatin** Produced in the pancreatic islet delta cells and in the hypothalamus, it suppresses insulin and glucagon and helps maintain normal blood sugar by acting as a general modulator of related metabolic activities.
3. **Steroid hormones** Originating from the adrenal cortex, they release glucose-forming carbon units from protein and act as insulin antagonists blocking the sugar-lowering effect of insulin.
4. **Epinephrine** Originating from the adrenal medulla, it stimulates the breakdown of liver glycogen to glucose, causing a quick release of readily available glucose for immediate use.
5. **Growth hormone (GH)** and **adrenocorticotropic hormone (ACTH)** Released from the anterior pituitary gland, they act as insulin antagonists.
6. **Thyroxine** Originating from the thyroid gland, it influences the rate of insulin destruction, increases glucose absorption from the intestine, and liberates epinephrine.

Lipid Metabolism
Fat Synthesis and Breakdown

Two organ tissues, the liver and adipose tissue, form an overall balanced axis of fat metabolism. Both function in fat synthesis and fat breakdown. The fatty acids released from fat are used by body cells as concentrated fuel to produce energy.

Lipoproteins

These lipid-protein complexes provide the major transport form of fat in the bloodstream. An excess amount in the blood produces a clinical condition called *hyperlipoproteinemia*. Lipoproteins are produced in the intestinal wall after initial absorption of dietary fat and in the liver (p. 457).

Hormonal Controls

Since fat and carbohydrate metabolism are closely interrelated, the same hormones that effect carbohydrate metabolism also affect fat metabolism:
1. **GH, ACTH,** and **thyroid-stimulating hormone (TSH)** All from the pituitary gland, they increase the release of free fatty acids from adipose tissue by imposing energy demands on the body.
2. **Cortisone** and **hydrocortisone** From the adrenal gland, they cause

the release of free fatty acids. *Epinephrine* and *norepinephrine* stimulate the breakdown of fat.

3. **Insulin** From the pancreas, this promotes fat synthesis, whereas *glucagon* has the opposite effect of increasing the breakdown of tissue to release free fatty acids.

4. **Thyroxine** From the thyroid gland, it stimulates adipose tissue release of free fatty acids. It also lowers blood cholesterol levels.

Protein Metabolism

Protein metabolism centers on the essential balance between *anabolism* and *catabolism*.

Anabolism or Tissue Building

Anabolism is the building up of protein tissue through the synthesis of new protein. This build-up is a specific process governed by a specific pattern—the "blueprint" provided by DNA in the cell nucleus—that requires specific amino acids (p. 89). This process follows what has characteristically been called the "all or none" law. This means that all the necessary amino acids for a given protein must be present at the same time or the protein will not be formed. Specific selection and supply of amino acids are necessary.

Several agents act as control factors for the intricate processes of protein synthesis. These control agents include specific cell enzymes and coenzymes. Also, specific hormones control or stimulate the building of tissue. These include: (1) the growth hormone, which stimulates extra tissue synthesis during the growth periods, (2) gonadotropins, especially testosterone, which stimulate tissue building associated with puberty, and (3) thyroxine (in normal amounts), which regulates the rate of basal metabolism.

Catabolism or Tissue Breakdown

Amino acids, which are released as the tissue protein is broken down and not used at that time for tissue synthesis, are further broken down and used for other purposes.[4] Two main elements of amino acids result: (1) the nitrogen containing group and (2) the remaining nonnitrogen residue.

Deamination Initial step in the metabolic breakdown (catabolism) of amino acids in which the amino group (NH₂) is split off. Deamination takes place chiefly in the liver.

Nitrogen group The first step in the breakdown of amino acids is the splitting off of the nitrogen portion. This process, which takes place chiefly in the liver, is called **deamination**. The nitrogen is converted to ammonia and may be excreted in the urine as urea or used to form other nitrogen-containing compounds.

Keto acid Amino acid residue left after deamination. Glycogenic keto acids are used to form carbohydrates. Ketogenic keto acids are used to form fats.

Nonnitrogen residue The nonnitrogen residues are called **keto acids.** These residues may be used to form either carbohydrates or fat substances. Certain amino acids tend to form carbohydrate substances, whereas other amino acids are used for fat substances. Intermediate products from carbohydrate, fat, and protein enter a common metabolic "pool." There is constant interplay between this pool and the amino acid pool. These residues may also be reaminated to form a new amino acid.

Control agents As in the case of tissue building, cell enzymes and coenzymes are constantly at work controlling tissue breakdown. Hormones also influence catabolism. These include (1) large amounts of thyroxine, which stimulate excessive catabolism of muscle tissue, and (2) adrenal steroids, which stimulate the breakdown of amino acids and the conversion of the residue to glucose or glycogen.

Metabolic Interrelationships

Each of these chemical processes of body metabolism is purposeful, and all are interdependent. The processes are designed to fill two essential needs: (1) to produce energy and (2) to maintain a dynamic equilibrium between the building up and breaking down of tissue. The controlling agents in the cells for these processes to be carried on in an orderly fashion are the cell enzymes, their coenzymes, many of which involve the vitamins and minerals, and hormones. Overall human metabolism is an exciting biochemical process, designed to develop, sustain, and protect our most precious possession—life itself.

To Sum Up

Nutrients are converted into usable forms via digestion and absorption. Metabolism is the means by which the body uses these nutrients to produce energy, build body tissues, and maintain normal body function.

Digestion consists of two basic activities: muscular and chemical. Muscular activity is responsible for (1) food's mechanical breakdown by such means as mastication and (2) movement of food along the gastrointestinal tract by such motions as peristalsis. Chemical activity involves enzymatic action that degrades food into smaller and smaller components for absorption.

Absorption involves the passage of food from the gut to the bloodstream across the intestinal wall. It occurs mainly in the small intestine via a number of efficient mechanisms. The vital work of cell metabolism handles all the absorbed nutrients. This cell metabolic work is the total of biochemical reactions that result in energy and maintain a dynamic equilibrium between catabolism and anabolism—tissue breakdown and buildup.

Questions for Review

1. Describe the five types of movement involved in mechanical digestion.
2. Identify digestive enzymes and any cofactors secreted by the following glands: salivary, mucosal, pancreas, and liver. What activity do they perform on fats, proteins, and carbohydrates? What stimulates their release? What inhibits their activity?
3. Describe four mechanisms of nutrient absorption from the small intestine. Describe the routes taken by the breakdown products of fats, proteins, and carbohydrates after absorption.
4. Describe in detail two major activities that occur in the large intestine.

References

1. Report: Gastric emptying of carbohydrate meals, Nutr. Rev. **40**(8):238, 1982.
2. Bach, A.C., and Babayan, V.K.: Medium-chain triglycerides: an update, Am. J. Clin. Nutr. **36**(5):950, 1982.
3. Holloway, W.D., Tasman-Jones, C., and Maher, K.: Pectin digestion in humans, Am. J. Clin. Nutr. **37**(2):253, 1983.
4. Mortimore, G.E.: Mechanisms of cellular protein catabolism, Nutr. Rev. **40**(1):1, 1982.

Further Readings

Phillips, S.F., and Stephen, A.M.: The structure and function of the large intestine, Nutr. Today **16**(6):4, 1981.

Good review of the role of the large intestine in water and other nutrient-related absorption and metabolic functions and of disease of this terminal GI organ. Views the colon not only as an organ for eliminating waste products of digestion but also as an important recycling plant for needed metabolites. Excellent graphics.

Ray, T.K., and others: Long-term effects of dietary fiber on glucose tolerance and gastric emptying in noninsulin-dependent diabetic patients, Am. J. Clin. Nutr. **37**(3):376, 1983.

This study reports effects of two forms of dietary fiber (guar gum and wheat bran) on gastric emptying time. Delayed gastric emptying was shown to have beneficial effect for long-term metabolic control in obese patients with Type II diabetes.

Issues and Answers

Lactose Intolerance—A Case Against Milk Subsidy Programs?

Hydrolysis Process by which a chemical compound is split into other compounds by taking up the elements of water. Common examples are the reactions of digestion in which the nutrients are split into simpler compounds by the digestive enzymes; that is, the conversion of starch to maltose, of fat to fatty acids and glycerol, and so on.

Picture this: a natural disaster strikes a poor nation, leaving thousands homeless and with very little food. CARE, UNICEF, and other international organizations work quickly to collect and ship foodstuffs to the area. Yet, the people find it difficult to be grateful: since the shipments began, they have found themselves not only without shelter but also in distress—gastrointestinal distress.

One of the most common foodstuffs shipped to impoverished areas is milk. One of the most common problems throughout the world is *lactose intolerance*—a condition that results in abdominal cramps, nausea, bloating, or diarrhea when milk is consumed. The problem stems from a deficiency in *lactase*, a digestive enzyme found in the microvilli of the small intestine that by **hydrolysis** converts marginal milk sugar (lactose) into its component monosaccharides, glucose and galactose, for absorption. All mammals are born with sufficient amounts of lactase to accommodate very high lactose levels in "mother's milk." In animal species, the amount of enzyme activity drops off significantly shortly after birth; in most humans, this occurs after age 5. A few among the human species do not experience this problem. Northern Europeans, a few African cattle-raisers, and residents of the northwestern sector of India manage to digest lactose very easily throughout adulthood. The remaining majority of the world's population experience symptoms on drinking as little as a half pint of milk.

Symptoms are similar to those seen in other food sensitivities. When there is any doubt regarding the cause, lactose intolerance tests are usually performed:

Lactose loading A 50-gram dose of lactose (approximately the amount provided by 4 cups of milk) is administered and symptoms evaluated.

Breath-hydrogen assay Hydrogen levels in the breath after a lactose load are measured to indicate the degree of intolerance.

Lactase assay Lactase levels in a jejunal biopsy are measured.

Once lactose intolerance has been identified and other clinical conditions with which it is associated are ruled out, treatment consists simply of cutting down on milk consumption. Most lactose-intolerant individuals digest fermented milk products (cheese, buttermilk, yogurt) very well and can use them as their primary source of calcium instead of milk. But these foods carry problems of transportation, storage, and cost. And yet the nutritional benefits of lactose-rich foods may become crucial in offsetting deficiency signs among those in dire need.

A possible solution to this problem is the use of recently developed low-lactose milk. Sweeter than regular milk, this lactose-hydrolyzed product has been not only acceptable but also more effective at reducing symptoms than another popular product often chosen by the

Continued.

Issues and Answers—cont'd

public to avoid symptoms: sweet acidophilus milk. Processing involves incubation with yeast lactose and increases the cost by a mere 2 to 3 cents/liter, keeping it inexpensive enough to be considered for mass distribution.

References
Ferguson, A.: Diagnosis and treatment of lactose intolerance, Br. Med. J. **283**(6304): 1423, 1981.
Payne, D.L., and others: Effectiveness of milk products in dietary management of lactose malabsorption, Am. J. Clin. Nutr. **34**:2711, 1981.

Chapter 3
Carbohydrates

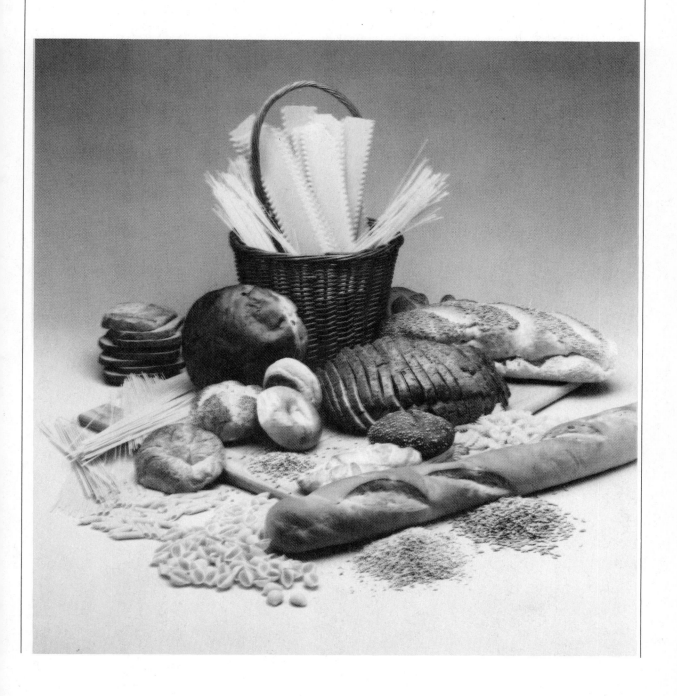

Preview

The human body has been uniquely designed and developed to solve three basic survival problems: (1) energy to do its work, (2) materials to build and maintain its form, and (3) agents to control these processes efficiently. Key nutrients in the food we eat have provided sensitive life-sustaining solutions.

All three of these problems are interrelated but we will look at them one at a time. In this chapter we consider the first of these basic problems—*energy production*—and the body's primary fuel—*carbohydrates*.

Chapter Objectives

After study of this chapter, the student should be able to:

1. Identify practical reasons for the prime position of carbohydrate in the human diet worldwide and name its two main dietary forms, giving examples of each.

2. Define carbohydrate in terms of its basic chemical structure and identify some of its major forms and functions that are important in human metabolism.

3. Describe the processes by which food carbohydrates are changed to a usable refined fuel and then carried to the cells for energy production.

Carbohydrates as Body Fuel

The Nature of Carbohydrates

The Problem of Energy

Energy is a primary necessity for life. It is the power an organism needs to do its work. Any energy system, to be successful, must provide four basic components: (1) a basic fuel, (2) a means of changing the basic fuel to a refined fuel that the machine is designed to use, (3) a means of carrying this refined fuel to the energy production sites, and (4) a means of burning the fuel at the production sites to produce energy. In the human energy system, this major basic fuel comes from carbohydrates.

Starches and Sugars

Photosynthesis Process by which plants containing chlorophyll are able to manufacture carbohydrate by combining carbon dioxide from the air and water from the soil. Sunlight is used as energy and chlorophyll is the catalyst.

The basic fuel forms of carbohydrates are starches and sugars that occur naturally in our foods. Since energy on this planet comes ultimately from the sun and its nuclear reactions, plants in the presence of sunlight and through the process of **photosynthesis** transform the sun's energy into plant form. They use carbon dioxide from the air and water from the soil, along with chlorophyll in green leaves as a chemical catalyst, to manufacture starches and sugars. Since the human body can rapidly break down these sugars and starches to yield energy, carbohydrates are called "quick energy" foods. They provide our major source of energy.

Dietary Importance

There are practical reasons for the large quantities of carbohydrates in diets all over the world. First, carbohydrates are widely available, easily grown in plants such as grains, vegetables, and fruits. In some countries, carbohydrate foods make up almost the entire diet of the people. In the American diet about 50% of the total calories is in the form of carbohydrates. Second, carbohydrates are relatively low in cost. Third, carbohydrates are practical because they may be stored easily. Compared with other types of foods, carbohydrate foods can be kept in dry storage for relatively long time periods without spoilage. Modern processing and packaging further extend the shelf life of carbohydrate products almost indefinitely.

Definition

The name *carbohydrate* comes from its chemical nature. It is composed of carbon, hydrogen, and oxygen, with the hydrogen/carbon ratio usually that of water—H_2O.[1]

Classification of Carbohydrates

Carbohydrates are classified according to the number of sugar, or *saccharide,* units making up their structure:

Monosaccharides

Monosaccharide Class of simple sugars composed of one saccharide (sugar) unit. Common members are glucose, fructose, and galactose.

The simplest form of carbohydrate is the **monosaccharide,** often called a simple (single) sugar. The three main monosaccharides important in human nutrition are glucose, fructose, and galactose.

Glucose A moderately sweet sugar, glucose is found naturally preformed in only a few foods, such as corn syrup. Mainly it is created in the body from starch digestion. In human metabolism all other types of sugar are

Dextrose Another name for glucose.

converted into glucose. It is the form, sometimes called **dextrose,** in which sugar circulates in the blood stream. It is oxidized to give energy.

Fructose The sweetest of the simple sugars, fructose is found in fruits and honey. In human metabolism it is converted to glucose for energy.

Galactose The simple sugar galactose is not found free in foods but is produced in human digestion from lactose (milk sugar) and is then changed to glucose for energy. This reaction is reversible, and during lactation, glucose may be reconverted to galactose for use in milk production.

Disaccharides

Disaccharides Class of compound sugars composed of two molecules of monosaccharide. The three common members are sucrose (table sugar), lactose (milk sugar), and maltose (grain sugar).

The **disaccharides** are simple (double) sugars composed of two monosaccharides linked together. The three main disaccharides of physiologic importance are sucrose, lactose, and maltose.

Sucrose Sucrose is common table sugar. It is the most prevalent disaccharide. With the increasing use of processed foods, sucrose contributes some 30% to 40% of the total carbohydrate kilocalories in the American diet. Sucrose can be found in all forms of sugar, molasses, pineapple, and carrots.

Lactose Lactose is the sugar in milk. It is formed in the body from glucose to supply the carbohydrate component of milk during lactation. The least sweet of the disaccharides, it is about one sixth as sweet as sucrose. When milk sours, as in the initial stages of cheese making, the lactose is changed to lactic acid and separates into the liquid whey from the remaining solid curd. The curd is then processed for cheese. Therefore, although milk has a relatively high carbohydrate content in the form of lactose, one of its main products—cheese—has relatively little or none.

Maltose Maltose occurs in malt products of starch breakdown and in germinating cereal grains. As such, it is a negligible *dietary* carbohydrate. But it is a highly significant *metabolic* factor in human nutrition as an intermediate product of starch digestion.

Polysaccharides

Polysaccharides Class of complex carbohydrates composed of many monosaccharide units. The common members are starch, dextrins, dietary fiber, and glycogen.

Polysaccharides are much more complex carbohydrates made up of many single sugar units. The most important polysaccharides in human nutrition include starch, glycogen, dextrins, and dietary fiber—cellulose and other noncellulose polysaccharides.

Starch Starch is by far the most significant polysaccharide in human nutrition. It is a relatively large complex compound made up of many coiled or branching chains of single sugar (glucose) units. It yields only glucose on digestion. The cooking of starch not only improves its flavor but also softens and ruptures the starch cells, which makes digestion easier. Starch mixtures thicken when cooked because the portion that encases the starch granules has a gel-like quality thickening it the same way that pectin causes jelly to set.

Starch is by far the most important source of dietary carbohydrate worldwide. Currently, the value of starch in human nutrition and health has received a great deal of recognition. The standard of the U.S. Dietary Goals (p. 397) recommends that about 50% to 55% of the total kilocalories come from carbohydrates, with a greater portion of that allowance coming from complex carbohydrate forms such as starch. In many other countries where starch is a staple food substance, it makes up an even higher portion of the diet. The major food sources of starch include cereal grains, legumes, potatoes, and other vegetables.

Glycogen Polysaccharide of animal body. It is formed in the body from glucose and stored in liver and muscle tissue.

Glycogen The animal storage compound comparable to starch in plants is **glycogen.** It is stored in relatively small amounts in the liver and muscle tissues. These stores help sustain normal blood sugar levels during fasting periods such as sleep hours and provide immediate fuel for muscle action. Dietary carbohydrate is essential to maintain these needed glycogen stores and prevent the symptoms of low carbohydrate intake—fatigue, dehydration, and energy loss, as well as other undesirable metabolic effects such as ketoacidosis (p. 395) and excessive protein breakdown. Sometimes a process called "glycogen-loading" is used by athletes to provide added fuel stores, but this diet manipulation can cause problems if used too often.

Dextrins Dextrins are polysaccaride compounds formed as intermediate products in the breakdown of starch. This starch breakdown occurs constantly in the process of digestion.

Dietary fiber The various forms of fiber are important in human nutrition:

1. **Cellulose** provides the chief constituent of the framework of plants. Human beings cannot digest cellulose because they lack the necessary digestive enzymes. Therefore, it remains in the digestive tract and contributes important bulk to the diet. This bulk helps move the digestive food mass along and stimulates peristalsis (p. 426). Cellulose makes up the principal structural material in plant cell walls and provides most of the substance labeled "crude fiber" (see box on pp. 46-47). The main sources are stems and leaves of vegetables, seed and grain coverings, skins, and hulls.
2. **Noncellulose polysaccharides** are carbohydrates that include hemicellulose, pectins, gums and mucilages, and algal substances. They absorb water, slow gastric emptying time, bind bile acids, and prevent intraluminal colon pressure by providing bulk for normal intestinal muscle action.
3. **Lignin** is the only noncarbohydrate type of fiber, a large compound forming the woody part of plants. It combines with bile acids to form insoluble compounds in the intestine, thus preventing their absorption. A summary of these dietary fiber classes is given in Table 3-1.

Dietary fiber produces various effects on the food mix consumed and its fate in the body. Most of these effects are caused by its physiologic properties: (1) *water absorption,* which contributes to its bulk-forming laxative effect and influences the transit time of the food mass through the digestive tract and consequent absorption of the various nutrients in the food mix, (2) *binding effect,* characteristic of certain fibers such as the non-

Clinical Application

The Semantics of Fiber: A Question of Definition

Much of the confusion concerning fiber in the human diet has centered on semantics. No term seems acceptable to cover all of the meanings involved. The older word *roughage* and the current term *fiber* denote a rough abrasive material of the physical character observed in plant cellulose, a woody type of material. However, a number of the undigestible materials in food are of a soft amorphous gel-like character. Other terms used—depending on the method for extracting the undigestible material from foods—are *acid-detergent fiber* and *neutral-detergent fiber*. As knowledge grows the problem of semantics grows likewise, and no investigator working in the field agrees that the term *fiber* is satisfactory.

The difficulties nutritionists and clinicians have met in determining a more precise nutritional and clinical significance for fiber in the human diet have not only stemmed from problems in defining the variety of food substances involved but also from difficulties surrounding the fact that not all of these undigestible materials in the human diet have the same properties. Further problems surround methods of accurately analyzing and measuring these substances in their variety of food sources.

General Definition

The word *fiber* as it is now used is a diffuse term commonly applied to a variety of nondigestible carbohydrate and carbohydrate-related substances for which specific hydrolytic enzymes are lacking in the human digestive system. Confusion arises from the erroneous interchangeable use of the two terms *dietary fiber* and *crude fiber*.

■ Dietary fiber This is the total amount of naturally occurring material in foods, mostly plant sources, that is not digested. This edible fiber in the diet includes: (1) plant dietary fiber, for which the term *plantix* has been proposed by some workers in the field, (2) undigested animal tissue polysaccharides, (3) undigested pharmaceutical products, and (4) undigested biosynthetic polysaccharides. Diets in Western countries usually contain little fiber in the energy foods such as starches, sugars, and fats. Diets in rural communities of developing countries, on the other hand, contain three to seven times more fiber in the energy foods. Current research suggests that the latter, higher fiber, diets are protective against a wide variety of Western civilization diseases.

■ Crude fiber This is the material remaining after vigorous treatment of the food sources with acid and alkali in the laboratory. Thus, it is derived from laboratory analysis and is the value given in most food value tables. These strong laboratory processes remove a good portion of the total dietary fiber that cannot withstand such treatment. Since the proportion of total dietary fiber and crude fiber varies widely among specific foods, depending on the fiber composition of a particular food, the fiber values given in food value tables have limited usefulness to the practitioner and must be used with qualification.

Clinical Application—cont'd

Enzymes Various complex proteins produced by living cells that act independently of these cells. Enzymes are catalysts capable of producing certain chemical changes in other substances without themselves being changed in the process.

Thus, in current usage, the term *crude fiber* expresses an antiquated concept and is being phased out. The term of choice, although not perfect, is *dietary fiber*. It refers to the nondigestible residues of plant foods in our diets—cellulose, hemicellulose, and lignin—that are resistant to digestion by human digestive **enzymes**, valuable to human nutrition, and shed some light on human disease.

References
Heaton, K.W., ed.: Dietary fiber: current developments in health, Westport, Conn., 1979, Technomic Pub. Co., Inc.
Inglet, G.E., and Falkehag, S.I., editors.: Dietary fibers and nutrition, New York, 1979, Academic Press.
Trowell, H.C.: Dietary fiber in human nutrition: a bibliography, London, 1979, John Libbey and Co., Ltd.

---

cellulose materials, which influences blood lipid levels through their capacity to bind bile salts and cholesterol and prevent their absorption, (3) *colon bacteria relation*, which provides fermentation substrates for bacterial action, producing volatile fatty acids and gas. Current research concerning possible clinical applications has centered largely on the relationship of fiber to gastrointestinal problems, cardiovascular disease, diabetes melli-

Table 3-1

Summary of Dietary Fiber Classes

	Source	Main Chain Structure	Function
Cellulose	Main cell-wall constituent of plants	Polyglycan, unbranched glucose polymer	Holds water; reduces elevated colonic intraluminal pressure; binds zinc
Noncellulose polysaccharides			
Gums	Secretions of plants	Galacturonic acid-mannose, galacturonic acid-rhamnose	Slows gastric emptying; provides fermentable material for colonic bacteria with production of gas and volatile fatty acids; binds bile acids
Mucilages	Plant secretions and seeds	Galactose-mannose, galacturonic acid-rhamnose, arabinose-xylose	
Algal polysaccharides	Algae, seaweeds	Mannose, xylose, glucuronic acid, glucose	
Pectin substances	Intercellular cement of plant material	Galacturonic acid	
Hemicellulose	Cell-wall plant material	Xylose, mannose, galactose, glucose (branching chains)	Holds water and increases stool bulk; reduces elevated colonic pressure; binds bile acids
Lignin	Woody part of plants	Phenylpropane polymer noncarbohydrate	Antioxidant; binds bile acids and metals

Table 3-2

Relationship Between Fiber and Various Health Problems

Problem	Effect of Fiber	Possible Mode of Action	Future Research Needs
Diabetes mellitus	Reduces fasting blood sugar levels	Slows carbohydrate absorption by	Influence of short-chain fatty acid (SCFA) production on metabolism of glucose and fats in the liver
	Reduces glycosuria	Delaying gastric emptying time	
	Reduces insulin requirements		Exact mechanisms by which fiber influences glucose metabolism
	Increases insulin sensitivity	Forming gels with pectin or guar gum in the intestine, thus impeding carbohydrate absorption	
		"Protecting" carbohydrates from enzymatic activity with a fibrous coat	
		Allowing "protected" carbohydrates to escape into large colon where they are digested by bacteria	
	Inhibits postprandial (after meals) hyperglycemia	Alters gut hormones (for example, glucagon) to enhance glucose metabolism in the liver	
Obesity	Increases satiety rate	Prolongs chewing and swallowing movements	Cause of increased satiety rate reported by subjects
	Reduces nutrient bioavailability	Increases fecal fat content	Effect on nutrient binding on nutritional status
	Reduces energy density	Inhibits absorption of carbohydrate in high fiber foods	Studies based on food composition and caloric density instead of fiber content alone
		Increases transit time	Effects of different types of fiber on gastric, small intestine, and colonic emptying time
	Alters hormonal reponse	Alters action of insulin, gut glucagon, and other intestinal hormones	
	Alters thermogenesis		

Satiety Feeling of fullness or satisfaction as after a meal or quenching one's thirst.

tus, and cancer.[2] About 15 to 20 g/day of fiber is wise for health. These clinical associations between fiber and various health problems are summarized in Table 3-2.

Functions of Carbohydrates

Energy

As indicated, the primary function of carbohydrates in human nutrition is to provide fuel for energy. Fat is also a fuel, but the body needs only a small amount of dietary fat, mainly to supply the essential fatty acids (p. 61). To function properly, however, the body tissues require a daily dietary supply of carbohydrate providing 50% to 55% of the total kilocalories.

Table 3-2 cont'd
Relationship between Fiber and Various Health Problems

Problem	Effect of Fiber	Possible Mode of Action	Future Research Needs
Coronary heart disease	Inhibits recirculation of bile acids	Alters bacterial metabolism of bile acids	Influence of fiber on cholesterol content of specific lipoprotein fractions (see Chapter 20)
		Alters bacterial flora, resulting in a change in metabolic activity	Influence on production of short-chain fatty acids
		Forms gels that bind bile acids	Role of dietary fiber as an independent variable in reducing risk of heart disease
		Alters the function of pancreatic and intestinal enzymes	
	Reduces triglyceride and cholesterol levels*	Reduces insulin levels†	Relationship between lipoprotein turnover and glucose turnover/ sensitivity to insulin
		Binds cholesterol, preventing absorption	Effect of higher concentration of bile salts on colon function
		Slows fat absorption by forming gel matrices in the intestine	
Colon cancer	Reduces incidence of disease‡	Bile acids or their bacterial metabolites may affect the structure of the colon, its cell turnover rate, and function	Testing of current hypotheses regarding the effects of dietary factors on the structure of the colon and cell turnover rate
Other gastrointestinal disorders	Reduces pressure from within the intestinal lumen	Increases transit time	
Diverticular disease	Increases diameter of the intestinal lumen, thus allowing intestinal tract to contract more, propelling contents more rapidly, and inhibiting segmentation§	Increases water absorption, resulting in a larger, softer stool	
Constipation			
Hiatal hernia			
Hemorrhoids			

*This effect is based on epidemiologic studies, usually observed in combination with reduced fat intake.
†Insulin is required for fat synthesis.
‡Preventive effect of fiber is assumed from epidemiologic studies that associate low-fiber, high-fat diets with an *increased* incidence of disease.
§Segmentation increases pressure and weakness along the walls of the intestinal tract.

The amount of carbohydrate in the body, though relatively small, is important to maintain energy reserves. For example, in an adult male about 300 to 350 g is "stored" in the liver and muscle tissues as glycogen, and about 10 g is present in circulating blood sugar. This total amount of available glucose provides energy sufficient for only about half a day of moderate activity. Therefore, carbohydrate foods must be eaten regularly and at moderately frequent intervals to meet the energy demands of the body.

Special Functions of Carbohydrates in Body Tissues

As part of their general function as the body's main energy source, carbohydrates serve special functions in many body tissues.

Glycogen Reserves

The liver and muscle glycogen reserves provide a constant interchange with the body's overall energy balance system and protect cells from depressed metabolic function and injury.

Protein-Sparing Action

Carbohydrate helps regulate protein metabolism. The presence of sufficient carbohydrates for energy demands of the body prevents the channeling of too much protein for this purpose. This protein-sparing action of carbohydrate allows a major portion of protein to be used for its basic structural purpose of tissue building.

Antiketogenic Effect

Carbohydrate also relates to fat metabolism. The amount of carbohydrate present in the diet determines how much fat will be broken down, thus affecting the formation and disposal rates of ketones. *Ketones* are intermediate products of fat metabolism, which normally are produced at a low level during fat oxidation. However, in extreme conditions such as starvation or uncontrolled diabetes, as well as with the unwise use of extremely low carbohydrate diets, carbohydrate is inadequate or unavailable for energy needs, so too much fat is oxidized. Ketones accummulate and the result is *ketoacidosis* (p. 395). Thus sufficient dietary carbohydrate helps prevent a damaging excess formation of ketones.

Heart

Heart action is a life-sustaining muscular excerise. Although fatty acids are the preferred regular fuel of the heart muscle, the glycogen in cardiac muscle is an important emergency source of contractile energy. In a damaged heart poor glycogen stores or low carbohydrate intake may cause cardiac symptoms and angina.

Central Nervous System

A constant amount of carbohydrate is necessary for the proper functioning of the central nervous system (CNS). The regulatory center of the CNS, the brain, contains no stored supply of glucose and is therefore especially dependent on a minute-to-minute supply of glucose from the blood. Sustained and profound hypoglycemic shock may cause irreversible brain damage. In all nerve tissue, carbohydrate is indispensable for functional integrity.

Digestion: Changing Basic Fuel to Usable Refined Fuel

Most carbohydrate foods, starches and sugars, cannot immediately be used by the cell to make energy available. They must be changed to a usable refined fuel for which the cell is designed—*glucose*. The process by which these vital changes are made is *digestion*. The digestion of carbohydrate foods proceeds through the successive parts of the gastrointestinal tract, accomplished by two types of actions: (1) mechanical or muscle functions that render the food mass into smaller particles and (2) chemical processes in which specific enzymes break down food nutrients into usable metabolic products.

Mouth

Mastication breaks food into fine particles and mixes it with the saliva. During this process, a salivary amylase (ptyalin) is secreted by the parotid gland. It acts on starch to begin its breakdown into dextrins and maltose.

Stomach

Successive wavelike contractions of the muscle fibers of the stomach wall continue the mechanical digestive process. This action is called *peristalsis*. It further mixes food particles with gastric secretions to allow the chemical activity of digestion to take place more readily. The gastric secretion contains no specific enzyme for the breakdown of carbohydrate. The hydrochloric acid in the stomach stops the action of salivary amylase. But before the food mixes completely with the acid gastric secretion, as much as 20% to 30% of the starch may have been changed into maltose. Muscle actions continue to bring the carbohydrate food mass to the lower part of the stomach and the *pyloric valve*. The food mass is now a thick creamy *chyme*, ready for emptying into the duodenum, the first portion of the small intestine.

Small Intestine

Lumen Space within a tube; e.g., gastrointestinal tract or a blood vessel.

Peristalsis continues to aid digestion in the small intestine by mixing and moving the chyme along the **lumen** in the length of the tube. Chemical digestion of carbohydrate is completed in the small intestine by enzymes from two sources: pancreas and intestines.

Pancreatic Secretions

These secretions from the pancreas enter the duodenum through the common bile duct. They contain a pancreatic amylase, which continues the breakdown of starch to maltose.

Intestinal Secretions

Lactose intolerance, a condition causing gastrointestinal problems, results from a deficiency of the enzyme lactase (p. 436).

These contain three disaccharidases, *sucrase, lactase,* and *maltase*. These disaccharidases act on their respective disaccharides to render the monosaccharides—glucose, galactose, and fructose—ready for absorption. These disaccharidases are integral proteins of the brush border of the small intestine and break down the disaccharides as absorption takes place. The digestive products, the monosaccharides, are then immediately absorbed into the *portal* blood circulation.

Table 3-3
Summary of Carbohydrate Digestion

Organ	Enzyme	Action
Mouth	Ptyalin	Starch → Dextrins → Maltose
Stomach	None	(Above action continued to minor degree)
Small intestine	Pancreatic amylopsin	Starch → Dextrins → Maltose
	Intestinal:	
	Sucrase	Sucrose → Glucose + Fructose
	Lactase	Lactose → Glucose + Galactose
	Maltase	Maltose → Glucose + Glucose

A summary of the major aspects of carbohydrate digestion through these successive parts of the gastrointestinal tract is given in Table 3-3.

Absorption: Carrying Refined Fuel to Energy Production Sites— Cells

The refined fuel glucose is now ready to be carried to the individual cells to produce energy. The process by which the body transports this basic end product of carbohydrate digestion to the cells throughout the body is called *absorption*. The major glucose absorption mechanism is an active transport system requiring sodium as a carrier substance.

Absorbing Structures

The absorbing surface area of the small intestine is uniquely designed to enhance this absorption process (Figure 2-1, p. 21). First, *mucosal folds* in the surface tissue enlarge the surface *area*. Second, millions of tiny finger-like projections called *villi* are located on the surface of these folds of the mucous membrane. Third, on the surface of each villus are still smaller projections, called *microvilli*, forming an extended brush border. Together, these structures provide a greatly increased absorbing surface that allows 90% of the digested food material to be absorbed in the small intestine. Only water absorption remains to be accomplished in the large intestine.

Route of Absorption

Portal Entryway, usually referring to the portal circulation of blood through the liver. Blood is brought into the liver by the portal vein and out by the hepatic vein.

By way of the capillaries of the villi, the simple sugars enter the **portal** circulation and are transported to the liver. Here fructose and galactose are converted to glucose, and glucose in turn is converted to glycogen for storage. Then glycogen is constantly being reconverted to glucose as needed by the body.

Metabolism: Burning Refined Fuel at Production Sites to Produce Energy

Cell Metabolism

Cells are the functional units of life in the human body. In cell nutrition the most important end product of the digestion of dietary carbohydrate is glucose, since the other two monosaccharides, fructose and galactose, are eventually converted to glucose. The liver is the major site of the intricate metabolic machinery that handles glucose. However, energy metabolism in general goes on in all cells. In these individual cells glucose is burned to produce energy through a series of chemical reactions involving specific cell enzymes. The final energy produced is then available to the cell to do its work. Extra glucose not immediately needed for energy may also be changed to fat and stored as a reserve supply of energy.

Metabolism Sum of all chemical changes that take place within an organism, by which it maintains itself and produces energy for its functioning.

Metabolism

This term refers to the sum of the various chemical processes in a living organism by which energy is made available for the functioning of the whole organism. It also includes processes by which protoplasm, the basic substance of cells and tissues, is produced, maintained, or broken down. Products of specific metabolic processes are called **metabolites.**

Metabolite Any substance that forms as a result of the breakdown (catabolism) or growth or maintenance (anabolism) of living tissue.

Blood Sugar Levels

In the previous chapter you saw how insulin and other balancing hormones work as control agents to maintain blood sugar levels within the normal range—approximately 70 to 120 mg/dl (p. 392). Foods vary according to their effect on blood sugar levels—their so-called **glycemic in-**

Glycemic index Blood sugar response value of a food in relation to that of glucose. It is an expression of the area under the blood glucose response curve for an individual food, stated as the percentage of the area after taking the same amount of carbohydrate as glucose.

dex (p. 398). *Hyperglycemia* means blood sugar levels above the normal range. *Hypoglycemia* indicates blood sugar levels below the normal range. (See Issues and Answers, pp. 55-56.)

Metabolic Concept of Unity

Here and in following discussions of other nutrients, a central significant scientific principle will emerge. This principle may be stated as the *unity of the human organism.* The human organism is a whole made up of many parts and processes that possess unequaled specificity and flexibility. Intimate metabolic relationships exist among all the basic nutrients and metabolites. Thus it is impossible to understand any one of the human body's many metabolic processes without viewing it in relationship to the whole.

Therefore, in all your work with patients and clients, you should remember this important fact: **All nutrients do their best work in partnership with other nutrients.** From this fact you can draw two practical conclusions: (1) the emphasis in health teaching and nutrition education should be on achieving a sound balanced nutritional basis for any dietary program, and (2) some deficiency states may be *iatrogenic* (induced by medical treatment), or may have their origin in a fad, or may be caused by long-term, over-zealous emphasis on one particular nutrient to the exclusion of other equally essential ones.

To Sum Up

Carbohydrate supplies most of the world's population with its primary source of energy. A product of photosynthesis, it is widely distributed in nature and its food products are easy to store and generally low in cost.

There are two basic types of carbohydrates: simple and complex. *Simple carbohydrates* consist of single and double sugar units (mono- and disaccharides) that are easily digested and provide quick energy. *Complex carbohydrates,* or polysaccharides, are less easily prepared for use. Though they vary somewhat in their effect on blood sugar, generally they provide energy more slowly and prevent large fluctuations in blood glucose levels.

In addition to providing general body energy, carbohydrates maintain liver, heart, brain, and nerve tissue function. They also prevent the breaking down of fats and proteins for energy, which results in excessive production of toxic metabolic byproducts. *Fiber,* a complex carbohydrate that forms the undigestable part of plants, also affects the digestion and absorption of foods in ways that have proved beneficial to good health.

Questions for Review

1. Refer to the RDA table to determine the daily caloric need of a 25-year-old woman who is 5 ft 4 in tall and weighs 125 lbs. How many kilocalories should be provided by carbohydrates in her diet? How much fiber is recommended?

2. Give a general description of the clinical effects of fiber in each of the following disease states: diverticular disease, hyperlipidemia, diabetes mellitus, and colon cancer.

3. Your client, Mr. Brown, wants desperately to lose 20 lbs before meeting his future in-laws next month. He purchased a month's worth of liquid protein and takes multivitamins daily. He seems adamant about not eating any starches or sweets. Based on your readings in this chapter, how would you explain the effects of a low-carbohydrate diet on carbohydrate functions so that he will know why carbohydrates are important even in a weight-loss program?

References

1. Sharon, N.: Carbohydrates, Sci. Am. **243**(5):90, 1980.
2. Vahouny, G.V.: Conclusions and recommendations of the Symposium on Dietary Fibers in Health and Disease, Washington, D.C., 1981, Am. J. Clin. Nutr. **35**:152, 1982.

Further Readings

Bohannon, N.V., Karam, J.H., and Forsham, P.H.: Endocrine responses to sugar ingestion in man, J. Am. Diet. Assoc. **76**(6):555, 1980.

These clinicians present their investigation of glucose, insulin, and glucagon responses to oral tolerance tests of three sugars—fructose, sucrose, and glucose. In comparison with the other two sugars, fructose caused less variation from baseline in all effects studied. It significantly blunted the plasma glucose rise.

Eastwood, M.A., and Passmore, R.: A new look at dietary fiber, Nutr. Today **19**:6, 1984.

This excellent article describes the place of fiber in modern nutrition and how it works; enhanced by many photographs and drawings.

Hannigan, K.J.: The sweetener report 1982-1987, Food Eng. **54**:75, 1982.

A revolution in the food industry is described, with increased use of corn syrup and high fructose corn syrup (HFCS) as a sugar (sucrose) replacement. This trend is expected to continue in the U.S. market, with fructose eventually becoming the number one sweetener by the end of this decade.

Mongeau, R., and Brassard, R.: Determination of neutral detergent fiber in breakfast cereals: pentose, hemicellulose, and lignin content, J. Food Sci. **47**(2):550, 1982.

Analysis is given for dietary fiber content in 91 breakfast cereals, showing that many of them contain less than 5% dietary fiber. Large chart summarizes analysis.

Powers, M.A., and Crapo, P.A.: The fructose story, Diabetes Educator **7**:22, 1982.

These research dietitians, both clinical research specialists, provide helpful answers to review fructose's structure, sources, uses, metabolism, effects on blood glucose and insulin, and its role in diabetes management and weight reduction.

Issues and Answers

Hypoglycemia   The lay public associates hypoglycemia primarily with an excessive amount of sugar in the diet. More specifically, however, the medical community has identified two general types of hypoglycemia and their known causes:

> **Reactive hypoglycemia** This type occurs after a meal and most frequently affects persons who have recently undergone abdominal surgery or who have diabetes.
>
> **Fasting hypoglycemia** This type occurs after extended periods without adequate food or from poor eating habits. It may also be caused by several drugs: (1) alcohol, which blocks glucose production by the liver, (2) hypoglycemic medications such as sulfonylureas used to treat diabetes, and (3) salicylate (aspirin). More serious conditions that may cause this effect include (1) tumors of the pancreas that stimulate excessive insulin secretion and (2) adrenal insufficiency, a rare condition that prevents the adrenal glands from responding to certain bodily needs, especially under stress.
>
> **Diagnosis** A normal blood glucose range is about 70 to 120 mg/dl. The traditional basis for medical diagnosis has usually been the oral glucose tolerance test (GTT). The patient drinks a beverage containing 75 to 100 g of glucose, and the blood sugar levels are measured at half-hour intervals for up to 5 hours. A glucose level of 40 to 60 mg/dl at 3 hours into the test is considered an indication of hypoglycemia. More recently, however, physicians have used blood tests at the time the patient is experiencing the characteristic symptoms to obtain a more realistic measure.
>
> **Treatment** In general, the lay public believes hypoglycemia should be treated with an extremely low-carbohydrate, high-protein diet. However, a very low-carbohydrate diet will make it difficult for the body to obtain sufficient amounts of glucose to achieve and maintain normal blood levels. It is evident now, from current carbohydrate research, that a diet of frequent small meals, rich in complex carbohydrates with a moderately low "glycemic index," a good fiber content, and fewer simple carbohydrates and sugars will maintain a more stable blood sugar level without dipping periods of low blood sugar. The only major dietary restriction is that of sugar and other simple carbohydrates.

The simple procedure for home blood glucose monitoring developed for persons with diabetes (pp. 409-410) can be used by persons with hypoglycemic symptoms to test their own blood sugar levels at the time they are experiencing symptoms and record results. This record will then provide an accurate profile of the blood glucose levels in the free home environment. This procedure can then provide a therapeutic tool for use in counseling and teaching. If the record provides no documented hypoglycemic periods, a sensitive

Continued.

Issues and Answers—cont'd

counselor can help provide the person with more insight into the problem, exploring other reasons for the symptoms experienced. On the other hand, if the record documents actual hypoglycemia in the home environment, then further diagnostic evaluation is required. This technique is simple, accurate, and effective for persons being evaluated for reactive or postprandial hypoglycemia.

References

American Diabetic Association Report: Statement on hyperglycemia, Diabetes Care **5**(1):72, 1982.

Sanders, L.R., and others: Refined carbohydrate as a contributing factor in reactive hypoglycemia, South. Med. J. **75**(9):1072, 1982.

Chapter 4
Fats

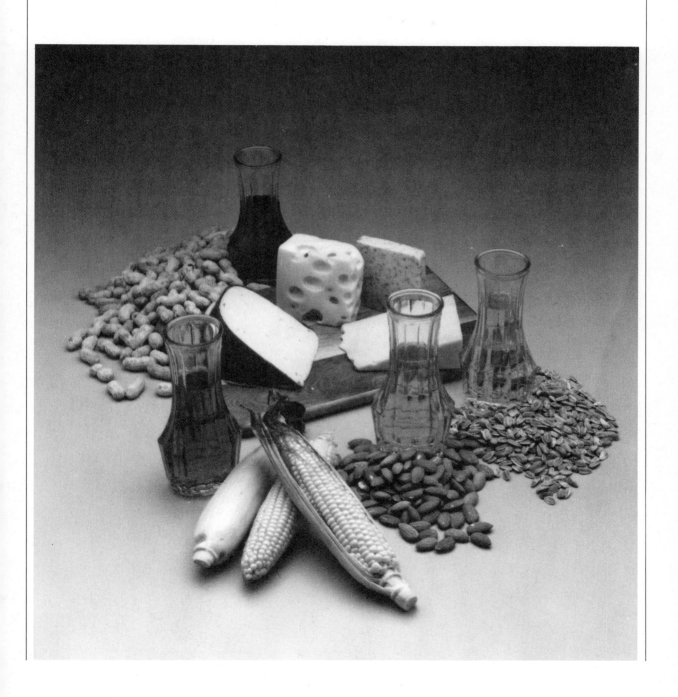

Preview

In addition to carbohydrate, to further solve its energy problem, the body turns to fat as another basic fuel source. Fat is a valuable fuel because it is highly concentrated, having about twice the energy value of carbohydrate.

Traditionally fat has held a prominent place in the American diet. We have maintained a relatively rich fare in our basic food patterns with approximately 45% of our total caloric intake coming from fat, more than that in any other developed country. However, spurred by our justified health concerns, our attitudes and usage patterns regarding fat have begun to change. Our general goal in this chapter is to help achieve some balance in our food habits and attitudes about fat and health based on our current knowledge of fat, its fate in our bodies, and its role in human nutrition.

Chapter Objectives

After study of this chapter, the student should be able to:

1. Identify forms of fat and other lipids essential in the human diet and describe their nature and functions in the human body.

2. Determine how much and what type of fats are necessary in our diet and in our bodies to maintain good health.

3. Identify sound guidelines to ensure the proper use of fat in the diet.

Fats as Basic Fuel

Lipids Group name for organic substances of fatty nature. The lipids include fats, oils, waxes, and related compounds.

Fats provide a concentrated storage form of basic fuel for the human energy system. They include substances such as fat, oil, and related compounds that are greasy to the touch and insoluble in water. Substances of this class are called **lipids**. Some basic food fuel forms of fat are easily seen as fat: butter, margarine, oil, salad dressings, bacon, and cream. Other food forms of fat are more hidden: egg yolk, meat fats, olives, avocados, and nuts and seeds. Even when all the visible fat has been trimmed from meat, about 6% of the fat surrounding the muscle fibers will still remain.

Many Americans eat a relatively large amount of fat, about 45% of the total kilocalories in their diet. However, questions are being raised about the amount and kind of fat we eat in relation to our health.

Relation of Fats to Health

Health Needs for Fat

We need fat in our food and in our bodies to keep us healthy. This need is indicated by the number of functions fat performs in nutrition, both in our diets and in our overall metabolism:

Food Fats

Linoleic acid Major essential fatty acid. It is polyunsaturated.

1. **Fuel source** Food fats supply a basic continuing source of fuel for the body to store and burn as needed for energy, yielding 9 kcal/g when oxidized, in comparison to carbohydrate, which yields 4 kcal/g.
2. **Essential nutrient supply** Food fats supply the essential fatty acids, especially **linoleic acid**, and cholesterol as needed to supplement the body's endogenous supply.
3. **Food satiety** Fats in the diet supply flavor to food, which contributes to a feeling of satisfaction that lasts longer after eating than does the feeling of satisfaction after eating carbohydrates. This satiety is enhanced by the fuller texture and body that fat contributes to food mixtures and the slower gastric emptying time it brings.

Body Fats

1. **Energy** A major function of fat in nutrition is to supply an efficient fuel to all tissues except the central nervous system and brain, which depend on glucose.
2. **Thermal insulation** The layer of fat directly underneath the skin controls body temperature within the range necessary for life.

Adipose Fat present in cells of adipose or fatty tissue.

3. **Vital organ protection** A web-like padding of **adipose** fat surrounds vital organs such as the kidneys, protecting from mechanical shock and providing a supporting structure.
4. **Nerve impulse transmission** Fat layers surrounding nerve fibers provide electrical insulation and transmit nerve impulses.
5. **Tissue membrane structure** Fat serves as a vital constituent of cell membrane structure, helping transport nutrient materials and metabolites across cell membranes.

Lipoproteins Noncovalent complexes of fat with protein. The lipoproteins probably function as major carriers of lipids in the plasma, since most of the plasma fat is associated with them. Such a combination makes possible the transport of fatty substances in a predominantly aqueous medium such as plasma.

6. **Cell metabolism** Combinations of fat and protein, **lipoproteins** carry fat in the blood to all cells.
7. **Essential precursor substances** Fat supplies necessary components such as fatty acids and cholesterol for synthesis of many materials required for metabolic functions and tissue integrity.

Health Problems with Fat

It is evident from the lists above that fat is an essential nutrient. But if fat is as vital to human health as indicated, what then is the problem about fat in the diet? Indeed, this is not a fully resolved question. Health problems with fat focus on two main issues: too much dietary fat and too much of that fat from animal food sources.[1]

Amount of Fat

Too much fat in the diet provides excessive kilocalories, more than required for immediate energy needs. The excess is stored as increasing adipose tissue and body weight. How much fat is in your own diet? You might try figuring it out for a day (see box, p. 61). This increased body weight has been associated with health problems such as diabetes, hypertension, and heart disease. Look for specific relationships in later chapters.

Kind of Fat

An excess of saturated fat in the diet, which comes from animal sources, has been associated with atherosclerosis, the underlying blood vessel disease (p. 455). This disease process contributes to heart attacks and strokes. However, the nature of this association is by no means resolved, and the diet-heart controversy is the basis of continuing research. (See Issues and Answers, pp. 69-71.)

The Nature of Lipids

The class name for fats and similar compounds is *lipids*. These are compounds defined by their common relationship to the fatty acids.

Fatty Acids

The same basic chemical elements that make up carbohydrates—carbon, hydrogen, and oxygen—also make up fatty acids and their related fats. Fatty acids are also refined fuel forms of fat that some cells such as heart muscle prefer over glucose.

Saturation of Fatty Acids

Saturation To cause to unite with the greatest possible amount of another substance through solution, chemical combination, or the like.

This state of **saturation** or unsaturation gives fat an important textural characteristic. Saturated fats are harder, less saturated ones are softer, and unsaturated ones are usually liquid oils. This differing state results from the ratio of hydrogen to carbon in the basic fatty acid structure. If a given fatty acid is filled with as much hydrogen as it can take, the fatty acid is said to be completely *saturated* with hydrogen. If, however, the fatty acid has less hydrogen it is obviously less saturated. Three terms for degrees of saturation are usually used:

1. **Saturated** Food fats composed mainly of such saturated fatty acids are called *saturated fats*. These fats are of animal origin.
2. **Monounsaturated** Food fats composed mainly of fatty acids with one less hydrogen atom are called *monounsaturated fats*.
3. **Polyunsaturated** Food fats composed mainly of fatty acids with two or more places unfilled with hydrogen are called *polyunsaturated* fats. Food fats composed mainly of unsaturated fatty acids are from plant sources. (Notable exceptions are coconut oil, palm oil, and cocoa butter.)

Clinical Application

How Much Fat are You Eating?

- Keep an accurate record of everything you eat or drink for 1 day. Be sure to estimate and add amounts of all fat or other nutrient seasonings used with your foods. (If you want a more representative picture and have a computer available with nutrient analysis programming, keep a 1-week record and calculate an average of the 7 days).

- Calculate the total kilocalories (kcal) and grams of each of the energy nutrients (carbohydrate, fat, and protein) in everything you eat. Multiply the total grams of each energy nutrient by its respective fuel value:

$$\text{fat} \underline{\hspace{2em}}g \times 9 = \underline{\hspace{2em}}kcal$$
$$\text{protein} \underline{\hspace{2em}}g \times 4 = \underline{\hspace{2em}}kcal$$
$$\text{carbohydrate} \underline{\hspace{2em}}g \times 4 = \underline{\hspace{2em}}kcal$$

- Calculate the percentage of each energy nutrient in your total diet:

$$\frac{\text{Fat kcal}}{\text{Total kcal}} \times 100 = \% \text{ fat kcal in diet}$$

- Compare with fat in American diet (40% to 45%); with the U.S. Dietary Goals (25% to 30%).

Essential Fatty Acids

Essential fatty acid (EFA) Fatty acid that is (1) necessary for body metabolism or function and (2) cannot be manufactured by the body and must therefore be supplied in the diet. The major essential fatty acid is linoleic acid ($C_{17}H_{31}COOH$). It is found principally in vegetable oils. Two other fatty acids usually classified as essential are linolenic acid and arachidonic acid.

The term *essential* or *nonessential* is applied to a nutrient according to its relative necessity in the diet. The nutrient is essential (1) if its absence will create a specific deficiency disease and/or (2) if the body cannot manufacture it and must obtain it from diet. If fat composes only 10% or less of the diet's kilocalories, adequate amounts of essential fatty acids aren't provided. Linoleic, linolenic, and arachidonic are the only fatty acids known to be essential for the complete nutrition of humans. Actually only linoleic acid is a true *dietary* **essential fatty acid (EFA)**, since the others may be naturally synthesized from it. **Linoleic acid,** along with linolenic and arachidonic acids, serve important functions in the body:

1. They strengthen capillary and cell membrane structure, which helps prevent an increase in skin and membrane permeability. A deficiency of linoleic acid leads to a breakdown in skin and other tissue membrane integrity with resulting eczema and other problems.
2. They combine with cholesterol for its transport in the blood.
3. They help to lower serum cholesterol. Linoleic acid plays a key role in the transport and metabolism of cholesterol.
4. They prolong blood-clotting time and increase fibrinolytic activity.
5. They help form a group of physiologically and pharmacologically active compounds known as prostaglandins. These substances are synthesized in the body from the essential fatty acids, especially arachidonic acid and its precursor, linoleic acid.

Prostaglandins Group of
naturally occurring long-chain
fatty acids having local
hormone-like actions of
widely diverse forms.

Prostaglandins

The **prostaglandins** are an interesting group of long-chain unsaturated fatty acids that the body synthesizes from the essential acids, mainly arachidonic acid. At present these substances are under intense investigation to determine their multiple physiologic roles in the body. They were first discovered by Swedish investigators in their study of reproductive physiology, identified initially in human semen, and named prostaglandins because they were thought to originate in the prostate gland. They are now known to exist in virtually all body tissues and to direct important widespread biologic activities. For example, they have been found in breast milk and give gastrointestinal protection to the infant.[2] They have been shown to be powerful modulators of vascular smooth muscle tone and platelet aggregation and hence have a relationship to cardiovascular disease.[3] Overall, these fascinating compounds affect their originating cell and neighboring cells in a number of bewildering and diverse ways and can be thought of as local hormones in their varied functions.

Chain Length of Fatty Acids

Another characteristic of fatty acids, important in their absorption, is the length of the carbon chain composing their structure. The long-chain fatty acids are more difficult to absorb and require a helping carrier. The medium- and short-chain fatty acids are more soluble in water and hence can be absorbed more easily directly into the blood stream. In malabsorptive disease of the intestine, when the absorbing surface is inflamed or infected, short- or medium-chain fat products are preferred. A commercial product called MCT (medium-chain triglycerides) is an oil made up of medium- and short-chain fatty acids that can be used in the diet in the same fashion as any ordinary vegetable oil.

Glycerides Group name for
fats, any of a group of esters
obtained from glycerol by the
replacement of one, two, or
three hydroxyl (OH) groups
with a fatty acid. Glycerides
are the principal constituent
of adipose tissue and are
found in animal and
vegetable fats and oils.

Glycerol Colorless, odorless,
syrupy, sweet liquid; a
constituent of fats usually
obtained by the hydrolysis of
fats. Chemically, glycerol is
an alcohol; it is esterified with
fatty acids to produce fats.

Triglycerides Compound of
three fatty acids esterified to
glycerol. A neutral fat,
synthesized from
carbohydrate, stored in
adipose tissue. It releases
free fatty acids into the blood
after being hydrolyzed by
enzymes.

Triglycerides
Structure

Fats are **glycerides** composed of **glycerol** and fatty acids. When glycerol is combined with one fatty acid it is called a *monoglyceride,* with two fatty acids a *diglyceride,* and with three fatty acids a *triglyceride.* Whether in food or in the body, fatty acids combine with glycerol to form glycerides. Most natural fats, whether from animal or vegetable sources, are triglycerides. These fats, the **triglycerides,** occur in body cells as oily droplets. They circulate in water-based blood serum sheathed with water-soluble protein in *lipoprotein* complexes and serve multiple functions throughout the body.

Dietary Fats

Food fats (as well as body fats) are composed of saturated or unsaturated fatty acids. If the food fat is made up mainly of unsaturated fatty acids, it is called an unsaturated fat. If the food fat is made up mainly of saturated fatty acids, it is called a saturated fat. Foods from animal sources such as meat, milk, and eggs contain saturated fats. Conversely, foods from vegetable sources such as the oils are unsaturated fats. A general saturated-unsaturated spectrum of food fats is shown in Figure 4-1. The animal food fats on the saturated end of the spectrum are solid; those toward the cen-

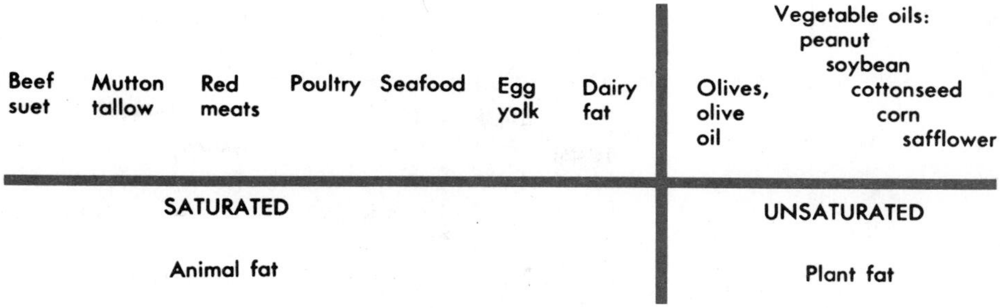

Figure 4-1
Spectrum of food fats
according to degree of
saturation of component fatty
acid.

Beef suet	Mutton tallow	Red meats	Poultry	Seafood	Egg yolk	Dairy fat		Olives, olive oil	Vegetable oils: peanut soybean cottonseed corn safflower

SATURATED	UNSATURATED
Animal fat	Plant fat

ter become somewhat less saturated and hence softer in texture. The plant fats on the unsaturated end of the spectrum are free-flowing vegetable oils that do not solidify even at low temperatures. Exceptions include coconut oil, palm oil, and cocoa butter which are saturated fats. Since these saturated plant fats are used extensively in commercial products because they are usually cheaper oils, it is important to read product labels carefully. There is a need for more label information about fat composition. This distinction in saturation is helpful in explaining to patients on modified fat diets the correct choices of food fats. Also, the unsaturated oils can be hardened commercially into products such as margarine and shortening by injection of hydrogen gas to saturate them. This process is called **hydrogenation**.

Hydrogenation Process of adding hydrogen to unsaturated fats to produce a solid, saturated fat. This process is used to produce vegetable shortening from vegetable oils.

Cholesterol
Structure

Cholesterol is often discussed in connection with dietary fat, but it is not a fat (triglyceride) itself. Many people confuse cholesterol with saturated fats. It is a fat-related compound that is structurally quite different from the triglycerides. Generally, cholesterol travels in the blood stream attached to long-chain fatty acids, forming cholesterol **esters.**

Cholesterol Fat-related compound, a sterol ($C_{27}H_{45}OH$). It is a normal constituent of bile and a principal constituent of gallstones. In body metabolism, cholesterol is important as a precursor of various steroid hormones, such as sex hormones and adrenal corticoids.

Functions

Cholesterol is a vital substance in human metabolism. It belongs to a family of substances called **steroids**, or sterols, and is a precursor to all steroid hormones. A derivative of cholesterol in the skin, *7-dehydrocholesterol,* is irradiated by sunlight's ultraviolet rays to produce vitamin D, a hormone. It is also essential in the formation of bile acids, which emulsify and prepare fats for enzymatic digestion and then help in their absorption. Cholesterol is widely distributed in all the cells of the body and is found in large amounts in brain and nerve tissue. It is an essential component of cell membranes. It is small wonder therefore that a constant supply of so vital a material for bodily processes would be made in body tissues, mainly in the liver. If a person consumed *no* cholesterol at all, the body would still synthesize a needed supply.

Ester A compound produced by the reaction between an acid and an alcohol with elimination of a molecule of water. For example, a triglyceride is an ester.

Steroids Any of a large group of fat-related organic compounds, including sterols, bile acids, sex hormones of the adrenal cortex, and D vitamins.

Food Sources

Cholesterol occurs naturally in all animal foods. There is none in plant foods. Its main food sources are egg yolks and organ meats such as liver and kidney. In fact, cholesterol occurs *only* in animal fats and animal tissue and not in plant fats or tissues. Therefore vegetable oils do not contain cholesterol. Although the plant oils vary in degree of saturation, *none* of them contain cholesterol.

Health Concerns

Most of the concern about cholesterol has resulted from studies over the last three decades indicating that a high blood cholesterol level—not necessarily a high dietary cholesterol—was one of the risk factors associated with atherosclerosis. This is the underlying disease process in cardiovascular disease in which fatty deposits or plaques containing cholesterol develop in and on the walls of the arteries (p. 455). A recent National Institute of Health's report of its 10-year study involving 3806 men (the Lipid Research Clinics Trial) did indicate a close relationship, but the subjects all had elevated serum cholesterol levels and a cholesterol-lowering drug was also used.[4] One of the factors that lowers blood cholesterol is the substitution in the diet of polyunsaturated fat for some of the saturated fat. It is still not clear just what the reason for this effect is. These fatty acids probably stimulate cholesterol excretion into the intestine and the oxidation of cholesterol to form bile acids.

Lipoproteins
Function

The lipoproteins are important combinations of fat with protein and other fat-related components that are highly significant in human nutrition. They are complexes of lipids and **apoproteins** (p. 459) that serve as the major vehicle for fat transport in the blood stream.

Apoprotein Protein part of a compound, as of a lipoprotein. For example, apoprotein C II, an apoprotein of HDL and VLDL that functions to activate the enzyme, lipoprotein lipase.

Fat Transport

Because fat is insoluble in water, a means of transporting fat throughout the body in a water-based circulatory system, the blood, presents a problem. The body has solved this problem through the development of the *lipoproteins,* packages of fat wrapped in water-soluble protein. These plasma lipoproteins contain triglycerides, cholesterol, fatty acids, **phospholipids,** and traces of other related materials such as fat-soluble vitamins and steroid hormones. The high or low density of the lipoprotein transport complex is determined by its relative loads of fat and protein. The higher the protein ratio, the higher the density:

Phospholipids Any of a class of fat-related substances that contain phosphorus, fatty acids, and a nitrogenous base. The phospholipids are essential elements in every cell.

1. **Chylomicrons** have the lowest density and are mostly triglycerides (90%) with a small amount of protein, delivering diet fat to liver cells.
2. **Very low–density lipoproteins (VLDL)** deliver endogenous triglycerides to tissue cells.
3. **Intermediate low–density lipoproteins (ILDL)** continue the delivery of endogenous triglycerides to tissue cells.
4. **Low-density lipoproteins (LDL)** deliver cholesterol to the peripheral tissue cells.
5. **High-density lipoproteins (HDL)** transfer free cholesterol from tissues to the liver for catabolism and excretion. All the lipoproteins are closely associated with lipid disorders related to cardiovascular disease, so look for details of their structures and functions in Chapter 20.

Digestion: Changing Basic Fuel to Usable Refined Fuel

Fatty acid Structural components of fats. See *glycerides*, p. 62.

The basic fat fuels—various animal and plant fats (triglycerides) that naturally occur in foods—are taken into the body with the diet. Then the task is to change these basic fuel fats into a refined fuel form of fat that the cells can burn for energy. These key refined fuel forms are the **fatty acids.** The body accomplishes this task through the process of fat digestion.

Mouth

No fat digestion takes place in the mouth. In this first portion of the gastrointestinal tract, fat is simply broken up into smaller particles through chewing and moistened for passage into the stomach with the general food mass.

Stomach

Little if any fat digestion takes place in the stomach. General peristalsis continues the mechanical mixing of fats with the stomach contents. No significant amount of enzymes specific for fats is present in the gastric secretions except a *gastric lipase* (tributyrinase), which acts on emulsified butterfat. As the main gastric enzymes act on other specific nutrients in the food mix, fat is separated from them and made more readily accessible to its own specific chemical breakdown in the small intestine.

Cholecystokinin Hormone that is secreted by the mucosa of the duodenum in response to the presence of fat. It causes the gallbladder to contract, which propels bile into the duodenum, where it is needed to emulsify the fat.

Small Intestine

Not until fat reaches the small intestine do the chemical changes necessary for fat digestion occur, with agents from two major sources.

Bile from the Liver and Gallbladder

The presence of fats in the duodenum stimulates the secretion of **cholecystokinin**, a local hormone from glands in the intestinal walls. In turn, cholecystokinin causes contraction of the gallbladder, relaxation of the sphincter, and subsequent secretion of **bile** into the intestine via the common bile duct. The liver produces a large amount of dilute bile, then the gallbladder concentrates and stores it, ready for use as needed. Its function is that of an **emulsifier.** *Emulsification* is not a digestive process itself, but is an important first step in the preparation of fat for digestion by the enzymes: (1) it breaks the fat into small particles, or globules, which greatly enlarges the surface area available for action of the enzyme, and (2) it serves to lower the surface tension of the finely dispersed and suspended fat globules, which allows the enzymes to penetrate more easily. This is similar to the wetting action of detergents. The bile also provides an alkaline medium for the action of lipase.

Bile Greenish yellow to golden brown alkaline fluid secreted by the liver and concentrated in the gallbladder. Made of bile salts, cholesterol, phospholipid, bilirubin diglucuronide, and electrolytes.

Emulsifier An agent that breaks down large fat globules to smaller, uniformly distributed particles.

Enzymes from the Pancreas

Pancreatic juice contains an enzyme for fat and one for cholesterol. First, *pancreatic* **lipase**, a powerful fat enzyme, breaks off one fatty acid at a time from the glycerol base of fats. One fatty acid and diglyceride, then another fatty acid and monoglyceride, are produced in turn. Each succeeding step of this breakdown occurs with increasing difficulty. In fact, separation of the final fatty acid from the remaining monoglyceride is such a slow process that less than one third of the total fat present actually reaches complete breakdown. The final products of fat digestion to be

Lipase Any of a class of enzymes that break down fats.

Table 4-1
Summary of Fat Digestion

Organ	Enzyme	Activity
Mouth	None	Mechanical, mastication
Stomach	No major enzyme	Mechanical separation of fats as protein and starch digested out
	Small amount of gastric lipase tributyrinase	Tributyrin (butterfat) to fatty acids and glycerol
Small intestine	Gallbladder bile salts (emulsifier)	Emulsifies fats
	Pancreatic lipase (steapsin)	Triglycerides to diglycerides and monoglycerides in turn, then fatty acids and glycerol

absorbed are fatty acids, diglycerides, monoglycerides, and glycerol. Some remaining fat may pass into the large intestine for fecal elimination. Second, the enzyme, *cholesterol esterase*, acts on cholesterol to form cholesterol esters by combining cholesterol and fatty acids in preparing free cholesterol for absorption.

Enzyme from the Small Intestine

The small intestine secretes an enzyme in the intestinal juice called *lecithinase*. It acts on lecithin to break it down into its components for absorption.

A summary of fat digestion in the successive parts of the gastrointestinal tract is given in Table 4-1.

Absorption: Carrying Refined Fuel to Energy Production Sites—Cells

The task of fat absorption is not easy. The problem is that fats are not soluble in water and blood is basically water. Hence fat always requires some type of solvent carrier. To accomplish this task of transporting fat from the intestine into the blood stream, the body has three basic stages of operation.

Stage I: Initial Fat Absorption

Micellar bile-fat complex A particle formed by the combination of bile salts with fat substances (fatty acids and glycerides) to achieve the absorption of fat across the intestinal mucosa. Bile salt micelles act as detergents to prepare lipids for digestion and absorption.

Bile combines with products of fat digestion in a **micellar bile-fat complex** (Figure 4-2) and carries fat into the intestinal wall.

Stage II: Absorption Within the Intestinal Wall

Bile separates again from the fat complex and is returned in circulation to accomplish its task over and over again. Two important actions on the fat products occur inside the intestinal wall: (1) *enteric lipase action:* an enteric lipase within the cells of the intestinal wall completes the digestion of remaining glycerides, and (2) *triglyceride synthesis:* with the resulting fatty acids and glycerol, new human triglycerides are formed as body fats.

Stage III: Final Absorption and Transport of Fat

Chylomicrons Particles of fat—lipoproteins—appearing in the lymph and blood after a meal rich in fat.

These newly formed human fats—triglycerides—and other fat materials present are combined with a small amount of protein to form lipoproteins called **chylomicrons**. These fat packages in a milk-like liquid called *chyle* cross the cell membrane intact into the lymphatic system and then into the portal blood. Here a final fat-clearing enzyme, *lipoprotein lipase*, helps

Figure 4-2
Micellar complex of fats with bile salts for transport of fats into intestinal mucosa.

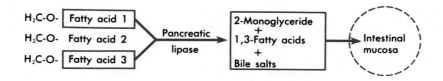

clear the large load of dietary fat from circulation. In the liver the fat is converted to other lipoproteins for transport to the cells for energy and for other structural functions.

Metabolism: Burning Refined Fuel at Production Sites to Produce Energy

In the cells, fatty acids are used as concentrated fuel to produce energy. These derived units of fat have about twice the energy value of glucose products. As you learned in Chapter 2, cell metabolism of fat is closely interrelated with that of the other nutrients.

To Sum Up

Fat is an essential nutrient which, in addition to supplying the highest density of energy among all the energy nutrients, protects against low temperatures and damage to vital organs. It also aids in the transmission of nerve impulses, production of metabolic precursors, formation of cell membrane structure, and transport of other molecules such as protein.

Fats are composed of glycerol and attached fatty acids of varying lengths and degrees of saturation. Essential fatty acids are long-chained unsaturated fatty acids that cannot be manufactured by the body. The major one is *linoleic acid.* Its functions include improving skin integrity, lowering serum cholesterol levels, prolonging blood-clotting time, and developing *prostaglandins,* or substances involved in many tissue activities including maintaining smooth mucle tone and platelet aggregation.

The type and amount of dietary fat can have an effect on health. Large amounts have been associated with cardiovascular disease and other general health problems. Too small an amount can result in a deficiency of the essential fatty acid, linoleic acid. Americans get about 45% of their total kilocalories from fat; the U.S. Dietary Goals recommends 30% to 35%. When fat provides 10% or less of total kilocalories, deficiency symptoms occur.

Questions for Review

1. Two clients with strong family histories of cardiovascular disease are concerned about avoiding heart problems. Both reduce their cholesterol intake and avoid butter. The first client replaces butter with stick margarine made from corn oil, the second with corn oil itself. Which client might have more success with avoiding heart disease? Identify and describe two characteristics of a lipid component that may affect this rate of success.
2. A woman runner concerned with her health dropped her total fat intake to an amount supplying about 10% of her total caloric intake. What health problems would you expect her to encounter?

References

1. National Research Council/National Academy of Science: Toward healthful diets, a statement of the Food and Nutrition Board, Division of Biological Sciences, Assembly of Life Sciences, National Research Council, National Academy of Sciences, Washington, D.C., 1980.

2. Reid, B., Smith, H., and Friedman, Z.: Prostaglandins in human milk, Pediatrics, **66**:870, 1980.

3. Hirsh, P.D., and others: Prostaglandins and ischemic heart disease, Am. J. Med. **71**:1009, 1981.

4. The Lipid Research Clinics Coronary Primary Prevention Trial Results, II. The relationship of reduction in incidence of coronary heart disease to cholesterol lowering, JAMA **251**(3):365, 1984.

Further Readings

Bassler, T.J.: Body build and mortality, JAMA **244**:1437, 1980.

Observations of sudden deaths among marathon runners from cardiac arrhythmia caused by linoleic acid deficiency and extremely reduced percentage of body fat. Their strict diet had consisted of 80% complex carbohydrate, 10% protein, and only 10% fat.

Langone, J.: Special report: I. Heart attack and cholesterol, II. Medical counterattacks, III. Early warning for strokes, Discover **5**(3):19, 28, 1984.

Excellent three-part series relating new concluding report of the NIH Lipid Research Clinics Coronary Primary Prevention Trial to medical advances in diagnosis and treatment of heart disease. Vivid photographs and drawings illustrating arteriosclerotic plaque buildup in arteries.

The Lipid Research Clinics Coronary Primary Prevention Trial Results. II. The relationship of reduction in incidence of coronary heart disease to cholesterol lowering, JAMA **251**(3):365, 1984.

Final report of this 10-year study involving 3806 men with elevated cholesterol. Results indicate that a low-cholesterol diet and drug (cholestyramine) significantly lowered serum cholesterol levels and incidence of heart attacks.

Issues and Answers

The Dietary Fat Controversy

Our initial question remains. What about fat in our diets? How much? What kind? Experts and consumers alike do not agree. They draw differing conclusions from the large body of research and recommendations that has been published. It is small wonder that the public is often confused. Consider this emerging list of recommendations over the last few years.

1977 The controversy began gathering steam, fanned by a government report. The U.S. Senate Committee on Nurtition and Human Health, justly alarmed by the extent of major disease in the population, developed a plan that included strategies for attacking the leading killer of American citizens—coronary heart disease. Its approach was direct and apparently simple: it would advise millions of Americans to follow a diet plan that would reduce their intake of total fats, cholesterol, and saturated fats. These recommendations were based on current research showing that people who eat large amounts of fat, as Americans do, tend to develop heart disease more than people who follow leaner diets. This sounds reasonable. But it is not as simple as it sounds. The fat-disease link still was tenuous. Moreover, Americans seem to love their fat and a great many sources with vested interests would like to whet those appetites. On the other hand, many concerned groups of health professionals and consumers remained uneasy about fat.

In the first place, getting Americans to reduce their fat intake is not going to be easy for several reasons:

- Fats make foods more tasteful and give them a pleasing texture. This is a taste cultivated over the past few years by our marketplace and is probably why some 40% to 45% of the kcal in the U.S. diet is made up of fats.
- Meats, milk, eggs, and cheese provide about half of the fat consumed in the United States, making the task of reducing such animal fat components as cholesterol and saturated fats *very* challenging, to say the least.

The task of making any dietary recomendations for the United States is further complicated by two additional concerns:

- Our population is such a heterogenous group, with a wide variety of food preferences dictated by culture, religion, food availability, and personal likes and dislikes that change is extremely difficult.
- We are such a large group, with persons requiring a wide range of dietary fat, depending on individual health and energy needs, that a "flat rate" for all wouldn't fit for all. So the initial guidelines were simple and general:
  1. Reduce total fat consumption to 30% of energy intake
  2. Reduce saturated fats and increase unsaturated fats instead
  3. Reduce cholesterol consumption

Continued.

Issues and Answers—cont'd

These initial guidelines also recommended that meat consumption be reduced to meet the recommendations. Obviously, this conflicts with the interests of meat-producing and marketing concerns. Many organizations were not comfortable with the initial dietary recommendations. The Senate committee was bombarded with comments, ranging from considered reflections to angry replies, initiated by a wide variety of organizations in both the scientific/medical communities and their adherents. The committee was not funded after 1978.

1978 A majority of nutrition experts serving on the American Society of Clinical Nutrition panels agreed, by a voting procedure on a scale of 0-100 (0: no association of nutrient and disease; 100: unquestionable association), that there was a relationship between fats and heart disease but disagreed on its importance.

1979 The American Medical Association declared that it could not accept the idea of specific amounts of fats, saturated fats, and cholesterol that would be ideal for the entire country. Instead, it suggested that healthy Americans use fat "in moderation."

1980 The Food and Nutrition Board of the National Research Council/National Academy of Sciences stated that the fat content of the American diet only needs to be adjusted to meet the individual's need for energy and not limited to any specific amount.

In essence, these organizations essentially stated that dietary guidelines must provide for a three-way balance between:
- Individual *need* for fat
- Effects of *excess* dietary fat
- Public *need* for education and guidance regarding basic preventive health issues

Apparently, these suggestions were taken to heart. New guidelines were issued:
- Eat a variety of foods
- Maintain an ideal weight
- Avoid too much fat, saturated fat, and cholesterol. The government has developed a booklet that explains these and other revised U.S. Dietary Goals to the public, identifying food sources of nutrients, recommended weights for heights, and other general nutrition information. The publication—"U.S. Dietary Guidelines for Americans"—advises persons who want more specific information (e.g., "How much fat and cholesterol is all right for *me?*") to contact their physician or clinical nutritionist/dietitian for personal counsel.

1985 And that's where we stand just now. Although a new 1984 NIH research report indicated strong diet-cholesterol ties, our knowledge is simply still incomplete—we wish it were otherwise. So we must act for ourselves and for our clients as wisely as possible in the light of

Issues and Answers—cont'd

current knowledge. The currently revised U.S. Dietary Goals seem to provide us with a reasonable basis for general nutrition counseling. Beyond that basic foundation, we will be guided by a careful assessment of each individual client or patient with diagnosed lipid disorders or disease and help work out food plans to meet these specific needs on an individual basis. And we will do this within the context of the *human condition,* recognizing personal desires and the need to live one's own life to the fullest. Too large an order, you say? No, just one that requires wisdom as well as knowledge, personal concern as well as professional skill. It is possible to *enjoy* food and still exercise considered judgment and selection within whatever variety may be available to us.

References
Ahrens, E.H., Jr., and others: The evidence relating six dietary factors to the nation's health, Am. J. Clin. Nutr. **32**:2621, 1979.
American Heart Association, Diet and coronary heart disease, Circulation **58**:762, 1978.
American Medical Association, Council on Scientific Affairs: Concepts of nutrition and health, 242:2335, 1979.
The Lipid Research Clinics Coronary Primary Prevention Trial Results, II. The relationship of reduction in incidence of coronary heart disease to cholesterol lowering, JAMA **251**(3):365, 1984.
Select Committee on Nutrition and Human Needs, U.S. Senate: Dietary goals for the United States, eds. 1 and 2, Washington, D.C., 1977, U.S. Government Printing Office.
Report: U.S. Department of Agriculture/Department of Health, Education, and Welfare/Health and Human Services: Dietary guidelines for Americans, Washington, D.C., 1980, U.S. Government Printing Office.

Chapter 5
Energy Balance

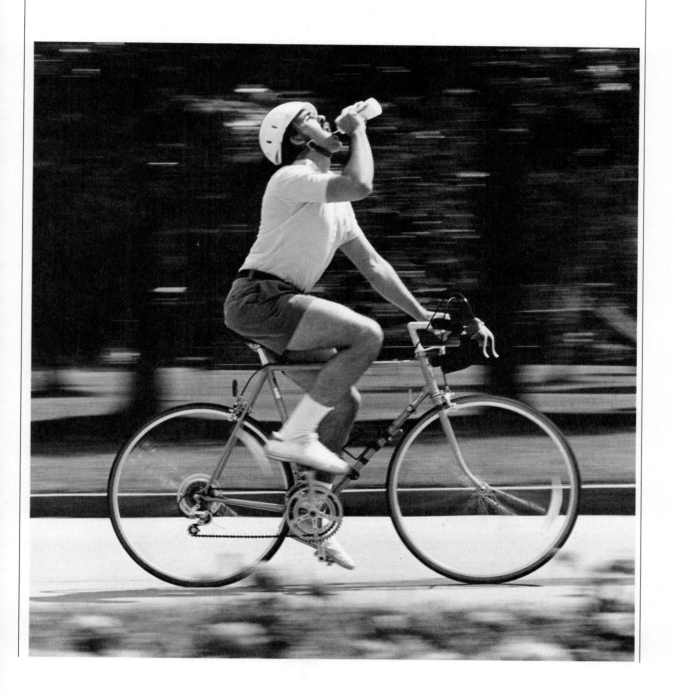

Preview

In human nutrition the fundamental question of how our efficiently designed bodies transform the elements in food we eat to energy is basic, for energy is our power to do all that we do. Carbohydrates and fats, as we have seen, provide the major fuel supply for power in the human energy system. *Energy metabolism* deals with real and dynamic facts underlying all life: *change* and *balance*. Many constant changes and balances in the food we eat and the body's physiologic constituents—its nutrients and their metabolites—produce energy for the body's work.

In fact, our study of energy metabolism reminds us that we live in two worlds. We discover anew that we exist in both a large energy cycle in our earth's environment and a microscopic one within our own body cells. Here in this warm, watery chemical environment, fuel is ignited and "burned," stored for continuous use as needed, yielding energy for all our pursuits, both work and play.

Chapter Objectives

After study of this chapter, the student should be able to:

1. Define energy and metabolism in terms of the dynamic changes and balances involved.

2. Identify and compare the basic units used in measuring energy in the human energy system.

3. Describe how the human body gets its energy and how this energy is controlled.

4. Identify procedures used to determine individual energy requirements and calculate own total energy balance.

Measurement of Energy

Calorie Measure of heat. The *energy* required to do the work of the body is measured as the amount of *heat* produced by the body's work.

Unit of Measure: Kilocalorie (kcal)

Since the body can perform work only as energy is released and since all work takes the form of heat production, energy may be measured in terms of heat equivalents. Such a heat measure is the **calorie**. In practice, to avoid using large numbers professional nutritionists and scientists use the term *kilocalorie* (1000 calories). This is the amount of heat required to raise 1 kg of water 1° C. The international unit for energy is the *joule* (J): one kilocalorie (kcal) equals 4.184 kilojoules (kJ); one *megajoule* (MJ) equals 239 kcal. Presently food and energy tables are given in kilocalories but as the metric system and precise scientific measures catch on, energy values will come to be expressed in joules.

Food Energy

The energy in various foods we eat is generally measured in two basic ways: calorimetry and proximate composition.

Calorimetry Measurement of heat loss.

Calorimetry

The caloric values of various foods listed in food value tables have usually been determined by the use of instruments called *calorimeters*. Remember when you use food value tables, however, that calorimetry averages of a number of samples of a given food tested and that a particular serving of that food will vary around that figure. According to nutrient composition foods have varying degrees of **caloric density.**

Caloric density Higher concentration of energy (kilocalories) in smaller amount of food.

Proximate Composition

Another way of measuring food energy is by computing the approximate nutrient composition of a given food using values in food value tables or databases. Today this task is done rapidly by a computer using a variety of databases. These values are based on the average kilocalorie value of each of the energy nutrients, which are known as their respective **fuel factors**: 1 g of carbohydrate yields 4 kcal, 1 g of protein yields 4 kcal, 1 g of alcohol yields 7 kcal, and 1 g of fat yields 9 kcal.

Fuel factor The kcal value (energy potential) of food nutrients; that is, the number of kcals 1 g of a nutrient yields when oxidized.

The Human Energy System

Energy Capacity of a system for doing work; power to affect changes in self and surroundings.

Energy Cycle and Transformation
Forms of Human Energy

It is clear that **energy**, like matter, is not created. When we speak of energy as being produced, what we really mean is that it is being transformed. It is being changed in form and cycled throughout a system. In the human body the various metabolic processes convert chemical energy to other forms of energy for the body's work. In our bodies energy is available in four basic forms for life processes: *chemical, electrical, mechanical,* and *thermal.* The ultimate source of power is the sun with its vast reservoir of nuclear reactions (Figure 5-1). Then through the process of photosynthesis, using water and carbon dioxide as raw materials, plants transform the sun's energy into food storage forms. In the body these food sources are converted to the basic energy unit, glucose, which together with fatty acids is burned to release energy. Water and carbon dioxide are the end products of this process of oxidation. And so the cycle goes on and on.

Figure 5-1
Transformation of energy
from its primary source (the
sun) to various forms for
biologic work by means of
metabolic processes
("transformers").

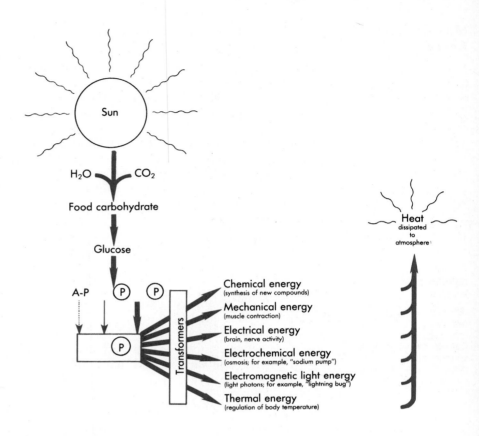

Transformation of Energy

Through the many processes of metabolism, after stored food energy is taken into the body, it is converted to chemical energy in other products to do the body's work. This chemical energy is then changed to other forms of energy as this work is performed. For example, chemical energy is changed to electrical energy in brain and nerve activity. It is changed to mechanical energy in muscle contraction. It is changed to thermal energy in the regulation of body temperature. It is changed to still other types of chemical energy in the synthesis of new compounds. In all these work activities of the body, heat is given off.

Metabolism Sum of all the chemical and physical processes that sustain life.

In human **metabolism** as in any energy system, energy is always present as either *free energy* or *potential energy*. Free energy is the energy involved at any given moment in the performance of a task. It is unbound and in motion. Potential energy is the energy that is stored or bound in various chemical compounds and is available for conversion to free energy as needed. For example, energy stored in sugar is potential energy. When we eat it and it is burned, free energy is released and work results. As work is done, energy in the form of heat is released.

Energy Balance: Input and Output

Whether the energy system is electrical, mechanical, thermal, or chemical, in the course of the many reactions that comprise its operation, free energy is decreased and the reservoir of potential energy is secondarily diminished. Therefore the system must be constantly refueled from some outside source. In the human energy system this basic input of fuel is our food.

The energy demands of the body require constantly available energy. These energy needs support the body's total basic metabolic needs, as well as its additional physical activity requirements. In the human energy system this basic energy output is evident in our activities. But it is also going on internally at all times to meet our basal needs.

Energy Control in Human Metabolism

In the human body the energy produced in its many chemical reactions, if "exploded" all at once, would be destructive. There must be some mechanism, therefore, by which energy is controlled in the human system so that it may support life and not destroy it. Several basic means of control are used to accomplish this task.

Chemical Bonding

Chemical bonding Mutual attachment of various chemical elements to form chemical compounds.

The main mechanism by which energy is controlled in the human system is **chemical bonding.** The chemical bonds that hold elements of compounds together consist of energy. As long as that compound remains constant, energy is being exerted to maintain it. When the compound is taken into the body and broken into its parts, this energy is released and available for the body's work. There are three basic types of chemical bonds by which energy is transferred in the body. First are *covalent bonds* such as those that hold carbon atoms together in the core of an organic compound. Second are *hydrogen bonds,* which are weaker than covalent bonds but significant in the body's metabolism because they can be formed in large numbers. Also, the very fact that they are less strong and can be broken easily makes them important because they can be transferred or passed readily from one substance to another to help form still another substance. The third type of chemical bond is the strong *high-energy phosphate bond,* the main example of which is **adenosine triphosphate (ATP).** This is the unique compound the human body uses to store energy for its cell work. Like storage batteries, these bonds become the controlling force for further energy needs.

Adenosine triphosphate (ATP) A high energy-phosphate compound important in energy exchange for cellular activity.

Controlled Reaction Rates

The many chemical reactions that make up the body's energy system must also have controls. Some of the reactions that break down proteins, for example, if left to themselves (as in sterile decomposition), would span several years. Such reactions must be accelerated or else it might take years to get the needed energy from a meal. At the same time, they must be regulated so that too fast a reaction will not produce a burst of energy in a single "explosion." Enzymes, coenzymes, and hormones are the control agents regulating these cell activities.

Enzyme Complex organic substance originating in living cells and capable of producing certain chemical changes in other organic substances by catalytic action.

Enzymes There are many specific **enzymes** in every cell that control specific reactions in the cell. All enzymes are protein substances. They are produced in the cells themselves under control of specific genes. One specific gene controls the making of one specific enzyme, and there are thousands of enzymes in each cell. Each enzyme works on a particular sub-

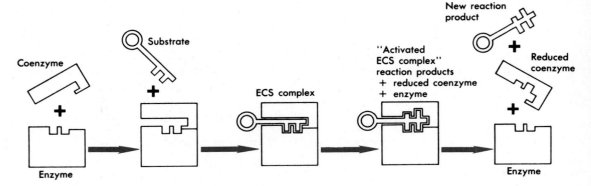

Figure 5-2
Lock and key concept of the action of enzyme, coenzyme, and substrate to produce a new reaction product.

Substrate Specific organic substance on which a particular enzyme acts.

Coenzymes Enzyme-activators required by some enzymes to produce their reactions.

Hormone A compound produced in an endocrine organ (an organ of internal secretion; a ductless gland), secreted by the endocrine organ into the bloodstream, and transported by body fluids to a specific receptor or target organ whose function the hormone controls.

stance called its **substrate.** The enzyme and its substrate lock together to produce a new reaction product, and the original enzyme remains unchanged, ready to do its work over and over again (Figure 5-2).

Coenzymes Many reactions require a partner to assist the enzyme in completing the reaction. These **coenzymes** in many instances involve several of the vitamins, especially the B vitamins, and some of the minerals. It may be helpful to think of the coenzyme as another substrate, for in receiving the material transferred, the coenzyme is changed or reduced.

Hormones In energy metabolism **hormones** act as messengers to trigger or control enzyme action. For example, the rate of oxidative reactions in the tissues, the body's metabolic rate, is controlled by *thyroxine* from the thyroid gland, which in turn is controlled by the *thyroid-stimulating hormone (TSH)* from the anterior pituitary gland. Another familiar example is the controlling action of insulin from the pancreas on the rate of glucose utilization in the tissues. Steroid hormones also have the capacity to regulate the cell's ability to synthesize enzymes.

Types of Metabolic Reaction

The two types of reaction constantly going on in energy metabolism are anabolism and catabolism. Each requires energy. *Anabolism* is the synthesis of a more complex substance. Energy is required to generate this synthesis. *Catabolism* is the breakdown of a more complex substance to simpler substances. This process releases free energy but also uses up some free energy in the work. Therefore there is a constant energy deficit, which must be supplied by food.

Sources of Stored Energy

When food is not available, as in periods of fasting or starvation, the body draws for energy on its own stores:
1. **Glycogen** Only a 12- to 48-hour reserve of glycogen exists in liver and muscle and is quickly depleted.
2. **Muscle mass** Storage of energy as protein exists in limited amounts in muscle mass, but in greater volume than glycogen stores.

3. **Adipose fat tissue** Although fat storage may be larger, the supply varies from person to person and from circumstance to circumstance.

Energy Requirements

Individual energy needs are based on requirements to maintain the body's internal work. This is called a measure of *basal metabolism energy needs*. Also, to these needs should be added the effect of food intake and physical activity needs to determine *total energy requirements*.

Basal Metabolic Needs

Basal Metabolic Rate (BMR)

Basal metabolism Amount of energy needed by the body for maintenance of life when the person is at digestive, physical, and emotional rest.

Basal metabolism is the sum of all internal chemical activities that maintain the body at rest. The basal metabolic rate (BMR) is a measure of the energy required by these activities of resting tissue. Certain small but vitally active tissues—brain, liver, gastrointestinal tract, heart, kidney—together make up less than 5% of the total body weight, yet they contribute about 60% of the total basal metabolic needs. Although resting muscle and adipose fat tissue are far larger in mass, they contribute much less to the body's BMR.

Measuring BMR

Respiratory quotient $= \dfrac{CO_2 \text{ produced}}{O_2 \text{ consumed}}$

Both direct and indirect methods of calorimetry have been used to measure BMR. In direct methods, a chamber large enough for a person to enter is used, and the body's heat production is measured. This instrument is large and costly and is therefore limited to research studies. Indirect calorimetry is seldom used now in clinic practice but is applied mainly in research. This method measures the exchange of gases in respiration (**respiratory quotient**—$CO_2 : O_2$) while the subject is at rest. Energy (BMR) calculated in this manner is equivalent to the body heat given off.

Today, however, in clinical practice newer methods employ measurements of glandular activities such as that of the thyroid gland. These tests serve as indirect measures of BMR. They include measures of serum protein-bound iodine (PBI), radioactive iodine uptake tests, and serum thyroxine levels. The free thyroxine index (FTI) is a common clinical test, which is based on the product of T_3 (triiodothyronine) and T_4 (thyroxine). These two compounds are produced in the final two stages of thyroid hormone synthesis in the thyroid gland. This product ($T_3 \times T_4$) reflects the relative functioning of the thyroid gland and the amount of circulating hormone activity influencing the BMR.

Factors Influencing BMR

A number of factors influence the BMR and should be considered when interpreting test results.

Lean body mass The major influencing factor of BMR is lean body mass.[1,2] This is because of the greater level of metabolic activity in lean tissues in comparison to relatively less active tissues such as bones and fat. Other factors such as surface areas, sex, and age are only influencing factors as they relate to the lean body mass. Energy requirement per unit body weight is higher when the weight is made up of a higher proportion of muscle mass. (See Issues and Answers, p. 85.) It is lower when body weight is made up of a higher proportion of fat or bone. Differences, for example, in metabolic requirements for women are primarily related to differences in lean body mass.

Growth During growth periods, the growth hormone stimulates cell metabolism and raises BMR 15% to 20%. Thus the BMR slowly rises during the first 5 years of life, levels off, rises again just before and during puberty, and then declines into old age.

During pregnancy, a rapid growth period, the BMR rises 20% to 25% because of the accelerated tissue growth process and the increased work of heart and lungs. The lactation period following pregnancy also increases the BMR about 60% or 1000 kcal (p. 197).

Fever and disease Fever increases the BMR about 7% for each .83° C (1° F) rise. Also, diseases involving increased cell activity such as cancer, cer-

Table 5-1
Energy Expenditure/Hour During Various Activities*

Light Activities: 120-150 kcal/hr	Light-moderate Activities: 150-300 kcal/hr	Moderate Activities: 300-420 kcal/hr	Heavy Activities: 420-600 kcal/hr
Personal care	Domestic work	Yard work	Yard work
Dressing	Making beds	Digging	Chopping wood
Washing	Sweeping floors	Mowing lawn (not motorized)	Digging holes
Shaving	Ironing	Pulling weeds	Shoveling snow
Sitting	Washing clothes	Walking	Walking
Rocking	Yard work	3½-4 mph on level surface	5 mph
Typing	Light gardening	Up and down small hills	Upstairs
Writing	Mowing lawn (power mower)	Recreation	Up hills
Playing cards	Light work	Badminton	Climbing
Peeling potatoes	Auto repair	Calisthenics	Recreation
Sewing	Painting	Ballet exercises	Bicycling 11-12 mph or up and down hills
Playing piano	Shoe repair	Canoeing 4 mph	Cross-country skiing
Standing or slowly moving around	Store clerk	Dancing (waltz, square)	Jogging 5 mph
Billiards	Washing car	Golf (no cart)	Swimming
	Walking	Ping-Pong	Tennis (singles)
	2-3 mph on level surface or down stairs	Tennis (doubles)	Water-skiing
	Recreation	Volleyball	
	Archery		
	Bicyling 5½ mph on level surface		
	Bowling		
	Canoeing 2½-3 mph		

*Energy expenditure will depend on the physical fitness (that is, amount of lean body mass) of the individual and continuity of exercise. Note that some of these activities can be used as aerobic activities to promote cardiovascular fitness. For more information, see Chapter 14.

tain anemias, cardiac failure, hypertension, and respiratory problems such as emphysema usually increase the BMR. In the abnormal states of starvation and malnutrition, the BMR is lowered, since the lean body mass is diminished.[3]

Cold climate BMR rises in response to lower temperatures as a compensatory mechanism to maintain body temperature.

Food Intake Effect

Food ingestion stimulates metabolism and requires energy to meet the many activities of digestion, absorption, and transport of the nutrients. This overall stimulating effect of food is called its *specific dynamic action (SDA),* or more recently *dietary thermogenesis.* About 10% of the body's total energy needs for metabolism is attributed to activities related to handling the food we eat. Since more metabolic work is involved with protein, protein-rich foods usually stimulate basal metabolism more than any other nutrient.

Physical Activity Needs

Exercise involved in work and recreation accounts for wide individual variation in energy requirement (see Chapter 14 on Physical Fitness). Some representative kilocalorie expenditures in various types of work and recreation are given in Table 5-1. Any mental effort as in studying demands few if any kilocalories. The feelings of fatigue following periods of study, for example, are caused by various amounts of muscle tension or

Table 5-2
Daily Energy Requirements*

	Age (yr)	Weight kg	Weight lb	Height cm	Height in	Calories (kcal)	Joules (MJ)
Infants	0.0-0.5	6	13	60	24	kg × 115	kg × 0.48
	0.5-1.0	9	20	71	28	kg × 105	kg × 0.44
Children	1-3	13	29	90	35	1,300	5.5
	4-6	20	44	112	44	1,700	7.1
	7-10	28	62	132	52	2,400	10.1
Males	11-14	45	99	157	62	2,700	11.3
	15-18	66	145	175	69	2,800	11.8
	19-22	70	154	177	70	2,900	12.2
	23-50	70	154	178	70	2,700	11.3
	51-75	70	154	178	70	2,400	10.1
	76+	70	154	178	70	2,050	8.6
Females	11-14	46	101	157	62	2,200	9.2
	15-18	55	120	163	64	2,100	8.8
	19-22	55	120	163	64	2,100	8.8
	23-50	55	120	163	64	2,000	8.4
	51-75	55	120	163	64	1,800	7.6
	76+	55	120	163	64	1,600	6.7
Pregnant						+300	1.3
Lactating						+500	2.1

*From Food and Nutrition Board, National Research Council, National Academy of Sciences: Recommended dietary allowances, ed. 9, Washington, D.C., 1980.

moving about. Heightened emotional states alone do not increase metabolic activity, but they may bring additional energy needs because they involve increased muscle tension, restlessness, and agitated movements.

Total Energy Requirements

The energy demands of basal metabolism combined with the effect of food and variable requirements of physical activity make up an individual's total energy requirement (Table 5-2). The energy requirements for the physical activity part may be measured by a 3-day activity record.[4] To maintain daily energy balance, the total energy requirement of an individual is the number of kilocalories necessary to replace daily basal metabolic loss plus loss from exercise and other physical activities. Obesity represents an energy imbalance resulting from an excess of energy input (fuel from food) over energy output (energy requirement or expenditure). Extreme weight loss as in anorexia nervosa (see p. 335) is a state of energy imbalance resulting from deficit energy input for energy output or requirement.

Where do you stand in your own energy balance? Try estimating your own energy requirement using the steps indicated in the box below. Compare your estimate with your general energy needs as indicated in the RDA standards.

Clinical Application

Estimate Your Own Daily Energy Requirement

- **Basal metabolism (BMR)**
  Use general formula: Women—0.9 kcal/kg body weight/hour
  Men—1.0 kcal/kg body weight/hour
  Convert weight (lbs) to kg: 1 kg = 2.2 lbs
  Multiply according to formula: 1 (or 0.9) × kg × 24 (hours in day)
- **Physical activity**
  Estimate your general average level of physical (muscular) activity.
  Find energy cost of activity (% of BMR) and add it to BMR.

Average Activity Level	Energy Cost: % of BMR
Sedentary	20%
Very light	30%
Moderate	40%
Heavy	50%

  For example, if you are sedentary (mostly sitting): BMR (step 1) + (20 × BMR).
- **Specific dynamic action (SDA) of food**
  Record food intake for day and calculate approximate energy (kcal) value.
  Find energy cost of food effect (10% of kcal in food consumed).
- **Total energy output**
  BMR + physical activity + SDA

To Sum Up

Energy is that force or power that enables the body to carry out its life-sustaining or metabolic activities. The energy provided by foods is measured in *kilocalories (kcal)* or *joules*.

Energy comes in various basic forms such such as chemical, electrical, mechanical, and thermal. *Metabolism* is the body's way of changing the *chemical* energy of food into the *electrical* energy of brain and nerve activity, *mechanical* energy of muscle contraction, *thermal* energy of body temperature control, and other forms of chemical energy in the body. Throughout the cycling of these energy forms, two types of balancing metabolic reactions constantly occur: *anabolism*, in which substances are synthesized and energy is stored and *catabolism*, in which substances are broken down and energy is released.

When food is not available, the body draws on its own stores to meet energy needs. *Carbohydrate* stores (glycogen) are most easily depleted and, therefore, the first to undergo catabolism. *Fat* stores (adipose tissue) are larger and catabolized once glycogen stores are depleted. *Protein* stores (body tissue) contain a fair amount of potential energy and are catabolized also after carbohydrate is depleted, along with fat stores.

Total energy needs are based on basal (maintenance) and nonbasal (exercise) requirements. The *basal metabolic rate (BMR)* reflects the amount of energy required to maintain the body at rest after a 12-hour fast. The best indicator of BMR is body composition, especially *lean body mass*. *Nonbasal requirement* for energy includes physical exercise and food intake.

Questions for Review

1. What are the fuel factors of protein, carbohydrate, fat, and alcohol?
2. Define "basal metabolism." What factor(s) influence basal energy needs? Which body tissues contribute most to the body's basal metabolic needs?
3. Which health conditions usually present a reduction in BMR? Which present a rise in BMR?
4. What factors influence nonbasal energy needs?
5. Calculate your own energy balance for 1 day, based on your energy input (food) and your energy output (BMR + SDA + physical activity).

References

1. Cunningham, J.J.: An individualization of dietary requirements for energy in adults, J. Am. Dietet. Assoc. **80**:335, 1982.
2. Webb, P.: Energy expenditure and fat-free mass in men and women, Am. J. Clin. Nutr. **34**:1816, 1981.
3. Moore, F.D.: Energy and the maintenance of the body cell mass, J. Parent. Enter. Nutr. **4**(3):228, 1980.
4. Bouchard, C., and others: A method to assess energy expenditure in children and adults, Am. J. Clin. Nutr. **37**:461, 1983.

Further Readings

Cunningham, J.J.: An individualization of dietary requirements for energy in adults, J. Am. Diet. Assoc. **80**(4):335, 1982.

Good article for students interested in more background on methods used in estimating energy needs of adults based on lean body mass (LBM). The author provides guidelines for using the LBM method in diet counseling to individualize nutrition therapy.

Rainey-Macdonald, C.G., Holliday, R.L., and Wells, G.A.: Nomograms for predicting resting energy expenditure of hospitalized patients, J. Parent. Enter. Nutr. **6**:59, 1982.

Two nomograms, based on the classic Harris and Benedict formula for standard metabolic rate, are used in estimating resting energy expenditure of hospital patients. Results obtained by this method compare favorably with calculated values.

Issues and Answers

The Difference Between Sam and Joe

Sam and Joe are both healthy, 35-year-old accountants who are 5 ft 10 in tall, weigh 165 lbs, and jog 2 miles a day. They need the same number of kcal to get through the day—right? Not necessarily.

Tradition dictates that energy requirements are based on basal needs plus physical activity. Since basal requirements are said to depend on the three factors of sex, age, and body composition, then Sam and Joe should have the same basal needs.

However, current researchers have taken a second look at an an old study that concluded that these three factors could predict basal energy needs and found that only one—body composition—really makes a difference. After analyzing data about the original 223 subjects, the current investigators found *lean body mass (LBM)* to be the *only* predictor of BMR.

Sam and Joe may weigh the same, but if Sam's weight is made up of more fatty tissue than lean, his requirements may be lower. But suppose Sam and Joe have the same amount of LBM, which you may suspect because of their similar activity levels. Would their energy levels be the same? The answer again is not necessarily. The assumptions that energy needs for physical activity are the same among individuals or stay the same within the same individual over time have both been questioned.

As far back as 1947, a study showed that workers performing similar tasks had a wider range of energy intake (kcal) than energy output, which means that some persons burn their kcal more efficiently than others. The same study, whose results have been repeated over the years by other researchers, also showed that individuals varied widely in the amount of energy spent doing the same work over a week's time, *even when changes in weight were accounted for,* which means that the individual might be more energy-efficient at certain times than at others. One study suggests that the differences might result from the body's attempt to regulate the amount of energy stored in the body.

Joe always seems to eat more than Sam. Sam wonders about this difference when they seem so much alike in their size and activity but does not know about the internal metabolism of his energy-efficient friend. Old and new energy balance studies are helping to provide some of the answers.

References
Cunningham, J.J.: A reanalysis of the factors influencing basal metabolic rate in normal adults, Am. J. Clin. Nutr. **33**(11):2372, 1980.
Cunningham, J.J.: An individualization of dietary requirements for energy in adults, J. Am. Diet. Assoc. **80**:335, 1982.
Sukhatme, P.V., and Margen, S.: Autoregulatory homestatic nature of energy balance, Am. J. Clin. Nutr. **35**(2):355, 1982.

Chapter 6
Protein

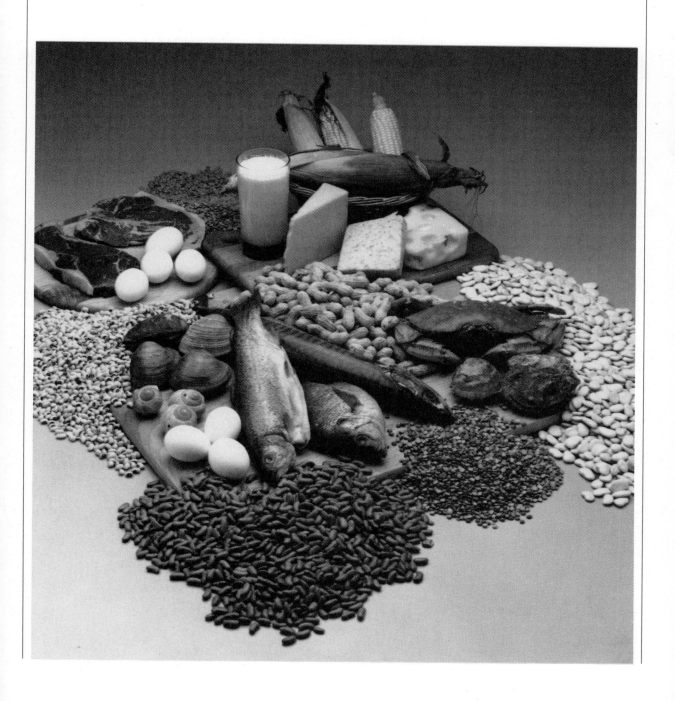

Preview

You are a unique marvel of structure and function. There are myriads of proteins in your body whose tremendous diversity makes your life possible. Your body contains thousands upon thousands of specific proteins, each one different to do its special job.

How can these proteins do their infinitely complex jobs? They accomplish their assigned tasks by their unique structure and packaging. But where do you get the necessary raw building materials to construct all of the thousands of specific proteins that make up your body? You get these essential construction units from the variety of food proteins you eat each day. Your body breaks these food proteins down to their unit-building materials—the amino acids—and builds the multitude of specific structures you need—the tissue proteins. It is this very specificity throughout the process that builds and maintains your body in its unique fashion and makes you *you*.

Chapter Objectives

After study of this chapter, the student should be able to:

1. Describe the general process by which tissue protein is built.

2. Identify and compare the building units that structure proteins.

3. Identify the types and amount of food proteins needed in our diets.

4. Describe the fate of dietary protein in our bodies.

Basic Tissue-Building Material

Amino acid These compounds form the structural units of protein. Out of a total of 20 or more, eight are considered *dietary essentials,* indispensable to life. (See *essential amino acid,* p. 90.) The various food proteins, when digested, yield their specific constituent amino acids. These amino acids are then available for use by the cells as the cells synthesize specific tissue proteins.

The story of protein must begin with its unique structural unit, the **amino acid**. In chemistry the word *amino* refers to a base (alkaline) substance, so we at once confront a paradox. How can a material be both a base and an acid at the same time and why is this important here? Consider the significance of this fact as you first examine the general and, then, the specific structure of amino acids.

The Nature of Amino Acids
General Pattern and Specific Structure

A general fundamental pattern holds for all amino acids. It is the unique side group attached to the common baseline pattern that makes each of the amino acids that make up proteins different. Amino acids are made of the same three elements—carbon, hydrogen, oxygen—that make up carbohydrates and fats. But amino acids and their proteins have an additional important element—*nitrogen*—as the base (alkaline) (NH_2) portion of their structure. There are some 22 amino acids, all of which are important in the body's metabolism. They all have the same basic pattern, but each is unique because it has a different side group attached.

Amphoteric Nature

This important chemical structure of amino acids, combining both acid and base (amino) factors, gives them a unique *amphoteric* nature. As a

---

Clinical Application

The Problem of Building Tissue

As you have discovered thus far in your study of nutrition, the first major problem of the body, securing a fuel source and converting it into a system to supply energy, is solved by using carbohydrates and fats for this purpose. These nutrients provide the fuel, and the body provides a balanced system of chemical changes to get energy from them.

The second major problem the body must solve to survive and maintain health is that of *building tissue.* Any successful construction system requires four basic components:

- Basic building materials
- A means of changing the basic building materials to ready-to-use building units.
- A means of carrying the finished building units to the construction site.
- A plan ("blueprint") and process for building and maintaining the specifically designed structures at the construction site.

Body growth and maintenance require constant building and rebuilding of body tissues. Healthy tissue is necessary for strength, vigor, and body functioning. The building material in food that enables us to accomplish this task is protein. These necessary components of any successful construction system can be applied to the body's use of protein for this vital task.

result of this dual nature, an amino acid in solution can behave either as an acid or as a base, depending on the pH of the solution. This means that amino acids have a *buffer capacity*, which is an important clinical characteristic.

Essential Amino Acids

Essential amino acid Amino acid that is indispensable to life and growth and that the body cannot manufacture; it must be supplied in the diet.

Eight of the amino acids are vital in our diets and have been termed **essential amino acids**. Note these eight amino acids carefully in Table 6-1. These eight amino acids are significant in our diets because they're the only ones that we cannot make. Over the years of human development, we have apparently lost the ability to synthesize these eight amino acids and so must get them in our foods. Thus the label "essential" means that they are *dietary* essentials. The remaining amino acids, which we can synthesize in our own bodies, are then labeled *nonessential* amino acids. Actually, this is a poor choice of labels in the sense that all of the amino acids are necessary for building the various body tissue proteins. However, the concept of *dietary essentiality* for these so-designated eight amino acids is important to remember in assessing food protein quality and protein-controlled diets such as vegetarian patterns (p. 99).

Table 6-1
Amino Acids Required in Human Nutrition, Grouped According to Nutritional (Dietary) Essentiality

Essential Amino Acids	Semiessential Amino Acids*	Nonessential Amino Acids
Isoleucine	Arginine	Alanine
Leucine	Histidine	Asparagine
Lysine		Aspartic acid
Methionine		Cystine (cysteine)
Phenylalanine		Glutamic acid
Threonine		Glutamine
Tryptophan		Glycine
Valine		Hydroxyproline
		Hydroxylysine
		Proline
		Serine
		Tyrosine

*These are considered semiessential because the rate of synthesis in the body is inadequate to support growth; therefore these are essential for children. Recent studies indicate that some histidine may also be required by adults.

The Nature of Proteins

The building units, amino acids, are used by the body to construct specific tissue proteins. This process is made possible by the nature of amino acids, which enables them to form peptide linkages and arrange themselves into peptide chains.

Tissue Protein Structure

The dual chemical nature of amino acids—the presence of an amino (base) group containing nitrogen on one end and an acid (carboxyl) group on the other—enables them to join in the characteristic chain structure of proteins. The amino group of one amino acid joins the acid group of another amino acid beside it. This characteristic chain structure of amino acids is called a **peptide linkage**. Long chains of amino acids linked in this manner are called *polypeptides*. To make a compact structure, the long polypeptide chains then coil or fold back on themselves in a spiral shape called a *helix* or in a "pleated sheet" arrangement.

Peptide linkage
Characteristic joining of amino acids to form proteins. Such a chain of amino acids is termed a "peptide."

Types of Protein

The proteins illustrate a huge diversity produced by specific amino acid linkages. As a result, according to their varied specific structures, tissue proteins perform many vital roles in body structure and metabolism. Some of these examples include: structural proteins such as collagen, contractile proteins such as muscle fibers, antibodies such as gammaglobulin, blood proteins such as fibrinogen, some hormones such as insulin, and all of the enzymes.

Complete and Incomplete Food Proteins

According to the amounts of essential amino acids that given protein foods possess, food proteins are generally classified as complete or incomplete. **Complete proteins** are those that contain all the essential amino acids listed in Table 6-1 (p. 90) in sufficient quantity and ratio to meet the body's needs. These proteins are of animal origin: egg, milk, cheese, and meat. *Incomplete proteins* are those deficient in one or more of the essential amino acids. These proteins are mostly of plant origin: grains, legumes, nuts, and seeds. In a mixed diet, however, animal and plant proteins supplement one another. Even a mixture of plant proteins may provide an adequate, balanced ratio of amino acids if planned carefully, especially to cover the "limiting" essential amino acid—the one occuring in the smallest amount and most likely to be deficient. The value of *variety* in the diet is therefore quite evident.

Complete protein Protein that contains the essential amino acids in quantities sufficient for maintenance of the body and for a normal rate of growth; includes egg, milk, cheese, and meat.

Functions of Protein

To sum up, proteins function in three main ways: building tissue, performing various specific additional physiologic roles, and sometimes providing energy.

Growth and Tissue-Building Maintenance

The primary function of dietary protein is the growth and maintenance of body tissue. It does this by furnishing amino acids of appropriate numbers and types for efficient synthesis of specific cellular tissue proteins. Also, protein supplies amino acids for other essential nitrogen-containing substances such as enzymes and hormones.

Specific Physiologic Roles

All amino acids supplied by protein participate in growth and tissue maintenance. But some also perform other important physiologic and metabolic roles. For example: *methionine* is an agent in the formation of choline, which is a precursor of acetylcholine, one of the major neurotransmitters in the brain. *Tryptophan* is the precursor of the B vitamin niacin and of the neurotransmitter serotonin. *Phenylalanine* is the precursor of the nonessential amino acid tyrosine, leading to formation of the hormones thyroxine and epinephrine. In addition, protein antibodies provide essential components of the body's immune system (p. 539) and plasma proteins protect water balance (p. 172).

Available Energy

Protein also contributes to the body's overall energy metabolism. This occurs as needed in the fasting state or in extended physical effort such as marathon running, but not in the fed state. After the removal of the nitrogenous portion of the constituent amino acid, the amino acid residue may be converted either to glucose or to fat. On the average, 58% of the total dietary protein may become available to be burned for energy. It is evident that sufficient amounts of nonprotein kilocalories from carbohydrate are always needed to spare protein for its primary building purpose and to prevent unnecessary protein breakdown in the process of yielding energy.

Digestion: Changing Basic Building Material to Usable Building Units

After the source of basic body building materials—the food protein—is secured, it must be changed into the needed ready-to-use building units: the amino acids. This work is done through the successive parts of the gastrointestinal tract by the mechanical and chemical processes of digestion.

Mouth

In the mouth only mechanical breaking up of the protein foods by chewing occurs. Here the food particles are mixed with saliva and are passed as a semisolid mass into the stomach.

Stomach

Because proteins are such large complex structures, a series of enzymes is necessary to finally break them down to produce the amino acids. These chemical changes, through a system of enzymes, begin in the stomach. In fact, the stomach's chief digestive function in relation to all foods is the partial enzymatic breakdown of protein. Three agents in the gastric secretions help begin this task: pepsin, hydrochloric acid, and rennin.

Pepsin

Pepsin is the main gastric enzyme specific for proteins. It is first produced as an inactive **proenzyme (zymogen),** *pepsinogen,* by a single layer of cells (the chief cells) in the mucosa of the stomach wall. Pepsinogen then requires hydrochloric acid for activation to the enzyme pepsin. The active pepsin then begins breaking the peptide linkages between the protein's amino acids, changing the large polypeptides into successively smaller peptides. If the protein were held in the stomach longer, pepsin could continue this breakdown until individual amino acids resulted. However, with normal gastric emptying time, only the beginning stage is completed by the action of pepsin.

Pepsin Main gastric enzyme specific for proteins that begins breaking large protein molecules into shorter chain polypeptides, proteoses, and peptones.

Proenzyme Inactive form of an enzyme as it is initially secreted. See *zymogen.*

Zymogen Inactive precursor converted to the active enzyme by the action of an acid, another enzyme, or other means. Also called proenzyme.

Hydrochloric Acid (HCl)

Gastric hydrochloride is an important catalyst in gastric protein digestion. It is necessary to convert the inactive *pepsinogen* to the active enzyme pepsin. Clinical problems result from lack of proper hydrochloric acid secretion.

Rennin

This gastric enzyme (not to be confused with the renal enzyme *renin* [see p. 173]) is important in the infant's digestion of milk. Rennin and calcium act on the casein of milk to produce a curd. By coagulating milk, rennin prevents too rapid a passage of the food from the stomach. In adults, however, rennin is an apparently absent secretion.

Small Intestine

Protein digestion begins in the acid medium of the stomach and continues in the alkaline medium of the small intestine. A number of enzymes take part:

Pancreatic Secretions

Three enzymes produced by the pancreas continue breaking down proteins to simpler and simpler substances:

Trypsin Protein-splitting (proteolytic) enzyme secreted by the pancreas that acts in the small intestine to reduce proteins to shorter chain polypeptides and dipeptides.

Chymotrypsin Protein-splitting (proteolytic) enzyme produced by the pancreas that acts in the intestine. Together with trypsin, it reduces proteins to shorter chain polypeptides and dipeptides.

1. **Trypsin** is secreted first as an inactive substance, trypsinogen, and is activated by a hormone, enterokinase, which is produced by glands in the duodenal wall. The active enzyme **trypsin** then acts on protein and the large polypeptide fragments carried over from the stomach to produce shorter chains of polypeptides and dipeptides.
2. **Chymotrypsin** is produced by special cells in the pancreas in its inactive precursor form chymotrypsinogen. It is then activated by the trypsin already present. **Chymotrypsin** continues the same protein-splitting action of trypsin.
3. **Carboxypeptidase,** as its name indicates, attacks the end of the peptide chain where there is a free acid (carboxyl) group. It produces, in turn, smaller peptides and some free amino acids.

Intestinal Secretions

Glands in the intestinal wall produce two additional protein-splitting enzymes in the peptidase group:

1. **Aminopeptidase** releases amino acids one at a time from the nitrogen-containing amino end of the peptide chain. Through this cleavage action, it produces smaller short-chained peptides and free amino acids.
2. **Dipeptidase,** the final enzyme in this protein-splitting system, b the remaining dipeptides into free amino acids.

Given this total system of protein-splitting enzymes, the large proteins are broken down into progressively smaller peptide amino acids are split off from the end of these chains. The of protein digestion are the amino acids, now ready for a intestinal mucosa. A summary of protein digestion is o 2.

Table 6-2
Summary of Protein Digestion

| Organ | Enzyme | | | Digestive Action |
	Inactive Precursor	Activator	Active Enzyme	
Mouth			None	Mechanical only
Stomach (acid)	Pepsinogen	Hydrochloric acid	Pepsin	Protein→polypeptides
			Rennin (infants) (calcium necessary for activity)	Casein→coagulated curd
Intestine (alkaline)				
Pancreas	Trypsinogen	Enterokinase	Trypsin	Protein, polypeptides→polypeptides, dipeptides
	Chymotrypsinogen	Active trypsin	Chymotrypsin	Protein, polypeptides→polypeptides, dipeptides
			Carboxypeptidase	Polypeptides→simpler peptides, dipeptides, amino acids
Intestine			Aminopeptidase	Polypeptides→peptides, dipeptides, amino acids
			Dipeptidase	Dipeptides→amino acids

Absorption: Carrying Building Units to Construction Sites

The construction sites in the body for building various kinds of necessary tissue protein are in the *cells*. Each cell, depending on its particular nature and function, has a specific job to do and so it must be specifically structured.

Absorption of Amino Acids

The end products of protein digestion are the water-soluble amino acids. These building units are rapidly absorbed from the small intestine directly into the portal blood system through the fine network of villus capillaries.

Active Transport System

Most of the amino acid absorption takes place in the first portion of the small intestine. An energy-dependent active transport system, using pyridoxine (vitamin B_6) as carrier, absorbs the amino acids into the blood circulation, delivering them into the cells for eventual metabolism.

Competition for Absorption

we eat a mixed diet with different amino acids in it, these amino
ompete with each other for absorption. The amino acid present in
rgest quantity retards the absorption of the others. In plasma, com-
on also exists among the circulating amino acids for entry into the

orption of Peptides and Whole Proteins

w larger fragments of short-chain peptides or intact proteins are ab-
ed as such and then by **hydrolysis** within the absorbing cells yield
ino acids. These larger protein molecules may play a part in the devel-

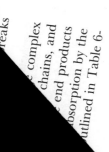
reaks
complex chains, and end products sorption by the outlined in Table 6-

opment of immunity and sensitivity. Antibodies in the mother's colostrum, the premilk breast secretion, are passed on to her nursing infant.

In human nutrition the amino acids are the metabolic currency of protein. It is with the fate of these vital compounds that the metabolism of protein is ultimately concerned. The many metabolic processes involved in protein metabolism form a fascinating array of complex activities that are intricately interwoven with those of carbohydrates and fats as you saw in Chapter 2. Here we will look briefly at the fundamental metabolic concept of protein and nitrogen balance. This will provide a base for relating tissue-building processes, **anabolism**, and breaking-down processes, **catabolism**, which maintain these important balances.

The Concept of Balance
Homeostasis

Many interdependent checks and balances exist throughout the body. There is a constant ebb and flow of materials, a building-up and breaking-down of parts, and a depositing and taking-up of components. The body has built-in controls that operate as finely tuned coordinated responses to meet any situation that tends to disturb its normal condition or function. This resultant state of dynamic equilibrium is called **homeostasis**, and the various mechanisms designed to preserve it are called *homeostatic mechanisms*. This sensitive balance between body parts and functions is life-sustaining.

Dynamic Equilibrium

As more and more is learned about human nutrition and physiology, older ideas of a rigid body structure are giving way to this important concept of dynamic equilibrium—balance amid constant change. All body constituents are in a constant state of flux, although some tissues are more actively engaged than others. This concept of dynamic equilibrium can be seen in all metabolism and is especially striking in protein metabolism.

Protein Balance
Protein Turnover

For a number of years the use of radioactive isotopes has clearly demonstrated that the body's protein tissues are continuously being broken down into amino acids and then resynthesized into tissue proteins.[1] When "labeled" amino acids are fed, they are rapidly incorporated into various body tissue proteins. The rate of this protein turnover varies in different tissues. It is highest in the intestinal mucosa, liver, pancreas, kidney, and plasma. It is lower in muscle, brain, and skin tissues. It is much slower in structural tissues such as collagen and bone.

Protein Compartments

Body protein exists in a balance between two compartments—tissue protein and plasma protein. These stores are further balanced with dietary protein intake. Protein from one compartment may be drawn to supply need in the other. For example, during fasting, resources from the body protein stores may be used for tissue synthesis. But even when the intake

Metabolism: Building and Maintaining Specific Body Tissues

Anabolism Constructive metabolic processes that build up the body substances by synthesizing more complex substances from simpler ones; the opposite of catabolism.

Catabolism Breaking-down phase of metabolism, the opposite of anabolism.

Homeostasis State of equilibrium of the body's internal environment.

of protein and other nutrients is adequate the tissue proteins are still being constantly broken down and reformed.

The adult body's state of stability then is the result of a **protein balance** between the rates of protein breakdown and protein resynthesis. In periods of growth the synthesis rate is higher so that new tissue can be formed. In conditions of starvation, wasting diseases, and more gradually as the aging process continues in the elderly, tissue breakdown exceeds that of synthesis, and the body gradually deteriorates.

Metabolic Amino Acid Pool

Amino acids derived from tissue breakdown and amino acids from dietary protein digestion and absorption both make up this common metabolic "pool" of amino acids. A balance of amino acids is maintained to supply the body's constant needs. Shifts in balances between tissue breakdown and dietary protein intake ensure a balanced mixture of amino acids. From this reserve pool (Figure 6-1), specific amino acids are supplied to meet the "all or none law" of specific protein synthesis (p. 91).

Nitrogen Balance

Another useful reference for indicating a person's state of protein balance is **nitrogen balance**, a test usually done in hospitals (p. 358). Total nitrogen balance involves all sources of nitrogen in the body—protein nitrogen as well as nonprotein nitrogen present in other compounds such as urea, uric acid, ammonia, and in other body tissues and fluids. It is the net result of all nitrogen gains and losses in all the body protein. A person is in a harmful state of negative nitrogen balance when the loss of body protein exceeds the input of food protein. Such a state exists in conditions such as starvation, a wasting disease, or long-term illness.

It is clear that protein is an essential nutrient. But just how much and what kind do we actuallly need? We know that some people get far less than they need. On a worldwide basis, protein-energy malnutrition is a major health concern in underdeveloped countries (p. 5). In contrast, however, in America and most other Western societies protein deficiency

---

Protein balance The word *balance* refers to relation between intake and output of a substance. Negative balance = output greater than intake. Positive balance = intake greater than output.

Nitrogen balance Difference between intake and output of nitrogen in the body. If intake is greater, a positive nitrogen balance exists. If output is greater, a negative nitrogen balance exists.

6.25 g protein = 1 g nitrogen

Protein Requirements

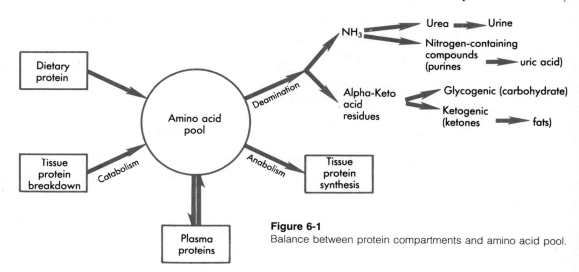

Figure 6-1
Balance between protein compartments and amino acid pool.

is not a problem. Actually most persons in America eat about twice as much protein as they really need, an intake often associated with excess body weight[2] because animal protein foods also carry fat. Clinicians have also begun to raise questions about the long-term effects of habitual excess protein intake on the human kidney designed in earlier ages to handle a different supply of protein.[3]

Factors Influencing Protein Requirement

Tissue Growth

The primary purpose of protein in the diet is to supply amino acids in the quantity and quality necessary for growth and maintenance of tissue. Thus any period of growth increases the need for protein. Growth-related factors include age, body size, and general physical status. There is evidence, for example, that the Recommended Dietary Allowances (RDA) for protein may be inadequate for elderly men and women[4] and for women during reproductive years.[5] Special periods of rapid growth, such as the growth of the fetus and maternal tissue during pregnancy, require additional increases in protein. An expectant mother may require as much as 70 to 100 g of protein a day.

Diet

Other factors include the nature of the protein in the diet and its ratio or pattern of amino acid structure. There must be sufficient nonprotein kilocalories in the diet to have a protein-sparing effect, so that the total amount of protein will not be diminished for energy requirements. Also, the digestibility and absorption of the protein is affected by the preparation and cooking of the food. Allowing the time intervals between ingestion of protein foods lowers the competition for absorption sites and enzymes.

Illness or Disease

The presence of any illness or disease will usually increase the requirement for protein. Diseases accompanied by fever especially increase the requirement for protein because of the increase in basal metabolic rate and the general destruction of tissue. Traumatic injury requires extensive tissue rebuilding. Postsurgical states require extra protein for wound healing and to replenish losses. Extensive tissue destruction as in burns requires a considerable increase in protein intake for the healing process.

Measure of Protein Requirements

It is evident, then, that two basic measures of protein requirement must be considered: quantity and quality.

Protein Quantity

The quantity of protein needed is the basis for establishing the total protein requirement. The RDA standard for adults is 0.8 g/kg (2.2 lb) of body weight. This amounts to about 56 g daily for a man weighing 70 kg (154 lb), and 44 g daily for a woman weighing 55 kg (120 lb). Increased protein is indicated during pregnancy and lactation. Requirements for infants and children vary according to age and growth patterns.

Protein Quality

Since the value of a protein depends on its content of essential amino acids, in the final analysis the measure of protein requirement must be based on its amino acid quality. Guidelines for protein needs, based on nitrogen balance studies determining specific amino acid requirements, have been developed (see Table 6-3).

Table 6-3

Required Amounts of Protein Per Day*

Individuals	Grams
Men (154 lb)†	56 g
Women (128 lb)†	44 g
Pregnancy, last 4½ mo	(+ 30 g)
Lactation	(+ 20 g)
Infants	
0 to 6 mo	Kg × 2.2 g
6 to 12 mo	Kg × 2.0 g
Children	
1 to 3 yr	23 g
4 to 6 yr	30 g
7 to 10 yr	34 g
Boys	
11 to 14 yr	45 g
15 to 18 yr	56 g
Girls	
11 to 14 yr	46 g
15 to 18 yr	46 g

*From Food and Nutrition Board: Recommended dietary allowances, ed. 9, Washington, D.C., 1980, National Academy of Sciences.

†0.422 g of protein per pound of ideal body weight.

Comparative Quality of Food Proteins

The nutritive value of a food protein is often expressed in terms of its *chemical score,* a value derived from its amino acid composition. Using the amino acid pattern of a high-quality protein food such as egg and giving it a value of 100, other foods are compared according to their comparative ratios of the essential amino acids. Other measures also determine protein quality:

1. **Biologic value (BV)** based on nitrogen balance.
2. **Net protein utilization (NPU)** based on biologic value and degree of the food protein's digestibility.
3. **Protein efficiency ratio (PER)** based on weight gain of a growing test animal divided by its protein intake.

A comparison of the scores of various protein foods with their nutritive values based on these measures is shown in Table 6-4. A sound diet is the

Food	Chemical Score	BV	NPU	PER
Egg	100	100	94	3.92
Cow's milk	95	93	82	3.09
Fish	71	76	—	3.55
Beef	69	74	67	2.30
Unpolished rice	67	86	59	—
Peanuts	65	55	55	1.65
Oats	57	65	—	2.19
Polished rice	57	64	57	2.18
Whole wheat	53	65	49	1.53
Corn	49	72	36	—
Soybeans	47	73	61	2.32
Sesame seeds	42	62	53	1.77
Peas	37	64	55	1.57

*Data adapted from Guthrie, H.: Introductory Nutrition, ed. 5, St. Louis, 1983, The C.V. Mosby Co., and
Food and Nutrition Board: Recommended dietary allowances, ed. 9, Washington, D.C., 1980, National
Academy of Sciences.

best way to obtain needed protein, eliminating the need for amino acid
supplements.

Vegetarian Diets
Complementary Food Proteins

Protein requirements in various vegetarian diets may be met by applying
the principle of combining complementary plant proteins to achieve the
necessary balance of essential amino acids. You may be working with persons following such food patterns who may be using one or more of the
following three basic types of vegetarian diets: (1) lactoovovegetarian, (2)
lactovegetarian, and (3) pure vegan (see Issues and Answers, pp. 102-104).
Guidelines for vegetable protein combinations and interesting recipes for
preparing these foods are available.[6] However, in relation to animal food
sources, larger amounts of vegetable protein foods must be consumed to
obtain comparable amounts of complete protein.

To Sum Up

Proteins build tissue, perform a variety of physiologic roles, and provide
energy. Amino acids are the structural components of proteins. There are
22 in total, 8 of which cannot be synthesized in adequate amounts by the
body. These are called essential amino acids (EAAs). Food proteins are
considered "complete" when they contain all 8 (or 9) EAAs. Animal proteins are complete. Vegetable proteins are incomplete but can be mixed
with complete proteins or with each other to provide all 8 EAAs in one
meal.

Amino acids participate in protein building (anabolism) or breakdown (catabolism). Both processes are dictated by genetic information and hormonal influence. *Anabolism* occurs when specific amino acids required for each protein are present. If one is missing, the protein is not formed—the law of "all or none." *Catabolism* occurs when the body tissues are broken down. The amino acid splits into its nitrogen group—which helps to form nonessential amino acids or other nitrogen compounds—and its nonnitrogen residue, which can form carbohydrates for energy or fat storage. In the unfed state, proteins are broken down for energy. Thus dietary carbohydrates have a protein-sparing effect.

Protein requirements are influenced by growth needs and rate of protein synthesis, food protein quality and digestibility dietary carbohydrate and fat levels, and timing of meals. Clinical factors affecting protein needs include fever, disease, medications, surgery or other trauma to body tissues.

Questions for Review

1. What is the difference between an *essential* and *nonessential* amino acid? List the names of the essential amino acids. Which one is required in the smallest quantity?
2. Explain the term "protein-sparing effect." What nutrients have this property?
3. List and describe what six factors affect dietary protein needs.
4. Calculate your own protein intake for a day and compare it with your need according to the RDA allowances.
5. A vegetarian couple decided to raise their 2-year-old daughter on a strict vegan diet. As expected, the child did not often finish meals and was allowed to snack on fruits and whole grain biscuits. Eventually, they noticed that she was not growing at the same rate as other children and was becoming thin. What food patterns would you expect in this family? What dietary factor may have been responsible for the child's poor growth? What advice would you offer this couple to improve their child's nutritional status? Plan one meal for this family that would meet one fourth of an adult man's dietary need for protein, while adhering to a typical vegan meal pattern.

References

1. Stein, T.P.: Nutrition and protein turnover: a review, J. Parent. Enter. Nutr. **6**(5):444, 1982.

2. Dietary protein and body fat distribution, Nutr. Rev. **40**:89, 1982.

3. Brenner, B.M., Meyer, T.W., and Hostetter, T.H.: Dietary protein intake and the progressive nature of kidney disease, N. Engl. J. Med. **307**(11):652, 1982.

4. Gersovitz, M., and others: Human protein requirements: assessment of the adequacy of the current Recommended Dietary Allowance for dietary protein in elderly men and women, Am. J. Clin. Nutr. **35**(1):6, 1982.

5. Calloway, D.H., and Kurger, M.S.: Menstrual cycle and protein requirements of women, J. Nutr. **112**:356, 1982.

6. Lappe, F.M.: Diet for a small planet, 10th anniversary ed., New York, 1982, Ballantine Books.

Further Readings

Guthrie, H.A.: Protein, Introductory nutrition, St. Louis, 1983, The C.V. Mosby Co., pp. 66-93.

Good section on evaluation of protein quality for students interested in further background development of methods of measurement.

Timmons, K.H., and others: Protein quality and the cost of selected commercial protein supplements, J. Am. Diet. Assoc. **78**:606, 1981.

Reviews the question of protein supplementation and the relative cost of a number of commercial products.

Wagner, M.: Ten years after *Diet For a Small Planet,* Med. Self-Care **21**:60, 1983.

Provides insights from an interview with social worker/author Frances Lappe as to why and how this well-known and useful little book on vegetarianism has influenced our food habits over the past decade.

Issues and Answers

The Vegetarian Revolution

At least 7 million Americans have become vegetarians, replacing meats as a main entree item with legumes, grains, and vegetables. Their meals follow a variety of patterns. Some groups call themselves "true" vegetarians because they allow no animal products in their diets. But their highly restrictive "dietary laws" have caused serious malnutrition problems. These problems are found among:

Zen macrobiotics, who eat only brown rice and herb tea to achieve a perfect balance of yin and yang in order to fend off disease.

Vegans, who rely on fruits, vegetables, nuts, and seeds, refusing any source of animal protein, fortified foods, or nutritional supplements.

Fruitarians, who eat only fresh and dried fruits, nuts, honey, and sometimes olive oil.

Other vegetarian diets, however, if well planned can be very nutritious. These include the "animal-product" vegetarians:

Lactovegetarians, who allow milk, cheese, yogurt, and other milk products as the only animal protein in their diets.

Ovovegetarians, who use eggs as their only source of animal protein.

Lactoovovegetarians, who consume milk and eggs, but no other animal products.

Pescovegetarians, who permit fish as their only animal product.

Pollovegetarians, who allow poultry.

"Red-meat abstainers," who eat any animal product except red meat and consider themselves to be vegetarians, too.

Reasons people give for becoming vegetarian are as varied as these diets:

Religion Religious communities, such as the Seventh-Day Adventists, use vegetarianism as a means of self-discipline as well as promoting good health. Other vegetarians may or may not be religious but feel it is "sinful" to kill a living animal for food.

Ecology Approximately half of the world's grain output is used to feed livestock. Some vegetarians feel it could be better used to feed people so that less land would be used to meet the world's protein needs. Some also feel that using less land would result in a reduction in the use of pesticides now used to ensure large crops.

Economics Beans, grains and vegetables are cheaper than meat. Some vegetarians are not only concerned with saving money for themselves but also finding a way to meet food shortages in poor nations throughout the world.

Health Another common reason for selecting vegetarianism is to achieve good health. By avoiding animal products, vegetarians manage to reduce their intake of cholesterol and saturated fats, thus perhaps gaining some protection against heart disease.

Issues and Answers—cont'd

Does a vegetarian diet offer other important nutrients besides protein?

Yes. Vegetarians can meet the recommended dietary allowance for most major nutrients without taking supplements. However, a few key nutrients create problems if the vegetarian is not careful:

Vitamin B_{12} This vitamin is found only in animal products. People who follow veganism or the macrobiotic diets are at the greatest risk for a deficiency. Vegans may be at special risk because they take in a large amount of folacin, another B vitamin that can mask signs of B_{12} deficiency. A deficiency can be avoided, however, by including fortified foods or taking a B_{12} supplement along with sufficient complete protein from complementary amino acids to ensure synthesis of the intrinsic factor (a mucoprotein) necessary for B_{12} absorption.

Vitamin A Vegetarians tend to get more provitamin A, carotene, than they need. This usually isn't a problem—unless they are also taking supplements that include vitamin A. One study shows that 85% of vegetarians take supplements. These may include as much as 10 times the RDA for vitamin A! As a fat-soluble vitamin, vitamin A can build up in body tissues and reach toxic levels. The result could be anorexia, irritability, dry skin, hair loss.

Iron Grains and legumes have iron but much of it is poorly absorbed from the gut. Absorption can be enhanced, however, by including a good source of vitamin C (p. 158) in the same meal.

Can vegetarian women get enough protein for a successful pregnancy?

Yes, though including animal products, as in lactoovovegetarianism, may become essential to meet extra nutritional needs. Supplements are recommended also for such hard-to-get nutrients as iron.

Is the vegetarian diet safe for children?

Children manage to grow and develop fairly well on a vegetarian diet that includes the nonmeat animal proteins milk, cheese, and eggs. They tend to be a little shorter than average but this may be the result of other genetic or environmental factors. Vegetarian children also tend to be mildly anemic, probably because of the poor availability of iron from grains and legumes. Again, including a source of vitamin C with meals may be helpful. The vegan and macrobiotic diets are too poor in required nutrients to sustain childhood growth needs.

Can you lose weight on a vegetarian diet?

Yes, definitely. Eliminating meats automatically removes a major source of fat in the diet. Since fats provide more than twice the number of kcal/g than carbohydrates or protein, the vegetarian diet is usually much lower in kcal than the "meat-and-potatoes" diet. In fact,

Continued.

Issues and Answers—cont'd

some vegetarians have to be careful to get *enough* kcal, especially pregnant women, children and athletes.

Thus, the well-planned vegetarian diet can be nutritious. If used wisely, especially in its lactoovo forms, it can offer many advantages in terms of health, economy, and ecology.

References

Dwyer, J.T., and others: Nutritional status of vegetarian children, Am. J. Clin. Nutr. **35**:204, 1982.

Gross, J., and Freifeld, K.: My child, the vegetarian, Fam. Health **13**(4):34, 1981.

Read, M.H., and Thomas, D.C.: Nutrient and food supplement practices of lactoovo vegetarians, J. Am. Dietet. Assoc. **82**(4):401, 1983.

Chapter 7
Vitamins

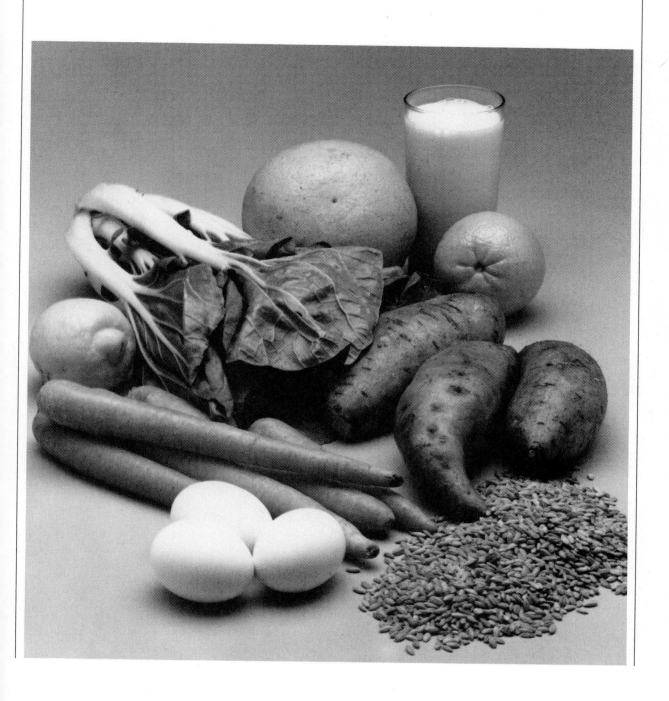

Preview

Probably no other group of
nutritional elements has so
captured the interest of scientists,
health professionals, and the
general public as has the vitamin
group. Attitudes toward vitamins
have varied widely. Concern
about them has run the gamut
from wise functional use to wild
flagrant abuse.

From 1900 to 1950 the
discovery of vitamins formed a
fascinating chapter in nutrition
history. During this time, the list
of vitamins grew one by one.
Some were first discovered in the
search for causes of certain age-
old diseases such as scurvy,
beriberi, pellagra, and rickets.
Others were discovered later as
the result of studies of various
body functions. In general, in
cases of malnutrition, not just one
but a number of vitamins may be
lacking. Current knowledge
indicates that at least one of the
organic substances we have been
calling a vitamin has been
actually misassigned to the
vitamin group. Vitamin D is now
known to behave as a hormone.
In this chapter we will look at
both fat- and water-soluble
vitamins and learn why we need
them and how we may obtain
them.

Chapter Objectives

After study of this chapter, the
student should be able to:

1. Define *vitamin* and describe the
general nature of each one.

2. Identify the functions of each
vitamin.

3. Relate the requirement for
each vitamin to health problems
from a deficiency and possible
dangers from an excess.

4. Identify food sources of each
vitamin and situations requiring
possible need for
supplementation.

The Study of Vitamins

Amine Organic compound containing nitrogen, formed from ammonia.

General Nature and Classification

Characteristics and Class Name

During the five decades of vitamin discovery occurring during the first half of the 1900s, the remarkable nature of these vital agents became more and more apparent. Three key characteristics were evident: (1) they were not "burned" to yield energy as were the energy nutrients carbohydrate, fat, and sometimes protein; (2) they were vital to life; and (3) often not a single substance but a group of related substances turned out to have the particular metabolic activity. The name *vitamin* developed during initial research years when one of the early scientists working with a nitrogen-containing substance called an **amine** thought that this was the nature of these vital agents. So he named it *vitamine (vital-amine)*. Later the final "e" was dropped when other similarly vital substances turned out to be a variety of organic compounds. The name *vitamin* has been retained to designate compounds of this class of essential substances. At first letter names were given to individual vitamins discovered. But as the number of them increased rapidly, this practice created confusion. So in recent years more specific names based on structure or function have developed. Today these scientific names are preferred and are commonly used.

Definition

Thus as the vitamins have been discovered one by one and the list of them has grown, two characteristics have clearly emerged to define a compound as a vitamin:

1. It must be a vital organic dietary substance that is not a carbohydrate, fat, protein, or mineral and is necessary in only very *small* quantities to perform a particular metabolic function or to prevent an associated deficiency disease.
2. It cannot be manufactured by the body and therefore must be supplied in food.

Classification

Vitamins are usually grouped and distinguished according to their solubility in either fat or water. The fat-soluble vitamins—A, D, E, and K—are closely associated with lipids in their fate in the body. They can be stored, and their functions are more related to structural activities. The water-soluble vitamins—B complex and C—have fewer problems in absorption and transport, cannot be stored except in the "tissue saturation" sense, and function more as coenzyme factors in cell metabolism.

Current Concepts and Key Questions

To clarify the current concepts concerning each known vitamin, consider these key questions as the basis for your study:

Nature What is the vitamin's general structural nature?

Absorption and transport How does the body handle this particular vitamin?

Function What does this vitamin *do?* This is, perhaps, the most significant question.

Requirement and sources How much of this vitamin do we need and where can we obtain it?

Fat-Soluble Vitamins

Vitamin A
General Nature of Vitamin A

Chemical and physical nature Vitamin A is a generic term for a group of compounds having similar biologic activity. These vitamin A compounds include retinol, retinal, and retinoic acid. The term *retinoids* refers to both the natural forms of retinol and its synthetic analogs. Because this substance has a specific function in the retina of the eye and because it is an alcohol, vitamin A has been given the name *retinol*. It is soluble in fat and in ordinary fat solvents. Because it is insoluble in water, it is fairly stable in cooking.

Forms There are two basic dietary forms of vitamin A. One of these is *preformed vitamin A (retinol)*. This substance, in its natural form, is found only in animal sources and is usually associated with fats. It is deposited primarily in the liver but also in small amounts in kidney, lung, and fat tissue. Thus, in this form, its dietary sources are found mainly in dairy products (the fat portion), egg yolk, and storage organs such as the liver. The other dietary form of vitamin A is *provitamin A (beta-carotene)*. The original source of retinol is a plant pigment substance—beta-carotene. It is called carotene because one of its main sources is the yellow pigment of carrots. Beta-carotene is the most common precursor of vitamin A and supplies about two thirds of the vitamin A necessary in human nutrition.

Absorption and Storage

Substances that aid absorption Vitamin A enters the body in the two forms, preformed vitamin A from animal sources and the precursor carotene from plant sources. Several substances aid in the absorption of vitamin A and carotene by the body.

1. **Bile** As with fat and other fat-related compounds, bile serves as a vehicle of vitamin A transport through the intestinal wall. Clinical conditions affecting the bilary system, such as obstruction of the bile ducts, infectious hepatitis, and cirrhosis of the liver, hinder vitamin A absorption.

2. **Pancreatic lipase** This fat-splitting enzyme is necessary for initial hydrolysis in the upper intestine of fat emulsions or oil solutions of the vitamin. In diseases of the pancreas where secretion of pancreatic lipase is curtailed, the water-soluble form would have to be used.

3. **Dietary fat** Some fat in the food mix, simultaneously absorbed, stimulates bile release for effective absorption of vitamin A.

Carotene conversion In the intestinal wall during absorption some of the carotene is converted to vitamin A. The remainder of the dietary carotene is absorbed as such and is dissolved in the fat part of lipoproteins.

Transport and storage The route of absorption of vitamin A and carotene parallels that of fat. In the intestinal mucosa all the retinol, from both preformed animal sources and from plant carotene conversion, is incorporated into the chylomicrons. In this form it enters the blood stream via the lymphatic system and is carried to the liver for storage and distribution to the cells. The liver, by far the most efficient storage organ for vitamin A, contains about 90% of the body's total quantity. This amount is sufficient to supply the body's needs for 6 to 12 months, and some persons have been known to store as much as a 4-year supply. These stores are reduced, however, during periods of infectious disease. Age is also a factor in vitamin A absorption. For example, in the newborn infant, especially the premature infant, absorption is poor. At the other end of the life cycle, with advancing age, elderly persons may experience increasing difficulties with absorption. Chronic use of mineral oil as a laxative hinders vitamin A absorption.

Functions of Vitamin A

Vitamin A's role in a person's visual adaptation to light and dark has been well established. It also has a number of more generalized functions that influence epithelial tissue integrity, growth, and reproductive function.

Vision The eye's ability to adapt to changes in light is dependent on the presence of a light-sensitive pigment, **rhodopsin** (commonly known as visual purple) in the rods of the retina (Figure 7-1). Rhodopsin is composed of the vitamin A substance, retinal, and the protein, opsin. When the body is deficient in vitamin A, the rods and cones become increasingly sensitive to light changes, which causes *night blindness*. This condition can usually be cured in a half-hour or so by an injection of vitamin A (retinol), which is readily converted into retinal and then into rhodopsin.

The vision cycle: light-dark adaptation role of vitamin A.

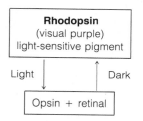

Figure 7-1
Structure of the eye.

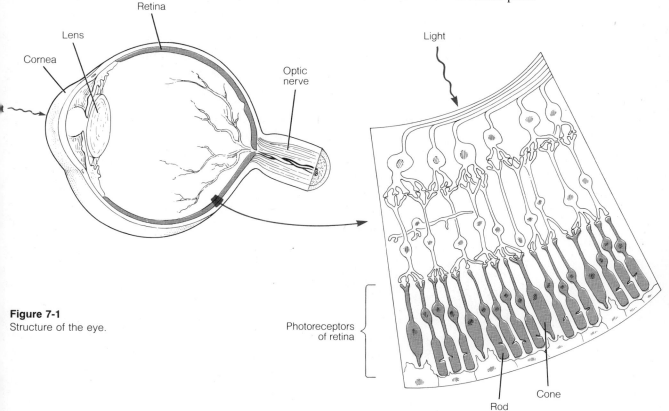

Epithelial tissue Vitamin A is necessary to build and maintain healthy epithelial tissue, which provides our primary barrier to infections. The epithelium includes not only the outer skin but also the inner mucous membranes. This function of vitamin A is the basis for current research relating vitamin A retinoids and carotene to cancers of epithelial origin.

Without vitamin A, the epithelial cells become dry and flat and gradually harden to form keratin, a process called **keratinization**. Keratin is a protein that forms dry, scalelike tissue such as nails and hair. When the body is deficient in vitamin A, many such epithelial tissue changes may occur:

Keratinization Process occurring in vitamin A deficiency states in which the epithelial cells either slough off or become dry and flattened, then gradually harden and form rough, horny scales.

1. **Eye** The cornea dries and hardens, a condition called *xerophthalmia*, progressing to blindness in extreme deficiencies. The teat ducts dry, robbing the eye of its cleansing and lubricating substance, and infection follows easily.
2. **Respiratory tract** Ciliated epithelium in the nasal passages dries and the cilia are lost, thereby removing a barrier to entry of infection. The salivary glands dry, and the mouth become dry and cracked, open to invading organisms.
3. **Gastrointestinal tract** The secretory function of mucous membranes is diminished so that the tissues slough off, affecting digestion and absorption.
4. **Genitourinary tract** As epithelial tissue breaks down, problems such as urinary tract infections, calculi, and vaginal infections become more common.
5. **Skin** As the skin becomes dry and scaly, small pustules or a hardened, pigmented, papular eruption may appear around the hair follicles, a condition called **follicular hyperkeratosis**.
6. **Tooth formation** Because of a lack of vitamin A, specific epithelial cells surrounding tooth buds in fetal gum tissue that become specialized cup-shaped organs called **ameloblasts** may not develop properly. These organs form the enamel structure of the developing tooth. Each cell carries out the task of producing and depositing minute prisms of enamel substance that eventually form the erupted tooth.

Follicular hyperkeratosis Vitamin A deficiency condition in which the skin becomes dry and scaly and small pustules or hardened, pigmented, papular eruptions form around the hair follicles.

Ameloblasts Special epithelial cells surrounding tooth buds in gum tissue, which form cup-shaped organs for producing the enamel structure of the developing teeth.

Growth Vitamin A is essential to the growth of skeletal and soft tissues. This effect is probably caused by its influence on protein synthesis, mitosis (cell division), or stability of cell membranes.

Reproduction The retinoids are necessary to support normal function of the reproductive system in both males and females. In tests with animals the lack of retinol and retinal produces sterility, testicular degeneration in males, and aborted or malformed offspring in females.

Vitamin A Requirement

Influencing factors A number of variables modify vitamin A needs. Although vitamin A is generally ample in most diets, many factors may alter its need in a given individual: (1) the amount stored in the liver, (2) the form in which it is taken (as carotene or vitamin A), (3) illness, and (4) gastrointestinal or hepatic defects. Vitamin A deficiency may occur for three basic reasons: (1) inadequate dietary intake, (2) poor absorption because of a lack of bile or a defective absorbing surface, and (3) inadequate conversion of carotene because of liver or intestinal disease.

Units of measure To cover such variables, the RDA standard recommends a margin of safety above minimal needs. Traditionally, vitamin A has been measured in international units (IU). Currently, the RDA uses the term **retinol equivalents (RE)**. This is a more accurate term because individual absorption and conversion of provitamin carotenoids are variable factors, and this variance is accounted for in the newer term. During this period of transition from international units to retinol equivalents as a measure of vitamin A activity, the RDA standard is given in both RE and IU.

Hypervitaminosis A Because the liver can store large amounts of vitamin A, and many persons take additional megadose supplements, it is clearly possible to consume a potentially toxic quantity. Hypervitaminosis A is manifested by joint pain, thickening of long bones, loss of hair, and jaundice. Excess vitamin A may also cause liver injury with resulting portal hypertension and ascites.

Food Sources of Vitamin A

There are few animal sources of preformed vitamin A. These include liver, kidney, cream, butter, and egg yolk. Our main dietary sources are the yellow and green vegetables and fruit sources of carotene, such as carrots, sweet potatoes, squash, apricots, cantalope, spinach, collards, broccoli, and cabbage. In addition, commercial products may be fortified with vitamin A. For example, margarine is fortified with 1500 IU of vitamin A per pound.

Vitamin D
General Nature of Vitamin D

Chemical and physical nature Early investigators wrongly classed this substance as a vitamin. It is now clear that it is really a *prohormone* of a sterol type and should be viewed as a hormone. The term *vitamin D activity* is somtimes useful in talking about the several substances that the body makes by ultraviolet irradiation of steroids, which are known collectively as vitamin D. Since the precursor base in human skin is the lipid material, 7-dehydrocholesterol, all forms of these compounds with vitamin D activity are soluble in fat but not in water. They are heat stable and are not easily oxidized.

Forms The two compounds with vitamin D activity involved in human nutrition are *ergocalciferol (vitamin D_2)* and *cholecalciferol (vitamin D_3)*. Vitamin D_2 is formed by irradiating ergosterol (provitamin D_2), which is found ergot and in yeast. The more important product is vitamin D_3, which is formed by irradiating 7-dehydrocholesterol (provitamin D_3) in the skin. Vitamin D_3 occurs also in fish liver oils.

Absorption, Transport, and Storage

Absorption Absorption of dietary vitamin D_3 occurs in the small intestine with the aid of bile. It mixes with the intestinal micelles (p. 30) and is

---

Retinol equivalent (RE)
Measure of vitamin A activity currently adopted by FAO/WHO and U.S. National Research Council's Food and Nutrition Board, replacing the term International Unit (IU). The measure accounts for dietary variances in preformed vitamin A (retinol) and its precursor, carotene. One retinol equivalent (RE) equals 3.33 IU or 1 mg retinol.

absorbed in these fat packets. Malabsorption diseases such as celiac syndrome, sprue, and colitis hinder vitamin D absorption.

Active hormone synthesis The synthesis of the active hormone form of **1,25-dihydroxycholecalciferol** is accomplished by the combined action of skin, liver, and kidneys:

1,25-Dihydroxycholecalciferol
Physiologically active
hormone form of vitamin D.

1. **Skin** In the skin the precursor cholesterol compound, 7-dehydrocholesterol, is irradiated by the sun's ultraviolet rays to produce vitamin D_3, which is then transported by a special protein carrier. The amount of vitamin D_3 formed by the action of sunlight on the skin depends on a number of variables, including length and intensity of exposure and color of the skin. For example, heavily pigmented skin can prevent up to 95% of ultraviolet radiation from reaching the deeper layer of the skin for adequate synthesis of the steroid hormone. Also, persons who lack exposure to sunlight—house-bound elderly persons or those living in crowded areas of urban cities with high air pollution rates, would be deprived of adequate skin irradiation.
2. **Liver** A special liver enzyme converts D_3 to the intermediate product 25-hydroxycholecalciferol.
3. **Kidneys** The vital function of final activation is accomplished here. Special enzymes form 1,25-dihyroxycholcalciferol, the physiologically active form of the hormone.[1]

Functions of Vitamin D

Absorption of calcium and phosphorus As indicated, the recently discovered vitamin D endocrine system is based in the kidney. In balance with the *parathyroid hormone* and the thyroid hormone *calcitonin,* the vitamin D hormone stimulates the active transport of calcium and phosphorus in the small intestine. Because vitamin D hormone has an active regulatory role as a balancing hormone and evident clinical use, it has been used to treat the bone disease caused by kidney failure—renal osteodystrophy (p. 489). It may also contribute to the treatment of osteoporosis, a bone loss common in older women that leads to fractures.[2]

Bone mineralization After it has aided calcium and phosphorus absorption, vitamin D hormones continue to work with these minerals to form bone tissue. They directly increase the rate of mineral deposit and resorption in bone, the process by which bone tissue is built and maintained. A deficiency of vitamin D causes *rickets,* a condition characterized by malformation of skeletal tissue in growing children (Figure 7-2).

Vitamin D Requirement

Influencing factors Difficulties exist in setting requirements for vitamin D. Variables arise from the limited number of food sources available, lack of knowledge of precise body needs, and degree of synthesis in the skin by irradiation. The amount needed may vary between winter and summer in northern climates. Also, a person's way of living determines the degree of exposure to sunlight and would therefore influence individual need. For example, a city dweller living in a high-rise apartment or in a tene-

Figure 7-2
Rachitic children. Note
knock-knees of child on left
and bowlegs of child on
right.
From Therapeutic notes.
Parke, Davis & Co., Detroit;
courtesy Dr. Tom Spies and
Dr. Orson D. Bird.

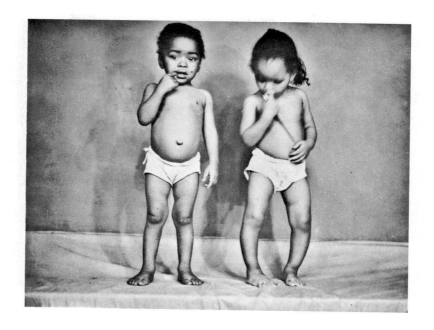

ment and working indoors needs more than a farmer. Growth demands
in childhood and in pregnancy and lactation necessitate increased intake.

RDA standard The RDA standard is 10 μg of cholecalciferol (400 IU)
daily for children and for women during pregnancy and lactation. The
daily recommendation for young adults is 7.5 μg and for older adults
5.0 μg.

Hypervitaminosis D As with vitamin A, it is possible to ingest excess
quantities of vitamin D and so produce toxicity. Intakes of vitamin D
above 50 μg cholecalciferol (2000 IU/day), which is five times the recommended daily allowance, for prolonged periods can produce hypercalcemia in infants and nephrocalcinosis in infants and adults. Infant feeding
poses a special problem. Excess intake is possible in infant feeding practices where fortified milk, fortified cereal, plus variable vitamin supplements are used. The infant needs only 10 μg (400 IU) daily, whereas the
amount in all of the above items can easily total 100 μg (4000 IU) or
more. The symptoms of vitamin D toxicity are calcification of the soft
tissues, such as lungs and kidney, as well as bone fragility. Renal tissue is
particularly prone to calcify, affecting glomerular filtration and overall
function.

Food Sources and Vitamin D

Few natural food sources of vitamin D exist. The two basic substances with
vitamin D activity, D_2 and D_3, occur only in yeast and fish liver oils. The
main food sources are those to which crystalline vitamin D has been
added. Milk, because it is a common food, has proved to be the most
practical carrier. It is now a widespread commercial practice to standardize
the added vitamin content of milk at 400 IU/qt. Milk is also a good carrier

for the vitamin, for it provides calcium and phosphorus as well. Butter substitutes such as margarines are also fortified.

Vitamin E
General Nature of Vitamin E

Tocopherol Vitamin E; from two Greek words meaning "childbirth" and "to bring forth"; so named because of its association with reproduction in rats.

Chemical and physical nature Vitamin E was discovered in connection with studies concerning the reproductive responses of rats and was identified as an alcohol. Because of this early function in rats and its chemical nature, it was named **tocopherol**. Since then, tocopherol has come to be commonly known as the antisterility vitamin, but this effect has been demonstrated only in rats and not in humans, despite all advertising claims for its contribution to sexual powers.

Forms Vitamin E is the generic name for a group of vitamins, one of which, alpha-tocopherol, is the most significant in human nutrition. Vitamin E is a pale yellow oil, stable to acids and heat and insoluble in water. It oxidizes very slowly, which gives it an important role as an **antioxidant** with significant clinical applications.

Antioxidant Substance added to a product to delay or prevent its breakdown by oxygen.

Absorption, Transport, and Storage

Vitamin E is absorbed with the aid of bile. With other lipids in the chylomicrons, it is transported out of the intestinal wall into the body circulation in the blood plasma lipoproteins. Storage takes place in different body tissues but especially in fat tissue.

Functions of Vitamin E

Antioxidant Vitamin E acts as nature's most potent fat-soluble antioxidant. The polyunsaturated fatty acids in structural lipid membranes in body tissues are particularly vulnerable to oxidative breakdown by free radicals in the cell. The tocopherols can interrupt this oxidation process, protecting the cell membrane fatty acids from the oxidative damage.

Selenium metabolism Even with adequate vitamin E intake, some damaging cell peroxides are formed, and a second line of defense is needed to destroy them before they can damage cell membranes. The agent providing this added defense is a selenium-containing enzyme (p. 165). Thus selenium spares vitamin E by reducing its requirement. Similarly, in this partnership role, vitamin E reduces the selenium requirements.

Vitamin E Requirement

RDA standard The requirements for vitamin E vary with the amount of polyunsaturated fatty acids in the diet. The RDA standard for adults in *alpha-tocopherol equivalents* (α-*TE*) is 10 mg for men and 8 mg for women. Needs during childhood growth periods range from 3 to 10 mg.

Special clinical needs Since vitamin E protects cellular and subcellular membranes and hence tissue integrity, it is an important nutrient in the diets of pregnant and lactating women, and especially newborn infants. Two medical problems found in infants, especially premature ones, have responded positively to vitamin E therapy: (1) *retrolental fibroplasia,* a condition of severely limited vision or complete blindness resulting from the effect of excess oxygen therapy following birth, and (2) *hymolytic anemia,* a condition in which fragile erythrocyte membranes break down because of high cell peroxide levels and the induced deficiency of vitamin E.[3] Also, vitamin E deficiencies have been demonstrated in intestinal malabsorption syndromes such as occur with surgical bowel resection. In general, older persons may require more vitamin E. It has been shown to be effective for those suffering circulatory disturbance such as pain in the legs after walking is begun but is of no help with varicose veins. Its effectiveness has not been shown in treating coronary heart disease.

Food Sources of Vitamin E

The richest sources of vitamin E are the vegetable oils. Curiously enough, these are also the richest sources of polyunsaturated fatty acids, which vitamin E protects from oxidation. Other food sources include milk, eggs, muscle meats, fish, cereals, and leafy vegetables.

Vitamin K
General Nature of Vitamin K

Chemical and physical nature The studies of a biochemist at the University of Copenhagen working with a hemorrhagic disease in chicks fed a fat-free diet led to the discovery of vitamin K. He determined that the absent factor responsible was a fat-soluble blood-clotting vitamin. He called it "koagulationsvitamin" or vitamin K, from the Swedish word for its function. Later he succeeded in isolating and identifying the agent from alfalfa, for which he received the Nobel Prize in physiology and medicine.

Forms As with most of the vitamins, not one but several forms of vitamin K comprise a group of substances with similar biologic activity in blood clotting. There are three main K vitamins:
1. K_1, which is the major form found in plants.
2. K_2, which is synthesized by intestinal bacterial flora, so vitamin K is not required directly in the diet.
3. K_3, a water-soluble analog, which does not require bile for absorption and goes directly into the portal blood system.

These water-soluble forms are available for clinical use.

Absorption, Transport, and Storage

K_1 and K_2 require bile for absorption as with other fat-related products. They are packaged in the chylomicrons and travel by way of the abdominal lacteals into the lymphatic system and then into the portal blood for transport to the liver. In the liver, vitamin K is stored in small amounts, though its concentration there declines rapidly. It is excreted in considerable quantity after administration of therapeutic doses.

Functions of Vitamin K

Prothrombin Protein (globulin) circulating in the plasma, essential to the clotting of blood. Prothrombin is produced by the liver.

Blood clotting The function of vitamin K is to catalyze the synthesis of blood-clotting factors by the liver. Vitamin K produces the active form of several precursors, mainly **prothrombin** (factor II), which combines with calcium (factor IV) to produce the clotting effect. In the absence of functioning liver tissue, vitamin K cannot act. When liver damage has caused the problem of hypoprothrombinemia, and this in turn has lead to hemorrhage, vitamin K is ineffective as a therapeutic agent.

Clinical problems Several clinical situations are related to vitamin K:

1. **Neonatology** The sterile intestinal tract of the newborn can supply no vitamin K during the first few days of life until normal bacterial flora develop. During this immediate postnatal period, *hemorrhagic disease of the newborn* may, therefore, occur. Thus a prophylactic dose of vitamin K is usually given to the infant soon after birth.

2. **Malabsorption disease** Any defect in fat absorption will cause a failure in vitamin K absorption, resulting in prolonged blood-clotting time. For example, patients with bile duct obstruction are routinely given vitamin K before surgery. Also, after a cholecystectomy, which hinders normal bile flow, vitamin K (which requires bile and fat for normal absorption) is not readily absorbed. The water-soluble form, vitamin K_3 (menadione) may be used instead.

3. **Drug therapy** Several drug-nutrient interactions involve vitamin K. An anticlotting drug such as bishydroxycoumarin (Dicumarol) acts as an antimetabolite or **antagonist**, thus inhibiting the action of vitamin K. When this drug is used for treating conditions such as pulmonary embolism or venous thrombosis, vitamin K may be used as a balancing "antidote" to the drug in the management of the blood-clotting time. Also, in extended use of antibiotics, the intestinal bacterial flora may be diminished, thus reducing the body's main source of vitamin K.

Antagonist Substance that counteracts the action of another substance. It gets in the way and prevents the reaction from taking place.

Vitamin K Requirement

No specific requirement for vitamin K is given because there is little information on which to base allowances. Instead, the RDA estimates a safe and adequate daily dietary intake for adults of 70 to 140 μg, with relatively small amounts for children. A deficiency of vitamin K is unlikely, except in the clinical conditions indicated. An adequate amount is usually ensured because (1) the intestinal bacteria constantly synthesize an adequate supply, and (2) the amount the body needs is apparently very small. The liver, however, must produce prothrombin and its related blood-clotting factors if vitamin K is to be effective.

Food Sources of Vitamin K

Dietary vitamin K is found in green leafy vegetables such as cabbage, spinach, kale, and cauliflower. Lesser amounts are found in tomatoes, cheese, egg yolk, and liver. However, the main source remains bacterial synthesis. A summary of the fat-soluble vitamins is given in Table 7-1.

Water-Soluble Vitamins

Vitamin C
General Nature of Vitamin C

Chemical and physical nature The recognition of vitamin C is associated with an unrelenting search for the cause of the ancient hemorrhagic disease, **scurvy**. Early observations, mostly among British sailors and explorers, led to the later American discovery of an acid in lemon juice that

Scurvy Hemorrhagic disease caused by lack of vitamin C.

Table 7-1
Summary of Fat-Soluble Vitamins

Vitamin	Physiologic Functions	Results of Deficiency	Requirement	Food Sources
Vitamin A Provitamin: beta-carotene Vitamin: retinol	Production of rhodopsin and other light-receptor pigments Formation and maintenance of epithelial tissue Growth Reproduction Toxic in large amounts	Poor dark adaptation, night blindness, xerosis, xerophthalmia Keratinization of epithelium Growth failure Reproductive failure	Adult male: 1000 μg RE (5000 IU) Adult female: 800 μg RE (4000 IU) Pregnancy: 1000 μg RE (5000 IU) Lactation 1200 μg RE (6000 IU) Children: 400 μg RE (2000 IU) to 800 μg RE (4000 IU)	Liver, cream, butter, whole milk, egg yolk Green and yellow vegetables, yellow fruits Fortified margarine
Vitamin D Provitamins: ergosterol (plants); 7-dehydro-cholesterol (skin) Vitamins: D_2 (ergocholecalciferol) and D_3 (cholecalciferol)	1,25-dihydroxycholecalciferol, a major hormone regulator of bone mineral (calcium and phosphorus) metabolism Calcium and phosphorus absorption Toxic in large amounts	Faulty bone growth: rickets, osteomalacia	Adult: 5-10 μg cholecalciferol (200-400 IU) Pregnancy and lactation: 10-12.5 μg (400-5000 IU), depending on age Children: 10 μg (400 IU)	Fortified milk Fortified margarine Fish oils Sunlight on skin
Vitamin E Tocopherols	Antioxidation Hemopoiesis Related to action of selenium	Anemia in premature infants	Adults: 8-10 mg αTE Pregnancy and lactation: 10-11 mg αTE Children: 3-10 mg αTE	Vegetable oils
Vitamin K K_1 (phylloquinone) K_2 (menaquinone) Analog: K_3 (menadione)	Activation of blood-clotting factors (for example, prothrombin) by α-carboxylating glutamic acid residues Toxicity can be induced by water-soluble analogs	Hemorrhagic disease of the newborn Defective blood clotting Deficiency symptoms, which can be produced by coumarin anticoagulants and by antibiotic therapy	Adult: 70-140 μg Children: 15-100 μg Infants: 12-20 μg	Cheese, egg yolk, liver Green leafy vegetables Synthesized by intestinal bacteria

prevented or cured scurvy. The name *ascorbic acid* was given to this substance because of its antiscorbutic, or "antiscurvy," properties. Vitamin C is soluble in water but not in fat. It is an unstable, easily oxidized acid. It can be destroyed by oxygen, alkalis, and high temperatures. Thus, vitamin C foods should be cooked in as little water as possible for brief period of time and kept covered. Also, soda should never be added as a coloring agent to foods during cooking. Vegetables should not be cut into small pieces until the time of cooking, since the more surface exposed to air, the greater the destruction of vitamin C. Also, juices should not be left out uncovered.

Absorption, Transport, and Storage

Vitamin C is easily absorbed from the small intestine, but this absorption is hindered by a lack of hydrochloric acid or by bleeding from the gastrointestinal tract. Vitamin C is not stored in single tissue depots as is vitamin A. Rather it is more generally distributed throughout body tissues, maintaining a tissue saturation level. Any excess is slowly excreted in the urine. The tissue levels relate to intake, and the size of the total body pool adjusts to maintain balances. The total amount in adults varies from about 4 g to as little as 0.3 g. Tissue levels diminish slowly, so, with no intake, deficiency symptoms would not appear for approximately 3 months. This explains why generally healthy people in more isolated living situations can survive the winter without eating many fresh fruits and vegetables. Sufficient vitamin C for needs in early infancy is present in breast milk if the mother has a good diet for lactation. Because cow's milk does not contain an adequate supply for the requirement of the human infant, formulas are supplemented with ascorbic acid.

Functions of Vitamin C

Intercellular cement substance We require vitamin C to build and maintain body tissues in general, including bone matrix, cartilage, dentin, collagen, and connective tissue. When vitamin C is absent, the important ground substance does not develop into collagen. When vitamin C is given, formation of cartilaginous tissue follows quickly. **Collagen** is a protein substance that exists in many tissues of the body, such as the white fibers of connective tissue. Blood vessel tissue particularly is weakened without the cementing substance of vitamin C to provide firm capillary walls. Therefore vitamin C deficiency is characterized by fragile, easily ruptured capillaries with resultant diffuse tissue bleeding. Deficiency signs include easy bruising, pinpoint hemorrhages of the skin, bone and joint hemorrhages, easy bone fracture, poor wound healing, and soft bleeding gums with loosened teeth (*gingivitis*).

> The word collagen is derived from two Greek words that mean "glue" and "to produce."

General body metabolism There is a greater concentration of vitamin C in the more metabolically active tissue such as the adrenal glands, brain, kidney, liver, pancreas, thymus, and spleen than in the less active tissues. There is also more vitamin C in a child's actively multiplying tissue than in adult tissue. Vitamin C also helps in the formation of hemoglobin and the development of red blood cells in two ways: (1) it aids in the absorption of iron, and (2) it influences the removal of iron from its transport complex so that it is available to tissues producing the hemoglobin.

Clinical Problems Clinical problems include:
1. **Wound healing** The significant role of vitamin C in cementing the ground substance of supportive tissue makes it an important agent in wound healing. This has evident implications for use in surgery, especially where extensive tissue regeneration is involved.
2. **Fevers and infections** Infectious processes deplete tissue stores of vitamin C. Optimal tissue stores of vitamin C help maintain resistance to infection. Just how large an amount may be required to maintain this prevention of infections is not known.
3. **Growth periods** Additional vitamin C is required during the growth periods of infancy and childhood. It is also required during pregnancy to supply demands for fetal growth and maternal tissues.

> Controversial claims have been made that massive doses of vitamin C have various therapeutic effects such as prevention of the common cold or treatment of cancer. Controlled studies have failed to support these claims.

Vitamin C Requirement

Difficulties in establishing requirements for vitamin C involve questions concerning individual tissue needs and whether minimum or optimum intakes are desired. Although studies indicate that a lower intake, from 20 to 30 mg daily, may suffice for the average adult, the RDA standard is 60 mg daily for an optimal margin to cover variances in tissue demand.

Food Sources of Vitamin C

Vitamin C can be oxidized easily. Thus the handling, preparation, cooking, and processing of any food source of the vitamin should be considered in evaluating that food's contribution of the vitamin to the diet. Well-known sources include citrus fruit and tomatoes. Less regarded, but good additional sources, include cabbage, sweet potatoes, white potatoes, and green and yellow vegetables. Other sources are seasonsal, local, or regional foods such as berries, melons, chili peppers, guavas, pineapple, chard, kale, turnip greens, broccoli, and asparagus.

A summary of vitamin C and its role in the body is given in Table 7-2. Some guidelines for vitamin supplementation are provided to help you in client counseling (box, pp. 120-121).

Table 7-2
Summary of Vitamin C
(Ascorbic Acid)

Physiologic Functions	Clinical Applications	Requirement	Food Sources
Antioxidation	Scurvy (deficiency)	60 mg	Fresh fruits, especially citrus
Collagen biosynthesis	Wound healing, tissue formation		Vegetables, such as tomatoes, cabbage, potatoes, chili peppers, and broccoli
General metabolism			
Makes iron available for hemoglobin synthesis	Fevers and infections		
	Stress reactions		
Influences conversion of folic acid to folinic acid	Growth		
Oxidation-reduction of the amino acids, phenylalanine and lyrosine			

B-Complex Vitamins

Deficiency Disease and Vitamin Discoveries

Deficiency disease The story of the B vitamins is a compelling one. It tells of persons dying of a puzzling, age-old disease for which there was no cure. It was eventually learned that common, everyday food held the answer. The paralyzing disease was **beriberi**, which had plagued the Orient for centuries and caused many men in many places to search for its solution. Early observations and studies provided important clues, but application of the "vitamine" connection to the human creeping sickness was needed. This was finally achieved when an American chemist with the Philippine Bureau of Science used extracts of rice polishings and cured the epidemic infantile beriberi. The food factor was named *water-soluble B*

Beriberi Disease of the peripheral nerves caused by a deficiency of thiamin (vitamin B_1).

Clinical Application

Nutrient or Drug?

In 1954, researchers found out that large doses, 10 to 1000 times the RDA, of specific nutrients helped alleviate symptoms in certain genetic disorders. Twenty years later, the general public began to think that this would be helpful for healthy people, too. So they started using nutrients as drugs.

A similarity does exist. Both nutrients and drugs are used by the body in specific amounts to control or improve a physiologic condition or illness, to prevent a disease, or to relieve symptoms. But for many persons, the similarity seems to end there. They know that too much of any drug can be harmful, but they fail to apply this same wise logic to nutrients.

Some Bad Effects

Toxic effects of vitamin megadoses. Physicians may prescribe large doses of water-soluble vitamins, believing they are safe because they are not stored in the body. However, they have recently discovered the potential toxicity of at least one such vitamin— pyridoxine (B_6). Gynecologists have been prescribing this vitamin at levels that were 1000 to 2700 times its RDA to help patients relieve the discomfort of edema during their menstrual cycle. The patients eventually developed unstable gaits, with such numbness in the hands that they were unable to walk or carry out their usual duties at work. To make matters worse, the prescription did nothing to relieve their discomfort.

"Artificially-induced" deficiency symptoms. These occur when blood levels of one nutrient rise above normal, resulting in an increased need for other nutrients with which it interacts. Deficiencies also occur when large doses are suddenly removed, creating a "rebound effect." This effect has been seen in infants born to mothers who took megadoses of vitamin C during pregnancy, yet developed scurvy after birth when their high nutrient supply was cut off.

Wise Warnings

The megavitamin lesson is not easily taught. Megadose salespersons frequently have more time, money, and better "selling" techniques with which they can misinform the public. Nonetheless, for your clients' welfare, you will still want warn them:

Vitamins, like drugs, can be harmful in large amounts. The only time megadoses are helpful is when the body already has a severe deficiency or is unable to absorb or metabolize the nutrient efficiently.

All nutrients work in harmony to promote good health. Adding large amounts of one only makes the body believe that it isn't getting enough of the others and increases the risk of developing deficiency symptoms.

Clinical Application—cont'd

Supplements should not be taken without first analyzing nutrient levels currently in the diet. This helps to avoid problems of excess, which may increase with an accumulative effect over time.

Food remains the best source of nutrients. Most food items provide a wide variety of nutrients, as opposed to the dozen or so found in a vitamin bottle. By itself a vitamin can do very little. Its action is catalytic and so it requires a substrate to work on. These necessary substrates are the energy nutrients—carbohydrate, protein, fat—and their metabolites. Food provides these necessities and a great deal of pleasure as well.

References

Houston, J.: The vitamin that conquered America, Family Health **12**(8):32, September, 1980.

Rudman, D.: Megadose vitamins: use and misuse, N. Engl. J. Med. **309**(8):489, 1983.

Schaumburg, H., and others: Sensory neuropathy from pyridoxine abuse, N. Engl. J. Med. **309**(3):445, 1983.

because it was thought to be a single vitamin. Now we know it to be a large family of many water-soluble vitamins having a variety of significant metabolic functions in human health.

Coenzyme Compound or molecule that must be present with an enzyme for a specific reaction to occur.

Enzyme Protein that acts as a catalyst by accelerating the chemical reactions of its often specific substrate.

Vital coenzyme role The B vitamins, originally believed to be important only in preventing the deficiency diseases that led to their discovery, have now been identified in relation to many important metabolic functions. As vital control agents, they serve in many reactions as **coenzyme** partners with key cell **enzymes** in energy metabolism and tissue building.

Here we will review briefly the eight basic B vitamins. First we will look at the three classic disease factor vitamins—thiamin, riboflavin, and niacin. Then we will explore more recently discovered coenzyme factors—pyridoxine (B$_6$), pantothenic acid, and biotin. Finally, we will examine the important blood-forming factors—folic acid and cobalamin (B$_{12}$).

Thiamin
General Nature of Thiamin

Deficiency disease related to discovery The search of many persons for the cause of beriberi led eventually to a successful conclusion with the identification of thiamin as the control agent involved. Its basic nature and metabolic functions were then clarified.

One of thiamin's major parts is a thiazole ring: *thi*(o + vit)*amin*.

Chemical and physical nature Thiamin is a water-soluble, fairly stable vitamin. However, it is destroyed by alkalis. The name "thiamin" comes from its chemical ringlike structure.

Absorption and Storage of Thiamin

Thiamin is absorbed more readily in the acid medium of the first section of the small intestine, the duodenum. In the lower duodenum the acidity of the food mass is counteracted by the alkaline intestinal secretions. Thiamin is not stored in large quantities in the tissue. The tissue content is highly relative to increased metabolic demand, as in fever, increased muscular activity, pregnancy, and lactation. The tissue stores also depend on the adequacy of the diet and on its general composition. For example, carbohydrate increases the need for thiamin, whereas fat and protein spare thiamin. Any excess unused thiamin is constantly excreted in the urine.

Function of Thiamin

Basic coenzyme role The main function of thiamin as a metabolic control agent is related to energy metabolism. It serves as a coenzyme in key reactions that produce energy from glucose or that convert glucose to fat for tissue storage. Thus the manifestations of beriberi (muscle weakness, gastrointestinal disturbances, and neuritis) can be traced to problems related to these basic functions of thiamin.

Clinical problems Inadequate thiamin to provide the key energizing coenzyme factor in the cells produces broad clinical effects:
  1. **Gastrointestinal system** Various symtpoms such as anorexia, indigestion, severe constipation, gastric atony, and deficient hydrochloric acid secretion may result from thiamin deficiency. When the cells of the smooth muscles and the secretory glands do not receive sufficient energy from glucose, they cannot do their work in digestion to provide still more glucose. A vicious cycle then ensues as the deficiency continues.
  2. **Nervous system** The central nervous system is extremely dependent on glucose for energy to do its work. Without sufficient thiamin to help provide this constant fuel, neuronal activity is impaired, alertness and reflex responses are diminished, and general apathy and fatigue result. If the deficiency continues, lipogenesis is hindered and damage or degeneration of *myelin sheaths*—lipid tissue covering the nerve fibers—follows. This causes increasing nerve irritation, pain, and prickly or deadening sensations. Paralysis gradually results if the process continues unchecked.
  3. **Cardiovascular system** With continuing thiamin deficiency, the heart muscle weakens and cardiac failure results. Also, smooth muscle of the vascular system may be involved, causing dilation of the peripheral blood vessels. As a result of cardiac failure, edema appears in the lower legs.

Thiamin Requirement

RDA standard The thiamin requirement in human nutrition is usually stated in terms of carbohydrate and energy metabolism needs, as expressed in caloric intake. Daily adult thiamin needs range from 0.23 to 0.5 mg/1000 kcal. The RDA standard is 0.5 mg/1000 kcal with a minimum of 1 mg for any intake between 1000 to 2000 kcal.

Special needs Several important factors influence thiamin requirements and should be recognized in the care of patients. Increased thiamin is required in the following situations:

1. **Alcoholism** Thiamin is most important in nutritional therapy for persons with alcoholism. Both a primary (lack of adequate diet) and a conditioned (effect of alcohol itself) malnutrition may develop and bring serious neurologic disorders.[4]
2. **Other disease** Fevers and infections increase cellular energy requirements. Geriatric patients and those with chronic illness require particular attention to prevent deficiencies.
3. **Growth and development** About a 50% increase in thiamin requirements accompanies pregnancy and lactation, demanded by the rapid fetal growth, the increased metabolic rate during pregnancy, and the production of milk. Continued growth during infancy, childhood, and adolescence requires attention to thiamin needs. At any point in the life cycle, the larger the body and its tissue volume, the greater its cellular energy requirements and thus thiamin needs.

Food Sources of Thiamin

Although thiamin is widespread in almost all plant and animal tissues commonly used as food, the content is usually small. Thus deficiency of thiamin is a distinct possibility when kilocalories are markedly curtailed, as in alcoholism, and when persons are following some highly inadequate special diet. In general good food sources include lean pork, beef, liver, whole or enriched grains (flour, bread, cereals), and legumes. Eggs, fish, and a few vegetables are fair sources.

Riboflavin
General Nature of Riboflavin

Discovery Although as early as 1897 a London chemist had observed in milk whey a water-soluble pigment with peculiar yellow-green fluorescence, it was not until 1932 that riboflavin was actually discovered by researchers in Germany. It was given the chemical group name *flavins* from the Latin word for *yellow*. Later, because the vitamin was found also to contain a sugar named *ribose*, the name *riboflavin* was officially adopted.

Chemical and physical nature Riboflavin is a yellow-green fluorescent pigment that forms yellowish brown, needlelike crystals. It is water-soluble and relatively stable to heat but is easily destroyed by light and irradiation. It is stable in acid media and is not easily oxidized. However, it is sensitive to strong alkalis.

Absorption and Storage of Riboflavin

Absorption of riboflavin occurs readily in the upper section of the small intestine, assisted by combination with phosphorus in the intestinal mucosa. Storage is limited, although small amounts are found in liver and kidney. Day-to-day tissue turnover needs must be supplied in the diet.

Functions of Riboflavin

Basic coenzyme role The cell enzymes of which riboflavin is an important part are called *flavoproteins*. Riboflavin enzymes operate at vital reaction points in the process of cellular energy metabolism and in *deamination*, the key reaction that removes the nitrogen-containing amino group from certain amino acids. Thus riboflavin acts as a control agent in both energy production and tissue building.

Clinical problems Clinical problems include the following:

Ariboflavinosis Riboflavin deficiency state.

1. **Ariboflavinosis** A deficiency of riboflavin, or **ariboflavinosis**, brings a combination of symptoms, which centers on tissue inflammation and breakdown and poor wound healing. Even minor injuries easily become aggravated and do not heal easily. The lips become swollen, cracking easily, and characteristic cracks develop at the corners of the mouth—a condition called *cheilosis*. Cracks and irritation develop at nasal angles. The tongue becomes swollen and reddened—a condition called **glossitis**. Extra blood vessels develop in the cornea—*corneal vascularization*—and the eyes burn, itch, and tear. A scaly, greasy skin condition—*seborrheic dermatitis*—may develop, especially in skin folds. Since nutritional deficiencies are usually multiple rather than single, riboflavin deficiencies seldom occur alone. They are especially likely to occur in conjunction with deficiencies of other B vitamins and protein.

Glossitis Swollen, reddened tongue; riboflavin deficiency symptom.

2. **Deficiency in newborns** Because riboflavin is light sensitive, newborn infants with hyperbilirubinemia treated with phototherapy have shown signs of riboflavin deficiencies even when supplements were provided.

Riboflavin Requirement

Influencing factors The body's riboflavin requirement is related to total energy needs, level of exercise,[5] body size, metabolic rate, and rate of growth.

RDA standard For practical purposes the general RDA standard for riboflavin is based on 0.6 mg/1000 kcal for all ages.

Risk groups Persons in certain risk groups or clinical situations may require increased riboflavin. These include persons living in poverty or following bizarre food habits, those with gastrointestinal disease or chronic illness where appetite is poor and malabsorption exists, people who have poor wound healing, and individuals during growth periods such as in childhood, pregnancy, and lactation.

Food Sources of Riboflavin

Lactoflavin Form in which riboflavin occurs in milk.

The most important food source of riboflavin is milk. One of the pigments in milk, **lactoflavin**, is the milk form of riboflavin. Each quart of milk contains 2 mg of riboflavin, which is more than the daily requirement. Other good sources are organ meats such as liver, kidney, and heart, whole or enriched grains, and vegetables. Since riboflavin is water-soluble and destroyed by light, considerable loss can occur in open, excess-water cooking.

Niacin
General Nature of Niacin

Pellagra Deficiency disease caused by a lack of niacin in the diet and an inadequate amount of protein containing the amino acid, tryptophan, which is a precursor of niacin.

Deficiency disease related to discovery The age-old disease related to niacin is **pellagra**. It is characterized by a typical dermatitis and often has fatal effects on the nervous system. Pellagra was first observed in 18th century Europe, where it was endemic in populations subsisting largely on corn. Later observations by an American physician studying the problem in an orphanage in rural southern United States gave further clues. He noticed that although the majority of the children in the orphanage had pellagra to some degree, a few of them did not. Finally he discovered that the few who did not have pellagra were sneaking into the pantries at night and eating from the orphanage's limited supply of milk and meat. His investigation established the relationship of the disease to a certain food factor. However, not until 1937, did a scientist at the University of Wisconsin definitely associate niacin with pellagra by using it to cure a related disease—black tongue in dogs.

Chemical and physical nature As further study of niacin and pellagra continued it became evident that the vitamin was closely connected to the essential amino acid tryptophan and had several forms.

1. **Relation to tryptophan** The initial mystery of the relation of niacin to the essential amino acid tryptophan grew with curious observations made by early investigators. Why was pellagra rare in some population groups whose diets were actually low in niacin, whereas the disease was common in other groups whose diets were higher in niacin? And why did milk, which is low in niacin, have the ability to cure or prevent pellagra? Why was pellagra so common in groups subsisting on diets high in corn? In 1945, workers at the University of Wisconsin finally made the key discovery: tryptophan can be used by the body to make niacin; it is a **precursor** of niacin. Here again was a vital link of a B vitamin with protein. Milk prevents pellagra because it is high in tryptophan. Almost exclusive use of corn contributes to pellagra because corn is low in tryptophan. Some populations subsisting on diets low in niacin may never have pellagra because they happen also to be consuming adequate amounts of tryptophan.

2. **Niacin equivalent** This tryptophan-niacin relationship led to the development of a unit of measure called **niacin equivalent (NE)**. In persons with average physiologic needs, approximately 60 mg of tryptophan produces 1 mg of niacin, the amount designated as a niacin equivalent. Dietary requirements are now given in terms of total mg of niacin and niacin equivalents.

Precursor Something that precedes; in biology, a substance from which another substance is derived.

Niacin equivalent (NE) Measure of the total dietary sources of niacin equivalent to 1 mg of niacin. Thus, a niacin equivalent (NE) is 1 mg of niacin or 60 mg of tryptophan.

Forms Two forms of niacin exist. Niacin (nicotinic acid) is easily converted to its amide form, *nicotinamide*, which is water-soluble, stable to acid and heat, and forms a white powder when crystallized.

Functions of Niacin

Basic coenzyme role Niacin is a partner with riboflavin in the cellular coenzyme system that converts protein to glucose and oxidizes glucose to release controlled energy.

Drug therapy High doses of nicotinic acid, but no nicotinamide, cause skin flushing, gastrointestinal distress, and itching. Such a dosage has been effective in lowering serum cholesterol levels, although the mechanisms for such action are unclear.

Clinical problems Generally niacin deficiency is manifested as weakness, lassitude, anorexia, indigestion, and various skin eruptions. More specific symptoms involve the skin and nervous system. Skin areas exposed to sunlight are especially affected and develop a dark, scaly dermatitis. If deficiency continues, the central nervous system becomes involved, and confusion, apathy, disorientation, and neuritis develop.

Niacin Requirement

Influencing factors Factors such as age and growth periods, pregnancy and lactation, illness, tissue trauma, body size, and physical activity affect the niacin requirement.

RDA standard The RDA standard is 6.6 mg/1000 kcal and not less than 13 niacin equivalents at intakes of less than 2000 kcal. This is about 50 mg higher than minimum requirements to provide a safety margin to cover variances in individual need. These recommendations also allow for the contribution of tryptophan in terms of niacin equivalents from the dietary protein sources.

Food Sources of Niacin

Meat is a major source of niacin. Other good sources include peanuts, beans, and peas. Enrichment makes good sources of all the grains. Otherwise corn and rice are poor food sources of niacin, because they are low in tryptophan. Oats are also low in niacin. Fruits and vegetables generally are relatively poor sources.

Pyridoxine (B$_6$)
General Nature of Pyridoxine

Discovery Continuing work with B vitamins suggested that this group of vitamins contained a factor that cured a particular dermatitis in rats. The vitamin factor was finally synthesized and its chemical structure identified as that of a pyridine ring. Thus it was named *pyridoxine*. Later the substance was isolated in animal tissue, related products were synthesized, and other phosphate forms were identified.

Chemical and physical nature Vitamin B$_6$ is a generic term for a group of vitamins with a similar function. Three forms occur in nature—pyridoxine, pyridoxal, and pyridoxamine. In the body all three forms are equally active as precursors of the potent pyridoxine coenzyme pyridoxalphosphate (B$_6$-PO$_4$). Pyridoxine is water-soluble, heat-stable, but sensitive to light and alkalis.

Absorption and Storage

Pyridoxine is easily absorbed in the upper portion of the small intestine. It is found throughout the body tissues, evidence of its many essential metabolic activities.

Functions of Pyridoxine

Coenzyme in protein metabolism In its active phosphate form (B$_6$-PO$_4$), pyridoxine is a coenzyme in many types of reactions related to use of amino acids in the body:

1. **Neurotransmitters** Helps produce gamma-aminobutyric acid and serotonin, vital regulatory substances in brain activity.
2. **New amino acids and energy** Transfers nitrogen from amino acids to form new ones and releases carbon residues for energy.
3. **Sulfur transfer** Moves sulfur from an essential sulfur-containing amino acid (methionine) to form other sulfur carrier ones.
4. **Niacin** Controls formation of niacin from tryptophan.
5. **Hemoglobin** Incorporates amino acids into *heme,* the essential non-protein core of hemoglobin.
6. **Amino acid transport** Actively transports amino acids from the intestine into circulation and across cell walls into the cells.

Coenzyme in carbohydrate and fat metabolism The active phosphate coenzyme provides metabolites for energy-producing fuel. It also converts the essential fatty acid, linoleic acid, to another fatty acid, arachidonic acid.

Clinical problems It is evident from such an impressive list of metabolic activities—and these are only a few examples—that pyridoxine holds a key to a number of clinical problems.

1. **Anemia** A hypochromic type of anemia related to role of pyridoxine in heme formation, occurs even in the presence of a high serum iron level in some patients. A deficiency of pyridoxine has been demonstrated in these persons by a special test and the anemia is cured by supplying the deficient vitamin.
2. **Central nervous system problems** Through its role in the formation of the two regulatory compounds in brain activity, serotonin and gamma-aminobutyric acid, pyridoxine controls related neurologic conditions. In infants deprived of the vitamin, there is increased hyperirritability that progresses to convulsive seizures. For example, a classic object lesson occurred early in the 1950s when a group of infants, who had been fed a commercial milk formula in which most of the pyridoxine content had inadvertantly been destroyed by high-temperature autoclaving, subsequently had convulsions. A vitamin B_6–supplemented formula stopped the seizures.
3. **Physiologic demands in pregnancy** Pyridoxine deficiencies during pregnancy have been demonstrated by special tests and subsequently alleviated by supplementation. Fetal growth, in addition to creating greater maternal metabolic needs, increases the pyridoxine requirement.
4. **Oral contraceptive use** Women taking estrogen-progesterone oral contraceptives require additional vitamin B_6. An abnormal state of tryptophan metabolism contributes to the increased need.
5. **Tuberculosis** The drug Isoniazid (isonicotinic acid hydrazide—INH), used as a chemotherapeutic agent for tuberculosis, is an antagonist to pyridoxine. Also, it inhibits the conversion of glutamic acid, the only amino acid the brain metabolizes, and causes a side effect of neuritis. Treatment with large doses, 50 to 100 mg daily, of pyridoxine prevents this effect.

Pyridoxine Requirement

RDA standard A deficiency of pyridoxine is unlikely because the amounts present in the general diet are large relative to the requirement. Since pyridoxine is involved in amino acid metabolism, the need varies with dietary protein intake. For adults approximately 1 mg/day is minimal. The RDA standard is 2 mg/day to ensure a safety margin for variances in need.

Toxic effects Descriptions of pyridoxine abuse have been reported in which megadoses of 1 g or more a day were used. Several adult cases have resulted from megadoses up to 5 g a day.[6] The primary symptoms were caused by severe nerve damage.

Food Sources of Pyridoxine

Pyridoxine is widespread in foods, but many sources provide only very small amounts. Good sources include grains, seeds, liver and kidney, and other meats. There are limited amounts in milk, eggs, and vegetables.

Pantothenic Acid
General Nature of Pantothenic Acid

Pantothenic comes from a Greek word that means "in every corner" or "from all sides."

Discovery Pantothenic acid was isolated and synthesized between 1938 and 1940. Its presence in all forms of living things and the amount of it throughout body tissues accounts for its name. It is widespread in nature and in body functions. Intestinal bacteria synthesize considerable amounts of pantothenic acid. This source, together with its widespread natural occurrence, makes deficiencies unlikely.

Chemical and physical nature Pantothenic acid is a white crystaline compound, is readily absorbed in the intestine, and combines with phosphorus to form the active coenzyme, *coenzyme A*. There is no known toxicity or a natural deficiency state.

Functions of Pantothenic Acid

Basic coenzyme role In its role as an essential constituent of the body's key activating agent, coenzyme A, pantothenic acid is vital to many key metabolic reactions throughout the body.

Pantothenic Acid Requirement

Deficiency is unknown, so a quantitative requirement for pantothenic acid has not been established. The RDA's "estimated safe and adequate" range for adults is 4 to 6 mg. The daily intake of pantothenic acid in an average American diet of from 2500 to 3000 kcal is about 10 to 20 mg. Thus a deficiency is unlikely because of its widespread occurrence in food.

Food Sources of Pantothenic Acid

Sources of pantothenic acid are equally as widespread as its occurrence in body tissue. Rich sources include metabolically active tissue such as liver and kidney. Egg yolk and milk contribute more. Fair additional sources include other meat, cheese, legumes, and vegetables.

Biotin
General Nature of Biotin

The minute traces of biotin in the body perform multiple metabolic tasks. Its potency is great and natural deficiency is unknown, but some cases of induced deficiency have occurred in patients on long-term total parenteral nutrition (TPN). There is no known toxicity.

Functions of Biotin

Biotin serves as a partner with acetyl-CoA in reactions that transfer carbon dioxide from one compound and fix it onto another. Examples of this combination of cofactors at work include: (1) initial steps in synthesis of some fatty acids, (2) conversion reactions involved in synthesis of some amino acids, and (3) carbon dioxide fixation in forming purines.

Biotin Requirement

Since the amount needed for metabolism is so small, the human requirement for biotin has not been established in specific terms. The RDA adult estimate is 100 to 200 µg daily. Most of the body's requirement is supplied from intestinal bacteria synthesis.

Food Sources of Biotin

Biotin is widely distributed in natural foods, but its bioavailability is highly variable in different foods. For example, the biotin of corn and soy meals is completely available, whereas that of wheat is almost completely unavailable. Excellent food sources include egg yolk, liver, kidney, and other animal tissues, as well as tomatoes (among the vegetables) and yeast.

Folic Acid
General Nature of Folic Acid

Discovery The isolation and identification of folic acid are associated with laboratory studies of anemias and growth factors in animals. In 1945 folic acid was obtained from liver and finally synthesized. The vitamin was given the name *folic acid* from the Latin word *folium,* meaning "leaf," because a major source of its extraction was dark-green leafy vegetables such as spinach. A reduced form of folic acid has since been discovered—*folinic acid.*

Chemical and physical nature Folic acid forms yellow crystals and is a conjugated substance made up of three acids, one of which is para-aminobenzoic acid (PABA). PABA is sometimes touted in nutrition supplement claims as a separate essential factor in human nutrition. It is not. Its only role in human nutrition is that of a component of the vitamin, folic acid. Animal and human cells are not capable of synthesizing PABA nor of attaching it to the rest of the vitamin molecule. Only plants and certain bacteria can do this. Thus dietary folic acid, preformed by plants, is the necessary ingredient in human nutrition, and the major source of this folic acid is leafy vegetables.

Functions of Folic Acid

Basic coenzyme role Folic acid coenzyme is a necessary agent in the important task of attaching single carbon to compounds. Several key compounds are examples:

1. **Purines** Nitrogen-containing compounds essential to all living cells, involved in cell division and in the transmission of inherited traits.
2. **Thymine** Essential compound forming a key part of deoxyribonucleic acid (DNA), the important material in the cell nucleus that transmits genetic characteristics.
3. **Hemoglobin** *Heme,* the iron-containing nonprotein portion of hemoglobin.

Clinical problems Some clinical problems connected with folic acid are:

1. **Anemia** A nutritional **megaloblastic anemia** occurs in simple folic acid deficiency. Since tissue growth requires additional folic acid, this anemia is a special risk in pregnant women, growing infants, and young children.
2. **Sprue** Folic acid is an effective agent in the treatment of sprue, a gastrointestinal disease characterized by intestinal lesions, malabsorption defects, diarrhea, macrocytic anemia, and general malnutrition. It corrects both the blood-forming and the gastrointestinal defects of the disease.
3. **Chemotherapy** The drug methotrexate (amethopterin), currently used in cancer chemotherapy, acts as a folic acid antagonist to reduce tumor growth (see p. 542). The effect of this action is to prevent synthesis of DNA and purines in the cell.
4. **Growth and stress** Increased folic acid is required during periods of growth, especially during rapid fetal development.

Folic Acid Requirement

The average American diet contains about 0.6 mg of total folic acid activity. The adult RDA standard is 400 µg daily. This amount covers variances in need and the amount of available folic acid in foods. A supplement of 400 µg/day is recommended during pregnancy to meet increased fetal demands.

Food Sources of Folic Acid

Green leafy vegetables, liver, kidney, and asparagus are rich sources of folic acid. Relatively poorer sources are found in milk, poultry, and eggs.

Cobalamin (B$_{12}$)
General Nature of Cobalamin (B$_{12}$)

Discovery The discovery of vitamin B$_{12}$ is associated with the search for a specific agent responsible for the control of pernicious anemia. At first the disease was thought to be associated with a deficiency of folic acid. However, although folic acid helped in initial red blood cell regeneration in patients with pernicious anemia, it was not permanently effective and did not control the nerve problems associated with the disease. When folic acid was found to be lacking in full effectiveness, the search continued for the remaining piece in the disease puzzle.

Megaloblastic anemia
Anemia characterized by formation of large immature red blood cells that are deficient carriers of oxygen; caused by deficiency of folic acid and hence faulty synthesis of heme.

In 1948 two groups of workers, one in American and one in England, crystallized a red compound from liver, which they numbered vitamin B_{12}. In the same year it was clearly shown that this new vitamin could control both the blood-forming defect and the neurologic involvement in pernicious anemia. Soon afterward, a method was discovered for producing the vitamin through a process of bacterial fermentation, which remains the main source of commercial supply today. The vitamin was named *cobalamin* because of its unique structure with a single red atom of cobalt at its center.

Chemical and physical nature Cobalamin is a complex red crystalline compound of high molecular weight, with a single cobalt atom at its core. It occurs as a protein complex in foods, so its food sources are mostly of animal origin. The ultimate source, however, might be designated as the synthesizing bacteria in the gastrointestinal tract of herbivorous animals. Some synthesis is done by human intestinal bacteria.

Absorption, Transport, and Storage

Absorption Intestinal absorption of vitamin B_{12} takes place in the ileum. Cobalamin is split from its protein complex by the gastric hydrochloric acid and is then bound to a specific glycoprotein *intrinsic factor,* secreted by the gastric mucosal cells. This cobalamin–intrinsic factor complex moves into the intestine where it is absorbed by special receptors in the ileal mucosa.

Storage Vitamin B_{12} is stored in active body tissues. Organs holding the greatest amounts are the liver, kidney, heart, muscle, pancreas, testes, brain, blood, spleen, and bone marrow. These amounts are very minute, but the body holds them tenaciously and the stores are only slowly depleted. For example, a typical postgastrectomy anemia does not become apparent until 3 to 5 years after removal of the organ and subsequent loss of its secretions.

Functions of Cobalamin (B_{12})

Basic coenzyme role As an essential coenzyme factor, vitamin B_{12} is closely related to amino acid metabolism and the formation of the heme portion of hemoglobin. Its requirement increases as protein intake increases.

Clinical problems Special needs for vitamin B_{12} occur in several blood-forming related problems:
  1. **Pernicious anemia** In the absence of the intrinsic factor—a component of gastric secretion required for vitamin B_{12} absorption—**pernicious anemia** develops. Vitamin B_{12} is then not available for its role in heme formation, and adequate hemoglobin cannot be synthesized.

     Conversely, however, folic acid is not a primary agent for treating pernicious anemia. Although folic acid results in blood cell regeneration in patients with pernicious anemia, its effect is not permanent, nor does it control degenerative neurologic problems associated with the disease. This is the critical distinction between vitamin B_{12} and

Pernicious anemia Chronic, macrocytic anemia occurring most commonly in Caucasians after age 40. It is caused by the absence of the intrinsic factor normally present in gastric juice and necessary for the absorption of vitamin B_{12}. Pernicious anemia is controlled by intramuscular injections of vitamin B_{12}.

Table 7-3
Summary of B-Complex Vitamins

Vitamin	Coenzymes: Physiologic Function	Clinical Applications	Requirement	Food Sources
Thiamin (B_1)	Carbohydrate metabolism Thiamin pyrophosphate (TPP): oxidative decarboxylation	Beriberi (deficiency) Neuropathy Wernicke-Korsakoff syndrome (alcoholism) Depressed muscular and secretory symptoms	5 mg/1000 kcal	Pork, beef, liver, whole or enriched grains, legumes
Riboflavin (B_2)	General metabolism Flavin adenine dinucleotide (FAD) Flavin mononucleotide (FMN)	Cheilosis, glossitis, seborrheic dermatitis	6 mg/1000 kcal	Milk, liver, enriched cereals
Niacin (nicotinic acid, nicotinamide)	General metabolism Nicotinamide adenine dinucleotide (NAD) Nicotinamide adenine dinucleotide phosphate (NADP)	Pellagra (deficiency) Weakness, anorexia Scaly dermititis Neuritis	14-20 mg (NE)	Meat, peanuts, enriched grains (protein foods containing tryptophan)
Vitamin B_6 (pyridoxine, pyridoxal, pyridoxamine)	General metabolism Pyridoxal phosphate (PLP): transamination and decarboxylation	Reduced serum levels associated with pregnancy and use of oral contraceptives Antagonized by isoniazid, penicillamine, and other drugs	2 mg	Wheat, corn, meat, liver
Pantothenic acid	General metabolism CoA (coenzyme A): acetylation	Many roles through acyl transfer reactions, (for example, lipogenesis, amino acid activation, and formation of cholesterol, steroid hormones, heme)	2-7 mg	Liver, egg, milk
Biotin	General metabolism N-carboxybiotinyl lysine: CO_2 transfer reactions	Deficiency induced by avidin (a protein in raw egg white) and by antibiotics Synthesis of some fatty acids and amino acids	35-200 μg	Egg yolk, liver Synthesized by intestinal microorganisms
Folic acid (folacin)	General metabolism Single carbon transfer reactions (for example, purine nucleotide, thymine, heme synthesis)	Megaloblastic anemia	Infants: 30-45 μg Children: 100-400 μg Adults: 400 μg	Liver, green leafy vegetables
Cobalamin (B_{12})	General metabolism Methylcobalamin: methylation reactions (for example, synthesis of amino acids, heme)	Pernicious anemia induced by lack of intrinsic factor Megaloblastic anemia Methylmalonic aciduria Homocystinuria Peripheral neuropathy (strict vegetarian diet)		Liver, meat, milk, egg, cheese

folic acid in the diagnosis and treatment of this disorder. The American Medical Association and the Food and Drug Administration have, therefore, recommended that no more than 0.4 mg of folic acid be included in multivitamin preparations, as this would suffice for common needs and not mask the development of pernicious anemia or prevent its diagnosis.

A patient with defective cobalamin absorption, and hence pernicious anemia, can be given from 15 to 30 μg of vitamin B_{12} daily in intramuscular injections during a relapse and can be maintained afterward by an injection of about 30 μg every 30 days. This treatment controls both the blood-forming disorder and the degenerative effects on the nervous system.

2. **Megaloblastic anemia** Since cobalamin shares close metabolic interrelationships with folic acid, a megaloblastic anemia develops when either of the vitamins is deficient. Cobalamin indirectly affects blood formation by providing an activated reduced form of folate.

3. **Sprue** Like folic acid, vitamin B_{12} is effective in the treatment of the intestinal syndrome of sprue. However, it is most effective when used in conjunction with folic acid. Therefore its role is indirect activation of folic acid.

Cobalamin (B_{12}) Requirement

The amount of dietary vitamin B_{12} needed for normal human metabolism is very small. Reported minimum requirements have been from 0.6 to 1.2 μg/day, with a range upward to approximately 2.8 μg to allow adequately for individual variances. The ordinary diet easily provides this much and more. For example, one cup milk, one egg, and 4 oz of meat provide 2.4 μg. The RDA standard recommends a daily intake of 3 μg for adults. This amounts allows a margin of safety to cover variances in individual need, absorption, and body stores.

Food Sources of Cobalamin (B_{12})

Vitamin B_{12} is supplied by animal foods. The richest sources are liver and kidney, lean meat, milk, egg, and cheese. Natural dietary deficiency is rare. It has only been observed in some groups of strict vegetarians (see p. 102). The general symptoms of a deficiency include nervous disorders, sore mouth and tongue, amenorrhea, and neuritis.

A summary of the B vitamins is given in Table 7-3.

To Sum Up

A vitamin is an organic, noncalorigenic food substance that is required in small amounts for certain metabolic functions and which cannot be manufactured by the body. Vitamins may be fat- or water-soluble, and their solubility affects their absorption and mode of transportation to target tissues.

The fat-soluble vitamins are A, D, E, and K. Their metabolic tasks are mainly structural in nature, and their fate in the body is associated with lipids. The possibility of toxicity is enhanced for fat-soluble vitamins because of the body's ability to store them. Such toxicity is no longer rare, because of the current popularity of vitamin A supplements.

The water-soluble vitamins are the eight B-complex vitamins and vitamin C. These vitamins share three characteristics: (1) synthesis by plants (except vitamin B_{12}), and (3) functioning as a coenzyme factor (except vitamin C). Toxicity levels are usually not associated with water-soluble vitamins because excess is easily excreted in the urine. However, two vitamins have shown toxic effects when taken in megadoses (i.e., in gram amounts): vitamin B_6 (pyridoxine), which can result in severe nerve damage, and vitamin C, which has been associated with gastrointestinal disturbances, renal calculi formation, and lowered resistance to infection. All water-soluble vitamins, especially vitamin C, are easily oxidized, and care must be taken in food storage and preparation practices.

Questions for Review

1. List and describe health problems caused by a vitamin A deficiency. Give three possible causes of a deficiency.
2. Describe the function of the vitamin D endocrine system. Who would be at risk for developing a deficiency? Why?
3. What three characteristics are shared by most water-soluble vitamins? Identify one exception to each.
4. Which B vitamins play significant roles in blood formation? Describe their roles and interactions.

References

1. Deluca, H.F.: New developments in the vitamin D endocrine system, J. Am. Dietet. Assoc. **80**:231, 1982.

2. Bone loss and vitamin D hormone deficiency, Science News **120**(9):133, 1981.

3. Bieri, J.G., Corash, L., and Hubbard, V.S.: Medical uses of vitamin E, N. Engl. J. Med. **308**(18):1063, 1983.

4. Roe, D.A.: Nutritional concerns in the alcoholic, J. Am. Diet. Assoc. **78**(1):17, 1981.

5. Roe, D.A.: Ribo-loading, Health **16**(12):5, 1984.

6. Schaumburg, H., and others: Sensory neuropathy from pyridoxine abuse, N. Engl. J. Med. **309**(8):445, 1983.

7. Innis, S.M., and Allardyce, D.B.: Possible biotin deficiency in adults receiving long-term total parenteral nutrition, Am. J. Clin. Nutr. **37**:185, 1983.

Further Readings

Fat-Soluble Vitamins

Liebman, B., Too much of a good thing is toxic, Nutri. Action **10**(4):6, 1983.

A sound, interesting review of vitamin A toxicity with several case studies. Also reports FDA's futile attempt to withstand vitamin manufacturers' trade association suit against FDA efforts to limit over-the-counter vitamin A sales to products with less than 10,000 IU.

Parfitt, A.M., and others: Vitamin D and bone health in the elderly, Am. J. Clin. Nutr. **30**(5):1014, 1982.

Comprehensive review of this increasing clinical problem and exploration of the two preventive approaches of diet and skin exposure to sunlight.

Wolf, G.: Is dietary beta-carotene an anticancer agent? Nutr. Rev. **40**(9):257, 1982, and Dietary carotene and the risk of lung cancer, Nutr. Rev. **40**(9):265, 1982.

Two companion articles in this single journal issue review the research relating dietary beta-carotene to cancer prevention. Wolf gives a positive reply, based on current studies. The second report reviews similar work in relation to lung cancer but with a sound disclaimer that unwary readers should not take these generally positive results to mean that large consumptions of carrots will *necessarily* protect against cancer. Additional work is needed and underway.

Water-Soluble Vitamins

Rudman, D., and Williams, P.J.: Megadose vitamins: use and misuse, N. Engl. J. Med. **309**(8):488, 1983, and Schaumburg, H., and others: Sensory neuropathy from pyridoxine abuse, N. Engl. J. Med. **309**(8):445, 1983.

Two articles in this single journal issue are on vitamin abuse: one, an editorial by a physician and a clinical nutritionist (RD) on the popular abuse of vitamins in self-imposed megadoses explains the basis for the dangers involved. In the other article, Schaumburg presents case reports of seven adults with ataxia and severe sensory neurotoxity from daily pyridoxine megadoses ranging from 2 to 6 g. Four were severely disabled but all improved after withdrawal. Demonstrates the dangers of such abuses.

Shapiro, L.R., and others: Patterns of vitamin C intake from food and supplements: survey of an adult population in Alameda County, California, Am. J. Pub. Health **73**(7):773, 1983.

This survey of a random sample of 3119 adults investigated the use of vitamin C in food and pills and its association with health habits and health status. Older adults tended to take vitamin C pills daily and those in poorer health took more.

Issues and Answers

Guidelines for Vitamin Supplementation

Conservative health workers often flatly declare that no one needs vitamin supplements. Pill-pushing, self-proclaimed "nutrition experts" push megadoses of everything from A through Z to cure anything.

Who's right? Probably someone who suggests something between these two extremist views. The Recommended Dietary Allowances (RDA) standards are based on the average needs of a healthy population, not on individual needs that can vary widely. But extremists may take these two concepts too far. Extreme "traditionalists" try to apply these standards rigidly to every individual. "Pill-pushers" recommend megadoses of everything "to cover all the bases" and increase their profits.

Biochemical individuality is a very real concept. It cannot be overlooked when assessing an individual client's nutritional needs. Since it is influenced by health status, personal habits, age, and other factors, the assessment process should consider *at least* the following conditions:

Pregnancy and lactation The RDA takes into account increased nutrient requirements for these situations. Meeting increased needs by diet alone may be difficult because of food preferences and availability. Reasonable supplements then ensure an adequate intake to meet the increased nutrient demands.

Oral contraceptive use This practice lowers serum levels of several B vitamins, including B_6 and niacin, as well as vitamin C. If nutrient intake levels are marginal, some supplements may be necessary. But the client should be encouraged to improve her diet or assisted in obtaining nutritious foods.

Aging Older adults often have decreased food intake and impaired nutrient absorption, storage, or usage. Marginal deficiencies of ascorbic acid, thiamin, riboflavin, and B_6 have been seen in the elderly, even among individuals using supplements. Current RDA standards may be too low to meet their particular needs.

Restricted diets Eternal "dieters" may find it difficult to meet any of the nutrient standards, particularly if their meals provide less than 1200 kcal/day. Very strict diets are not recommended. Anyone on a weight reduction regimen should be carefully assessed.

Exercise Exercise increases the need for riboflavin. The combination of a reducing diet and exercise increases this need and may indicate supplement use, especially in women who do not tolerate milk (the major source of riboflavin).

Smoking This unhealthful addictive habit can reduce vitamin C levels by as much as 30%. If dietary intake is marginal, a small supplement (100 mg/day) may help compensate. Of course, kicking the habit will help even more.

Issues and Answers—cont'd

Alcohol Chronic or abusive use of alcohol impedes absorption and use of the B vitamins, especially thiamin, and even destroys folic acid. Supplements of multivitamins rich in B-complex vitamins will help. But alcohol reduction must accompany nutritional therapy to prevent recurrence of deficiency signs.

Caffeine In large quantities, caffeine will flush water-soluble vitamins out of the body faster than usual. Small supplements of B-complex vitamins and ascorbic acid may help. Reduced caffeine intake will help even more.

Disease Carefully assess patients with disease, malnutrition, debilitation, or hypermetabolic demands to determine the degree of overall nutrient supplementation and diet modification needed for clinical purposes. These needs are particularly evident in long-term illness.

Once all of these conditions are carefully evaluated, help your client with a wise nutrition program. In many situations supplementation can be avoided by a change in personal habits. Best of all, the general public will be better served. They will be able to maintain good health while avoiding "artificially-induced" deficiencies and expensive health food store bills.

References
Andresky, J.H.: The ABCs of vitamins, Consumers Digest **20**(5):46, 1981.
Belko, A.Z., and others: Effects of exercise on riboflavin requirements of young women, Am. J. Clin. Nutr. **35**:509, 1983.
Love, A.H.G.: Nutritional assessment in the elderly. In Assessing the Nutritional Status of the Elderly—State of the Art, Columbus, Ohio, July, 1982, Ross Laboratories.

Chapter 8
Minerals

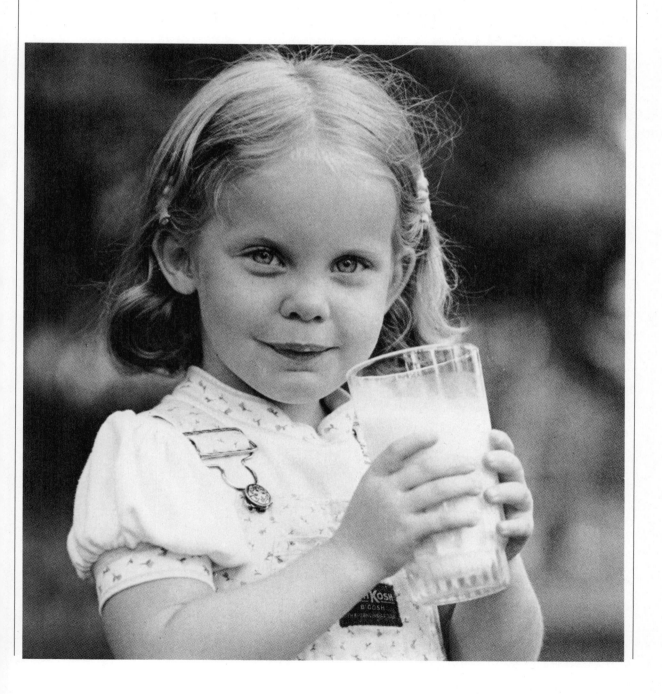

Preview

We live within an extended cycle of minerals essential to our existence. Over eons of time in our planet's development, shifting oceans and mountains have deposited an array of elements that move from rock to soil to plant to animals and humans. These minerals may seen simple in comparison to the complex, organic vitamin compounds. Nonetheless, they fulfill an impressive variety of metabolic functions.

Elements for which the human dietary requirement is greater than 100 mg/day are usually called *minerals*. Those needed in much smaller amounts are called *trace elements*.

Chapter Objectives

After study of this chapter, the student should be able to:

1. Identify the comparative amounts of the various body minerals and the forms in which they occur.

2. Describe the function of each mineral in the body and relate these functions to health and disease.

3. Compare the amount of each mineral we need and give some main food sources of each one.

4. Identify the role of minerals and other solutes in helping to maintain body water balance.

Minerals in Human Nutrition

Metabolic Roles
Variety of Functions

Minerals are inorganic elements widely distributed in nature. They have vital roles in metabolism that are as varied as are the minerals themselves. These substances, which appear so inert in comparison with the complex organic vitamin compounds, fulfill an impressive variety of metabolic functions: building, activating, regulating, transmitting, and controlling. For example, ionized sodium and potassium exercise all-important control over shifts in body water. Dynamic calcium and phosphorus provide structure for the framework of the body. Oxygen-hungry iron gives a core to heme in hemoglobin. Brilliant red cobalt is the atom at the core of vitamin B_{12}. Iodine is the necessary constituent of thyroid hormone, which in turn controls the overall rate of body metabolism. Far from being static and inert, minerals are active participants, helping to control many of the overall metabolic processes in the body.

Variety in Amount Needed

Minerals differ from vitamins also in that widely varying amounts are required in the body to perform their many functions, whereas vitamins occur in extremely small amounts in the body. For example, calcium forms a relatively large amount of body weight—about 2%. Most of this calcium is in skeletal tissue. An adult weighing 150 lbs has about 3 lbs of calcium in the body. On the other hand, iron is present in very small amounts. This same adult has only about 3 g (about $\frac{1}{10}$ oz) of iron in the body.

Classification

In your study here, you will find these important mineral elements grouped in three main sections. These commonly used divisions are based on two factors: (1) how much mineral is required by the body and (2) how essential it is for human life. On this basis, then, we will look in turn at the major minerals and trace elements.

Major Minerals

Seven minerals present in the body in large amounts are called the *major minerals*. These include: calcium, magnesium, sodium, potassium, phosphorus, sulfur, and chlorine.

Trace Elements

The remaining minerals are present in smaller amounts and are called *trace elements*. The essential nature of a large number of these trace elements has already been determined. However, for a few remaining ones, their need is as yet unclear.

In Table 8-1, as a study guide, you will find a listing of the minerals in each group.

Major Minerals

Calcium

Of all the minerals in the human body, calcium by far is present in the largest amount. The total amount of body calcium is in constant balance with food sources of calcium from outside as well as with tissue calcium

Table 8-1
Major Minerals and Trace
Elements in Human Nutrition

Major Minerals (required intake over 100 mg/day)	Trace Elements	
	Essential (required intake under 100 mg/day)	Essentiality Unclear
Calcium (Ca)	Iron (Fe)	Silicon (Si)
Phosphorus (P)	Iodine (I)	Vanadium (V)
Magnesium (Mg)	Zinc (Zn)	Nickel (Ni)
Sodium (Na)	Copper (Cu)	Tin (Sn)
Potassium (K)	Manganese (Mn)	Cadmium (Cd)
Chloride (Cl)	Chromium (Cr)	Arsenic (As)
Sulfur (S)	Cobalt (Co)	Aluminum (Al)
	Selenium (Se)	Boron (B)
	Molybdenum (Mo)	
	Fluorine (Fl)	

from within the body (among its various parts). A number of balance mechanisms are constantly at work to maintain these levels within normal ranges. The balance concept can be applied, therefore, at three basic levels: (1) the intake-absorption-output balance, (2) the bone-blood balance, and (3) the calcium-phosphorus blood serum balance.

Intake-Absorption-Output Balance

Calcium intake The average adult American diet contains about 700 to 1200 mg of calcium. Most of this comes from dairy products and some from green leafy vegetables and grains. However, all of the dietary intake of any given mineral is not necessarily available to the body. The term **bioavailability** refers to the degree to which the body uses a particular nutrient such as calcium in this case, which depends on many factors that may influence its absorption-excretion balance or its balance in body tissue.[1] This is one of the basic facts that makes the setting of precise requirements for minerals difficult. Stated requirements for many of these elements are given as estimated ranges of need rather than as precise figures.

Bioavailability Degree to which the amount of a nutrient ingested actually gets absorbed and is available to the body.

Absorption of calcium Only about 10% to 30% of the calcium in an average diet is absorbed. Most food calcium occurs in complexes with other dietary components. These complexes must be broken down and the calcium released in a soluble form before it can be absorbed. Absorption takes place in the small intestine, chiefly in the duodenum, where the pH is lower than in the distal portion of the intestine.

Factors increasing calcium absorption The following factors increase calcium absorption:
1. **Vitamin D** An optimum amount of this control agent is necessary for calcium absorption.
2. **Body need** During periods of greater body demand, such as growth or depletion states, more calcium is absorbed. Physiologic states in

Each of the following food items contributes about 300 mg of calcium:
1 cup milk
1 ounce cheese
1 cup dark greens (except spinach, chard, beet greens)
1 serving of oysters
1 serving of salmon (with bones)
2 servings of ice cream

the life cycle—growth, pregnancy and lactation, and old age—have a strong influence on the amount of absorption needed to meet body requirements.[2] In the elderly, in general, and postmenopausal women, in particular, there is a reduced ability to absorb calcium.

3. **Dietary protein and carbohydrate** A greater percentage of calcium is absorbed when the diet is high in protein. This larger amount absorbed results in increased renal excretion, with a negative calcium balance following.[3] Thus high protein diets induce increased calcium requirements to maintain calcium balance. Lactose enhances the absorption of calcium through the action of the lactobacilli which produce lactic acid that in turn lowers intestinal pH. Thus nature's packaging of both lactose and calcium in milk makes a fortunate combination.

4. **Acidity** Lower pH (increased acidity) favors solubility of calcium and consequently its absorption.

Factors decreasing calcium absorption The following factors decrease calcium absorption:

1. **Vitamin D deficiency** Vitamin D hormone, along with parathyroid hormone, is essential for calcium absorption.

2. **Dietary fat** Excess dietary fat or poor absorption of fats results in an excess of fat in the intestine. This fat inhibits calcium absorption through formation of insoluble calcium soaps. These insoluble soaps are excreted, with the consequent loss of the incorporated calcium.

3. **Fiber and other binding agents** An excess of fiber in the diet binds calcium and hinders its absorption. Other binding agents include oxalic acid, which combines with calcium to produce calcium oxalate, and phytic acid, which forms calcium phytate. Oxalic acid is a constituent of green leafy vegetables, but the amount of oxalate varies in these vegetables so that some are better sources of calcium than others. Phytic acid is found in the outer hull of many cereal grains, especially wheat.

4. **Alkalinity** Calcium is insoluble in an alkaline medium.

Calcium Output

The overall body calcium balance is maintained first, therefore, at the point of absorption. A large unabsorbed amount—some 70% to 90% varying according to body need—is excreted in the feces. A small amount of calcium may be excreted in the urine, about 200 mg daily. This urine excretion depends on the levels of calcium in the body fluid.

Bone-Blood Balance

Calcium in the bones In a healthy state the body maintains a constant turnover of the calcium in the bone tissue, which is the major cite of calcium storage. (Calcium in the bones and teeth is about 99% of that in the entire body.) However, this is not a static storage. Bone tissue is constantly being reshaped according to various body needs and stresses, with as much as 700 mg calcium entering and leaving the bones each day. All the while a dynamic equilibrium is maintained. In certain conditions or disease, the withdrawals may exceed the deposits, and a state of calcium imbalance occurs. Conditions such as immobility because of a body cast or diseases such as osteoporosis would cause such excess bone withdrawals.

Calcium in the blood The remaining small amount of calcium not in bone tissue (about 1% of the total) is circulating in the blood and body fluids. Although this is a relatively small amount, it plays a vital role in controlling body functions. This calcium in the blood occurs in two main forms:

1. **Bound calcium** About half the calcium in the blood is bound in the plasma proteins and hence is not free or diffusable, that is, able to move about or to enter into other activities.
2. **Free ionized calcium** Free particles of calcium, carrying electrical charges and hence in an active form, move freely about and diffuse through membranes to control a number of body functions, including blood clotting, transmission of nerve impulses, muscle contraction and relaxation, membrane permeability, and activation of enzymes. This is a good illustration of a small amount of a nutrient doing a great deal of metabolic work beause it is in an activated form.

Calcium-Phosphorus Serum Balance

Calcium-to-phosphorus (Ca:P) ratio Inverse ratio affecting the absorption rate of each mineral. The *dietary ratio* of 1:1 is ideal for periods of rapid growth; 1:1½ for normal adult functions.

A final level of calcium balance is that which calcium maintains with phosphorus in the blood serum. Amounts of these minerals in the blood serum are normally maintained in a definite relationship because of their relative solubility. This relationship is called the serum **calcium-to-phosphorus (Ca:P) ratio**. This ratio is the solubility product of calcium × phosphorus, expressed in milligrams of each mineral per deciliter (100 ml) of serum. This is an important ratio in the blood. Any situation that causes an increase in the phosphorus level would cause a resulting decrease in the calcium level. Such a condition of decreased calcium brings on signs of *tetany*.

Synergism is an important biologic concept. It is the cooperative action of two or more factors acting together to produce a total effect greater than the sum of their separate effects.

Control agents for calcium balance All of these vital levels of calcium balance in the body are carefully regulated by two main control agents working together: *parathyroid hormone (PH)* and *vitamin D hormone*. The cooperative action of these two factors is a good example of the **synergistic** behavior of metabolic controls. Consider the interdependent relationship of these agents:

1. **Parathyroid hormone** The parathyroid gland is particularly sensitive to changes in the circulating plasma level of free ionized calcium. When this level drops, the parathyroid gland releases its hormone, which acts in three ways to restore the normal calcium level: (1) it stimulates the intestinal mucosa to increase the absorption of calcium, (2) it withdraws more calcium rapidly from the **bone compartment**, and (3) it causes the kidney to excrete more phosphate. These combined activities then restore calcium and phosphorus to their correctly balanced ratio in the blood.

Bone compartment Body's total content of skeletal tissue. The bone compartment contains 99% of the body's total metabolic calcium pool.

2. **Vitamin D hormone** Vitamin D hormone in general controls the absorption of calcium. However it also affects the deposit of calcium and phosphorus in bone tissue. Thus these two agents balance each other, with vitamin D acting more to control calcium absorption and

bone deposit and parathyroid hormone acting more to control calcium withdrawal from bone and kidney excretion of its partner, phosphorus.

A third hormonal agent, **calcitonin**, is also involved in calcium balance. It is produced by special C cells in the thyroid gland. It prevents abnormal rises in serum calcium by decreasing the release of calcium from bone. Thus its action counterbalances the action of parathyroid hormone to regulate serum calcium at normal levels in balance with bone calcium.

The overall relationship of all of these various factors involved in calcium absorption and metabolism is illustrated in Figure 8-1.

Calcitonin Quick-acting hormone secreted by the parathyroids in response to hypercalcemia; it acts to induce hypocalcemia.

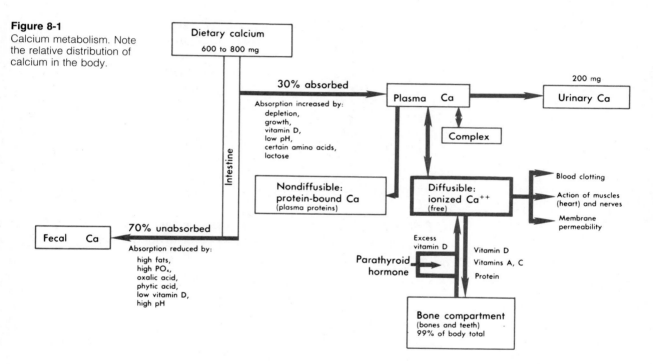

Figure 8-1
Calcium metabolism. Note the relative distribution of calcium in the body.

Physiologic Functions of Calcium

Bone formation The physiologic function of 99% of the calcium in the body is to build and maintain skeletal tissue. This is done by special cells that are in a constant balance between depositing and withdrawing bone calcium.

Tooth formation Special tooth-forming organs in the gums deposit calcium to form teeth. The mineral exchange continues as in bone. This exchange in dental tissue occurs mainly in the dentin and cementum. Very little deposit occurs in the enamel once the tooth is formed.

General metabolic functions The remaining 1% of the body's calcium performs a number of vital physiologic functions:

1. **Blood clotting** In blood clotting, calcium ions are required for cross-linking of fibrin, giving stability to the fibrin threads.

2. **Nerve transmission** Calcium is required for normal transmission of nerve impulses. A current of calcium ions triggers the flow of signals from one nerve cell to another and on to the waiting target muscles.[4]

3. **Muscle contraction and relaxation** Ionized serum calcium helps to initiate muscle contraction and control the relaxation following. This catalyzing action of calcium ions on the muscle protein filaments allows the sliding contraction between them to occur (p. 315) and is particularly vital in the contraction-relaxation cycle of the heart muscle.

4. **Cell membrane permeability** Ionized calcium controls the passage of fluid through the cell membranes by affecting cell wall permeability. It influences the integrity of the intercellular cement substance.

5. **Enzyme activation** Calcium ions are important activators of specific enzymes, especially one that releases energy for muscle contraction. They play a similar role with other enzymes, including lipase, which digests fat, and with some members of the protein-splitting enzyme system.

Clinical Problems

A number of clinical problems may develop from imbalances that interfere with the varied physiologic and metabolic functions of calcium.

Tetany A decrease in ionized serum calcium causes **tetany,** a state marked by severe, intermittent spastic contractions of the muscle and by muscular pain.

Tetany Disorder caused by abnormal calcium metabolism.

Rickets A deficiency of vitamin D hormone causes rickets. When inadequate calcium and phosphorus are absorbed, proper bone formation cannot take place.

Osteoporosis The usual form of **osteoporosis**, which is characterized by loss of bone mineral, occurs mainly in the aged, especially in postmenopausal women. The cause is not clear. In most patients it is not corrected by increased calcium alone but is often improved by exercise coupled with supplements. An idiopathic osteoporosis occurring in young adults does not respond to calcium therapy.

Osteoporosis Abnormal thinning of bone tissue caused by calcium loss.

Resorptive hypercalciuria and renal calculi When the usually fine-tuned calcium deposition–mobilization balance maintained by the controlling hormones is disturbed, resorption of calcium from bone and subsequent elevated calcium excretion in the urine occurs. A condition that causes this imbalance is prolonged immobilization such as occurs from a full body cast after orthopedic surgery or a spinal cord injury or a body brace following a back injury. In such cases, the normal muscle tension on the bones that is necessary for calcium balance is diminished, and the risk of renal stone formation is increased. By far the majority of kidney stones are composed of calcium. A second example is the hypercalciuria observed in astronauts on the Skylab and Apollo flights, a problem that may become a barrier to prolonged manned space flights in the future.[5]

Calcium Requirement

To meet these varied body functions of calcium, the RDA standard for adults is set at 800 mg daily, with increases to 1200 mg for women during pregnancy and lactation. The recommendation for infants younger than 1 year is 360 to 540 mg and for children is 800 to 1200 mg.

Calcium need in older adults There is growing evidence that the recommendation for adults in middle and later years is insufficient. There has been a general assumption in the past that the efficiency of calcium absorption would easily "adapt" to lower calcium intakes on the part of some adults and that the issue of optimal intake and availability was of little concern. Many clinicians and investigators no longer accept this assumption as tenable in the light of recent evidence that this adaptive mechanism is inadequate to support calcium balance and optimum bone mineralization at the levels of dietary calcium consumed by many individuals.[2] Current studies indicate that extra calcium increases bone density and that a daily calcium intake of 1500 mg is needed to help slow down bone loss in middle-aged and older adults.[6,7]

Food Sources of Calcium

Dairy products provide the bulk of dietary calcium. For example, 1 quart of milk and/or about 4 oz brick-type cheese contains about 1 g of calcium. Other nondairy sources, including eggs, green leafy vegetables, broccoli, legumes, nuts, and whole grains, contribute smaller amounts.

Phosphorus

Phosphorus makes up about 1% of total body weight. It is closely associated with calcium in human nutrition and has been called its "metabolic twin." However, it has some unique characteristics and functions of its own.

Absorption-Excretion Balance

Absorption The same factors that control calcium absorption also regulate phosphorus. Free phosphate is absorbed in the jejunum of the small intestine in relation to calcium and is also regulated by active vitamin D hormone (p. 112). Equal amounts of calcium and phosphorus should exist in the diet in an optimal ratio. Since phosphorus occurs in food as a phosphate compound, mainly with calcium, the first step for its absorption is its splitting off as the free mineral. Factors similar to those that influence calcium absorption also affect phosphorus absorption. For example, an excess of calcium or other binding material, such as aluminum or iron, inhibits phosphorus absorption.

Excretion The kidneys provide the main excretion route for regulation of the serum phosphorus level. Usually, 85% to 95% of plasma phosphate is filtered at the renal glomeruli and largely reabsorbed at the tubules, along with calcium, under the influence of vitamin D hormone. But when increased phosphate excretion is needed to maintain the normal Ca:P serum ratio, parathyroid hormone acts to override the effect of vitamin D hormone. The amount of phosphorus excreted in the urine of a person ingesting an average diet is from 0.6 to 1.8 g/day.

Bone-Blood-Cell Balance

Bone From 80% to 90% of the body's phosphorus is in the skeleton, including the teeth, compounded with calcium. This bone compartment of

Calcium supplements should be monitored carefully. The ground dolomite popular in health food circles has been found to contain lead, mercury, arsenic, and aluminum. Elevated concentrations of these metals have been found in the hair of neurologic patients who had been taking large amounts of dolomite.

In the typical feedback mechanism of hormone action, when the serum phosphate level is low, the kidney is stimulated to produce vitamin D hormone, which in turn increases phosphorus absorption from the intestine.

Renal threshold for phosphate means that the amount of phosphate excreted by the kidney is relative to the serum phosphorus level.

phosphorus is in constant interchange with the rest of the body's phosphorus, which is circulating in the blood and in the body fluids.

Blood The serum phosphorus level normally ranges from 3 to 4.5 mg/dl in adults and is somewhat higher, 4 to 7 mg/dl, in children. The higher range during growth years is a significant clue to its role in cell metabolism.

Cells In its active phosphate form phosphorus plays a major role in the structure and function of all living cells. Here it works with proteins, lipids, and carbohydrates to produce energy, build and repair tissues, and to act as a buffer.

Hormonal controls Since calcium and phosphorus work closely together, phosphorus balance is under the direct control of the same two hormones controlling calcium—vitamin D hormone and parathyroid hormone. A deficiency or depletion of phosphate occurs from a dietary lack, diminished absorption from the intestine, or excessive wasting through the kidney.

Physiologic Functions of Phosphorus

Bone and tooth formation From 80% to 90% of body phosphorus helps make bones and teeth. As a component of calcium phosphate, it is constantly being deposited and reabsorbed in the process of bone formation.

General metabolic activities Far out of proportion to the relatively small amount of the remaining substance, phosphorus is intimately involved in overall human metabolism in every living cell. It has several vital roles:

1. **Absorption of glucose and glycerol** Phosphorus combines with glucose and glycerol to assist their intestinal absorption. It also promotes renal tubular reabsorption of glucose to return this sugar to the blood.
2. **Transport of fatty acids** Phospholipids provide a form of fat transport.
3. **Energy metabolism** Phosphorus-containing compounds, for example, adenosine triphosphate (ATP), are key cell substances in energy metabolism (p. 315).
4. **Buffer system** The phosphate buffer system of phosphoric acid and phosphate helps control acid-base balance in the blood.

Physiologic changes Situations involving physiologic and clinical changes in serum phosphorus level include:

1. **Recovery from diabetic acidosis** Active carbohydrate absorption and metabolism uses much phosphorus, depositing it with glycogen, thus causing temporary hypophosphatemia.
2. **Growth** Growing children usually have higher serum phosphate levels, resulting from high levels of growth hormone.
3. **Hypophosphatemia** Low serum phosphorus levels occur in intestinal diseases such as sprue and celiac disease, which hinder phosphorus absorption; in bone disease such as rickets or osteomalacia, which upset the calcium/phosphorus serum ratio; and in primary hyperparathyroidism, in which the excess quantity of parathyroid hormone secreted causes in excess renal tubular excretion of phospho-

rus. Symptoms of hypophosphatemia include muscle weakness, because the muscle cells are deprived of phosphorus essential for energy metabolism.

4. **Hyperphosphatemia** Both renal insufficiency or hypoparathyroidism cause excess accumulation of serum phosphate. As a result, the calcium side of the calcium/phosphorus serum ratio is low, causing tetany.

Phosphorus Requirement

Dietary ratio During growth, pregnancy, and lactation, the ratio of dietary phosphorus-calcium should ideally be 1:1. In ordinary adult life the intake of phosphorus is about 1½ times that of calcium. In general, since these two minerals are found in the same food sources, if calcium needs are met, adequate phosphorus will be ensured.

RDA standard The RDA standard for phosphorus is the same as that of calcium for all ages (800 to 1200 mg) except for the young infant when it is lower—from birth to 6 months, 240 to 360 mg/day for calcium and from 6 months to 12 months, 360 to 540 mg/day for calcium.

Food Sources of Phosphorus

Milk and milk products are the most significant sources of phosphorus as they are for calcium. However, because phosphorus plays such a large role in cell metabolism, it is also found in lean meats. There is growing concern that we may be getting an excess of phosphorus in our diet because of its increasing use in the dairy industry and in processed foods, especially in soft drinks.[8-10]

Sodium

Sodium is one of the more plentiful minerals in the body. About 120 mg (4 oz) is in the body of an adult, with one third present in the skeleton as inorganic bound material. The remaining two thirds is free ionized sodium, the major electrolyte in body fluids outside cells.

Absorption-Excretion Balance

Absorption Sodium intake is readily absorbed from the intestine; normally only about 5% remains for elimination in the feces. Larger amounts are lost in abnormal states such as diarrhea.

Aldosterone Potent hormone secreted by the cortex of the adrenal glands, which acts on the distal renal tubule to cause reabsorption of sodium in an ion exchange with potassium.

Excretion The major route of excretion is through the kidney, under the powerful hormonal control of **aldosterone**, a sodium-conserving hormone from the adrenal gland (p. 172).

Physiologic Functions of Sodium

Osmosis Passage of a solvent such as water through a membrane that separates solutions of different concentrations. The water passes through the membrane from the area of lower concentration of solute to the area of higher concentration, which tends to equalize the concentrations of the two solutions.

Water balance Ionized sodium is the major guardian of body water outside of cells. Variations in its body fluid concentrations largely determine the distribution of water by **osmosis** from one body area to another.

Acid-base balance In association with chloride and bicarbonate ions, ionized sodium helps regulate the acid-base balance.

Cell permeability The sodium pump in cell membranes helps exchange sodium and potassium and other cellular materials. A major substance carried into cells by this active transport mechanism is glucose.

Muscle action Sodium ions play a large part in transmitting electrochemical impulses along nerve and muscle membranes and help maintain normal muscle action. Potassium and sodium ions balance the response of nerves to stimulation, the travel of nerve impulses to muscles, and the resulting contraction of the muscle fibers.

Sodium Requirement

RDA standard The body can function on a rather wide range of dietary sodium by mechanisms designed to conserve or excrete the mineral. Thus there is no specific stated requirement. The RDA standard estimates an adequate daily intake for adults of 1100 to 3300 mg.

General dietary intake Sodium in the average American diet usually far exceeds the RDA estimate of intake. About 4 g of sodium is in the average 10 g of table salt consumed daily. A wiser adult intake of about 2 g sodium would equal about 5 g salt.

Food Sources of Sodium

The main dietary source of sodium is common salt used in cooking and seasoning. Increased amounts of sodium compounds used in processed foods contribute still more. Natural food sources include milk, meat, egg, and certain vegetables such as carrots, beets, leafy greens, and celery.

Potassium

Potassium is about twice as plentiful as sodium in the body. An adult body contains about 270 mg (9 oz, 4000 mEq). By far the greater portion is found inside the cells, since potassium is the major guardian of the body water inside cells (p. 170). However, the relatively small amount in fluid outside cells has a significant effect on muscle activity, especially heart muscle.

Absorption-Excretion Balance

Absorption Dietary potassium is easily absorbed in the small intestine. Potassium also constantly circulates in the gastrointestinal secretions, being reabsorbed in the digestive process. However, diseases such as prolonged diarrhea cause dangerous losses.

Excretion Urinary excretion is the principal route of potassium loss. Since maintenance of serum potassium within the narrow normal range is vital to heart muscle action and is an indicator of electrolyte balance, the kidney guards potassium carefully. However, it cannot guard potassium as effectively as it can sodium. In the renal aldosterone mechanism for sodium conservation, potassium is lost in exchange for sodium (p. 172). The normal obligatory loss amounts to about 160 mg (40 mEq)/day.

Physiologic Functions of Potassium

Water and acid-base balance As the major guardian of cell water, potassium balances with sodium outside cells to maintain normal osmotic pres-

Continuous use of some *diuretic drugs* (though not all) increases potassium loss, requiring adequate replacement, primarily in food sources. Heart failure and subsequent depletion of ionized potassium in heart muscle make the myocardial tissue more sensitive to *digitalis toxicity* and *arrhythmia* or irregular contractions (p. 170). Recent studies indicate that inadequate intake of potassium contributes to the development of essential hypertension while a high potassium intake may lower blood pressure, probably because potassium antagonizes the biologic effects of sodium.

sures and water balance to protect cellular fluid. Potassium also works with sodium and hydrogen to maintain acid-base balance.

Muscle activity Potassium plays a significant role in the activity of skeletal and cardiac muscle. Together with sodium and calcium, potassium regulates neuromuscular stimulation, transmission of electrochemical impulses, and contraction of muscle fibers. This effect is particularly notable in the action of *heart muscle.* Even small variations in serum potassium concentration are reflected in electrocardiographic (ECG) changes. Variances in serum levels or low serum potassium may cause muscle irritability and paralysis; the heart may even develop a gallop rhythm and finally cardiac arrest.

Carbohydrate metabolism When blood glucose is converted to glycogen for storage, 0.36 mmol of potassium is stored for each 1 g of glycogen. When a patient in diabetic acidosis is treated by insulin and glucose, rapid glycogen production draws potassium from the serum. Serious hypokalemia can result unless adequate potassium replacement accompanies treatment.

Protein synthesis Potassium is required for the storage of nitrogen in muscle protein and general cell protein. When tissue is broken down, potassium is lost together with the nitrogen. Amino acid replacement therapy usually includes potassium to ensure nitrogen retention.

Decreased serum potassium of a dangerous degree may be caused by prolonged wasting disease with tissue destruction and malnutrition. This condition may also result from prolonged gastrointestinal loss of potassium such as occurs in diarrhea, vomiting, or gastric suction.

Potassium Requirement

No specific dietary requirement is given for potassium. The RDA standard estimates a safe daily intake for adults of 1875 to 5625 mg. The usual diet contains from 2000 to 4000 mg daily, which is ample for common need.

Food Sources of Potassium

Potassium is widely distributed in natural foods. Legumes, whole grains, fruits such as oranges and bananas, leafy vegetables, broccoli, potatoes, and meats supply considerable amounts. Many other foods are supplementary sources.

Other Major Minerals

Three additional minerals are assigned to the major minerals group because of the extent of their occurrence in the body. These are magnesium, chloride, and sulfur.

Magnesium Magnesium has widespread metabolic functions and is present in all body cells. An adult body contains about 25 g of magnesium or a little less than an ounce. About 70% of this small but vital amount is combined with calcium and phosphorus in the bone. The remaining 30% is distributed in various tissues and body fluids, where it has widespread metabolic use and is present in all body cells as a metabolic control agent. It acts as an enzyme activator for energy production and building tissue protein. It also aids in normal muscle action. The RDA standard is 350 mg/day for men and 300 mg for women. Magnesium is relatively widespread in nature. Its main sources are nuts, soybeans, cocoa, seafood, whole grains, dried beans, and peas.

Table 8-2
Summary of Major Minerals (required intake over 100 mg/day)

Mineral	Metabolism	Physiologic Functions	Clinical Applications	Requirement	Food Sources
Calcium (Ca)	Absorption according to body need; requires Ca-binding protein and regulated by vitamin D, parathyroid hormone, and calcitonin; absorption favored by protein, lactose, acidity Excretion chiefly in feces: 70%-90% of amount ingested Deposition-mobilization in bone tissue constant, regulated by vitamin D and parathyroid hormone	Constituent of bones and teeth Participates in blood clotting, nerve transmission, muscle action, cell membrane permeability, enzyme activation	Tetany (decrease in serum Ca) Rickets, osteomalacia Osteoporosis Resorptive hypercalcinuria, renal calculi Hyperthyroidism and hypothyroidism	Adults: 800 mg Pregnancy and lactation: 1200 mg Infants: 360-540 mg Children: 800-1200 mg	Milk, cheese Green, leafy vegetables Whole grains Egg yolk Legumes, nuts
Phosphorus (P)	Absorption with Ca aided by vitamin D and parathyroid hormone as above; hindered by binding agents Excretion chiefly by kidney according to serum level, regulated by parathyroid hormone Deposition-mobilization in bone compartment constant	Constituent of bones and teeth, ATP, phosphorylated intermediary metabolites Participates in absorption of glucose and glycerol, transport of fatty acids, energy metabolism, and buffer system	Growth Recovery from diabetic acidosis Hypophosphatemia: bone disease, malabsorption syndromes, primary hyperparathyroidism Hyperphosphatemia: renal insufficiency, hypothyroidism, tetany	Adults: 800 mg Pregnancy and lactation: 1200 mg Infants: 240-360 mg Children: 800-1200 mg	Milk, cheese Meat, egg yolk Whole grains Legumes, nuts
Magnesium (Mg)	Absorption according to intake load; hindered by excess fat, phosphate, calcium, protein Excretion regulated by kidney	Constituent of bones and teeth Coenzyme in general metabolism, smooth muscle action, neuromuscular irritability Cation in intracellular fluid	Low serum level following gastrointestinal losses Tremor, spasm in deficiency induced by malnutrition, alcoholism	Adults: 300-350 mg Pregnancy and lactation: 450 mg Infants: 50-70 mg Children: 150-400 mg	Milk, cheese Meat, seafood Whole grains Legumes, nuts

Table 8-2, cont'd
Summary of Major Minerals (required intake over 100 mg/day)

Mineral	Metabolism	Physiologic Functions	Clinical Applications	Requirement	Food Sources
Sodium (Na)	Readily absorbed Excretion chiefly by kidney, controlled by aldosterone	Major cation in extracellular fluid, water balance, acid-base balance Cell membrane permeability, absorption of glucose Normal muscle irritability	Losses in gastrointestinal disorders, diarrhea Fluid-electrolyte and acid-base balance problems Muscle action	Adults: 1100-3300 mg Infants: 115-350 mg Children: 325-2700 mg	Salt (NaCl) Sodium compounds in baking and processing Milk, cheese Meat, egg Carrots, beets, spinach, celery
Potassium (K)	Readily absorbed Secreted and reabsorbed in gastrointestinal circulation Excretion chiefly by kidney, regulated by aldosterone	Major cation in intracellular fluid, water balance, acid-base balance Normal muscle irritability Glycogen formation Protein synthesis	Losses in gastrointestinal disorders, diarrhea Fluid-electrolyte, acid-base balance problems Muscle action, especially heart action Losses in tissue catabolism Treatment of diabetic acidosis: rapid glycogen production reduces serum potassium level Losses with diuretic therapy	Adults: 1875-5625 mg Infants: 350-1275 mg Children: 550-4575 mg	Fruits Vegetables Legumes, nuts Whole grains Meat
Chlorine (Cl)	Readily absorbed Excretion controlled by kidney	Major anion in extracellular fluid, water balance, acid-base balance, chloride-bicarbonate shift Gastric hydrochloride—digestion	Losses in gastrointestinal disorders, vomiting, diarrhea, tube drainage Hypochloremic alkalosis	Adults: 1700-5100 mg Infants: 275-1200 mg Children: 500-4200 mg	Salt (NaCl)
Sulfur (S)	Elemental form absorbed as such; split from amino acid sources (methionine and cystine) in digestion and absorbed into portal circulation Excreted by kidney in relation to protein intake and tissue catabolism	Essential constituent of protein structure Enzyme activity and energy metabolism through free sulfhydryl group ($-SH$) Detoxification reactions	Cystine renal calculi Cystinuria	Diet adequate in protein contains adequate sulfur	Meat, egg Milk, cheese Legumes, nuts

Chlorine (chloride) Chloride accounts for about 3 % of the body's total mineral content, mainly as a part of fluids outside the cells where it helps control water and acid-base balances. Spinal fluid has the highest concentration of chloride. A relatively large amount of ionized chloride is found in the gastrointestinal secretions, especially as a component of gastric hydrochloric acid (HCl).

Sulfur Sulfur is present is all body cells, usually as a constituent of cell protein. Elemental sulfur occurs in sulfate compounds with sodium, potassium, and magnesium. Organic forms occur mainly with other protein compounds: (1) *sulfur-containing amino acids,* such as methionine and cystine, (2) *glycoproteins* in cartilage, tendon, and bone matrix, (3) *detoxification products* formed in part by bacterial activity in the intestine, (4) *other organic compounds* such as heparin, insulin, coenzyme A, lipoic acid, and the B vitamins thiamin and biotin, and (5) *keratin* in hair and skin.

The major minerals are summarized in Table 8-2.

Trace Elements

The Concept of Essentiality
The Study of Major Elements

Definition By the simplest definition, an essential element is one required for existence; conversely, its absence brings death. However, for things that occur in very small amounts in the body, this determination of essentiality is not easy to make. Of the 54 known chemical elements in the major part of the periodic table, 27 have been determined to be essential to our life and function.

Main components of living matter By far most living matter as we know it is made up of five fundamental elements: hydrogen (H), carbon (C), nitrogen (N), oxygen (O), and sulfur (S). We know these elements well because their concentrations are relatively large, hence more easily studied and the requirements can be stated for human function. The major minerals you have just reviewed here also occur in relatively large quantities in the body, so their essentiality has been more easily studied and determined.

The Study of Microelements

However, a much larger number of elements—microelements—occur in biologic matter in very small amounts, and we know little about them and understand even less. It it much harder to determine the essentiality of these trace elements because we require so little of them even though they exist in large amounts in our diet and environment.

Essential Function

Definition Despite these difficulties in determining the essentiality of these small amounts of trace elements in our bodies, studies have indicated that essentiality can be determined on the basis of function and effect of deficiency. In general, trace elements have been defined as those having a required intake of less than 100 mg/day.

Functions of trace elements An element is essential when a deficiency causes an impairment of function and supplementation with that substance but not with others prevents or cures this impairment. Studies in this field have identified the function of trace elements in terms of *catalytic* and *structural* components of larger molecules.

Deficiency and requirement Because these small amounts of trace elements are not easily measured, specific requirements have been stated only for the following: (1) iron (Fe) because it has a long history, (2) zinc (Zn) because it occurs in higher concentration than some of the others, and (3) iodine (I) because it has only a specific single known function. Thus far, the RDA standard only estimates requirements for the others in terms of a general range of need.

Essential Trace Elements: Definite and Probable

On the basis of current knowledge, these small trace elements may be placed in two groups: those that are definitely essential and those that are probably essential.

Definitely essential elements Ten trace elements have been assigned the role of essential elements in human nutrition based on defined function and need determined from research. This group includes iron (Fe), iodine (I), zinc (Zn), copper (Cu), manganese (Mn), chromium (Cr), cobalt (Co), selenium (Se), molybdenum (Mo), and fluorine (Fl).

Probably essential elements A remaining group of six and possibly eight trace elements are probably essential, but a more complete understanding of their marginal status awaits the development of better means of analysis and tests for function. These elements include silicon (Si), vanadium (V), nickel (Ni), tin (Sn), cadmium (Cd), arsenic (As), aluminum (Al), and boron (B).

We will look first at iron and iodine because of their long history and clearly defined specific function. Then in turn we will briefly review the remainder. These essential trace elements are summarized in Table 8-3.

Essential Trace Elements
Iron

Forms of iron in the body The human body contains only about 45 mg iron/kg body weight. This iron is distributed in the body in four forms that point to its basic metabolic function:

1. **Transport iron** A trace of iron, 0.05 to 0.018 mg/dl, is in plasma bound to its transport carrier protein, *transferrin*.
2. **Hemoglobin** Most of the body's iron, about 70%, is in red blood cells as a vital constituent of the heme portion of **hemoglobin**. Another 5% is a part of the muscle hemoglobin—*myoglobin*.
3. **Storage iron** About 20% of the body iron is stored as the protein-iron compound **ferritin**, mainly in liver, spleen, and bone marrow.
4. **Cellular tissue iron** The remaining 5% of body iron is distributed throughout all cells as a major component of oxidative enzyme systems for the production of energy.

Absorption-transport-storage-excretion balance In the body, iron follows a unique system of interrelated absorption-transport-storage-excretion. Optimal levels of body iron are not maintained by urinary excretion as is the case with most plasma constituents. Rather, the mechanisms of iron control lie in an absorption-transport-storage complex.

Hemoglobin Protein that gives the color to red blood cells. A conjugated protein composed of an iron-containing pigment called heme and a simple protein, globin. Carries oxygen in the blood; combines with oxygen to form oxyhemoglobin.

Ferritin Protein-iron compound in which iron is stored in the tissues; the storage form of iron in the body.

Table 8-3
Summary of Trace Elements (required intake less than 100 mg/day)

Element	Metabolism	Physiologic Functions	Clinical Applications	Requirement	Food Sources
Iron (Fe)	Absorption controls bioavailability; favored by body need, acidity, and reduction agents such as vitamins; hindered by binding agents, reduced gastric HCl, infection, gastrointestinal losses Transported as transferrin, stored as ferritin or hemosiderin Excreted in sloughed cells, bleeding	Hemoglobin synthesis, oxygen transport Cell oxidation, heme enzymes	Anemia: hypochromic, microcytic Excess: hemosiderosis, hemochromatosis Growth and pregnancy needs	Adults: men—10 mg, women—18 mg Pregnancy and lactation: 30-60 mg supplement Infants: 10-15 mg Children: 15-18 mg	Liver, meats, egg Whole grains Enriched breads and cereals Dark green vegetables Legumes, nuts (iron cookware)
Iodine (I)	Absorbed as iodides, taken up by thyroid gland under control of thyroid-stimulating hormone (TSH) Excretion by kidney	Synthesis of thyroxine, which regulates cell metabolism, BMR	Endemic colloid goiter, cretinism Hypothyroidism and hyperthyroidism	Adults: 150 μg Infants: 40-50 μg Children: 70-150 μg	Iodized salt Seafood
Zinc (Zn)	Absorbed with zinc-binding ligand (ZBL) from pancreas Transported in blood by albumin; stored in many sites Excretion largely intestinal	Essential coenzyme constituent: carbonic anhydrase, carboxypeptidase, lactic dehydrogenase	Growth: hypogonadism Sensory impairment: taste and smell Wound healing Malabsorption disease	Adults: 15 mg Infants: 3-5 mg Children: 10-15 mg	Widely distributed: Seafood, oysters Liver, meat Milk, cheese, egg Whole grains
Copper (Cu)	Absorbed with copper-binding protein metallothionein Transported in blood by histidine and albumin Stored in many tissues	Associated with iron in enzyme systems, hemoglobin synthesis Metalloprotein enzymes constituent	Hypocupremia: nephrosis and malabsorption Wilson's disease, excess copper storage	Adults: 2-3 mg Infants: 0.5-1.0 mg Children: 1-3 mg	Widely distributed: Liver, meat Seafood Whole grains Legumes, nuts (Copper cookware)

Table 8-3, cont'd
Summary of Trace Elements (required intake less than 100 mg/day)

Element	Metabolism	Physiologic Functions	Clinical Applications	Requirement	Food Sources
Manganese (Mn)	Absorbed poorly Excretion mainly by intestine	Enzyme component in general metabolism	Low serum levels in diabetes, protein-energy malnutrition Inhalation toxicity	Adults: 2.5-5.0 mg Infants: .05-1.0 mg Children: 1-5 mg	Cereals, whole grains Legumes, soybeans Leafy vegetables
Chromium (Cr)	Absorbed in association with zinc Excretion mainly by kidney	Associated with glucose metabolism; improves faulty glucose uptake by tissues; glucose tolerance factor	Potentiates action of insulin in persons with diabetes Lowers serum cholesterol, LDL-cholesterol Increases HDL	Adults: 0.05-0.2 mg Infants: 0.01-0.06 mg Children: 0.02-0.2 mg	Cereals Whole grains Brewer's yeast Animal proteins
Cobalt (Co)	Absorbed as component of food source, vitamin B_{12} Elemental form shares transport with iron Stored in liver	Constituent of vitamin B_{12}, functions with vitamin	Deficiency only associated with deficiency of B_{12}	Unknown; evidently minute	Vitamin B_{12} source
Selenium (Se)	Absorption depends on solubility of compound form Excreted mainly by kidney	Constituent of enzyme glutathione perioxidase Synergistic antioxidant with vitamin E Structural component of teeth	Marginal deficiency when soil content is low Deficiency secondary to parenteral nutrition (TPN), malnutrition Toxicity observed in livestock	Adults: 0.05-0.2 mg Infants: 0.01-0.04 mg Children: 0.02-0.2 mg	Varies with soil Seafood Legumes Whole grains Low-fat meats and dairy products Vegetables
Molybdenum (Mo)	Readily absorbed Excreted rapidly by kidney Small amount excreted in bile	Constituent of oxidase enzymes, xanthine oxidase	Deficiency unknown in humans	Adults: 0.15-0.5 mg Infants: 0.03-0.08 mg Children: 0.05-0.5 mg	Legumes Whole grains Milk Organ meats Leafy vegetables
Fluorine (Fl)	Absorption in small intestine; little known of bioavailability Excreted by kidney—80%	Accumulates in bones and teeth, increasing hardness	Dental caries inhibited Osteoporosis: may help control Excess: dental fluorosis	Adults: 1.5-4.0 mg Infants: 0.1-1.0 mg Children: 0.5-2.5 mg	Fish Fish products Tea Foods cooked in fluoridated water Drinking water

Table 8-4
Characteristics of Heme and
Nonheme Portions of
Dietary Iron

	Dietary Iron	
	Heme **Smallest Portion**	**Nonheme** **Largest Portion**
Food Sources	None in plant sources; 40% of iron in animal sources	All iron in plant sources; 60% of iron in animal sources
Absorption Rate	Rapid; transported and absorbed intact	Slow; tightly bound in organic molecules

Heme Iron-containing,
nonprotein portion of
hemoglobin.

Nonheme Protein portion of
hemoglobin that does not
contain the heme.

Apoferritin Protein base
found in intestinal mucosa
cells, which will bind with ion
(from food) to form ferritin,
the storage form of iron.

Absorption The main control of the body's iron balance is at the point of intestinal absorption. Dietary iron enters the body in two forms: **heme** and **nonheme** (Table 8-4). By far the larger portion is nonheme—all plant sources plus 60% of animal sources. But it is absorbed at a much slower rate than the smaller heme portion, a source of nutritional concern because of nonheme's greater quantity in the diet.[12] A protein receptor in the intestinal mucosal cells, **apoferritin**, receives iron to form ferritin. The amount of ferritin already present in the intestinal mucosa determines the amount of ingested iron that is absorbed or rejected. When all available apoferritin has been bound to iron to form ferritin, any additional iron that arrives at the binding site is rejected, returned to the lumen of the intestine, and passed on for excretion in the feces. In all, only 10% to 30% of the ingested iron is absorbed, mostly in the duodenum. The remaining 70% to 90% is eliminated in the feces.

Factors favoring absorption The following factors favor absorption:
1. **Body need** In deficiency states or in periods of extra demand as in growth or pregnancy, mucosal ferritin is lower and more iron is absorbed. When tissue reserves are ample or saturated, iron is rejected and excreted.
2. **Acidity and reduction agents** Vitamin C aids in absorption of iron by its reducing action and effect on acidity. Other agents have similar effects, as does the hydrochloric acid of the gastric secretions, which provides the optimal acid medium for the preparation of iron.
3. **Calcium** An adequate amount of calcium helps bind and remove agents such as phosphate and phytate, which if not removed would combine with iron and inhibit its absorption.

Factors hindering absorption The following factors hinder absorption:
1. **Binding agents** Materials such as phosphate, phytate, and oxalate bind iron and remove it from the body; tea and coffee inhibit nonheme iron absorption.
2. **Reduced gastric acid secretion** Surgical removal of stomach tissue (gastrectomy) reduces the number of cells that secrete hydrochloric acid, which provides the acid medium necessary for iron reduction.
3. **Infection** Severe infection hinders iron absorption.
4. **Gastrointestinal disease** Malabsorption or any disturbance that causes diarrhea will hinder iron absorption.

Transport In the mucosal cells of the duodenum and proximal jejunum, iron is oxidized and bound with the plasma *transferrin* for transport to the body cells. Normally, only about 20% to 35% of the iron-binding ca-

Figure 8-2
Summary of iron metabolism,
showing its absorption,
transport, main use in
hemoglobin formation, and its
storage forms (ferritin and
hemosiderin).

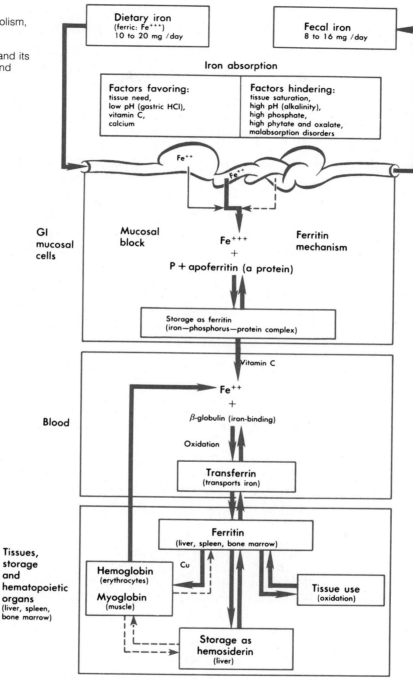

pacity of transferrin is filled. The remaining capacity forms an unsaturated plasma reserve for handling variances in iron intake.

Storage Bound to plasma transferrin, iron is delivered to its storage sites in the bone marrow and to some extent in the liver. Here it is transferred to the storage form, ferritin, and drawn on as needed for hemoglobin in red blood cells and for general tissue metabolism. A secondary, less soluble storage compound, **hemosiderin**, is used as a reserve storage in the liver; an excess storage causes the condition called **hemosiderosis.** From these storage compounds, iron is mobilized for hemoglobin synthesis as needed, from 20 to 25 mg/day in an adult. The body avidly conserves the iron in hemoglobin, recycling the iron when red cells are destroyed after their average life span of about 120 days. Study carefully these interrelationships of body iron as diagrammed in Figure 8-2.

Excretion Since the main mechanism controlling iron levels in the body occurs at the point of absorption, only minute amounts are lost by renal excretion. Essentially none is in the urine, as is usually the case with other circulating minerals. Rather, the small amounts of iron excreted normally come from the sloughing off of skin tissue, gastrointestinal cells, and normal gastrointestinal and menstrual blood loss. Unusual blood loss such as that from heavy menstrual flow, childbirth, surgery, acute or chronic hemorrhage, or gastrointestinal disease may bring severe iron loss.[12]

Physiologic functions of iron There are two main physiologic functions of iron:

1. **Oxygen transport** Iron is the core of the *heme* molecule, the fundamental nonprotein part of hemoglobin in the red blood cell. As such, iron functions as a major transporter of vital oxygen to the cells for respiration and metabolism.
2. **Cellular oxidation** Although iron exists in smaller amounts in cells, it also functions there as a vital component of enzyme systems for oxidation of glucose to produce energy.

Clinical needs Iron contributes to rapid growth and the prevention of anemia.

Normal life cycle During rapid growth, positive iron balance is imperative. At birth, the infant has about a 4 to 6 months supply of iron stored in the liver during fetal development. Breast-fed infants obtain some iron in breast milk. However, since cow's milk does not supply iron, it is added to commercial infant formulas, and supplementary iron-rich foods are added subsequently to the diet at about 4 to 6 months of age. Iron is also needed for continued growth and the building up of reserves for the physiologic stress of adolescence, especially the onset of menses in girls. The woman's need for iron is increased markedly during pregnancy, and normal blood loss during delivery reduces iron stores further.

Anemias Iron deficiency occurs in both developed and undeveloped countries for two main reasons: (1) the small dietary supply is not readily absorbed, and (2) it is not conserved by the kidney but is excreted through a number of avenues of potential loss. Iron deficiency results in a hypo-

Hemosiderin Insoluble iron oxide–protein compound in which iron is stored in the liver when the amount of iron in the blood exceeds the storage capacity of ferritin, e.g., during rapid destruction of red blood cells (malaria, hemolytic anemia).

Hemosiderosis Condition in which large amounts of hemosiderin are deposited, especially in the liver and spleen. Occurs with the excessive breakdown of red blood cells, as in malaria and hemolytic anemia, or after multiple blood transfusions.

Anemia Blood condition characterized by decrease in number of circulating red blood cells, hemoglobin, or both.

chromic microcytic **anemia**. This deficiency may occur from several causes:

1. **Nutritional anemia** or an inadequate dietary supply of iron.
2. **Hemorrhagic anemia** or excessive blood iron loss.
3. **Postgastrectomy anemia** or lack of gastric hydrochloric acid necessary to liberate iron for absorption.
4. **Malabsorption anemia** or the presence of iron-binding agents that prevent its absorption or mucosal lesions that affect the absorbing surface.

Iron requirement The RDA standard is 10 mg/day for men, and a larger amount—18 mg/day—for women during the childbearing years. This larger amount is needed to cover menstrual losses. During pregnancy, an added 30 to 60 mg supplement is required. Individual iron needs vary with age and situation, and growth allowances for infants and children are designed to provide margins for safety.

Food sources of iron By far the best sources of iron are organ meats, especially liver. Other food sources include meats, seafood, egg yolk, whole grains, legumes, green leafy vegetables, and nuts.

Iodine

The body of an average adult contains a small amount of iodine, from 20 to 50 mg. Approximately 50% of this is in the muscles, 20% in the thyroid gland, 10% in the skin, and 6% in the skeleton. The remaining 14% is scattered in other endocrine tissue, in the central nervous system, and in plasma transport. By far, however, the greatest iodine tissue concentration is in the thyroid gland, where its one function is to participate in the synthesis of the hormone *thyroxine* by the thyroid gland.

Absorption-excretion balance In the body, iodine balance is maintained by the following controls:

1. **Absorption** Dietary iodine is absorbed in the small intestine in the form of iodides. These are loosely bound with proteins and are carried by the blood to the thyroid gland. About one third of this iodide is selectively absorbed by the thyroid cells and removed from circulation.
2. **Excretion** The remaining two thirds of the iodide is usually excreted in the urine within 2 to 3 days after ingestion.
3. **Hormonal control** A pituitary hormone, **thyroid-stimulating hormone (TSH),** stimulates the uptake of iodine by the thyroid cells in direct feedback response to the plasma levels of the hormone. This normal physiologic **feedback mechanism** maintains a healthy balance between supply and demand.

Feedback mechanism Mechanism that regulates production and secretion by an endocrine gland (A_g) of its hormone (A_h), which stimulates another endocrine gland (T_g—the *target gland*) to produce its hormone (T_h). As sufficient T_h is produced, blood levels of T_h signal A_g to stop secreting A_h.

Physiologic function of iodine Iodine has the following physiologic functions:

Thyroid hormone synthesis Iodine participates in the synthesis of thyroid hormone as its only known function in human metabolism. The thyroid hormone, thyroxine, in turn stimulates cell oxidation and regulates basal metabolic rate, apparently by increasing oxygen uptake and reaction rates of enzyme systems handling glucose. In this role iodine indirectly exerts a tremendous influence on the body's overall total metabolism.

Plasma thyroxine The free thyroxine is secreted into the blood stream and bound to plasma protein for transport to body cells as needed. After being used to stimulate oxidation in the cell, the hormone is degraded in the liver and the iodine is excreted in bile as inorganic iodine.

Tests for iodine metabolism Three tests are commonly used:

1. **Protein-bound iodine (PBI)** This test measures the amount of iodine bound to thyroxine and in transit in the plasma. The normal range is from 4 to 8 mg/dl. Values below 4 indicate hypothyroidism and those above 8 indicate hyperthyroidism.
2. **Radioactive iodine uptake** Tests of thyroid gland function may be done through the use of **radioactive** ^{131}**I** uptake. This procedure measures the uptake and use of the tagged iodine by the thyroid gland.
3. **Thyroid function tests** The level of circulating thyroid hormone in the blood stream also indicates iodine metabolism. In the synthesis of the hormone, three prestages (T_1, T_2, and T_3) of iodine addition to the tyrosine base produce the final active hormone (T_4). Both T_3 and T_4 (thyroxine) have hormonal activity. T_3 has the greater activity and the free thyroxine index (FTI) is the product of the two.

Clinical needs Clinical needs provided for by iodine are:

Abnormal thyroid function Both hyperthyroidism and hypothyroidism affect the rate of iodine uptake and use and subsequently influence the body's overall metabolic rate.

Goiter Endemic colloid **goiter**, characterized by great enlargement of the thyroid gland, occurs in persons living where water and soil and, therefore, locally grown foods contain little iodine. When iodine is insufficient in the diet, the gland cannot produce a normal quantity of thyroxine, and the blood level of the hormone remains low. In response, the pituitary continues to put out TSH. These large quantities of TSH constantly stimulate the thyroid gland to produce the needed thyroxine, but without iodine it cannot. The only response that the iodine-starved gland can make is to increase the amount of colloid tissue of which it is composed, and the gland becomes increasingly engorged. It may attain a tremendous size, weighing 500 to 700 g (1 to 1½ lb) or more (Figure 8-3). Unusual "goiter zones" have also been reported in various parts of the world where, despite iodine supplementation, large numbers of persons have developed goiter as a result of contamination of the drinking water with goiter-producing chemicals such as resorcinol and phthalate esters.[13]

Iodine overload Current concern centers upon the relatively new problem of increased incidental intake of iodine by adults, infants, and children. Most of this excess comes through dairy products. These dairy sources include iodized salt licks for the animals and the use of iodine-containing chemicals to sanitize and disinfect udders, milking machines, and milk tanks. Other iodine-containing compounds are used as dough conditioners in breads, food coloring, and supplements for animal feeds.

Protein-bound iodine (PBI) The PBI test is used to measure thyroid activity by determining the amount of iodine bound to thyroxine and in transit in the plasma.

Radioactive ^{131}I tests Tests of thyroid function using a radioactive isotope of iodine, ^{131}I.

Goiter Enlargement of the thyroid gland caused by lack of sufficient available iodine to produce the thyroid hormone, thyroxine.

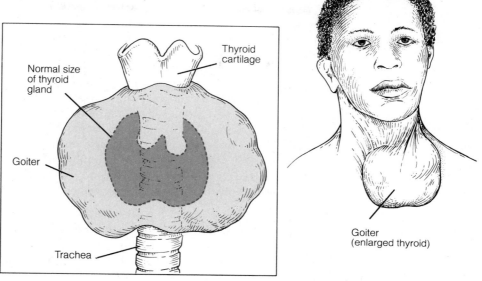

Figure 8-3
Goiter. The extreme enlargement shown here is a result of extended duration of iodine deficiency.

Excess iodine may result first in acnelike skin lesions or may worsen preexisting acne of adolescents or young adults.[14,15] Excessive amounts may also cause "iodine goiter," which could be misdiagnosed as goiter caused by insufficient iodine.

Iodine requirement The RDA standard is 140 µg/day for young men and 100 µg for young women. These needs normally increase during periods of accelerated growth such as adolescence and pregnancy and decrease in older adulthood.

Food sources of iodine Seafood provides a considerable amount of iodine. The quantity in natural sources varies widely depending on the iodine content of the soil and the iodine compounds used in food processing. The commercial iodizing of table salt (1 mg to every 10 g of salt) provides a main dietary source.

Other Essential Trace Elements

Zinc Recently, zinc has come to nutritional prominence as an essential trace element with wide clinical significance. However, much is still to be learned about the details of its metabolism. Its wide tissue distribution relfects its broad metabolic function as a component of key cell enzymes. It is distributed in many tissues including the pancreas, liver, kidney, lung, muscle, bone, eye (cornea, iris, retina, and lens), endocrine glands, prostate secretions, and spermatozoa. Because of its widespread metabolic use, a number of clinical problems are caused by zinc deficiency. Some examples of these conditions include:

1. **Hypogonadism** Diminished function of the gonads and dwarfism result from pronounced human zinc deficiency during growth periods.

2. **Taste and smell defects** Hypogeusia and hyposmia in a number of clinical situations are improved with zinc supplementation.
3. **Wound healing defects** Such defects occur in zinc-deficient persons, an effect common in the average hospital, where many patients can benefit from zinc supplementation.
4. **Chronic illness in aging** Older patients with poor appetites who subsist on marginal diets in the face of unhealed wounds and illness also need zinc supplementation.
5. **Malabsorption disease** Zinc deficiency can occur, especially with malabsorption diseases such as Crohn's disease.

As with iron, an optimal intake of zinc in the U.S. population cannot be assumed. The RDA adult standard is 15 mg/day with 10 mg for children and 3 to 5 mg for infants. The best sources of dietary zinc are seafood (especially oysters), meat, and eggs. Additional less rich sources are legumes and whole grains. Since animal food sources supply the major portion of dietary zinc, pure vegetarians, especially women, may be at risk for development of marginal zinc deficiency.

Copper This element has frequently been called the "iron twin." The two are metabolized in much the same way and share functions as cell enzyme components. Both are related to energy production and hemoglobin synthesis. The average American diet provides about 2 to 4 mg of copper each day, which is sufficient for adults. It is widely distributed in natural foods, so a general dietary deficiency is rare. Its main sources include meat, shellfish, nuts, seeds, legumes, and whole grains.

Manganese The total adult manganese body content is about 20 mg, occurring mainly in the liver, bone, pancreas, and pituitary. It functions like other trace elements as an essential part of cell enzymes that catalyze a number of important metabolic reactions. Manganese deficiency, manifested by low serum manganese levels, has been reported in diabetes and pancreatic insufficiency as well as in protein-calorie malnutrition states such as *kwashiorkor*. Toxicity occurs as an industrial disease syndrome, *inhalation toxicity*, in miners and other workers who undergo prolonged exposure to manganese dust. Excess manganese accumulates in the liver and central nervous system, producing severe neuromuscular symptoms that resemble those of Parkinson's disease. The RDA adult standard is 2.5 to 5.0 mg/day with 1.0 to 2.0 mg/kg for children. The best food sources of manganese are of plant origin: cereal grains, legumes, seeds, nuts, leafy vegetables, tea, and coffee. Animal foods are poor sources.

Chromium The precise amount of chromium present in body tissues is not well defined, because of difficulties in analysis. Although large geographic variations occur, the total body content is low, less than 6 mg. The highest concentrations have been found in skin, adrenal glands, brain, muscle, and fat. Serum levels are extremely low, less than 10 mg/ml. Chromium functions as an essential component of the organic complex **glucose tolerance factor (GTF)**, which stimulates the action of insulin. Insulin resistance manifested by impaired glucose tolerance has responded positively to chromium supplementation by restoring normal blood sugar. Also, significant reduction of elevated serum cholesterol has been observed in persons treated with chromium supplementation, with a lower-

Glucose tolerance factor (GTF) Chromium compound associated with glucose and lipid metabolism and insulin activity.

ing of LDL cholesterol and a simultaneous increase in the HDL cholesterol. The RDA standard estimates an adequate adult requirement for chromium at 50 to 200 µg/day. Brewer's yeast is a rich source of chromium. Most grain and cereal products contain significant quantities.

Cobalt Cobalt occurs in only minute traces in body tissues, and the main storage area is the liver. As an essential constituent of vitamin B_{12} (cobalamin), cobalt's only known function is associated with red blood cell formation. The normal cobalt blood level, representing the element in transit and in red blood cells, is about 1 µg/dl. Cobalt is provided in the human diet only by vitamin B_{12}. The human requirement is unknown but is evidently minute. For example, as little as 0.045 to 0.09 µg daily maintains bone marrow function in patients with pernicious anemia. Cobalt is widely distributed in nature. However, for our needs—as an essential component of vitamin B_{12}—cobalt is obtained in the preformed vitamin, which is synthesized in animals by intestinal bacteria.

Selenium Selenium is deposited in all body tissues except fat. Its highest concentrations in the body are found in liver, kidney, heart, and spleen. Selenium functions as an integral component of an antioxidant enzyme that protects cells and lipid membranes against oxidative damage. In this role, selenium balances with vitamin E, each sparing the other (p. 114). Selenium's protective function is widespread, since the enzyme is found in most body tissues. Selenium also acts as structural component. It is incorporated into the protein matrix of the teeth. The RDA standard estimates an adult intake of selenium at about 50 to 200 µg. Food sources vary with the selenium soil content. Usually good sources include seafood, legumes, whole grains, low-fat meats and dairy products, with additional amounts in vegetables.

Molybdenum The precise occurrence of molybdenum in human tissue and its clear role is still under investigation. The amount in animal tissue is exceedingly small, 0.1 to 3 parts per million (ppm), based on dry tissue weight. The largest amounts are deposited in the liver, kidney, bone, and skin. Malybdenum is required as a catalytic component of the metalloenzymes: xanthine oxidase, aldahyde oxidase, and sulfite oxidase. As such, it is essential for a number of metabolic reactions. The RDA standard estimates an adequate daily adult intake of molybdenum of 0.15 to 0.5 mg. Food sources include legumes, whole grains, milk, leafy vegetables, and organ meats.

Fluorine Fluorine accumulates in all tissue in the body showing calcification. It is found mostly in bones and teeth. In human nutrition fluoride functions mainly to inhibit *dental caries*. The principal cause of caries is acid dissolution of tooth enamel. This acid is produced by microorganisms feeding on fermentable carbohydrates, especially sucrose, adhering to the teeth after a meal or snack. Fluoride therapy enhances the ability of the tooth structure to withstand the erosive effect of the bacterial acid. Establishment of a fluoride requirement is difficult because it appears to be retained in the bones regardless of the level of intake. The RDA adult standard is 1.5 to 4.0 mg/day. Fish, fish products, and tea contain the highest concentration of fluorine. Cooking in fluoridated water raises the levels in many foods. Artificial *fluoridation* of water supply to 1 ppm provides adequate amounts. Total daily intakes, excluding water, generally range between 0.5 to 3.0 mg.

The clearly established role of fluorine in controlling dental caries is evident in the declining prevalence of caries as a public health problem.[16] Maximal benefits in tooth structure are achieved if the fluoride is present during tooth formation. Three factors have contributed to the decreased incidence of caries in young children: (1) the use of fluoridated tooth paste (0.1% fluoride), (2) fluoridation of public water supplies, and (3) improved dental hygiene habits. Less well defined, but promising, is fluoride's possible role in helping to control the development of *osteoporosis*, which is under study. It may provide protection from the bone mineralization that characterizes this condition. Osteoporosis has been reported to be less frequent in high-fluoride areas. However, treatment of patients with osteoporosis and other demineralizing diseases has brought inconsistent results.[17]

Probably Essential Trace Elements

The ten remaining trace minerals that have been found in human tissue and are currently under intense study are silicon, vanadium, nickel, tin, cadmium, arsenic, aluminum, and boron. Most of these have been found to be essential in animal nutrition and are probably essential in human nutrition as well, although their metabolism and function in humans is not yet defined. At this point, their practical roles in human health are unclear. If these elements are shown to be essential, they are needed in such minute amounts that primary dietary deficiency is highly unlikely. However, with increased use of long-term total parenteral nutrition (TPN) therapy, they may be of increasing clinical concern.

Water Balance

A number of the major minerals described previously have basic functions in controlling the body's vital water balance. Since this collective function is fundamental to health and often a vital part of patient care, we will briefly summarize the principles of this balance here. The main aspects of water balance involve three interdependent factors: (1) the water itself, (2) the particles in solution in the water, and (3) the separating membranes that control flow.

Water-Electrolyte Balance
Body Water Distribution

If you are a woman, your body is about 50% to 55% water. If you are a man, your body is about 55% to 60% water. The higher water content in most men is a result of their greater muscle mass. *Striated* muscle contains more water than any body tissue other than blood. The remaining 40% of a man's weight is about 18% protein and related substances, 15% fat, and 7% minerals. A woman's remaining body content is about the same, except for a somewhat similar muscle mass and a larger fat deposit.

Water functions Body water performs three functions essential to life: (1) it helps gives structure and form to the body through the turgor it provides for tissue, (2) it creates the water environment necessary for cell metabolism, and (3) it provides the means for maintaining a stable body temperature.

Figure 8-4
Body fluid compartments.
Note the relative total
quantities of water in the
intracellular compartment and
in the extracellular
compartment.

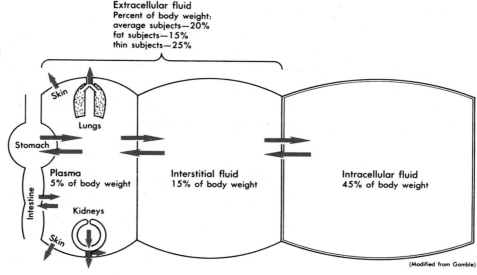

Extracellular fluid
Percent of body weight:
average subjects—20%
fat subjects—15%
thin subjects—25%

Skin

Lungs

Stomach

Plasma
5% of body weight

Interstitial fluid
15% of body weight

Intracellular fluid
45% of body weight

Intestine

Kidneys

Skin

(Modified from Gamble)

Compartment Collective
quantity of material in a given
type of tissue space in the
body.

Interstitial Refers to spaces
or interstices between the
essential parts of an organ
that comprise its tissue.

Water compartments Consider the water in your body in two **compartments,** as shown in Figure 8-4: (1) the total amount of water outside of cells or the *extracellular fluid compartment (ECF),* and (2) the total water inside cells or the *intracellular fluid compartment (ICF).*

1. **ECF** Water outside the cells makes up about 20% of the total body weight. It consists of four parts: (1) *blood plasma,* which accounts for approximately 25% of the ECF and 5% of body weight; (2) **interstitial** *fluid,* the water surrounding the cells; (3) *secretory fluid,* the water in transit; and (4) *dense tissue fluid,* water in dense connective tissue, cartilage, and bone.

2. **ICF** Water inside the cells makes up about 40% to 45% of the total body weight. Since the body cells handle our vast basic metabolic activity, it is no surprise that the total water inside the cells is about twice the amount outside the cells.

Overall Water Balance: Intake and Output

The average adult metabolizes from 2.5 to 3 L of water/day in a constant turnover balanced between intake and output. Normally water enters and leaves the body by various routes, controlled by basic mechanisms such as thirst and hormonal controls:

1. **Intake** Water enters the body in three main forms: (1) as preformed water and other liquids that are consumed, (2) as preformed water in foods that are eaten, and (3) as a product of cell oxidation.

2. **Output** Water leaves the body through the kidneys, the skin, the lungs, and the feces.

These routes of water intake and output must be in constant balance. This balance is summarized in Table 8-5. Abnormal conditions, such as diarrhea or dysentery, produce much greater losses, causing serious clinical problems if they continue.[18] Extensive loss of body fluids can be especially dangerous in infants and children. Their bodies contain a greater percentage of total body water, and much more of that water is outside of cells and thus easily available for loss.

Table 8-5
Approximate Daily Adult
Intake and Output of Water

	Intake (replacement) ml/day		Output (loss)	
			Obligatory (insensible) ml/day	Additional (according to need) ml/day
Preformed		Lungs	350	
Liquids	1200-1500	Skin		
In foods	700-1000	Diffusion	350	
Metabolism (oxidation of food)	200- 300	Sweat	100	±250
		Kidneys	900	±500
		Feces	150	
TOTAL	2100-2800	TOTAL	1850	750
	(approx. 2600 ml/day)		(approx. 2600 ml/day)	

Forces Influencing Water Distribution

Forces that influence and control the distribution of water in the body revolve around two factors: (1) the **solutes**, particles in solution in body water, and (2) the *separating membranes* between the water compartments.

Solute Dissolved substance; particles in solution.

Solutes A variety of particles with varying concentrations occur in the body. Two main types, electrolytes and plasma protein, control water balance:

Electrolyte Chemical element or compound, which in solution dissociates by releasing ions. The process of dissociating into ions is termed ionization.

Electrolytes Several minerals provide major electrolytes for the body. **Electrolytes** are small inorganic substances that are free in solution and carry an electrical charge. These free particles are called *ions*. They are atoms or elements (such as minerals) or groups of atoms that carry electrical charges, either positive or negative. An ion carrying a positive charge is called a *cation*: examples are sodium (Na^+)—major cation of water outside cells, potassium (K^+)—major cation of water inside cells, calcium (Ca^{++}), and magnesium (Mg^{++}). An ion carrying a negative charge is called an *anion*: examples are chloride (Cl^-), carbonate (HCO_3^-), phosphate (HPO_4^{--}), and sulfate (SO_4^{--}). Because of their small size, these ions or electrolytes can diffuse freely across body membranes. Thus they produce a major force controlling movement of water within the body.

Colloidal osmotic pressure (COP) Pressure produced by the protein molecules in the plasma and in the cell.

Plasma proteins Organic substances of large molecular size, mainly albumin and globulin of the plasma proteins, influence the shift of water from one compartment to another. They are called *colloids* (Gr. *kolla*, glue) and form *colloidal solutions*. Because of their large size, these particles or molecules do not readily pass through separating membranes. Therefore they normally remain in the blood vessels, where they exert **colloidal osmotic pressure (COP)** to maintain the integrity of the blood volume.

Organic compounds of small molecular size Other organic compounds of small size such as glucose, urea, and amino acids diffuse freely but do not influence shifts of water unless they occur in abnormally large concen-

Figure 8-5
Movement of molecules, water, and solutes by osmosis and diffusion.

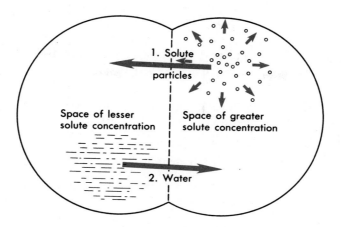

trations. For example, the large amount of glucose in the urine of a patient with uncontrolled diabetes causes an abnormal osmotic diuresis or excess water output.

Separating membranes Two basic types of membranes are involved in the movements of water and solutes within the body: (1) the capillary membrane and (2) the cell membrane. The capillary membrane is thin and porous, thus relatively "free," allowing rapid passage of substances. On the other hand, the cell membrane is a more complex, semipermeable (not as easily penetrated) structure. It is composed essentially of lipid material embedded with protein molecules. The metabolic processes within the cell usually govern the passage of electrolytes and, therefore, water across this barrier.

Mechanism Moving Water and Solutes Across Membranes

According to the type of membrane and the number of particles in the involved solution, water and solutes move across membranes by one or more of five mechanisms:

Osmosis Because of the pressure created by osmosis, water molecules move from a space of greater concentration of water molecules to a space of lesser concentration of water molecules. The effect of this movement is to distribute water molecules more evenly throughout the body and thus provide a solvent base for materials the water must carry.

Filtration Passage of a fluid through a semipermeable membrane (a membrane permeable to water and small solutes, but not to large molecules) as a result of a difference in pressures on the two sides of the membrane.

Active transport Movement of solutes in solution (for example, products of digestion such as glucose) across a membrane *against* the usual opposing forces.

Diffusion Diffusion is similar to osmosis but applies to the particles in solution in the water. It is the force by which these particles move outward in all directions from a space of greater concentration to a space of lesser concentration of particles. Compare the relative movements of water molecules and solute particles by osmosis and diffusion (Figure 8-5).

Filtration Water is forced or filtered through membranes when these is a difference in pressure on the two sides of the membrane. This difference in pressure is the result of differences in concentration of particles.

Active transport Particles in solution vital to body processes must move across membranes throughout the body even when the pressures are against their flow. Thus some means of energy-driven **active transport** is necessary to carry these particles across the separating membranes. Usually these active transport mechanisms require some kind of carrier partner to help them across.

Pinocytosis Sometimes larger particles such as proteins and fats enter cells by the interesting process of *pinocytosis*. The word means "cell drinking." Larger molecules are engulfed by the cell and carried into and across it as needed.

Controls of Water Balance
Influence of Electrolytes

Measurement of electrolytes The activity of a solution is determined by the concentration of electrolytes in a given volume of the solution. It is the *number* of particles in a solution that is the important factor in determining chemical combining power. Thus electrolytes are measured according to the total number of particles in solution, each one of which contributes chemical combining power according to its **valence,** rather than their total weight. The unit of measure commonly used is an *equivalent.* Since small amounts are usually in question, most physiologic measurements are expressed in terms of *milliequivalents.* The term refers to the *number* of ions—cations and anions—in solution, as determined by their concentration in a given volume. This measure is expressed as the number of *milliequivalents per liter (mEq/L).*

The relation of equivalents (Eg), milliequivalents (mEq), and milligrams of electrolytes can be determined in the following manner:

$$1 \text{ Eq} = \frac{1 \text{ mol of a substance}}{\text{valence of that substance}}$$

Sodium (Na⁺)

$$1 \text{ Eq Na}^+ = \frac{23 \text{ g (mol wt of sodium)}}{1 \text{ (valence of sodium)}} = 23 \text{ g}$$

$$1 \text{ mEq Na}^+ = 23 \text{ mg}$$

Calcium (Ca⁺⁺)

$$1 \text{ Eq Ca}^{++} = \frac{40 \text{ g (mol wt of calcium)}}{2 \text{ (valence of calcium)}} = 20 \text{ g}$$

$$1 \text{ mEq Ca}^{++} = 20 \text{ mg}$$

Electrolyte balance Electrolytes are distributed in the body water compartments in a definite pattern, which has great physiologic significance. This distribution pattern maintains stable *electrochemical neutrality* in body fluid solutions. According to biochemical and electrophysical laws, a stable solution must have equal numbers of positive and negative particles. In other words, the solution must be electrically neutral. When shifts and losses occur, compensating shifts and gains follow to maintain this essential *electroneutrality.*

Electrolyte control of body hydration As indicated, ionized sodium is the chief cation of ECF, and ionized potassium is the chief cation of ICF.

Valence Power of an element or a radical to combine with (or to replace) other elements or radicals. Atoms of various elements combine in definite proportions. The valence number of an element is the number of atoms of hydrogen with which one atom of the element can combine.

Clinical Application

Clinical Management of Edema

Tissue water imbalance—edema—is often considered a sign of an abnormal condition and not as a separate condition requiring evaluation itself. In some situations, as in normal pregnancy it is benign, simply a result of the woman's normal changed physiology (p. 548). In any situation it requires wise monitoring, but in clinical conditions it should receive special attention.

Edema can be a sign of congestive heart failure, pericardial effusion, or thrombophlebitis. It may also accompany anemia, hyperalbuminemia, malnutrition, blockage or damage to blood vessels or the lymphatic system, as is seen sometimes in patients with cancer. It may also lead to psychological depression or anxiety in patients, who are upset by yet another assault on their body image or who view the physical change as a sign of further deterioration in health. Thus failure to relieve **edema** may lead to a worsened condition because of psychological as well as physical factors.

Edema Large, abnormal amounts of fluid filling the intercellar tissue spaces; may be either localized or systemic.

Edema relief is achieved by one or more of three methods:

Nutritional Modifying fluid and nutrient intakes can affect some of the clinical conditions leading to pedal edema in cancer patients.

Positional Lying in the supine position redistributes fluids throughout the body, allowing venous return to increase.

Pharmacologic Using diuretics reduces the tissue fluid volume. Because of their potential side effects, however, these drugs are recommended as a last resort, to be used only when the other two methods prove ineffective.

Nutritional control of edema is achieved by monitoring:

- **Proteins** Such monitoring may help relieve hypoalbuminemia and cachexia. Adequate amounts of essential amino acids (p. 545) are required to increase plasma protein levels and reduce plasma oncotic pressure.
- **Sodium** This element must be monitored to reduce fluid retention. Mild sodium restriction (2 to 4 g/day) can be achieved by eliminating table salt, seasoned salts, salted foods, and salty processed foods.
- **Potassium** This element is monitored to achieve some "antisodium" effect on the body (p. 168). Potassium intake can be increased with a wide variety of fruits and vegetables (especially bananas and oranges) in the diet. Salt substitutes (KCl) providing 10 to 13 mEq/g may also be helpful in acute cases.
- **Fluids** Monitoring is needed to maintain a reasonable intake, especially in patients whose edema is caused by cardiac or renal problems. Extreme restrictions should be avoided, however, in ambulatory cancer patients whose fluid volume may be low because of low serum protein levels.

References
Maxwell, M.B.: Pedal edema in the cancer patient, Am. J. Nursing, **82**:1225, 1982.

These two electrolytes control the amount of water retained in any given compartment. The usual bases for these shifts in water from one compartment to another are ECF changes in concentration of these electrolytes. The terms *hypertonic dehydration* and *hypotonic dehydration* refer to the electrolyte concentration of the water *outside* the cell, which in turn causes a shift of water into or out of the cell.

Influence of Plasma Protein

Capillary fluid shift mechanism Water is constantly circulated throughout the body by the blood vessels. It must, however, get out of the blood vessels to service the tissues and then be drawn back into circulation to maintain the normal flow. Two opposing pressures—**colloidal osmotic pressure (COP)** from plasma protein (mainly albumin) and **hydrostatic pressure** (blood pressure) of the capillary blood flow—provide balanced control of water and solute movement across capillary membranes. The body maintains this constant flow of water and the materials it is carrying to and from the cell by means of a balance of these two main pressures. It is a filtration process operating according to differences in osmotic pressure on either side of the capillary wall.

When blood first enters the capillary system, blood pressure forces water and small solutes (glucose, for example) out into the tissues to bathe and nourish the cells. The plasma protein particles, however, are too large to go through the pores of capillary walls. Hence the protein remains in the vessel to exert the necessary pressure to draw the fluid back into circulation after it has bathed the cells. This process is called the **capillary fluid shift mechanism**. It provides one of the body's most important homeostatic mechanisms to maintain fluid balance.

Cell fluid control Much as plasma proteins provide colloidal osmotic pressure (COP) to maintain the integrity of extracellular fluid (ECF), cell protein helps to provide the osmotic pressure that maintains integrity of the fluid inside the cell. In addition to the osmotic pressure from the cell protein, there is the osmotic pressure provided by the intracellular ionized potassium. Balanced against the total intracellular pressure from these two forces is the osmotic pressure outside the cell, which is maintained by ionized sodium. As a result of the balance between the intracellular and extracellular osmotic pressures, water and nutrients flow in and water and metabolic products flow out through the cell membrane.

Hormonal Controls

ADH mechanism Antidiuretic hormone (ADH) (vasopressin) is secreted by the posterior lobe of the pituitary gland. Its major function is to cause reabsorption of water by the kidney according to body need. Thus it is a water-conserving mechanism. In any stress situation with threatened or real loss of body water, this hormone is triggered to conserve precious body water.

Aldosterone mechanism Aldosterone is primarily a sodium-conserving hormone, related in its operation to the renin-angiotensin system, but in doing this job it also exerts a secondary control over water loss. This mechanism is more precisely called the *renin-angiotensin-aldosterone mecha-*

Colloidal osmotic pressure (COP) Pressure produced by protein molecules in the plasma and in the cell.

Hydrostatic pressure Pressure exerted by a liquid on the surfaces of the walls that contain it. Such pressure is equal in the direction of all containing walls.

Capillary fluid shift mechanism Process that controls the movement of water and small molecules in solution (electrolytes, nutrients) between the blood in the capillaries and the surrounding interstitial area.

Antidiuretic hormone (ADH) or nasopressin Hormone secreted by the posterior pituitary gland in response to body stress. It acts on the renal tubules (chiefly the distal tubule) to cause reabsorption of water.

Angiotensin Pressor substance produced in the body by interaction of the enzyme, **renin,** produced by the renal cortex and a serum globulin fraction, angiotensinogen, produced by the liver.

nism because **renin** and **angiotensin** as intermediate substances are used to trigger the adrenal glands to produce the aldosterone hormone. Both ADH and aldosterone may be activated by stress situations such as body injury or surgery. However, they also compound problems of water balance in such disease conditions as congestive heart failure, when the failing heart muscle cannot maintain the normal amount of blood output.

To Sum Up

Minerals are inorganic substances that are widely distributed in nature. They build body tissues; activate, regulate, and control metabolic processes; and transmit neurologic messages.

Minerals are classified as (1) *major minerals,* required in relatively large quantities, which make up 60% to 80% of all the inorganic material in the body; and (2) *trace elements,* required in quantities as small as a microgram, which make up less than 1% of the body's inorganic material. Seven major and ten trace minerals are known to be essential, with others probably essential, and still others constantly being examined for potential essentiality.

Electrolyte Chemical compound, which in solution dissociates by releasing ions.

Overall water balance in the body is controlled by fluid intake and output. The distribution of body fluids is mainly controlled by two types of solutes: (1) electrolytes, charged mineral elements and other particles derived from inorganic compounds; and (2) *plasma protein,* mainly albumin, consisting of particles too large to pass through capillary membranes but capable of influencing the flow of fluid from one compartment to another. These solute particles influence the distribution of fluid passing across cell or capillary membranes, separating fluid into its two compartments.

Questions for Review

1. List the seven major minerals, describing physiologic function and problems created by dietary deficiency or excess.
2. List the ten trace elements with proven essentiality for humans. Which have established Recommended Dietary Allowances (RDA)? Which have "safe and adequate intake" limits established? Why is it difficult to establish RDA for everyone?
3. What accounts for the edema of starvation?
4. Why does potassium depletion occur in prolonged diarrhea?

References

1. Rosenberg, I.H., and Soloman, N.W.: Biological availability of minerals and trace elements: a nutritional overview, Am. J. Clin. Nutr. **35**:781, 1982.

2. Allen, L.H., and Lindsay, H.: Calcium bioavailability and absorption: a review, Am. J. Clin. Nutr. **35**:783, 1982.

3. Lutz, J., and Linkswiler, H.M.: Calcium metabolism in postmenopausal women consuming two levels of dietary protein, Am. J. Clin. Nutr. **34**(10):2178, 1981.

4. Llinas, R.R.: Calcium in synaptic transmission, Sci. Am. **247**(4):56, 1982.

5. Stewart, A.F., and others: Calcium homeostatis in immobilization: an example of resorptive hypercalciuria, N. Engl. J. Med. **306**(19):1136, 1982.

6. Marcus, R.: The relationship of dietary calcium to the maintenance of skeletal integrity in man—an interface of endocrinology and nutrition, Metabolism **31**(1):257, 1982.

7. Benzaia, D.: The calcium connection, Health **14**(2):20, 1982.

8. Greger, J.L., and Krystofiak, M.: Phosphorus intake of Americans, Food Tech. **36**:78, 1982.

9. Massey, L.K., and Strang, M.M.: Soft drink consumption, phosphorus intake, and osteoporosis, J. Am. Dietet. Assoc. **80**(6):581, 1982.

10. Zemel, M.B.: Phosphates and calcium, J. Am. Diet. Assc. **81**(5):606, 1982.

11. Mertz, W.: The essential trace elements, Science **213**:1332, 1981.

12. Monsen, E.R., and Balintfy, J.L.: Calculating dietary iron bioavailability: refinement and computerization, J. Am. Diet. Assc. **80**(4):307, 1982.

13. Garmon, L.: Zones of goiter: drinking water connection? Sci. News **123**(15):230, 1983.

14. Erdman, J.: Excess dietary iodine, Cereal Foods World **27**(9):417, 1982.

15. Monagan, D.: The iodine scare, Am. Health **1**(4):26, 1982.

16. Casey, C.E., and Hambidge, K.M.: Trace element deficiencies in man, Adv. Nutr. Res. **3**:23, 1980.

17. Levertt, D.H.: Fluorides and the changing prevalence of dental caries, Science **217**:26, 1982.

18. Hirschhorn, N.: Oral rehydration therapy for diarrhea in children—a basic primer, Nutr. Rev. **40**(4):97, 1982.

Further readings

Albanese, A.A., and Osborn, M.: Older women and health: The problem of brittle bones, The Professional Nutritionist **14**(2):11, 1982.

Heaney, R.P., et al.: Calcium nutrition and bone health in the elderly, Am. J. Clin. Nutr. **36**(5):986, 1982.

Spencer, H., Kramer, L., and Osis, D.: Factors contributing to calcium loss in aging, Am. J. Clin. Nutr. **36**(4):776, 1982.

   With the population of older adults increasing, the problem of bone loss with aging and associated health concerns such as osteoporosis are also increasing. These three articles explore the problem and related factors in our food and exercise patterns and the effects of aging on calcium balance.

Mertz, W.: Our most unique nutrients, Nutr. Today **18**(2):6, 1983.

   Very readable, well-illustrated article by a leading trace element researcher, which relates these important elements in human nutrition to our geologic environment.

Prasad, A.S.: Nutritional zinc today, Nutr. Today **16**(2):4, 1981.

   From his extended studies, including those in the Middle East, Prasad reviews clinical problems associated with zinc deficiency. Excellent illustrations.

Tanne, J.H.: Vital traces, Am. Health **2**(1):62, 1983.

   Reviews the ten essential elements and presents a good summary chart.

Issues and Answers

Guidelines for Trace Element Supplementation

Currently in the consumer marketplace, trace elements have become popular in both sales and discussions of supplementation. Are there any reasonable guidelines for supplementation based on reliable and current research?

Ten trace elements have generally been identified as essential for optimum health. These elements are chromium, cobalt, copper, fluorine, iodine, iron, manganese, molybdenum, selenium, and zinc. Nutritionists are concerned about toxicity, in terms of dietary and supplemental contributions leading to excess intake, as well as deficiency, in terms of eliminating factors interfering with bioavailability and evaluating the possible need for supplements.

The following list may serve as a basic guide for examining the need for supplementing the U.S. diet with trace minerals.

Iron is provided by organ meats, dried fruits, whole grains, fortified breakfast cereals, legumes, and dark green leafy vegetables. Men require 10 mg/day; women 18 mg. The need for supplements has long been established for pregnant and breast-feeding women, who require *daily supplements of 30 to 60 mg*. Other high-risk groups may also need to supplement their diets: adolescent girls, low-income adolescent boys, athletes, and elderly Blacks. Before recommending a supplement to these individuals, however, you should evaluate their intake of iron antagonists such as fiber and caffeine.

Iodine is provided by foods grown in iodine-rich soil, seafood, and iodized salt. Daily requirements are 75 to 150 µg/day, although the average intake is several times that amount because of the widespread use of iodine-containing compounds in the dairy and baking industries. Since greater levels can result in thyrotoxicosis, *supplementation is not recommended*.

Zinc is supplied by oysters, whole grains, legumes, nuts, and meats. The recommended intake is 15 mg/day. Pregnancy and lactation increase the need by 5 and 10 mg, respectively, to avoid deficiency signs of slow growth, impaired taste and smell, poor wound healing, and skin problems. Others at risk include alcoholics and individuals on long-term, low-calorie diets. It takes 3 to 24 weeks for symptoms to appear, but *supplementation relieves deficiency symptoms* in a matter of days. To avoid an overdose, characterized by gastrointestinal upset, nausea, and bleeding, check the client's eating habits for zinc antagonists, for example, an excessive intake of fiber or iron.

Copper is widely available in liver, oysters, shellfish, nuts, whole grains, and legumes. The average diet was previously believed to provide 2 to 5 mg/day, easily meeting the minimum RDA recommendation of 2 to 3 mg/day. Intake levels are now believed to range from less than 1 mg to no more than 2 mg/day, based on new analysis methods, thus placing a larger segment of the population at risk for developing a mild deficiency. Before recommending

Continued.

Issues and Answers—cont'd

supplementation, however, examine factors that reduce copper bioavailability, such as a low protein intake, or high levels of zinc, cadmium, fiber, or ascorbic acid.

Chromium is provided by brewer's yeast, animal products, and whole grains. Daily requirements have been estimated between 50 to 200 μg. Deficiency signs include resistance to insulin and other signs of diabetes. Supplementation not only reduces insulin resistance but also increases HDL cholesterol, thereby offering some protection against coronary heart disease. While reliable diagnostic tests have not been developed yet, it is estimated that current intakes fall below recommended levels. However, because it has only shown effectiveness in small, controlled studies, *supplementation recommendations have not been made yet for any population groups.*

Selenium is provided for by fish, whole wheat, and plants grown in selenium-rich soil. Intakes of 50 to 200 μg/day are considered safe after the age of 7, with the average diet providing 50 to 150 μg/day. Selenium is believed to offer protection against breast cancer. One group of researchers believes that "optimal cancer protection" is provided at levels of 150 to 300 μg/day, although the connection between blood levels and cancer patients and cancer-free individuals has not been established. In addition to cancer, selenium is believed to protect against heart disease, arthritis, heavy metal poisoning, sexual dysfunction, and aging. As there is no current evidence of selenium deficiency in the general population, *supplementation is not recommended.*

Manganese is provided by whole grains, green vegetables, and dried beans. Safe intakes are estimated in the range of 2.5 to 5.0 mg/day. Deficiency signs in humans have not been reported, but signs of toxicity have. These signs include weakness and psychologic problems. Toxicity is associated mainly with industrial exposure. However, the possibility of an excess suggests that *supplementation is not recommended.*

Silicon requirements for humans are not known, nor are reliable food sources. Deficiency has been associated with poor bone growth in chicks and statistically correlated with cardiovascular disease in humans. However, *the need for supplementation has not been established.*

Nickel is provided by legumes, cocoa, wheat, shellfish, milk, meats, and a variety of vegetables and fresh fruits. Requirements are estimated at about 75 μg/day, though U.S. intakes have been estimated between 300 to 600 μg/day. In light of this excessive intake, plus the existence of at least one sign of toxicity, a nickel-sensitive dermatitis, *supplementation is not recommended.*

Vanadium requirements are unknown, as are reliable food sources. However, it is estimated that the average American diet provides 1 to 2 mg/day. Some individuals are apparently sensitive to this amount,

Issues and Answers—cont'd

exhibiting severe depression. They improve when given megadoses of vitamin C, which blocks vanadium activity. *The need for supplementation is not indicated* because of its potential for toxicity in at least this one sensitive population group.

References

Ehn, L., Carlmark, B., and Hoglund, S.: Iron status in athletes involved in intense physical activity, Med. Sci. Sports Exerc. **12**(1):61, 1980.

Lamberg, L.: Zinc deficiency: when skin sends signals, Am. Health **1**(4):26, 1982.

Lynch, S.R., and others: Iron status of elderly Americans, Am. J. Clin. Nutr. **36**(5):1032, 1982.

Mertz, W.: The essential trace elements, Science **213:**1332, 1982.

Nickerson, H.J., and Tripp, A.D.: Iron deficiency in adolescent cross-country runners, Phys. Sports Med. **11**(6):60, 1983.

Sandstead, H.H.: Copper bioavailability and requirements, Am. J. Clin. Nutr. **35:**809, 1982.

Shultz, T.D., and Leklem, J.E.: Selenium status of vegetarians, nonvegetarians, and hormone-dependent cancer patients, Am. J. Clin. Nutr. **37:**114, 1983.

Solomons, N.W., and others: Bioavailability of nickel in men: effects of foods and chemically-defined dietary constituents on the absorption of inorganic nickel, J. Nutr. **112:**39, 1982.

Report: Vanadium, vitamin C, and depression, Nutr. Rev. **40**(10):293, 1982.

Part Two
Community Nutrition: The Life Cycle

Chapter 9
The Food Environment and Food Habits

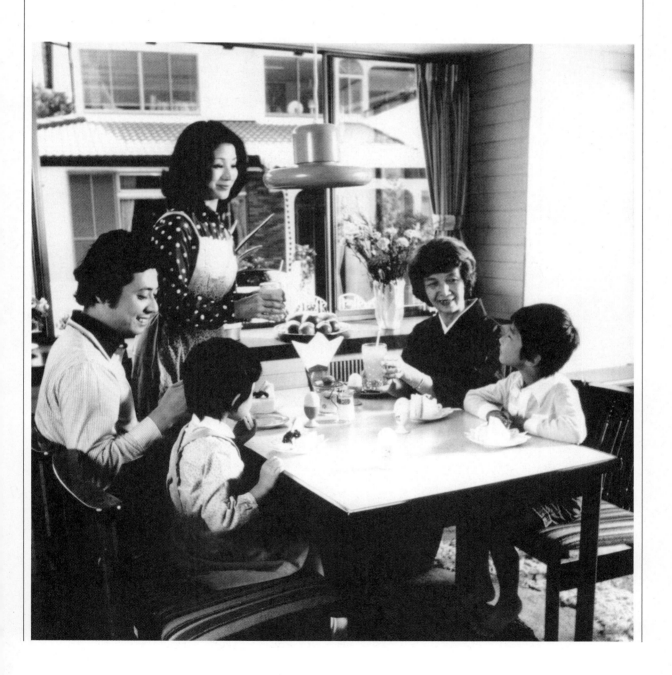

Preview

We live in a rapidly changing environment. As a result, health care is changing in method, in setting, and in the needs of the people it seeks to serve. Also changing is the nature of health workers providing the care. It is inevitable in the face of such change that the real needs of people must be learned and met, if good health care is to be provided. Nutrition is basic to such health care.

In the first part of your study, you have reviewed some basic principles of the science of human nutrition. But these can only come alive in terms of *personal need*. Knowledge alone is not enough to meet these health care needs. Human compassion and concern are necessary, as well as practical guides and skills, for you to apply knowledge in a useful and helpful manner. The chapters in this section of your study will provide a background on which you can build as you help to fulfill some of these human needs in your own clinical and community practice.

Chapter Objectives

After study of this chapter, the student should be able to:

1. Identify personal and environmental forces that determine food choices and nutritional status.

2. Relate social, psychologic, and cultural factors to the development of personal food habits.

3. Examine personal food beliefs and habits of clients and patients in helping them plan nutritional food patterns.

4. Identify ways our food safety and quality is protected.

5. Describe changing food pattern trends in the United States today and account for their development.

The Ecology of Human Nutrition

Ecology Relations between organisms and their environment.

Malnutrition Faulty nutrition resulting from poor diet, malassimilation, or overeating.

Epidemiology Branch of medicine dealing with the study of various factors that determine the frequency and distribution of disease in given populations.

The Food Environment and Malnutrition

Out of necessity, our food habits and patterns are inevitably linked to our environment. As a result, our rapidly changing human environment, with its problems of environmental imbalance such as pollution and malnutrition, sometimes threatens health. The word **ecology** comes from a Greek word meaning "house." Just as many factors and forces within a family interact to influence the members, so even greater forces in our physical environment and social system interact to produce disease.

The public health significance of **malnutrition**, local to worldwide in scope, continues to grow. Observation and experience have brought deepened awareness of two important interrelated facts: (1) having adequate food *alone* is not the complete answer, although it fulfills a fundamental need for all persons, and (2) a national high standard of living does not necessarily eliminate the problem of malnutrition. Even in the midst of plenty here in America, malnutrition exists. It is found among vulnerable groups such as hospitalized elderly persons and among persons suffering from alcoholism. It is associated with poverty on the one hand and our distorted obsession with thinness on the other. Human misery and human waste of life from malnutrition, more stark in some regions of our country and the world than in others, occurs nonetheless in both world hemispheres. The extent of this human suffering is impossible to quantify.

At its fundamental biologic level, malnutrition results from an inadequate supply of nutrients to the cell. However, this lack of essential nutrients at the cell level is by no means a simple problem. It is caused by a complex web of factors: psychologic, personal, social, cultural, economic, political, and educational.[1] Each of these factors is more or less important at a given time and place for a given individual. If these factors are only temporarily adverse, the malnutrition may be short term, alleviated rapidly, and will cause no long-standing results or harm to life. But if they continue unrelieved, malnutrition becomes chronic. Irreparable harm to life follows and eventually death ensues. For the **epidemiologist** a triad of variables influences disease: (1) agent, (2) host, and (3) environment. These three factors may be used to describe malnutrition.

Agent

The fundamental agent or factor in malnutrition is *lack of food*. Because of this lack, certain nutrients in food that are essential to maintaining cell activity are missing. As indicated, many factors may interact to cause or modify this lack of food: inadequate quantity and quality of food, insufficient amounts for children during critical growth periods, loss of supply through famine or poverty or maldistribution, or unwise choices made from foods available.

Host

The host is the person—infant, child, or adult—who suffers from malnutrition. Various personal characteristics may influence the disease: presence of other diseases, increased need for food during times of growth, pregnancy, or heavy labor, congenital defects or prematurity, and personal factors such as emotional problems and poverty.

Figure 9-1
Multiple etiology of
malnutrition.
Modified from Williams, C.D.:
Lancet **2**:342, 1962.

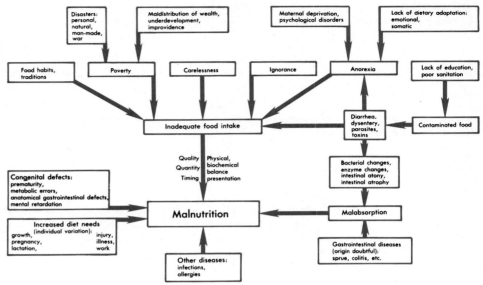

Environment

Many environmental factors influence malnutrition. These include sanitation, culture, social problems, economic and political structure, and agriculture. The interaction of some of these factors leading to malnutrition is shown in Figure 9-1.

Economic and Political Environment

In any society, at both governmental levels and personal levels, food availability and use involves both money and politics. It is plainly evident that money is a basic necessity for getting an adequate food supply. Sometimes, however, the role of politics and government structure and policies are not always as evident. Nonetheless, both are always intertwined in securing human nutrition.

Government Food and Agriculture Programs

In any country, food and agricultural programs at any level of government influence food availability and distribution. A number of factors may be involved, such as land management practices and erosion, water distribution and its consequent pollution from long-term use of questionable pesticides, food production and distribution policies, and food assistance programs for individual persons in need (see pp. 229-230).

Problem of Poverty

We are all made increasingly aware through the daily news that malnutrition, even famine and death, exists in countries such as India, parts of Africa, and the mid-Eastern nations.[2] Closer home, peoples of Central and South America are hard-pressed by social conditions such as revolution, inequity, and desperate poverty. But hunger does not stop at our border. Here, in the United States, the wealthiest country on earth, many studies document widespread hunger and malnutrition among the poor. For example, in a study of 1000 households of extremely low-income Black fam-

The national infant mortality rate for Blacks is about 22/1000 live births. For whites the rate is about 11.5/1000.

ilies in a Mississippi county, half the families showed an annual income of less than $1000.[3] There was a correspondingly high level of malnutrition. Black infants in the United States still have twice the chance of dying in their first year than white infants do.

Tremendous problems exist among the poor and at times they seem almost insurmountable. Often a "culture of poverty" develops and is reinforced and perpetuated by a society's values and attitudes, which wall off such persons more completely than do physical barriers. As a result of extreme pressures caused by living conditions, poverty-stricken persons become victims of negative attitudes and characteristics that influence their use of community health services:

Isolation Strong feelings of alienation are common among the poor. In many communities few if any channels of communication are open between the lowest income groups and the rest of society. In most instances a poor person responds to such feelings of alienation by further withdrawal. Each person feels isolated and alone and concludes that no one is really concerned. Hazards to health are inherent in poor housing and poor nutrition and are often compounded by distance from the sources of health care.

Powerlessness It is ironic that often those persons most exposed to risks and emergencies have the fewest coping resources. Extreme frustration is inevitable and persons become overwhelmed. Why try, they conclude, if they have no control over the situation? Why plan, if there is no future different from today? In such a day-to-day struggle to exist, the poor person often sees little value in long-range preventive health measures.

Insecurity Subjected to forces outside their control, poor individuals and families have little or no security. Insecurity and anxiety often incapacitate them. In such a setting, where hunger may be a constant companion, food—which has for poor people the same deep psychologic and emotional meaning that it has for all people—assumes even greater meaning than it has for persons who rarely know hunger.

Role of the Health Worker

How can a concerned health worker help individuals and families conditioned by years of poverty or crushed by new poverty? In the face of such overpowering feelings of isolation, helplessness, and insecurity, what attitudes are necessary to help them? What methods and approaches are most likely to reach clients and patients and supply their needs? Some basic principles can be helpful:

Self-awareness First, we must explore our own feelings about the poor. We must be aware of our own class values and attitudes. If we are to be agents of constructive change, true "helping vehicles," we must first have some understanding of the person's situation and its broad social setting. We must also understand ourselves better and our own cultural conditioning and biases.

Genuine *rapport* between persons is born of mutual respect and trust.

Rapport Genuine warmth, interest, friendliness, and kindness grow from within. **Rapport** is that feeling of relationship between persons that is born of mutual respect, regard, and trust. This sense of relationship gives both helper and helped a deep feeling of working *together*. Its most basic ingredient is a concern for people and for persons—a positive orientation toward human beings in general and a love and concern for individuals in particular.

Acceptance This term is another way of stating the principle that one must begin where the client or patient is. Each person's own concerns should be the primary consideration. Often we work with other team specialists to cut through the maze of factors involved in a given situation before the client or patient is ready to accept or even consider the health practice or the diet counsel that is needed or desired. Much time may have to be spent, for example, in coming to understand the meaning of food to this person, before practical dietary matters can begin to be explored.

Listening Here, more than elsewhere, the art of listening—positive, active, creative listening—is vital. Clients must tell their story in their own way, with no interruption by distracting statements or questions and no deflecting of the conversation to another's problems. This listening must also be observant. Sequence of statements, subjects introduced, areas of intense feeling, and areas ignored give clues to needs. Throughout we must proceed with sensitivity and create a relaxed, nonthreatening atmosphere, in which persons feel free to talk—*and we must listen*. The reason that some frustrated persons finally take their problems to the streets may well be that *no one listens to them unless they do*.

Worldwide Factors

The world's affluent countries consume 70% of the world's grain. But only about 7% of that amount is consumed directly as human fare in the form of grains or flour. Most of it is used to feed livestock, and a sizeable portion is used to make alcoholic beverages.

On a broader level, international problems of population increase and export-import policies compound problems of malnutrition for two reasons: (1) the world population is rising at an alarming rate—a matter of great concern; (2) as to who feeds whom, it is a common conception that the rich world feeds the poor world. But this is not always the case. In fact, our grain exports go predominantly to other industrialized nations.[4] Only one fifth of the exports go to developing nations. Developed countries export nearly four times as much food to other developed countries as they do to the developing world. Less developed countries also export three times as much to the industrialized countries as they do to other less developed nations.

Development of Food Habits

In addition to these factors of poverty and politics, other aspects of our lives influence our food patterns. Food habits, like other forms of human behavior, do not develop in a vacuum. They result from many personal, cultural, social, and psychologic influences. For each of us these factors are interwoven to develop a whole individual. To study these influences on food habits, we will look at each one of them separately.

Cultural influences
Strength of Personal Culture

Culture System of customs, habits, and values developed over time by a people, usually resulting from adaptation to environment, interpretation of life experiences, and religious beliefs.

Often the most significant thing about a society's **culture** is what it takes for granted in daily life. Culture involves not only the more obvious and historical aspects of a person's communal life—that is, language, religion, politics, technology, and so on—but also all the little habits of everyday living, such as preparing and serving food and caring for children, feeding them, and lulling them to sleep. These facets of a person's culture are *learned* gradually as a child grows up in a given society. Through a slow process of conscious and unconscious learning, we take on our culture's values, attitudes, habits, and practices through the influence of our parents, teachers, and others. Whatever is invented, transmitted, and perpetuated—socially acquired knowledge and habits—we learn as part of our culture. These elements become internalized and entrenched.

Food in a Culture

Food habits are among the oldest and most deeply rooted aspects of many cultures and exert deep influence on the behavior of the people. The cultural or subcultural background determines what shall be eaten as well as when and how it shall be eaten. There is, of course, considerable variation. But rational or irrational, beneficial and injurious customs are found in every part of the world. Nevertheless food habits are primarily based on food availability, economics, and personal food meanings and beliefs. Included among these influential factors are the geography of the land, the agriculture practiced by the people, their economic and marketing practices, their view about healthy or safe food, and their history and traditions. Within every culture there are certain foods that are deeply infused with symbolic meaning. These symbolic foods are related to major life experiences from birth through death, religion, politics, and general social organization. From early times ceremonies and religious rites have surrounded certain events and seasons. Food gathering, preparing, and serving has followed specific customs and commemorated special events of religious significance. Many of these customs remain today.

Some Traditional Cultural Food Patterns

A number of different cultural food patterns are represented in American community life. Many have contributed characteristic dishes or modes of cooking to American eating habits, and, in turn, many food habits of subcultures have been Americanized. Traditional foods tend to be used more consistently by the older members of the family, whereas younger members may use such foods only on special occasions or holidays. Nevertheless, these traditional food patterns have strong meanings and serve to bind families and cultural communities in close fellowship. A few representative cultural food patterns are discussed here. However, among persons of different cultures, individual tastes and geographic patterns vary. Economic factors cause wide differences, as does educational level. For various food patterns the type of food may be unique with special dishes and methods of preparation. These special food patterns are representative of certain ethnic or regional groups and make use of foods that are easily available. Other food patterns develop in relation to religious beliefs or festivals. Whatever the origin, such food practices are usually deeply ingrained in the lives of the people and require respect.

Jewish Food Patterns

Jewish dietary food laws are different for the three basic groups within Judaism: (1) Orthodox—strict observance, (2) Conservative—nominal observance, and (3) Reform—less ceremonial emphasis and minimum observance of the general dietary laws.

The Jewish body of dietary laws is called the *Rules of Kashruth* and foods selected and prepared accordingly are called *kosher* foods. The basis of these laws is primarily self-purification and a means of service to God, although they probably also had some hygienic or ethical foundation in the beginning. Most of these rules relate to ordinances given the ancient Hebrews, as recorded in the Old Testament books of the Law (Leviticus and Deuteronomy), and to the Jewish traditions accumulated over the centuries. These traditions were collected and interpreted in the Talmud, a body of laws set down in the fourth to the sixth centuries BC. Since the original Hebrew religion was centered in practices of animal sacrifice and the blood had special ritual significance, the present Jewish dietary laws apply specifically to the slaughter, preparation, and service of meat, to the combining of meat and milk, to fish, and to eggs.

Food restrictions Food restrictions include:
1. **Meat** Only meat from cloven-hoofed quadrupeds that chew a cud (cattle, sheep, goats, and deer) is used, and only the forequarters of these animals is allowed. The hindquarters may be eaten only if the sinew of Jacob (hind sinew of the thigh) is removed (Leviticus 11:1-8). Chickens, turkeys, geese, pheasants, and ducks may also be eaten (Leviticus 11:13-19).
2. **Blood** Ritual slaughter follows rigid rules based on minimum pain to the animal and maximum blood drainage and involves several steps. The meat is water soaked in a special vessel, then rinsed, and thoroughly salted with coarse salt. It is placed on a perforated board and left to stand for an hour. After draining thoroughly, it is washed three times before being cooked. No blood may be eaten as food in any form. Blood is considered synonymous with life (Genesis 9:4; Leviticus 3:17).
3. **Meat and milk** No combining of meat and milk is allowed (Exodus 23:19). Milk or food made from milk, such as cheese and ice cream, may be eaten just before a meal, but not for 6 hours after eating a meal that contains meat. In the Orthodox Jewish household, the custom is to maintain two sets of dishes, one for serving meat and the other for serving dairy meals.
4. **Fish** Only those fish with fins and scales are allowed. No shellfish or eels may be eaten (Leviticus 11:9-12). Fish of the type permitted may be eaten with either dairy or meat meals.
5. **Eggs** No egg that contains a blood spot may be eaten. Eggs may be taken with either dairy or meat meals.

Foods for special occasions Many of the traditional Jewish foods are related to festivals of the Jewish calendar. These holidays commemorate events in Jewish history (Table 9-1). Often special Sabbath dishes are used. In Orthodox Jewish homes, no food is prepared on the Sabbath, which begins at sundown on Friday and ends when the first star becomes visible Saturday evening. Foods are prepared on Friday and held for use on the Sabbath. A long-honored custom is that of inviting a guest to share the Sabbath meal as a remembrance of the biblical statement, "For you

Both words come from the Hebrew word *kashar,* meaning "right" or "fit".

Table 9-1

Jewish Holidays and Associated Foods

Holiday	Month	Event	Traditional Foods
Rosh Hashanah (New Year)	September or October	Beginning of Jewish New Year (Tishri 1)	Honey, honey cake, carrot tzimmes
Yom Kippur	September or October	Day of Atonement	Fast day (total)
Sukkoth	October	Feast of Booths, Harvest festival; symbolizes booths in which Israelites lived on flight from Egypt and Wilderness wanderings	Kreplach or holishkes (chopped meat wrapped in cabbage leaves) Strudel
Chanukah	December	Feast of Lights; celebrates heroic battle of the Maccabees for Jewish independence (165 BC) Home festival with candles	Grated potato latkes, potato kugel
Chamise Oser b'Sh'vat	January	Festival of the Trees (Arbor Day); blossoming time of trees in Palestine	Bokser (St. John's Bread) fruits, nuts, raisins, cakes
Purim	March	Feast of Esther, celebrates downfall of Haman and deliverance of Hebrews by influence of Queen Esther to King Xerxes of Persia	Hamantaschen (three-cornered pastry), apples, nuts, raisins
Passover (Pesach)	April	Festival of Freedom, celebrates escape of Israelites from Egyptian slavery	Seder meal, matzoth and matzoth dishes, wine, nuts
Shevuoth	May	Feast of Weeks (Pentecost); celebrates the day Moses received Ten Commandments on Mt. Sinai	Cheese blintzes, cheese kreplach, dairy foods

were once strangers in the land of Egypt" (Exodus 22:20). A few representative Jewish foods include:

1. **Challah** A special Sabbath loaf of white bread, shaped as a twist or a beehive coil, used at the beginning of the meal after the kiddush (the blessing over wine)
2. **Gefüllte (gefilte) fish** From a German word that means stuffed fish, usually the first course of the Sabbath evening meal and made of fish filet, chopped, seasoned, and stuffed back into the skin or minced and rolled into balls
3. **Bagels** Doughnut-shaped, hard yeast rolls
4. **Blintzes** Thin, filled, and rolled pancakes
5. **Borscht (borsch)** Soup of meat stock and beaten egg or sour cream made with beets, cabbage, or spinach (served hot or cold)
6. **Kasha** Buckwheat groats (hulled kernels), used as a cooked cereal or as a potato substitute with gravy
7. **Knishes** Pastry filled with ground meat or cheese
8. **Lox** Smoked, salted salmon
9. **Matzo** Flat unleavened bread
10. **Strudel** Thin pastry, filled with fruit and nuts, rolled, and then baked

Mexican Food Patterns

A blending of the food habits of Spanish settlers and native Indian tribes forms the basis of the present food patterns of persons of Mexican heritage who now live in the United States, chiefly in the Southwest. Three foods are basic to this pattern—dried beans, chili peppers, and corn. Variations and additions may be found in different localities or among those of different income levels. Food use habits include:

1. **Milk** Little milk is used. A small amount of evaporated milk may be purchased for babies.
2. **Meat** Because of its cost, little meat is taken. Beef or chicken may be eaten two or three times a week. Eggs are also used occasionally, but fish is rarely eaten.
3. **Vegetables** Corn, fresh or canned, and chili peppers are the main vegetables. *Chicos* is steamed green corn dried on the cob. *Pasole* is similar to whole-grain hominy (lime-treated, hulled whole kernels). Chili peppers provide a good source of vitamin C; they are usually dried and ground into a powder. Pinto or chalice beans are used daily; they may be reheated by frying (refried beans) or cooked with beef, garlic, and chili peppers (chili con carne).
4. **Fruits** Depending on availability and cost, oranges, apples, bananas, and canned peaches are used.
5. **Bread and cereals** For centuries corn has been the basic grain used as bread and cereal by the Mexican people. *Masa* (dough) is made from dry corn that has been heated, soaked in lime water, washed, and ground wet to form a mass with the consistency of putty. This dough is then formed into thin, unleavened cakes and baked on a hot griddle to make the typical tortilla. Wheat is now replacing corn for making some tortillas. Unless the wheat flour is enriched, however, the calcium in the previously used treated corn is lost. Cornmeal gruel, or *atole,* is served with hot milk. Rice cooked in milk may be used as a dessert. Oatmeal is a popular breakfast cereal.
6. **Beverages** Large amounts of coffee are generally used. In some families coffee is also given to young children.
7. **Seasonings** Chili pepper, onions, and garlic are used most frequently; occasionally other herbs may be added. Lard is the basic fat.

Puerto Rican Food Patterns

The Puerto Rican people share a common Spanish heritage with the Mexicans. A large part of their food pattern is similar. However, the use of tropical fruits and vegetables that grow on the island have formed the base of the Puerto Rican food pattern. Some of these habits are carried over to Puerto Ricans living in this country when the foods are available in the neighborhood markets. Almost everyone eats the main food, *viandas,* which are starchy vegetables and fruits, such as plantain and green bananas. The two other staples of the diet are rice and beans. Milk, meat, yellow and green vegetables, and other fruits are used in limited quantities. Food use habits include:

1. **Viandas** The many kinds of viandas eaten every day include green bananas, green and ripe plantains, white and yellow sweet potatoes, white yams, breadfruit, and cassava. These foods are cooked in many

ways. Usually codfish and onion are added. If income permits, some avocados and hard-boiled eggs are also added. This dish is called *serenata*. A soup containing vianda and meat is called *sancocho*.

2. **Rice** A large portion of daily kilocalories is obtained from rice. Most Puerto Ricans eat about 7 ounces daily, usually cooked in salted water and seasoned with lard. Other rice dishes include a rice stewed with beans and *sofrito* (a sauce of tomatoes, green pepper, onion, garlic, salt pork, lard, and herbs); rice with chicken, seasoned with olives, red pepper, and sofrito; a dessert made with rice, sugar, and spices; and a thick soup of chicken and rice.

3. **Other cereal grains** Some wheat is used in the form of bread, noodles, and spaghetti. Oatmeal and cornmeal mush may be added if income permits.

4. **Beans** Legumes used include chickpeas (garbanzos), navy beans, red kidney beans (preferred), and dried peas. Usually they are boiled until tender and cooked with sofrito.

5. **Meat** Most families cannot afford meat, although pork and chicken are used when income allows. The only animal protein that the majority can buy is dried codfish.

6. **Milk** Low-income groups can afford little milk. Most of what is taken is boiled and used with coffee; some cocoa and chocolate are used the same way.

7. **Vegetables and fruits** Small amounts of other vegetables are used by the Puerto Rican people. Many tropical fruits are available on the island. Puerto Rico is the home of the *acerola*, the tiny, sour, West Indian cherry, which looks like a miniature apple and has the highest quantity of ascorbic acid known to be contained in any food (about 1000/mg/100 g). Other fruits include oranges, pineapples, grapefruits, papayas, and mangoes.

Meal pattern In most households a typical day's food pattern would include coffee with milk for breakfast; a large plate of viandas with codfish for lunch; and rice, beans, and viandas for dinner. If income permits, egg or oatmeal may be added to the breakfast, some meat to dinner, and fruit between meals. This simple daily diet contrasts with a holiday meal such as that enjoyed at Christmas time. This feast would include whole pig roasted on a spit, blood sausage, green bananas or plantains cooked in the ashes, rice, *pasteles* (plantain dough filled with chopped pork, sofrito, olives, raisins, and boiled peas), rice pudding, and wine, beer, or brandy.

Community health workers are making efforts to improve this diet: (1) the basic foods that everyone eats are listed (rice, beans, viandas, codfish, lard, sugar, and coffee); (2) then suggestions are made for items that need to be added, such as either dry or goat's milk, meat and eggs, yellow and green vegetables, and fresh native fruit.

Chinese Food Patterns

Traditional Chinese cooking is based on three principles: (1) natural flavors must be developed, (2) texture and color must be maintained, and (3) the undesirable qualities of foods must be masked or modified. Like the French, Chinese cooks believe that refrigeration diminishes natural flavors. They select the freshest possible foods, hold them the shortest possible time, and then cook them quickly at a high temperature in small amounts of liquid or fat. This is called *stir-frying*. By these means natural flavor, color, and texture are preserved. Vegetables are cooked just before serving, so that they are still crisp and flavorful when eaten. The only sauce that may be served with them is a thin, translucent one usually made with cornstarch. A thick gravy is never used. Foods that have been dried, salted, pickled, spiced, candied, or canned may be added as garnishes or relishes to mask some flavors or textures or to enhance others. Food use habits include:

1. **Milk** Little milk and limited amounts of cheese are used.
2. **Meat** Pork, lamb, chicken, duck, fish, and shellfish are used in many ways. Usually they are cooked in combination with vegetables, thus extending the amount of meat. Eggs and soybeans in the form of soybean curd and milk add to the protein content of the Chinese diet. Some characteristic dishes include *egg roll*—a thin dough spread with meat and vegetable filling, rolled and fried in deep fat; *egg foo yung*—an omelet of egg, chopped chicken, mushrooms, scallions, celery, and bean sprouts; and *sweet and sour pork*—pork cubes fried and then simmered in a sweet-sour sauce of brown sugar, vinegar, and other seasonings. Chow mein, or chop suey, is purely an American invention. It is a mixture of meat, celery, and bean sprouts, served over rice or noodles and seasoned with soy sauce.
3. **Vegetables** Cooked by the characteristic method just described—stir frying—vegetables such as cabbage, cucumbers, snow peas, melons, squashes, greens, mushrooms, bean sprouts, and sweet potatoes are made into many fine dishes.
4. **Fruit** Usually fruits are eaten fresh. Pineapple and a few others are sometimes used in combination dishes.
5. **Bread and cereals** Rice is the staple grain used at most meals.
6. **Seasoning** Soy sauce is a basic seasoning. Almonds, ginger, and sesame seed are also used. The most frequently used cooking fats are lard and peanut oil.
7. **Beverage** The traditional beverage is unsweetened green tea.

Japanese Food Patterns

Japanese food patterns are in some ways similar to Chinese. Rice is a basic constituent of the diet, soy sauce is used for seasoning, and tea is the main beverage. However, some characteristic differences occur. The Japanese diet contains more seafood, especially raw fish. A number of taboos prohibit certain food combinations or the use of certain foods in specific localities or at specific times. Some of these taboos are associated with religious practices such as ancestor veneration. Food use habits include:

1. **Milk** Little milk or cheese is used. Some evaporated or dried milk may be added in cooking or given to babies.
2. **Meat** The main animal protein source is seafood. Many varieties of fish and shellfish such as raw squid or octopus are served. Other unusual saltwater fare are eels, abalone, and globe fish (puffer fish—deadly if the chef's knife slips in cutting out a certain poisonous gland). More familiar to the Westerner are crab, shrimp, mackerel, carp, and salmon. Families living inland especially may also eat rab-

bit, chicken, and occasionally beef or lamb. Eggs are a source of additional protein.

3. **Vegetables** Japanese menus include many vegetables, usually steamed and served with soy sauce. Pickled vegetables are also well liked.

4. **Fruit** Fresh fruit is eaten in season, a tray of fruit being a regular course of the main meal.

5. **Bread and cereals** Although rice is the staple grain, some corn, barley, and oats are served, and white wheat bread is coming into increasing use in Japanese cities.

Meal pattern A specific sequence of courses is usually followed at most traditional Japanese dinners: green tea, unsweetened; some appetizer, such as soy cake or red bean cake, a raw fish (sashimi) or radish (komono) relish; broiled fish or omelet; vegetables with soy sauce; plain steamed rice; herb relish; fruits in season; a broth-based soup; and perhaps more unsweetened green tea. Typical dishes include *tempura* (batter-fried shrimp) and *aborakge* (fried soybean curd). *Sukiyaki,* a mixture of sauteed beef and vegetables served with soy sauce, is as American as chow mein. Soybean oil is the main cooking fat.

Italian Food Patterns

The sharing of food and companionship is an important part of the Italian life pattern. Meals are associated with much warmth and fellowship, and special occasions are marked by the sharing of food with families and friends. Leisurely meals are customary, with a light breakfast, dinner in the middle of the day, and a small evening meal. Bread and pasta are basic Italian foods. On religious fast days, such as Fridays, Lent, and the period of Advent before Christmas, pasta is prepared with meatless sauces or with fish. Food use habits include:

1. **Milk** Milk is seldom used alone as a beverage but is frequently consumed with coffee in a mixture of about half and half. Cheese, however, is a favorite food. Parmesan and Romano are hard, grating cheeses used in cooking; ricotta and mozzarella are two soft cheeses used in cooking or with bread.

2. **Meat** Chicken baked with oil or in tomato sauce is often used. Beef and veal are eaten as meatballs, meat loaf, cutlets, stews, roasts, and chops. Roasted or fried Italian pork sausage is common. A number of Italian cold cuts are famous—*salami, mortadella* (bologna-type sausage), *coppa* (peppered sausage), and *prosciutto* (Italian cured ham). Many kinds of fish are used. Fresh fish are preferred, but some canned fish such as tuna, sardines, anchovies, and special salted codfish are used also. Some characteristic meat dishes are chicken browned in olive oil, then simmered in wine and tomato sauce, and thin floured strips of veal browned in olive oil and simmered in a sauce flavored with wine and herbs. Italian meatballs are served with spaghetti, and dry salted codfish, soaked several days and browned in olive oil, is simmered with tomato sauce and herbs.

3. **Vegetables** Favorite vegetables include zucchini and other types of squash, broccoli, spinach, eggplant, salad greens, green beans, peppers, and tomatoes. The latter are used in many ways—in sauces,

either whole or as paste, or pureed. Vegetables are usually cooked in water, drained, and seasoned with olive oil or with oil and vinegar. A combination salad of salad greens, with a simple dressing of olive oil, vinegar, garlic, salt, and pepper, is called *insalata*.

4. **Fruit** Fresh fruit in season is eaten for dessert.
5. **Bread and cereals** Bread is present at every Italian meal as a highly regarded principal food. It is made into loaves of many shapes, each one characterisitic of a different Italian province. All breads are made of wheat flour and are white, crusty, and substantial. Some rice and cornmeal are used in special dishes; for example, *polenta* is a thick, yellow cornmeal mush, somtime made into a casserole with sausage, tomato sauce, and cheese. *Pasta* is a basic food item. This term is used for a variety of wheat products made into various forms such as spaghetti, macaroni, and egg noodles. Pasta is served in many ways. Spaghetti is commonly used with a characteristic tomato sauce and cheese or with meatballs or fish. Special dishes of pasta filled with meat mixtures are served on holidays—ravioli, lasagna, manicotti, tortellini, and cannelloni. A dry red or white wine is usually served also.
6. **Soups** Thick soups often serve as a main food for lighter meals. Minestrone is made with vegetables, chickpeas, and pasta. Often a substantial bean soup is used.
7. **Seasonings and basic cooking method** Herbs and spices characteristically used in Italian dishes include oregano, rosemary, basil, saffron, parsley, and nutmeg. Garlic is used often, as are wine, olive oil, tomato puree, salt pork, and cheese. The basic cooking process for main dishes is the initial browning of the vegetables and seasonings in olive oil, adding of meat or fish for browning also, then covering with liquid such as wine, tomato sauce, or broth, and simmering slowly on low heat for several hours.

Greek Food Patterns

In the close-knit, traditionally organized life of the Greek family, food and ceremonial aspects of meals constitute primary values. In many Greek homes the meal is a family ritual. A blessing is said or sung, and hospitality is extended to guests. Everyday meals are simple, but holiday ones are the occasion for serving a great variety of delicacies. Bread is always the center of every meal—indeed it *is* the meal—with other foods considered accompaniments to it: bread is eaten between bites of other food. During religious holidays such as Lent, there are fast days of meatless meals with large use of vegetables. Food use habits include:

1. **Milk** A relatively small amount of milk is used as a beverage by adults, who usually take this food in the form of yogurt. Children drink hot boiled milk sweetened with sugar. Cheese is a favorite food, however. Varieties include *feta*, a special white cheese made from sheep's milk and preserved in brine, and two hard salty cheeses, *caceri* and *cephalotyri*.
2. **Meat** Lamb is the favorite meat. Little beef and some pork and chicken are eaten. Frequent use is made of organ meats or fresh fish. Eggs are sometimes used as a main dish, but not at breakfast.

3. **Vegetables** Vegetables are usually cooked until soft and are seasoned with meat broth or tomato with onions, olive oil, and parsley. Vegetables are often the main dish. Large amounts of many varieties are eaten, with fresh ones preferred. Combination salad of thinly cut raw vegetables with a simple dressing of olive oil and vinegar or lemon juice is often used. Many legumes (beans, peas, lentils, and chickpeas) are eaten. Often a meal consists of cooked dried beans served with olives and pickles. A characteristic dish is *dolmathes,* a meat and rice mixture rolled in cabbage or vine leaves, steamed, and served with egg sauce.

4. **Fruits** Large amounts of fruit are eaten. Peeled raw fruit is an everyday dessert.

5. **Bread and cereals** Bread is made of plain wheat flour, water, salt, and yeast. An indispensable part of every meal, it is preferred plain without butter, jam, or jelly. Dark breads are used by some families. Wheat products such as noodles, macaroni, and spaghetti may be used plain or with meat and tomato sauce. Rice is commonly served. A characteristic rice dish is *pilaf,* which is rice, first browned in butter, covered with broth or water, and simmered until the liquid is absorbed.

6. **Desserts** Desserts other than raw fruit are usually served on special occasions such as holiday meals. Such a characteristic dessert is *baklava,* made of many layers of very thin pastry, brushed with butter, sprinkled with nuts, sugar, and spices, cut in diamond shapes, baked, and then served with honey or syrup.

Social Influences

Social Organization

The study of human group behavior reveals numerous activities, processes, and structures by which social life goes on. Human behavior can be understood in terms of social phenomena and problems—social change, urbanism, rural life, the family, the community, race relations, crime, or delinquency. These influences have many implications for nutrition. Two aspects of social organization concern health professionals:

Class structure The structure of a society is largely formed by groupings according to such factors as economic status, education, residence, occupation, or family. Within a given society many of these groups exist, and their values and habits vary. Subgroups develop on the basis of region, religion, age, sex, social class, health concerns, occupation, or political affiliation. Within these subgroups there may be still smaller groupings with distinguishing attitudes, values, and habits. A person may be a member of several subcultural groups, each of which influences values, attitudes, and habits. Our democratic philosophy, as well as the humanitarian ideals on which the health professions have been nurtured, combine to make the reality of class differences difficult for us to accept. Yet differences do exist, and they probably influence our approach to patients, relationships with them, and the outcome of these relationships more than we may be aware of or care to admit.

Value systems A society's value systems develop as a result of its history and heritage. Traditionally four basic premises have influenced American value systems and have affected attitudes toward health care and food habits:

1. **Equality** The placement of a high value on equality leads health workers to establish standards of quality health care for all people, although in reality this does not always work out.
2. **Sociality** The high respect accorded to a social nature builds peer group pressures and status-seeking within social groups. Foods may be accepted because they are high-status foods or rejected because they are low-prestige foods.
3. **Success** The esteem in which success is held often leads persons to measure life in terms of competitive superlatives. They want to set the best table, to provide the most abundant supply of food for the family, or to have the biggest eater and the fattest baby of any in the neighborhood.
4. **Change** The value that is placed on change leads families and individuals to seek constant variety in their diets, to be geared for action, to be a mobile society, and to seek quick-cooking, conveniently prepared foods. In response to such marketing demands, food technologists continually produce an array of new food products.

Food and Social Factors

Food habits in any setting are highly socialized. These habits perform significant social functions, some of which may not always be evident:

Social relationships Food is a symbol of social acceptance, warmth, and friendliness. People tend to accept food more readily from those persons they view as friends or allies. They accept advice about food from persons they consider to be authorities or with whom they feel warm relationships. Persons tend to distrust food given to them by strangers and outsiders. Emotional feelings about persons are transferred to their food. The more alien the authority figure, the more that person is considered to be unconcerned and his/her food suggestions will be considered outlandish or perhaps even harmful.

Food in family relationships Food habits that are most closely associated with family sentiments are the most tenacious throughout life. Long into adulthood, certain foods trigger a flood of childhood memories and are valued for reasons totally apart from any nutritional value. Strong religious factors associated with food tend to have their origin and reinforcement within the family meal circle. Also, family income, community sources of food, and market conditions influence food habits and ultimately food choices. Persons eat foods that are readily available to them and that they can afford.

Psychologic Influences
Social Psychology: Understanding Dietary Patterns

Social psychology is concerned with: (1) social interaction in terms of its effect on individual behavior, and (2) the social influences of individual perception, motivation, and action. How does a particular individual perceive a given situation? What basic needs motivate action and response? What social factors surround a particular action? Issues of particular concern include the effect of culture on personality, the socialization of the child, differences in individuals in groups, group dynamics, group attitudes and opinions, and leadership. The methods of social psychology have made important contributions to nutrition, medicine, nursing, and allied health care, especially to problems of human behavior under stress.

Food and Psychologic Factors

Individual behavior patterns, including those related to eating, are the result of many interrelated psychosocial influences.[5] Factors that are particularly pertinent to the shaping of food habits are motivation and perception:

Motivation People are not the same the world over. Those of differing cultures are not motivated by the same needs and goals. Even primary biologic drives such as hunger and sex are modified in their interpretation, expression, and fulfillment by many cultural, social, and personal influences. The kinds of food sought, prized, or accepted by one individual at one time and place are rejected by another living in different circumstances. For the person existing in a state of basic hunger or semistarvation, food is the whole perception and motivation. Such a person thinks, talks, and dreams about food. Under less severe circumstances, however, the concern for food may be on a relatively abstract level and may involve symbolism that is associated with other levels of need. For example, the classic hierarchy of human needs developed by Maslow illustrates these human strivings.[6] He described five levels that operate in turn, each building on the prior ones:

1. **Basic physiologic needs**—hunger, thirst
2. **Safety needs**—physical comfort, security, protection
3. **"Belongingness" needs**—love, giving and receiving affection
4. **Recognition needs**—self-esteem, status, sense of self-worth, strength, self-confidence, capability, adequacy
5. **Self-actualization needs**—self-fulfillment and creative growth

Although these levels of need overlap and vary with time and circumstance, we can use them to help us understand the needs of our clients and plan care accordingly.

Perception To make sense out of an otherwise chaotic assortment of impressions, we perceive our environment in different ways. These perceptions enable us to live in an environment that feels relatively stable. However, perception also limits understanding. Every phenomenon that the outer world offers is understood through our own social and personal lenses. In every experience of our lives, we perceive a blend of three factors: (1) the *external reality*, (2) the *message* of the stimulus that is conveyed by the nervous system to the integrative centers where thinking and evaluation go on, and (3) the *interpretation* that we put on every part of our personal experience. A host of subjective elements—such as hunger, thirst, hate, fear, self-interest, values, and temperament—influence our response to the outer world's phenomena.

Personal learning This very personal human dimension makes a health professional's work profound. We cannot impose on our clients and patients mechanical routines of sanitation, hygiene, and nutrition born of our own antiseptic cultural values. Patients will not carry them out if they are presented in this way. Glib answers fail. In the last analysis, persons learn because they sense an urgent need to know. They learn because their curiosity is aroused. They learn because they want to make meaning out of their lives. They learn by exploring, making mistakes and correcting them, testing, and verifying. *All of these things individuals must do for themselves.* This is true of everyone's learning. It is true of the learning we desire for our patients. The process cannot be changed or shortened or avoided.

Current Confusions Influencing Food Habits

Food Misinformation

Unscientific statements about food often mislead the public and contribute to poor food habits. False information may come from folklore, or it may be built on subtle half-truths, innuendos, and outright deception. In contrast, nutritional science is a growing body of knowledge built on vigorously examined scientific evidence. Concern for food safety and wholesomeness clearly existed long before the scientific method was known. Nonetheless, it is only on a sound basis of scientific knowledge that we may make wise food choices and recognize misinformation as such.

Types of Food Faddist Claims

Food faddists make exaggerated claims for certain types of food. These claims fall into four basic groups: (1) certain foods will cure specific conditions, (2) certain foods are harmful and should be omitted from the diet, (3) special food combinations are very effective as reducing diets and have special therapeutic effects, and (4) only **"natural" foods** can meet bodily needs and prevent disease.

"Natural" food Popular term for food said to be "as grown" without any food additives.

Basic Error

Examine these claims carefully. You will notice that each one focuses on foods per se, not on the chemical components in them—the nutrients—which are the actual physiologic agents of life and health. Certain individuals may be allergic to specific foods and should obviously avoid them. Also, certain foods may have particularly high concentrations of certain nutrients and are therefore good sources of such nutrients. But it is the *nutrients,* not the specific foods, that have specific functions in the body. Each of these nutrients may be found in a number of different foods. Remember, persons require specific nutrients, never specific foods.

Dangers of Food Fads

Why should the health worker be concerned about food faddism and its effect on food habits? What harm may it do? Essentially food fads involve four basic dangers:

Dangers to health Responsibility for care of one's health is fundamental. However, self-diagnosis and self-treatment can be dangerous. When such action is based on questionable sources, the dangers are multiplied. By following such a course, a person with real illness may fail to seek appropriate medical care. Many ill and anxious patients have been misled by fraudulent claims of cures and postposed effective therapy.

Money spent needlessly Some of these foods and supplements used by faddists are harmless, but many are expensive. Money spent for useless food or supplements is wasted. When dollars are scarce, the family may neglect to buy foods that will fill its basic needs to purchase a "guaranteed cure."

Lack of knowledge of scientific progress Misinformation hinders the development of society along lines opened by scientific progress. Superstitions that are perpetuated can counteract sound health teaching.

Distrust of food market Our food environment is rapidly changing. We need intelligent concern and rational approaches to meet nutritional requirements. A wise course is to select a variety of primary foods "closer to the source"—having minimal processing—adding a few carefully selected processed items for specific uses. Blanket erroneous teaching concerning food and health breeds public suspicion and distrust of the common food market and of food technology and agriculture in general. Many food products are responsible for the multitude and variety of standard quality food items. Each food product, however, must be evaluated on its own merits in terms of individual needs—nutrient contribution, aesthetic values, and cost.

Vulnerable Groups

Food fads appeal especially to certain groups of people with particular needs and concerns:

Older persons Fear of changes that come with aging leads many middle-aged persons to grasp at exaggerated claims that some product will restore vigor. Older persons in pain and discomfort, perhaps facing chronic illness, reach out for the "special supplement" that promises a sure cure. Desperately ill and lonely individuals are an easy prey for a cruel hoax.

Young people Figure-conscious girls and muscle-minded boys frequently respond to advertisements that offer a crash program to attain the perfect body. Young people, those who are lonely or have exaggerated ideas of glamour, hope to achieve peer-group acceptance by these means.

Obese persons One of the most disturbing personal concerns and frustrating health problems in America today is obesity. Obese persons, faced with a bewildering barrage of propaganda advocating diets, pills, candies, wafers, and devices, are likely to succumb to fads.

Athletes and coaches This group is a prime target for those who push miracle supplements. Always looking for the added something to give them that "competitive edge," athletes tend to fall prey to nutrition myths and hoaxs.

Entertainers Persons in the public eye, such as entertainers, are often prey to those who make false claims that certain foods, drugs, or dietary combinations will enable them to attain the physical appearance and strength on which their careers depend.

These various groups are vulnerable for obvious reasons. But there seems to be no segment of the population that is completely free from food faddism's appeal. Particularly in metropolitan areas, large groups of persons present a constant array of misinformation that hinders the efforts of members of the legitimate health professions to raise the community's standards in nutrition.

What is the Answer?

What can be done to counter food habits associated with food faddism, misinformation, or outright deception? What can workers in the health professions do? What *should* they do? Several courses of action merit consideration:

Assess your own attitudes and habits We cannot counsel or teach other persons until we have first examined our own position. Instruction based on personal conviction, practice, and enthusiasm will achieve far more than teaching that says, in effect, "do as I say, not as I do."

Use reliable sources Two types of background knowledge are vital: (1) knowledge of the product and the persons behind it and (2) knowledge of human nutritional physiology and the scientific method of problem-solving.

Recognize human needs Consider the emotional needs that are symbolically fulfilled by the eating of foods and by the rituals surrounding the process. Respect these needs. Everyone has them. They are a part of life. Welcome the positive power that food and eating rituals possess in fulfilling these needs. Use this knowledge wisely and work it into the nutrition program. Food should not be disparaged as a mere "crutch." Even when there is reason to believe that the client is using foods as a crutch for emotional adjustment, the value of such an adjustment must be considered. A wise teacher of mine once put if well, "We must avoid 'breaking crutches' without offering alternative support."

Be alert to community opportunities Grasp any opportunity that arises to present sound health information to groups or individuals, formally or informally. Learn of available community resources, such as local or state university agricultural extension services; volunteer agencies; clinic and hospital facilities; federal, state, county, and city public health departments; and professional health organizations. Develop communication skills. Avoid monotony. Use a well-disciplined imagination. Without these things, the message will not convince.

Think scientifically We can teach even very young children to use the problem-solving approach to everyday situations. Children are naturally curious. With their eternal *why*, they often seek evidence to support statements they hear. Far to often our system of education fails to develop this natural spirit of inquiry. We need to teach them, and ourselves, the value of asking three significant questions: "What do you mean?" "How do you know?" and "What is your evidence?"

Know responsible authorities The Food and Drug Administration (FDA) has the legal responsibility of controlling the quality and safety of food and drug products marketed in the United States (see p. 204). But this is a monumental task and needs the help of vigilant consumers. Other governmental, professional, and private organizations can provide additional resources.

Food Safety

A number of chemicals have been developed by the agricultural and food processing industries to increase and preserve our food supply. They have rapidly changed the character of America's present food supply and its environment into a complex "feeding web," which has increasingly raised issues about nutritional ecology.[1] Critics voice concerns about the rapid changes these effects have brought to our overall food environment.

Intentional Food Additives

In the past three decades chemicals intentionally added to foods have increasingly become components of the food supply. Our present variety of marketed items would be impossible without them. They have been a major factor in the rapid evolution of the corner grocery store into the giant supermarket chain. These changes, which have swept the food-marketing system during the last 25 years, are rooted in a deeper social revolution and in scientific advance.

Reasons for development and use of food additives include the following factors:

Enriched Food with added nutrients, usually to replace some of those lost in processing, such as addition of several B vitamins and iron to white flour.

Fortified Food with added nutrients to make it a comparable substitute for a similar regular food, such as vitamin A fortified margarine used for butter; or food having a needed nutrient added, such as vitamin D fortified milk.

1. **Population growth** requires increased food production.
2. **Publicized scientific discoveries** have increased consumers' awareness of nutritional needs and impressed them with the importance to health of a well-balanced diet. Specific foods are **enriched** or **fortified** to help supply these needs.
3. **Desire for variety** in foods and creativity in cooking has increased. Foods from local and distant places provide great variety and choice.
4. **Complexity of family life** and the number of working wives and mothers have created a desire for convenience foods that require little or no preparation.
5. **Safe, quality food** is a public desire. Americans are becoming more aware that their health depends on an adequate supply of fresh or properly preserved foods. Efforts of the consumer to purchase quality foods are backed by laws governing food production, processing, and sale. However, the rapidly changing food environment requires constant reevaluation of these regulations to ensure their adequacy to meet needs.

Food additives serve a variety of purposes in modern food products. They (1) add specific nutrients to enrich products; (2) produce uniform properties such as color, flavor, aroma, texture, and general appearance; (3) standardize many functional properties, such as thickening or stabilization; (4) preserve foods by preventing oxidation; and (5) control acidity or alkalinity to improve flavor, texture, and the cooked product. Some examples of intentional food additives are listed in Table 9-2.

Table 9-2

Some Examples of Intentional
Food Additives

Function	Chemical Compound	Common Food Uses
Acids, alkalis, buffers	Sodium bicarbonate Tartaric acid	Baking powder Fruit sherbets Cheese spreads
Antibiotics	Chlortetracycline	Dip for dressed poultry
Anticaking agents	Aluminum calcium silicate	Table salt
Antimycotics	Calcium propionate Sodium propionate Sorbic acid	Bread Bread Cheese
Antioxidants	Butylated hydroxyanisole (BHA) Butylated hydroxytoluene (BHT)	Fats Fats
Bleaching agents	Benzoyl peroxide Chlorine dioxide Oxides of nitrogen	Wheat flour
Color preservative	Sodium benzoate	Green peas Maraschino cherries
Coloring agents	Annotto Carotene	Butter, margarine
Emulsifiers	Lecithin Monoglycerides and diglycerides Propylene glycol alginate	Bakery goods Dairy products Confections
Flavoring agents	Amyl acetate Benzaldehyde Methyl salicylate Essential oils; natural extractives Monosodium glutamate	Soft drinks Bakery goods Candy; ice cream Canned meats
Nonnutritive sweeteners	Saccharin Aspartame	Diet packed canned fruit Low-calorie soft drinks
Nutrient supplements	Potassium iodide Vitamin C Vitamin D Vitamin A B vitamins, iron	Iodized salt Fruit juices Milk Margarine Bread and cereal
Sequestrants	Sodium citrate Calcium pyrophosphoric acid	Dairy products
Stabilizers and thickeners	Pectin Vegetable gums (carob bean, carrageenan, guar) Gelatin Agar-agar	Jellies Dairy desserts and chocolate milk Confections "Low-calorie" salad dressings
Yeast foods and dough conditioners	Ammonium chloride Calcium sulfate Calcium phosphate	Bread, rolls

Problems with Food Additives

Although food additives have served many useful purposes in the development of the modern food industry, problems have accrued along with these gains. These problems are of increasing concern to consumers and producers.

Food Additives Amendment and Delany Clause The Food Additives Amendment of the Federal Food, Drug, and Cosmetic Act of 1938 was passed on September 7, 1958. This amendment, which took effect on March 6, 1960, completely altered the U.S. government's method of regulating the use of additives in food. The law provided for the first time that no additive could be used in food unless the FDA, after careful review of the test data, agreed that the compound was safe at the intended levels of use. An exception was made for all additives in use at that time, which, because of years of widespread use without bad effects reported, were "generally recognized as safe" (GRAS) by experts in the field. This approach was a compromise between giving blanket approval to all additives then in use or banning all untested food additives until several years of laboratory safety studies could be conducted. The Delany Clause was attached in the final hours of congressional debate on the legislation. This clause to the Food Additives Amendment states that "no additive shall be deemed safe if it is found to induce cancer when ingested by man or animal, or if it is found, after tests which are appropriate for the evaluation of the safety of food additives, to induce cancer in man or animal."

GRAS list The result of this amendment has been to establish what is now known as the GRAS list—large numbers of food additives "generally recognized as safe" but not having undergone rigid testing requirements. This list includes several thousand common food additives, including salt, sugar, baking powder, spices, flavorings, vitamins, minerals, preservatives, emulsifiers, and nonnutritive sweeteners. Some of them are restricted to uses in certain foods and at certain levels, but most are limited only to their "intended use" and to "good manufacturing practice."

Problems, however, exist with the GRAS list. First, there has been uncertainty as to how many GRAS items there are, and only now with computer aid has this large list been tabulated.[7] Second, in the years since the GRAS list was formulated, two developments challenge the soundness of its original concept: (1) we know much more now about toxicity testing, so relying merely on a lack of reported human adverse effect as the sole measure of safety is inadequate; and (2) we see the demands of modern technology increase the uses of certain GRAS items well beyond our original exposure patterns. In short, the total food environment has changed radically, creating new problems.

Need for Review

As a result, in 1977 the U.S. government directed the FDA to reevaluate all the items on the GRAS list for safety. This large task is still in progress, and all persons involved agree that there is a pressing need to establish priorities for review.

The Delany Clause is now considered by many scientists to be too rigid.[8] It is seen as an example of Congressional opinion during the 1950s that there was no way to tell safe levels for carcinogens. Now the FDA is moving toward a policy of *risk assessment*. The options being considered by the FDA include what is called *constituent policy,* which proposes two requirements for an additive to trigger the Delany Clause: (1) the additive *as such* would have to be carcinogenic in tests, not just the particular constituents of it; and (2) if the constituent *is* carcinogenic, it would have to be judged to be a significant risk by a quantified risk assessment test. Under such an agreement, the FDA could reinstate some substances now banned, such as yellow food dye No. 1 and red food colors Nos. 10, 11, 12, and 13. But how do we assess a degree of risk? This is particularly perplexing in the area of human health, where errors of judgment can result in tragedy.

Incidental Food Additives: Pesticides

Today's farmers use chemicals to control a wide variety of destructive insects, kill weeds, control plant disease, stop fruit from dropping prematurely, make leaves drop so that harvesting will be easier, make seeds sprout, keep seeds from rotting before they sprout, increase yield, and improve marketing qualities. Concerns and confusion continue about pesticide *residues* in food. Farm workers, consumers, and the general public have increasing questions about the effect of current levels of agricultural chemicals used to increase needed food production. These practices have led to our present "pesticide dilemma," for agricultural chemicals bring hazards as well as gains. Today the FDA directs a pesticide control program in two phases: (1) requirement for initial approval, and (2) continued surveilance.

Control Agencies

Numerous government and private agencies and professional organizations are charged with the responsibility of ensuring the safety and high quality of our food. Concerned groups in the U.S. Department of Health and Human Services (HHS) are the FDA and the Public Health Service (PHS) while in the U.S. Department of Agriculture, there is the Agricultural Research Service and the Consumer Marketing Service. Also protecting the consumer are the Federal Trade Commission (FTC) and the National Bureau of Standards (NBS).

FDA

The broad work of the FDA serves as an example of the U.S. government's effort to protect and control our food supply. In essence the FDA is a law enforcement agency charged by Congress to ensure, among other things, that the food supply is safe, pure, and wholesome. The agency enforces federal regulations through a number of basic projects related to food safety. This work includes activities such as food sanitation and quality control, control of chemical contaminents and pesticides, control of food additives, regulating movement of foods across state lines, nutrition and nutrition labeling of foods, safety of food service, meat, and milk. The methods of enforcement available to the FDA are recalls, seizure, injunction, and prosecution. The use of recalls is the most common method, with seizures of contaminated foods second.

Food Labeling

Nutritional labeling is currently a controversial area. Although the FDA passed "truth-in-packaging" laws in the mid-1960s, many persons are concerned that nutritional labeling is inadequate. Sodium leads the list of labeling topics. Other nutrients and constituents of foods that consumer groups believe should be listed on labels include macronutrients, cholesterol, saturated fat, and additives such as sulfiting agents, to which some persons are dangerously allergic. The FDA is currently reviewing different approaches to labeling to develop a labeling system that adequately describes the food, while not being overwhelming or incomprehensible to the consumer.[9] Various label arrangements and use of symbols are being tested.

Food Standards

Section 401 of the Federal Food, Drug, and Cosmetic Act was designed to "promote honesty and fair dealing in the interest of consumers." The FDA has the responsibility for establishing and enforcing uniform national food standards. The label must indicate these standards and tell what is in the package. It must not be false of "misleading" in any particular.

Standards of identity Reference standards have been established for a number of common foods. On such identified foods there is no requirement to list the ingredients, since they are named in the standard. For many less common foods with no standard of identity, the label must list all the ingredients in the order of their predominance in the food product.

Standards of quality For a number of canned fruits and vegetables, minimum standards have been set concerning such properties as tenderness, color, and freedom from defects. If the food is safe to eat but does not meet these standards, it must specifically indicate this on the label.

Standards of fill of container For many foods, standards have been set to protect the consumer against slack fillings. These are specially necessary for products that settle after filling, such as cereals, or products that consist of a number of pieces packed in liquid such as fruit cocktail.

Standards for enriched products Standards are set for enrichment of flour, cereals, margarine, and other foods with specific quantities of vitamins and minerals. Any product labeled "enriched" or "fortified" must contain precisely the specified amount of added nutrients.

Consumer Education

The FDA Division of Consumer Education conducts an active program of consumer protection through education and public information. Special attention is given to nutrition misinformation. Sound materials are prepared and distributed to individuals and students and community groups. Consumer specialists work through all FDA district offices.

Food Contamination in Disasters

In cooperation with local and state officials, the FDA inspects food that has been damaged by flood, hurricane, fire, or other disasters and removes contaminated items from the market.

Figure 9-2
Research in food chemistry.
A chemist in the U.S.
Department of Agriculture's
Agricultural Research Service
makes an adjustment on a
molecular still used in a
project to aid in the
manufacture of dry milk.

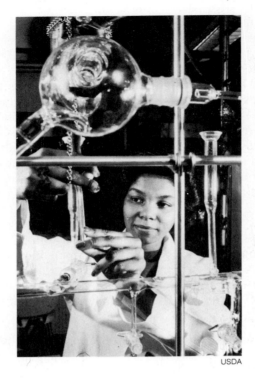

USDA

Scientific Research

As a basis for all its activities in a world of burgeoning technology, **FDA** scientists continually seek to provide a background of evaluation through their own research (Figure 9-2). Precise policies have varied with different administrators and bureaucratic entanglements occur. Nevertheless, the declared intent of persons in charge of the FDA is that food safety must be interpreted not only in the traditional sense that food must be free from danger but also in the more positive sense that its nutritional value must be clear. It is reasonable for consumers to insist that additives introducing possible hazard without adding any benefits to food must be avoided. An attempt is being made to develop nutritional guidelines for a variety of food products, including formulated main dishes, new foods such as meat analogs, foods important as groups for having high malnutrition risks, fruit juices and drinks, and snack foods. This is a broad jump from the former attitude of a purely regulatory function and should go far in meeting changing needs in these changing times.

Changes In American Food Habits

Determinants of Food Choice
Basic Determinants

Clearly some of the basic and universal determinants of food choice focus on physical, social, and physiologic factors (Table 9-3). We have discussed the broad areas of culture, sociology, and psychology in terms of their influence on food habits. Attempting to change our own eating patterns or helping our clients to make needed changes in their patterns is difficult. It requires a sensitive, flexible understanding of the complex factors that influence choices persons make when they eat what they do.

Table 9-3
Factors Determining
Food Choices

Physical Factors	Social Factors	Physiologic Factors
Food supply available	Advertising	Allergy
Food technology	Culture	Disability
Geography, agriculture, distribution	Education, nutrition and general	Health-disease status
Personal economics, income	Political and economic policies	Heredity
Sanitation, housing	Religion and social custom	Personal food acceptance
Season, climate	Social class, role	Needs, energy, or nutrients
Storage and cooking facilities	Social problems, poverty, or alcoholism	Therapeutic diets

Conservative and Dynamic Influences

Two sets of factors—conservative and dynamic—influence our eating habits in opposite directions. The group processes of ethnic patterns and regional and cultural habits precondition our food choices and exert a conservative influence on our inclination to change. On the other hand, new dynamic factors arise when we no longer have to spend most of our time getting food. We are thrust in the direction of diversity and change and also into dissatisfaction with out current situation. These new factors include:

1. **Wealth** A sufficient income affords us increasing amounts of both choice and time.
2. **Technology** Our expanding technology has vastly increased what is available to us from our food supply.
3. **Environment** We are reassessing our relationship with our world, realizing that we cannot endlessly exploit it.
4. **Vision** Mass media and greatly improved communications have made us aware of multiple options, changed our expectations, and developed a new sense of perspective.

Changing American Food Patterns

The stereotype of the all-American family with parents and two children eating three meals a day with a ban on snacking is no longer the common pattern. In the last decade we have experienced far-reaching changes in our way of living and subsequently in our food patterns.

Households

There has been a 50% increase in single-person households in the last 5 years.

Between 1970 and 1980 there was a 25% increase (or 15.7 million) in the number of American households. Most of these are groups of unrelated persons or persons living alone—an increase of 73%—whereas family households have climbed only 13%. The average size of the American household is now 2.75 persons instead of 3.17 in 1970.[10] These trends indicate a very significant change in the American social picture—sometimes lamented as the "deterioration" of the American family—but more appropriately seen as one facet of a dynamic and rapidly changing society.

Working Women

The number of women in the work force continues to increase rapidly, a trend that is not likely to reverse.[11] This increase results from increased educational opportunities for women: 51% of college undergraduates are now women. Women account for 30% of the enrollment in law schools, 25% in medical schools, 30% in business schools, and 12% in technical graduate schools. This phenomenon of working women is not restricted to one social, economic, or ethnic group. It is a widespread societal change, bringing with it changes in the functioning of the family. Working mothers rely increasingly on food items and cooking methods that save time, space, and labor.

Family Meals

Half the American people between the ages of 22 and 40 skip breakfast on a regular basis and 25% skip lunch.

Family meals as we have known them in the past are becoming increasingly obsolete. Breakfasts and lunches are no longer eaten in a family setting by many American family members. Also, as many as 25% of American households do not have a sit-down dinner as often as five nights a week.

Meal Times

Americans are increasing the number of times a day they eat, sometimes having as many as 11 "eating occasions" a day, a pattern recently termed "grazing."

There has been a dramatic increase in flexibility concerning when we eat and whether it is with our families or not. Midmorning snacks are now commonplace, a midafternoon snack similar to a European "tea" is popular, with snacks over television and a midnight refrigerator raid at the day's end. Nutrition hardliners from the old school decry this snacking behavior, but Americans are moving toward a concept of "balanced days" instead of "balanced meals." In fact, studies indicate that frequent, small meals are better for the body than three larger meals a day, depending on what snacks are included. (See box p. 209.)

Health and Fitness

The interest of Americans in physical fitness seems here to stay. This has taken primarily two forms:

1. **Nutrition awareness** Americans are becoming increasingly aware of the nutritional content of their foods and are demanding a wholesome, safe, nutritious food supply. This is reflected in the desire for **"natural"** or **"organic"** foods and many similar items.

"Organic" food Popular term for food said to be grown without pesticides.

2. **Weight concern** Our weight consciousness has affected the foods we choose to eat, and foods perceived as lower in kilocalories, including whole new lines of "light" foods, are popular.

Economical Buying

More and more Americans are economizing on food. In a recent survey of supermarket shoppers, 64% said they had made changes in their diet primarily to save money.[12] Consumers are stocking up on bargains and cutting back on expensive "convenience" foods. They are buying items in larger packages and in bulk and doing much less "store-hopping" for bargains, staying with a store they consider to have the lowest overall prices. They are less loyal to brand names and purchase more generic products. They are using food labels both for unit pricing and for "calorie-counting."

Clinical Application

Snacking: An All-American Food Habit

The snack market in the United States is growing at a rate of over 10% a year. The Consumer Price index increase in cost for all foods in 1981, due to inflation, was 8.6%. But the Index shows a rise of 11.5% for salty snacks, 11% for cookies, and 9% for crackers. Studies of college students show the popularity of soft drinks, candies, gum, and fresh fruit as snacks, followed by bakery items, milk, and chips.

Snacking is said to "ruin your appetite," and we certainly consume far too many soft drinks. But is snacking all bad? Not necessarily. A recent report shows a direct association of more complete nutrition with an increase in snacking—those who snack more show higher percentages in the "adequate" range of the RDAs. Researchers also found that many people snack on foods that aren't "empty extras" but essential contributions to nutritional adequacy. These items include fruit, cheese, eggs, bread, crackers.

Snacking is clearly a significant components of food behavior. Health workers need to remain aware of consumer behavior. Rather than rule against the practice of snacking, we need to promote snack foods that enhance nutritional wellbeing.

References
Crocetti, P.F., and Guthrie, H.A.: Food consumption patterns and nutritional quality of U.S. diets: a preliminary report, Food Tech. **35**:40, 1981.
Khan, M.A., and Lipke, L.K.: Snacking and its contribution to food and nutrient intake of college students, J. Am. Diet. Assoc. **81**(5):583, 1982.
Scales, H.: The U.S. snack food market, Cereal Foods World **27**(5):203, 1982.

Gourmet Cooking

There has been a rise in demand for gourmet foods, and food speciality shops have sprung up in every shopping center. Gourmet cooking has become a popular hobby, and entertaining guests at home over a gourmet meal has been called a "new elitism." This phenomenon parallels the general trend toward meals that are easy to fix, take little time, and fulfill the consumers' nutritional needs. As a result, two new food industry markets have developed: (1) nutritional products, and (2) entertainment products or fun foods.

Fast Foods

Over the last decade sales of fast-food products rose 300%, from $6.5 billion to $23 billion per year.

At one time or another, 90% of all Americans eat in a fast-food restaurant; 10% more than five times a week.[13] As family income rises, so does the consumption of fast foods, especially among the upper-middle class.

Report from Industry

Profits in the food industry are rising.[14] Cereal products are selling better, since more persons are seeing them as nutritious items. Sales have increased in frozen vegetables, low-fat milk, cheese, yogurt, and decaffeinated coffee. Sales have dropped in whole milk and canned goods, and sales of white bread have dropped 44% in the last 20 years. There has been a spectacular rise in ethnic packaged foods in "fast-foods," and in new lines of "light foods," from beer to pizza, in response to the fitness movement. There are more pure fruit juices, yogurts, and decaffeinated products, including soft drinks. There are many new spreads, sauces, processed meats, and snack foods. Leading the list of popular snack foods is tortilla chips. Nuts and dried fruit are popular, and the market is seeing a variety of new breads and brands of bottled water.

To Sum Up

We all grow up and live our lives in a social context. We each inherit at least one cultural background and live in our particular society's social structure, complete with food habits and attitudes about eating. It is from a social perspective that we can best examine changes in food habits. We need to understand the effects on health that are associated with major social and economic shifts. We also need to understand current social forces to best help persons make new dietary changes that will benefit their health; we must meet concerns about food misinformation and food safety.

America is changing a number of its food patterns. We increasingly rely on food technology in our fast, complex life. More women are working, households are getting smaller, more and more persons are living alone, and our meal patterns are different. We search for less fancy, lower-cost food items, and also creative gourmet cooking. In general we are more nutrition and health conscious. Fast food outlets and snacking are social habits here to stay.

Questions for Review

1. What is the meaning of culture? How does it affect our food patterns?
2. What are social and psychologic factors that influence our food habits? Give examples of personal meanings related to food.
3. Why does the public tend to accept nutrition misinformation so easily? What groups of people are more susceptible? Select one such group and give some effective approaches you might use in reaching them.
4. What is the basis of concern about food additives and pesticide residues?
5. Name seven trends in the American mainstream of food patterns and discuss their implications for nutrition and health.

References

1. Gussow, J.D.: The feeding web: issues in nutritional ecology, Palo Alto, Calif., 1978, Bull Publishing Co.

2. World hunger: grim accounting, Nutr. Week **13**(22):4, 1983.

3. Koh, E.T., and Chi, M.S.: Clinical signs found in association with nutritional deficiencies as related to race, sex, and age for adults, Am. J. Clin. Nutr. **34**(8):1562, 1981.

4. Kent, G.: Food trade: the poor feed the rich, Food Nutr. Bull. **4**:25, 1982.

5. Gibson, L.D.: The psychology of food: why we eat what we eat when we eat it, Food Tech. **35**(2):54, 1981.

6. Maslow, A.H.: Motivation and personality, New York, 1954, Harper & Bros.

7. Smith, M.V., and Rulis, A.M.: FDA's GRAS review and priority-based assessment of food additives, Food Tech. **35**:71, 1981.

8. Seligsohn, M.: Delaney: FDA searches for a way out, Food Eng. **54**:23, 1982.

9. Seligsohn, M.: Nutrition labeling: search for a new format, Food Eng. **55**:20, 1982.

10. Report: Will there be more households and fewer families in the 1980s? J. Am. Diet. Assoc. **81**(6):738, 1982.

11. Kastens, M.L.: Revolution in the food system, Food Eng. **54**:105, 1982.

12. Chou, M.: The impact of the economy on food habits, Cereal Food Worker **27**:570, 1982.

13. Report: "Fast foods" and the American consumer, J. Am. Diet. Assoc. **81**(5):579, 1982.

Further readings

Food habits
Baker, C.M.: One approach to teaching cultural similarities and differences, J. Nursing Ed. **21**(4):17, 1982.

This nursing educator provides helpful background for learning about different cultures in relation to health practices.

Schwerin, H.S., and others: Food, eating habits, and health: a further examination of the relationship between food eating patterns and nutritional health, Am. J. Clin. Nutr. **35**(5):1319, 1982.

Findings of this follow-up examination of national food intake surveys provide knowledge of how people actually eat rather than what they should eat. This provides a helpful background for planning more successful food habit changes by involving the base of the person's existing food behavior and attitudes.

Food misinformation
Herbert, V.: Will questionable nutrition overwhelm nutrition science? Am. J. Clin. Nutr. **34**(12):2848, 1981.

Morris, C.E.: The food industry's role in diet and health, Food Eng. **54**:57, 1982.

Stephenson, M.G.: FDA view of nutrition regulations, Cereal Foods World **28**(2):143, 1983.

Three articles addressing varying points of view on the controversy between questionable popular nutrition practices and scientific nutrition. Herbert expresses sound medical-legal view of its physician-lawyer author. The other authors present views of food industry and the FDA.

Heyn, D.: The nutrition free-for-all, Health **13**(1):24, 1981.

LaChance, P.A.: Do you belong in a health food store? Health **14**(8):26, 1982.

Mayer, J.: Megavitamin madness, Health **12**(2):48, 1980.

Three very readable and informative articles from the public press on current consumer practices and problems.

Food safety

ADA Reports: ADA comments on FDA's proposal for sodium labeling, J. Am. Diet. Assoc. **81**(6):732, 1982.

ADA Reports: ADA comments on nutrition labeling formats, J. Am. Diet. Assoc. **82**(4):414, 1983.

Seligsohn, M.: Nutrition labeling: search for new format, Food Eng. **55**:20, 1983.

These articles provide background about the problems involved in developing improved food labels to meet consumer needs and the changing food market.

Issues and Answers

Proposed Changes in FDA Regulations: The Hatch Bill

The Hatch Bill, first introduced in the 1981 U.S. Congress, would make key changes in FDA regulations. It represents one approach to resolving some of the problems that have recently arisen in applying the Federal Food, Drug, and Cosmetic Act, especially the Delaney Clause. The Hatch Bill's food safety provisions cover four categories: natural constituents of agricultural commodities, environmental contaminants, substances used intentionally as food ingredients, and substances that become part of food through their intentional use for other purposes. We will look at three of these:

Natural Food Constituents

According to Section 402 (a)(1) of the Federal Food, Drug, and Cosmetic Act, if a naturally occurring substance is harmful, it isn't looked on as "added" and the food is not said to be adulterated unless the substance is present in a large enough dose to be "injurious to health." This exempts common spices such as black pepper. The Hatch Bill attempts to ensure that spices and familiar foods will continue to be considered under Section 402 (a)(1) of the act and thus be exempt from the strict anti-cancer rules of the Delaney clause. But the problem is one of definition. What is a "familiar food?" Should we include processed foods? If so, how much processing, or changing, of the food should we allow?

Environmental Contaminants

These are substances introduced into foods as a result of human activities. Examples include **aflatoxin**, PCBs (polychlorinated biphenyls), mercury, and lead. A food is considered adulterated if the added substance may render it injurious to health, that is, if there is a reasonable possibility of harm. These substances are not regulated as food additives because they are not deliberately part of foods. The anti-cancer regulations do not technically apply. They are regulated under Section 406 of the Food, Drug, and Cosmetic Act and are allowed if they "cannot be avoided by good manufacturing practice." The Hatch Bill would allow the FDA to judge the importance of the food as well as the toxicity of the substance in setting tolerance levels for the unavoidable contaminants, for example, pesticides. But several of these provisions raise questions:

■ Rule-making, as a consequence, would be informal, rather than the formal hearing now required for setting tolerance levels. But if the rules are informal, what would that do to FDA's enforcement authority?

■ FDA would take into account the cost and availability of the food in setting tolerance levels. Does this mean that the FDA should move out of the arena of scientific objectivity and consider social issues as well?

■ If FDA initiates action against a contaminant, the agency would

Aflatoxin Food poison produced in stored agricultural products by strains of a common storage mold *Aspergillus flavus,* usually abbreviated to *A. flavus.*

Continued.

Issues and Answers—cont'd

be required to set formal tolerance levels for it. Would this make FDA reluctant to initiate action?

Intentionally Added Ingredients

This category includes the GRAS foods, those "generally recognized as safe." In 1977, in the wake of the cyclamate controversy, the federal administration directed the FDA to review the safety of the GRAS list, which also includes "direct food additives." Unless a substance deliberately added to foods is covered by the GRAS list, by "prior sanctions" (food approved by the FDA before 1958), or by legislation regulating pesticides, animal drugs, and color additives, it is subject to the food additives regulations, which include the Delaney Clause of 1960. The Hatch Bill would make it substantially harder for a GRAS item to be reviewed. The Delaney Clause prohibits use of any substance that has been found to induce cancer in animals or humans. Instead the Hatch Bill proposes: (1) to streamline the review process (which many fear would inhibit thorough scientific research of a substance's possible danger), and (2) to prevent banning a food additive on the basis of insignificant risk. This second point is perhaps the pivot of the ongoing unresolved debate. Is this an obvious, commonsense approach? Or would it seriously undermine the FDA's ability to safeguard our food supply?

Questions for Further Thought

1. Does the concept of "risk/benefit" make sense in relation to carcinogens in our food supply? If so, on what basis are the decisions to be made? Who should make them?

2. If the FDA considers a food's economic or cultural benefits to society, won't it be moving into the sphere of public policy? Is that the role it should take?

3. What problems do you see with the Delaney Clause? With the Hatch Bill? What would you propose?

References
Dunkelberger, E.: The Hatch Bill: how it would modify the Food, Drug, and Cosmetic Act, Cereal Foods World 27(6):271, 1982.
Senate Bill 1441: Sections 106, 108, 97th Congress, First Session, 1981 (The Hatch Bill).

Chapter 10
Family Nutrition Counseling: Food Needs and Costs

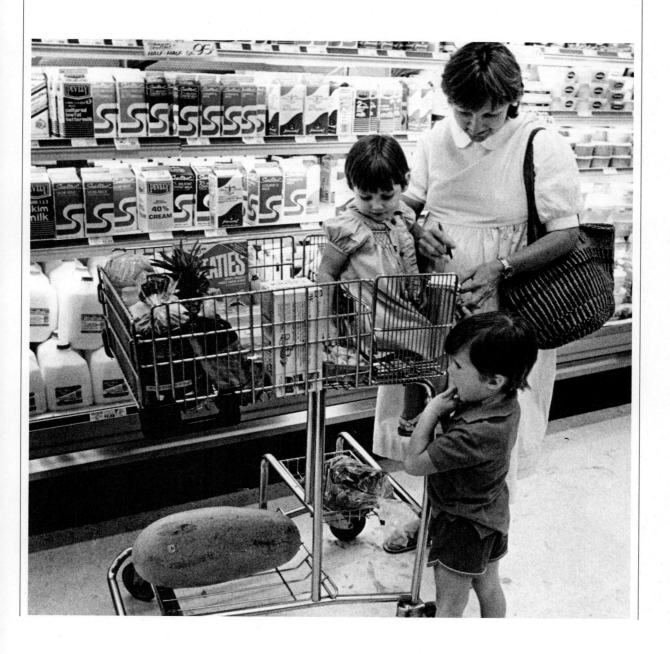

Preview

Health care that is helpful and useful to the client or patient must always be based on the individual's particular health needs. For this reason, finding out what those needs are and planning with the client the best way of meeting these needs is a necessary beginning and continuing part of all health care and education. Health counseling in its broad sense centers upon this basic type of activity—helping the client to meet personal health needs. Good health depends on good nutrition. Therefore a basic part of meeting health needs always involves attention to nutritional needs. In a variety of situations health workers will be closely involved with the health team—the general health team, the nursing team, or the nutritional care team—in helping to meet each patient's nutritional care and education needs.

Chapter Objectives

After study of this chapter, the student should be able to:

1. Describe the role of the nutrition counselor-educator in health care settings.

2. Identify the primary focus and components of the counseling or teaching-learning process and apply these components to the nutrition interview.

3. Identify available community food-assistance resources for families with economic problems and assist them with wise buying approaches.

Family Nutrition Counseling

Realistic family diet counseling must be *person-centered*. It involves close attention to personal and family needs, nutrition and health problems, and food choices and costs. As health care workers all of us will be involved at some time to some degree with the nutritional needs and concerns of our patients and clients. In our work we should have three main goals: (1) to obtain basic information about the patient and his/her living situation that relates to nutrition and health needs, (2) to provide basic health teaching to help meet these needs, and (3) to support the patient in all personal efforts to meet needs through encouragement, reinforcement, and general concern and caring. A basic skill that all health workers must learn, therefore, is the skill of talking with patients in a helpful manner. Skills in *interviewing* are essential in health care.

Interviewing

Interviewing does not necessarily mean only the more formal or structured diet history or other history-taking activity. Frequently it means a purposeful "planned conversation" either in the hospital or clinic setting or a telephone call to the home to determine ongoing needs or progress. Several general principles of interviewing should guide such activity.

Focus and Purpose

As indicated, the focus of all health care is the individual patient and personal health needs. Our ultimate purpose is to provide whatever help the patient may need to determine personal health needs and goals and to provide the means of meeting those needs and goals.

Means

Several means are used by health workers to accomplish these purposes:

Dynamic Pertaining to change. A dynamic process is one that is constantly changing.

Relationship Counseling is a **dynamic** person-centered process built upon a helping relationship. The most important means of helping a person is establishing a relationship of mutual trust and respect. The most significant tool we ever have for helping others is *ourselves*. Our role is that of a "helping vehicle." Within this kind of relationship, true healing can take place.

Climate The kind of climate that we create involves both the physical setting and the psychologic feelings involved. The circumstances surrounding the interview should be as comfortable as possible with regard to the physical conditions of ventilation, heating, lighting, and sitting or lying down. Other important factors include providing sufficient time for the interview, in a quiet setting free from interruptions and with sufficient privacy to assure confidentiality—preferably in an office setting with a desk to the side, not between the therapist and client.

Attitudes The word "attitude" refers to that aspect of personality that accounts for a consistent behavior toward persons, situations, or objects. Our attitudes are *learned*. Hence they are the result of total life experiences and influences. Because they are learned, they can be examined. We can become more aware of them. We can try to strengthen those attitudes that are desirable and at the same time seek to change those that are less desirable. Certain attitudes are necessary components of a health worker's capacity to meet patients' needs:

1. **Warmth** A genuine concern for the patient is displayed by interest, friendliness, and kindness. We convey warmth by being human and thoughtful.
2. **Acceptance** We must meet the patient "as he is, where he is." To accept the patient does not necessarily mean approval of behavior. It does mean a realization that patients usually regard their behavior as purposeful and meaningful. It may well be for them a means of handling stress. An attitude of acceptance conveys that a person's thoughts, ideas, and actions are important and worth attention simply because a person—a human being—has the right to be treated as a person of worth and dignity.
3. **Objectivity** To be objective is to be free of bias. It is having a nonjudgmental attitude. Of course, complete objectivity is impossible, but reasonable objectivity is certainly a goal that can be obtained. We must be aware of our own feelings and biases and we should attempt to control them. Evaluation of a situation must be based on what is actually happening, the facts as we perceive them. It cannot be based on mere opinions, assumptions, or inferences lacking evaluation.
4. **Compassion** This attitude enables us to feel with and for another person or oneself. It means accepting the impact of an emotion, holding it long enough with sufficient absorption to accept its meaning, and entering into a kind of "fellowship of feeling" with the person who is moved by that emotion. There is nothing soft or easy in developing the attitude of compassion. It requires emotional maturity.

Measure

Continuous and terminal evaluations of our interviews must always be a part of our activity. Evaluation is measuring how behavioral changes in the patient and in ourselves are related to the needs and goals that were originally identified. In summary, therefore, the health worker will always be dealing with the following sequence of questions in interviewing:

1. What is wrong? What is the health problem or *need* of the patient?
2. What does the patient want to do about it? What is the patient's immediate *goal?* What is the long-range goal?
3. What *information* do I need to know to help the patient? What does the patient need to know to help take care of personal needs? What knowledge and skills are necessary to solve the health problem?
4. What has to be done to help meet the need? What *plan of action* is best for solving the health problem and meeting the patient's personal goals?
5. What happened? What was the *result* of the action planned? Did it solve the problem or meet the need? If not, why not? What change in plan is indicated?

Important Aspects of the Interview

Several important actions during the interview can be identified that deserve study and development of skills.

Observation

Ordinarily we do not deliberately and minutely look at all the persons we meet. However, in the care of persons with health needs the helping role requires such behavior. Our purpose is to gather information that will guide us in understanding patients and their environment. Observation is a skill that is developed through concentration, study, and practice. Areas of observation include the following:

Physiologic functioning and features Refer back to Table 1-1, p. 13 and review the list of clinical signs of nutritional status. Such features as these may be used as a basis for making detailed observations concering the patient's physical features. Learning to take an organized look at the person may help us develop greater accuracy and objectivity. It is true that we see what we have the "mindset," sensitivity, or awareness to see. Therefore, we need to develop certain sensitivities that can detect details that may provide important clues to help identify needs.

Behavior patterns Observe closely not only the physical features of the patient but also the immediate behavior in the health care situation. Attempt to look at behavior in terms of its meaning to the patient and in terms of the patient's self-concept and the illness. From these observations of patient behavior, certain assumptions—"educated guesses"—concerning immediate and long-term needs and goals can be made, always recognizing that these are assumptions and will have to be clarified with the patient to determine whether they are indeed factual. This action helps us to understand our own feelings and to rule out our own biases, prejudices, or distortions of the situation.

Environment Observing the patient's immediate environment in an organized manner is also helpful. This may be the home environment on a visit or the immediate environment in a clinic or hospital setting.

Listening

The eye can handle about 5 million bits of information per second, but the resolving power of the brain is only about 500 bits per second.

Hearing and listening are not the same thing. Hearing is only the first phase of the listening process. The function of listening is to hear, to identify the sound, to understand its meaning, and to learn by it.

Although the senses have amazing powers of perception, they are limited. The nervous system must constantly select and discriminate among those bits of information it confronts. Listening is also limited. A large part of communication time is spent in listening, but the average person without special training has only 25% listening efficiency. In other words, one "hears" only a small percent of the total surrounding communication.

Creative listening—listening with a sincere effort to see matters from the patient's point of view.

The task of the health worker is to learn the art of "creative listening." First of all, we must learn to be comfortable as a listener. Usually our lives are so filled with activity and *noise* that to sit and listen quietly is often difficult. Moreover, we have had little experience during our own development of being listend to, so that listening to others must be learned. We practice "how to listen" by staying close by, assuming a comfortable position, and giving our full attention to the person who is speaking. We show genuine interest by indicating agreement or understanding with a nod of the head or making such sounds as "uh-huh," "I see," or "And then?" at the appropriate moments in the conversation. We must learn to remain silent when the other person's comment jogs some personal memory or parallel experience of our own. We learn to listen not only to words the patient uses but also to the repetition of key words, to the rise and fall in the tone of voice, to hesitant or aggressive expression of words and ideas, and to the softness or harshness of tone. We listen to the overall content of what is being said, to the main ideas being expressed, and to the topics chosen for discussion. We listen for the feelings, needs, and goals that are being expressed. We also listen for clues, sometimes not so openly expressed, to these feelings, needs, and goals. We learn to listen to the silences and to be comfortable with them, giving the patient time to frame thoughts and give expression to them.

Responding

The responses we give to the patient may be verbal or nonverbal. Nonverbal responses include signs and actions, such as gestures and movements, silences, facial expressions, and touch. Verbal responses make use of language—words and meanings (Table 10-1). But we must remember that we give our own meanings to the words that we use. A word is only a symbol, not the thing itself. Thus we must give attention to our choice of words—we must "begin where the patient is" and provide a supportive environment for responses (see p. 221). We must watch the level and pace of our speaking. Questions should be clear, concise, free from bias, and nonthreatening. Sometimes a verbal response may be a simple restatement of what the patient has said. This enables the patient to hear the statement again and thus reinforce, expand, or correct it. At other times

Table 10-1
Verbal Responses Used by the Helping Professions

Purpose of Response	Type of Response	Description
Clarification	Content	Counselor summarizes content of conversation up to that point
	Affective	Counselor paraphrases or defines concern that client has implied but not actually stated
Leading	Closed question	Question that can be responded to with "yes" or "no," or with very few words
	Open question	Question that cannot be answered briefly; often triggers discussion or a flow of information
	Advice	Provision of an alternative type of behavior by counselor for client; may be an activity or thought
	Teaching	Information presented by counselor with intention of helping client acquire knowledge, skills, and so on to perform appropriate nutrition-related behaviors
Self-revealing	Self-involving	Response made to client's statements that reflects the personal feelings of counselor
	Self-disclosing	Response made to client's statements that reflects factual information about counselor
	Aside	Statement counselor makes to self

the response may be a reflection of what the expressed feelings seem to be. This will enable the patient to respond, to verify or deny that this was indeed the feeling. We must never act on assumptions about the patient's feelings without verifying them first.

Terminating the Interview

The close of the interview should meet several needs. It may be used to summarize the main points covered or to reinforce learning. If contact with the patient is to continue, it can include plans for the follow-up appointments or activities. It should always leave the patient with the sense

---

Clinical Application

Creating a Supportive Nutrition-Counseling Environment

Nutrition counselors may inadvertently close communication channels by (1) failing to ask questions or otherwise verbally discouraging the client from expressing concerns and expectations, or (2) using "body language" that is distracting, inappropriate, or misinterpreted by the client because of cultural differences.

Questions or statements that encourage the client to be expressive are usually *open-ended* (i.e., a simple yes-or-no response will not be adequate) or *affective,* reflecting feelings that the client may have implied but not expressed directly. Closed questions and self-referent statements do little to encourage the client to "open up" (Table 10-1).

Body language can be distracting or intimidating, or it can make the client feel "at home." The key is to understand the client's concept of:

- **Personal space** Americans like lots of room. Try sitting next to the only passenger on a city bus and note the amount of anxiety created! In other cultures (e.g., the Middle East) closeness, even to the point of pushing and shoving, is considered acceptable behavior. Thus, your *distance* from clients may affect their sense of comfort.
- **Eye contact** Americans show respect by looking each other straight in the eye; Asians, by looking downward. Attempts to interchange these two behaviors can be interpreted as rude.
- **Speech inflection** The tone of voice, its loudness and inflection, may be interpreted as threatening or comforting, depending on the region or country of origin of the listener.

You cannot always be aware of your client's attitudes towards body language ahead of time. Note any signs of uneasiness and at least invite the client to discuss anything about the interview that may be causing concern.

References
Spencer, H.: The hidden meaning of body language, Am. Pharm. **NS21**(7):416, 1981.
Danish, S.J., and others: The anatomy of a dietetic counseling interview, J. Am. Diet. Assoc. **75**:626, 1979.

that the health worker's concern has been sincere and that the door is always open for further communication, should the patient so desire.

Recording

Some means of recording the important points of the interview should be arranged. This should be as unobtrusive as possible, with little note-taking during the interview itself and completion of the record afterward. If some mechanical device is used, such as a recorder, the patient's permission must always be obtained. There needs to be full assurance that identity will be erased and that the recording is to be used for a specific purpose, such as to help the health worker improve interviewing skills or to learn the health needs of a particular group of people.

Various members of the health team contribute information about the patient in a system of written reports: this is the patient's chart, a legal document which in case of litigation could be used in court. There is an obligation to the patient to respect confidentiality of the communication and to screen what and how much information is shared and with whom. At the same time health workers have a responsibility for relaying to other members of the health team pertinent information to aid in the total planning of care.

What aspects of the patient interview should be recorded then? Data from two basic areas of communication are needed: (1) a description of the patient's general physical and emotional status, followed in some instances by judgment of the immediate and ongoing care needs, and (2) whatever care and teaching was administered, with a description of the results. In addition, we may sometimes wish to include appointments made with the patient or notes of information concerning needs that were passed on to other members of the health team or to other agencies. Similar information is often communicated through oral team reports and various case conferences.

Nutrition History and Analysis
Personal Life Situation and Food Patterns

First, learn the family's situation and values and identify health and nutrition needs through a nutrition history and its analysis. Several methods for such interviewing may be used:

1. **Twenty-four–hour recall** Ask the pateint to recall all food and drink consumed during the previous day.
2. **Food records** Have the patient record all items eaten or drunk over a 3- to 7-day period.
3. **Schedule of meal pattern or food use** Use a structured questionaire that lists common food items or food groups to obtain information about quantity and frequency of use.
4. **General food habits** Use a guided interview structure to learn the individual's basic food habits. Perhaps one of the simplest and most helpful methods for both the interviewer and the client is using the *activity-associated general day's food pattern* (Tool A, p. 223). Since for most people eating is related to activity or work throughout the day, making use of this pattern gives both the interviewer and the patient a structure—beginning, middle, and end—and provides a series of "memory jogs" to flesh out the interview with greater detail to permit

---

Tool A

**Nutrition History:
Activity-Associated
General Day's
Food Pattern**

Name _____ Date _____

Height _____ Weight (lb) _____ (kg) _____ Age _____

Ideal weight _____

Referral
Diagnosis
Diet order
Members of household
Occupation
Recreation, physical activity

Present food intake

	Place	Hour	Frequency, form, and amount checklist
Breakfast			Milk
			Cheese
			Meat
			Fish
Noon meal			Poultry
			Eggs
			Cream
			Butter, margarine
Evening meal			Other fats
			Vegetables, green
Extra meals			Vegetables, other
			Fruits (citrus)
			Legumes
Summary			Potato
			Bread—kind
			Sugar
			Desserts
			Beverages
			Alcohol
			Vitamins
			Candy

---

constructive counseling. With respect to each item, the questions are asked in terms of general habits—food item, form, frequency, preparation, portion, and seasoning—not in terms of a specific day's intake. Throughout such an interview, important clues to food attitudes and values can be communicated. Note these for later thought and exploration. If your manner throughout is interested and accepting, the information you receive should be valid and straightforward. On the other hand, if you are judgmental and authoritarian, patients will probably only tell you what they think you want to hear, not what the true situation may be.

Plan of Care

On the basis of the diet history and review of any needed health conditions requiring diet modification, develop a realistic personal food plan with the patient and the family. Then plan any related follow-up care as needed. This may take the form of return visits to the clinic, home visits, consultation and referral with other members of the health care team, or use of community resources. Follow-up work requires patience, persistence, and a steady focus on the goal. Imagination and good humor are invaluable. Take one step at a time. Guide the patient and family in applied nutrition principles, give support as needed, help with adjustments of the plan, provide reinforcement of prior learning, and continue to add new learning opportunities as the family's needs develop. Tool B (p. 225) and Tool C (pp. 226-228) provide general guides for determining nutritional needs of patients and helping to plan their care.

The Teaching-Learning Process

There is far more to teaching and learning than merely dispensing information. But the myth still prevails in much of health education that if enough information is provided, harmful health practices will be changed. This is not the case. There is a vast difference between a person who has learned and a person who has only been informed. Learning must ultimately be measured in terms of *changed behavior*. As with counseling, valid education focuses not on the practitioner-teacher or the content, but on the *patient-learner*. The health teacher's major task is to create situations in which patients and families can learn, succeed, and develop self-direction, self-motivation, and self-care (see Issues and Answers, pp. 240-241).

Aspects of Human Personality Involved in Learning

The teaching-learning experience involves three fundamental aspects of human personality—thinking, feeling, and the will to act.

Thinking

We grasp information through our personal thinking process. We take in information selectively, then process and shape it according to our needs. The total thought process provides the background knowledge that is the basis for reasoning and analysis. The learner senses the contribution of this thinking to the learning process as "I know how to do it."

Feeling

In each of us specific feelings and responses are associated with given items of knowledge and given situations. These emotions reflect desires and needs that are aroused. Emotions provide impetus, creating the tensions that spur us to act. The learner senses the contribution of emotion to the learning process as "I want to do it."

Will to Act

The will to act arises from the conviction that the knowledge discovered can fulfill the felt need and relieve the symptoms of tension. The will

Tool B

Guide for Assessment and Care of Nutrition Needs

I. Assess nutrition needs
   A. Define the person
      1. Who the person is: age, sex, family, occupational role, cultural background, socioeconomic status, personal characteristics, limitations, strengths
      2. Where the person is: physical setting—place of care, its possibilities and limitations and personal setting—mental, psychologic, emotional, and physical, in relation to health or disease, adaptation
      3. Nutritional status: food habits and general nutritional analysis (p. 269); clinical observations and signs (Table 16-1, p. 271)
   B. Determine the disease or normal physiologic stress (such as pregnancy and growth)
      1. The general disease or physiologic process: anatomy and physiology, signs and symptoms, general treatment or management, pathology, course, prognosis
      2. Patient's unique experience with the disease or physiologic stress: duration, intensity, medical management, prior diet therapy, adaptation, problems and solutions, knowledge of disease and its care—source, form, attitude, behavior response
II. Identify and define problems and develop plan of care
   A. Explore present needs
      1. Day-to-day nutritional support: maintenance, optimum intake, basic nutritional requirements
      2. Nutritional therapy: treatment by modified diet
      3. Teaching: basic nutrition knowledge or principles of special diet modification
   B. Explore future needs
      1. Continuity of care: home, responsible significant others, extended-care facility
      2. Plan for medical management: health team conferences, nursing team conferences
      3. Plan for nutritional care: diet modifications, practical food management (family situation, living alone, degree of disability, etc.), follow-up diet counseling and nutrition education, community resources
III. Carry out plan of care
   A. Physical, psychosocial responses: diet and its meaning
   B. Teaching plan: materials needed, content, sequence, methods, approaches, plan for evaluation
   C. Records of action for study
IV. Check results
   A. Follow-up care: planned with patient, family, and health team
   B. Reinforcement to strengthen learning
   C. Revision: as needed

Tool C

Stages of Nutrition Interview

I. The patient as a person
   A. Introduction
      1. Developing a relationship — Establishing rapport; putting the patient at ease; gaining the patient's confidence and trust; mutual trust
      2. Defining roles — Selling health worker's role as helper, health counselor, teacher; determining patient's role as learner and active participant in taking increasing responsibility for own learning and care according to individual capacity
      3. Determining the patient's health need or problem and related personal goals — Discovering whether the patient's goals are different from what was expected; deciding whether underlying objectives exist other than those concerning the immediate dietary problem
      4. Redefining objectives in light of patient's goals — Seeing counseling goals in terms of those of patient
   B. Patient profile — Who and what kind of person is the patient?
      1. Gathering physical data — How do these data affect the dietary problem? How long has the problem existed? Has the patient known anyone with a similar problem?
         a. Age
         b. Height
         c. Weight—present and past history
         d. Experience with disease or weight problem
      2. Understanding the patient's setting — The patient's environment: social and economic factors involved
         a. Family — Identity of family (ethnic); number in family; who cooks, markets, etc.
         b. Work — Hours; extent of activity; effect on eating habits; education
         c. Social activity — Recreation; physical exercise

Tool C—cont'd

3. Interpreting the patient's attitudes toward disease or weight problem	How has the patient's experience with the problem influenced personal belief about it? Have family members or friends influenced the patient? Fears, misconceptions, understanding

II. The patient's food habits
  A. Nutrition history

1. Determining present food intake	What does the patient usually eat? Flavorings, seasonings, condiments, beverages, other relevant additions
2. Learning place and time	Where and when does the patient eat? How do these affect what is eaten? Can any times or places be changed or eliminated?
3. Referring to checklist of various food groups and some individual foods	Keeping some form of reminder for the counselor to make sure that relevant foods have been covered
4. Determining who prepares the food and how	Possible consultation with wife or mother
B. Physical exercise and reaction: activities associated with the patient's food habits	Work, school, social gatherings, travel
C. Food reactions: patient's likes, dislikes, intolerances, allergies	Could food be accepted in a different form or by using another method of preparation? Possible substitutes?

III. Diet counseling

A. Choosing the diet	What is the diet ordered by the physician or the nutritionist? What form will be best understood by the patient?
B. Explaining the reasons for the diet	Why the increases in certain foods or restrictions on others; the effect of the disease on food; the effect of food on the disease

Continued.

Tool C—cont'd

	C. Planning a daily food pattern with the patient	Considering the patient's likes and dislikes, usual habits, and restrictions because of dietary problem; developing a dietary plan that fits into daily activity
	D. Reviewing the diet and answering questions	Answering inquiries throughout interview but asking specifically for questions or feedback toward the end
		Does the patient understand?
IV.	Termination of the interview	
	A. Planning for follow-up	When will the patient be seen again? Encouraging recording of questions or problems that may develop to discuss next time
		Should the patient keep food records of any kind?
	B. Recording the interview	Completing any needed charting of the interview
		Keeping any needed notes in records

focuses decision to act on the knowledge received so attitude, value, thought, or pattern of behavior can be changed. The learner senses the contribution of the will to the learning process as "I will do it."

Principles of Learning

Learning follows three basic laws: (1) learning is *personal,* occurring in relation to perceived needs; (2) learning is *developmental,* building on prior information; and (3) learning means change, resulting in *changed behavior.*

Individuality

Learning can only be individual. In the final analysis we must learn for ourselves, according to our own needs, in our own way and time, and for our own purpose. The teacher must discover who the learner is by asking questions that clarify the learner's relationship to the problem.

Need Fulfillment

Motivation Providing something that prompts an individual to act in a certain way.

Motivation is important to learning. Persons learn only what they believe will be useful to them, and they retain only what they think they need or shall need. The more immediately persons can put new learning to use, the more readily they grasp it. The more it satisfies their immediate goals, the more effective the learning will be.

Contact

Learning starts from a point of contact between prior experience and knowledge, an overlap of the new with the familiar. Find out what the individual already knows and to what past experience the present situation can be related. Start the process of learning at that point. Search for the areas of association that are present in the individual learner, then relate your teaching to that point of contact.

Active Participation

Since learning is an active process through which behavior changes, learners must become personally involved. One means of securing participation is through *planned feedback*. Feedback may take several forms: (1) Ask questions that require more than a "yes" or "no" answer and that reveal a degree of understanding and motivation (Table 10-1). (2) Use guided return demonstrations, which are brief periods in which procedures are practiced or skills discussed. Such guided practice develops ability, self-confidence, and security. It enables the learner to clarify the principles involved (see Issues and Answers, pp. 240-241). (3) Have the learner try out the new learning in personal experience outside the teacher-directed situation. Alternate such trials with return visits to review these experiences. Answer, or help the person to answer, any questions raised and provide continued support and reinforcement.

Appraisal

At appropriate intervals take stock of the changes that your patients have made in outlook, attitude, and actions toward their specific goals in health and nutrition education. Careful, sympathetic questioning may reveal any blocks to learning. In addition to speeding the learning process, such concern will show you whether you are communicating successfully, making contact, or making the best choices of method. It may help you recall principles that you may have glossed over. In the final analysis the measure of success in teaching lies not in the number of facts transferred, but in the change for the better that has been initiated in the client.

In all, the nutrition educator who imparts a strong knowledge and interest in the subject, shows respect and concern for each individual in the program, and projects self-confidence has the greatest chance for success. A number of sources for educational materials on sound nutrition is provided in the Appendixes.

Food Needs and Costs

Food Assistance Programs

In situations of economic stress your clients and their families may need financial help. You may need to discuss available food assistance programs and make appropriate referrals.

Commodity Distribution Program

In the post-Depression years, legislation was initiated to stabilize agricultural prices. This legislation provided for the federal government to purchase market surpluses of perishable goods. Later the resulting accumulation of food stocks led to the creation of distribution programs as a means of disposing of the stored products (Figure 10-1). Such surplus has been defined as either physical (exceeding requirements) or economic (prices below desired levels). Foods coming under these regulations include meat and poultry, fruits and vegetables, eggs, dried beans and peas. Most of these items purchased under this program have been donated by

Figure 10-1
Warehouse for food surplus
goods used in Commodity
Distribution Program.

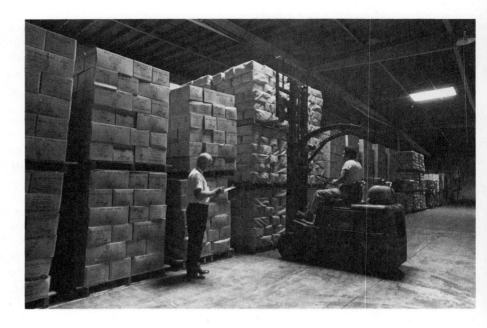

the Food and Nutrition Service of the U.S. Department of Agriculture
(USDA) to schools through the National School Lunch and School Breakfast Programs. Foods accumulated through other aspects of the legislation
are price-supported basic and nonperishable items. These foods have
been donated to child-feeding programs, summer camps, Indian reserva-
tions, trust territories, nutrition programs for the elderly, charities, disas-
ter-feeding programs, and the Commodities Supplemental Food Program
(Figure 10-2).

Figure 10-2
Pregnant mother and her
child participating in the
supplemental Commodities
Distribution Program.

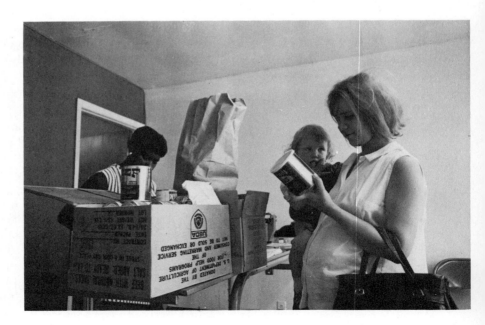

Food Stamp Program

Also growing out of the post-Depression years, the Food Stamp Program was founded to help low-income families purchase needed food. Under this program the participant is issued coupons or "food stamps." The coupons are distributed to participating "households," defined by the program as a group of people living in the same house who buy, store, and eat food together. The coupons are supposed to be sufficient to cover the household's food needs for 1 month. These households must have a net monthly income below the program's eligibility limit in order to qualify. This limit is quite low, and usually families who qualify simply aren't making enough money to buy food. Eligibility is based on gross income (Table 10-2).

Table 10-2
Eligibility Standards for the
Food Stamp Program

| | Household Size | | | | | | | | Each Additional |
	1	2	3	4	5	6	7	8	
Maximum net income level	$360	$475	$590	$705	$820	$935	$1050	$1165	+115
Maximum gross income level	$467	$617	$766	$916	$1065	$1215	$1364	$1514	+150

*Data compiled from USDA Human Nutrition Information Service, Consumer Nutrition Division, Hyattsville, Md. 20782.

NOTE: Alaska, Hawaii, and the territories have higher eligibility figures.

Child Nutrition Programs

After the Surplus Commodities Program was started, the government faced a glut of accumulated food items and needed a means of disposing of them. Then during World War II the military discovered a distressing rate of nutrition-related disorders that prevented its draftees from serving in the army. Out of these two situations the National School Lunch Program of 1946 was born.[1] From this initial program came all of the child nutrition programs of today.

National School Lunch and Breakfast Programs These programs provide financial assistance to schools to enable them to provide nutritious lunches and breakfasts to all their students. The programs allow poor children to eat free meals or meals at reduced price whereas other students pay somewhat less than the full cost of the meal. Commodity foods are available to participating schools, and the programs usually entail minimal costs to the school district. All public and private nonprofit schools are eligible to participate in the programs if their average tuition per student does not exceed $1500. Children's residential institutions, preschools, and Head Start programs run as part of a school system are also eligible. Lunches served must fulfill approximately one third of the child's Recommended Dietary Allowance (RDA) for nutrients.[2]

Child care food program This program provides USDA food commodities, cash equivalents, and meal reimbursements for most or all of the meal and administration costs of feeding children up to 12 years of age who are enrolled in organized child care programs. These settings include day care centers, recreation centers, settlement houses, and some Head Start programs. The children's eligibility for free and reduced-price meals is the same as for the school lunch and breakfast programs.

WIC The Special Supplemental Food Program for Women, Infants, and Children (WIC) provides nutritious foods to low-income women who are pregnant or breast-feeding and to their infants and children under age 5. The food is either distributed free or purchased by free vouchers (Figure 10-3). It is designed to supplement the diet with rich sources of iron, protein, and certain vitamins. The vouchers are good for such foods as milk, eggs, cheese, juice, fortified cereals, and infant formulas. The program includes funding for clinic visits for medical check-ups and for nutrition education and counseling of participants. It is administered by the USDA through state health departments and Native American tribes, bands, or groups, run locally by public or nonprofit health facilities or organizations. Participants must be pregnant or postpartum mothers (up to 6 months), lactating mothers (up to 12 months), or women having children under age 5; they must be at nutritional risk and must have an income under the reduced-price meal guidelines for the school lunch program. Factors indicating nutritional risk include evidence of an inadequate diet, poor growth patterns, a lack of nutrition understanding, or a medical history of

For a family of two to participate in the WIC program, the family income must be less than $10,530 annually.

Figure 10-3
Mother in WIC program using program vouchers at a supermarket to buy groceries.

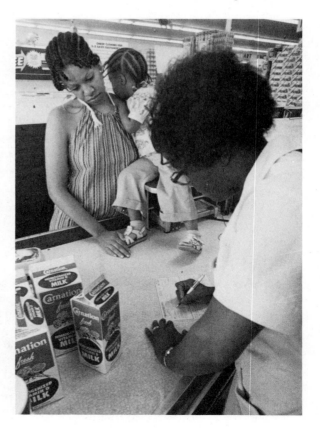

By the early 1980s, the WIC program served the needs of about 2 million persons who received benefits at just over 1000 clinics across the United States.

nutrition-related problems, such as low birthweight or premature infants, toxemia, miscarriages, and anemia. Unlike the Food Stamp or School Food Program, WIC is not an "entitlement" program. This means that eligibility does not automatically entitle one to benefits. There is an absolute ceiling each year on funding and therefore on participation.

Nutrition Program for Elderly Persons

Congress has provided two types of food programs to benefit the growing numbers of elderly citizens in the United States. Regardless of their income level, all persons over 60 years of age are eligible to receive meals from the Congregate Meals Program or the Home-Delivered Meals Program. Elderly persons often face many social, physical, and economic difficulties and do not or cannot eat adequately to fulfill their nutritional needs. Many of them suffer from isolation and social deprivation. The main difference in these two programs is their setting and social aspect: (1) the *Congregate Meals Program* provides ambulatory elderly persons with a hot nourishing meal at a community center where they can share food once a day, 5 days a week, with a group of their peers. Free transportation is often provided. Social events and nutrition information accompany the meals. (2) In comparison, the *Home-Delivered Meals Program,* sometimes called Meals-on-Wheels, provides homebound elderly persons who have difficulty preparing their own meals with at least one nutritious meal delivered to them in their home Monday through Friday. Both programs are allowed to accept voluntary contributions for meals.

Food Buying Guides

Family nutrition counseling may also involve guidance in planning for control of family food costs.

USDA Food Plans

The USDA has developed food plans at four different levels of cost: liberal, moderate, low, and thrifty. The thrifty food plan (USDA 1983)[3] was developed by nutritionists, economists, and computer experts at USDA on the basis of a predetermined level of spending appropriate to the **poverty** threshold. This plan is used to determine allotments of Food Stamp coupons to eligible households.

Poverty Having little or no money, goods, or means of support; scantiness, insufficiency; meagerness. The 1981 federal government definition of the poverty level was an annual income of less than $9,287 for a family of four.

Family food costs

A number of factors influence the way in which a family divides its food dollar. You will want to explore these factors with your client's family in helping them outline their family food plan:

1. Family income
2. Number, sex, ages, and general activities of family members
3. Whether any part of the family food is produced or preserved at home (gardening, canning, freezing)
4. Likes and dislikes of family members and special family dishes
5. Special dietary needs of any family member
6. Time, transportation, and energy available for shopping and food preparation
7. Skill and experience in family food management (planning, shopping, storing, preparing)

8. Storage and cooking facilities in the home
9. Amount and kind of entertaining, if any
10. Number of meals eaten away from home
11. Value the family places on food and eating

Good Shopping and Food Handling Practices

Today's American family spends more time shopping for food than cooking it. Food marketing is big business, and buying food for a family may seem to be a more intricate affair than the preparation of food at home. A large American supermarket may stock some 8000 or more different food items, and more are being added daily. A single food item may be marketed a dozen different ways at as many different prices. Frequently in family diet counseling and in talking with clients about special modified diets, you will observe that the family places greater stress on their need for help in food buying. Four shopping and food handling practices will help to control cost:

1. **Plan ahead** Use market guides in newspapers, plan general menus, keep a kitchen supply checklist, and make out a market list ahead of time according to location of items in a regularly visited market. Such planning helps to avert "impulse buying" and extra trips.

2. **Buy wisely** Know the market, market items, packaging, grades, brands, portion yields, measures, and food value in a market unit. Watch for sale items and buy in quantity if it results in savings and the food can be adequately stored or used. Be cautious in selecting "convenience foods." The added timesaving may not be worth the added cost.

3. **Store food safely** The kitchen waste that results from food spoilage and misuse can be controlled. Conserve food by storing items according to their nature and use, using dry storage, covered containers, and refrigeration as needed. After a food package has been opened and part of its contents consumed, keep the opened package at the front of a shelf for early use. Avoid plate waste by preparing only the amount needed by the family and use leftovers intelligently.

4. **Cook food well** Retain maximum food value in cooking processes and prepare food with imagination and good sense. Zest and appeal can be given to dishes by using a variety of seasonings and combinations. However, as much as the client and the family may have learned about nutrition, members of a family usually eat because they are hungry or because the food looks and tastes good—not necessarily because it is nutritious.

The Best Food Buys

Vegetables and Fruits

In addition to minerals, these foods supply vitamins A and C, two nutrients found in surveys to be most often lacking in the average American diet. Counsel your clients with the following guidelines:

1. Buy fresh vegetables and fruits in season. The price usually goes through seasonal cycles according to supply. For example, citrus fruits usually cost less during the winter, and fresh garden vegetables cost less during the summer. Winter garden vegetables include cabbage, winter squash, and sweet potatoes.

Completely unplanned purchases account for more than half of the items usually bought in supermarkets.

2. Select fresh produce that is firm, crisp, and heavy for size. Fresh vegetables and fruits that are of medium size are usually better buys than large, most of which may need to be discarded.

3. Distinguish between types of fresh produce defects. Small surface defects do not affect the eating quality or food value, and pieces so blemished may cost less. Many or deep defects cause more waste, as does decay that is even slightly evident.

4. Compare cost of fresh produce sold by weight or count. The resulting price per item can be computed by each method of sale to find the one that costs less.

5. Avoid fancy grades in canned vegetables and fruits. Grading is based on shape, size, and perfection of pieces. Lower grades contain small, broken, or imperfect pieces but are equal to higher grades in food value and are therefore good buys.

6. If family size warrants, buy vegetables and fruits in large cans.

7. Select low-cost dried foods. Dehydrated foods vary in price. Dried beans, peas, and lentils are excellent food buys. Specialty dried foods, however, such as potatoes, are usually more expensive than the fresh product.

8. Compare cost of frozen, canned and fresh vegetables and fruits. Frozen vegetables and fruits are usually more expensive than fresh or canned. However, specials and large family-sized packages can be compared weight for weight with canned or fresh produce in season.

9. Cook vegetables with care. Excess cooking water and time destroy or eliminate vitamins and minerals and rob the vegetable of color and texture and taste. Such unappetizing food often goes uneaten by the family and causes costly waste.

Breads and Cereals

Most bread and cereal products are well liked, inexpensive, and fit easily into meal plans. This group of foods, along with potatoes and other vegetables and fruits, provides complex carbohydrate, which nutritionists advise should be the basic staple food of most persons' diets. Whole-grain foods are good sources of dietary fiber and are high in important vitamins and minerals. They're also important sources of amino acids and, in combination with legumes, form complete or "complementary" proteins. Many foods in this group can be excellent bargains in nutrition:

1. Whole-grain or enriched products are much more nutritious than refined grains and products and are usually no more expensive.

2. Enriched specialty breads, such as French or Italian, cost up to three times more than whole-grain bread with similar or better nutritive value.

3. Precooked rice is much more expensive than unprocessed and often lacks many of the nutrients of the unprocessed rice.

4. Many cereals have nutrients added. Cereals that advertise 100% of the RDA for vitamins and minerals are usually more expensive. If the diet is adequate, such levels of fortification are unnecessary.

5. Ready-to-eat cereals and instant hot cereals and those packaged for individual servings are usually much more expensive. Buy grains in bulk if adequate storage can be provided.

6. Baked goods made at home, from scratch or even from some mixes, are usually much cheaper than bakery goods.

7. A large loaf of bread may not weigh more than a small loaf. Compare prices of equal weights of bread to find the better buy. The weight is shown on the wrapper.

8. Try unusual forms of grains. For example, bulgur, buckwheat groats, barley, and millet are excellent grains and can be the basis for delicious, nutritious new meals. Bulgur, which is cooked dried wheat, keeps well in a porous container in a cool place. It is cooked like rice, has a toastlike color, is rich in wheat flavor, and is equal in food value to whole wheat.

Protein Foods

Plant proteins Beans, peas, nuts, and grains are inexpensive sources of complementary proteins. Legumes and grains contribute different ratios of needed amino acids to provide the entire complement needed by the human body for the synthesis of body proteins (see p. 90). These foods store well, are versatile in preparation, and low in fat. They are also a good source of vitamins and minerals, including iron, zinc, and the B vitamins. Tofu, a curd made from soybeans, has been the low-cost protein backbone of the East Asian diet for more than 2000 years. Since tofu is a plant product, it has no cholesterol. It is a fair source of iron and is a good source of calcium.

A quarter pound of tofu has about 85 kcal, 8 to 10 g of protein, and 5 g of fat, most of which is unsaturated.

Eggs Eggs are sold according to grade and size, neither of which is related to food value. Usually it is best to buy the least expensive. Egg grades are based on qualities such as firmness of the egg white, appearance, and delicacy of flavor. They have no relation to food value or quality. Shell color varies with poultry species and has no effect on egg quality.

Milk and cheese Dairy products are good sources of protein, but it is important to distinguish among them for the better sources of protein that are lower in fat as well as lower in price:

1. Fluid nonfat milk, buttermilk, and canned evaporated milk cost less than whole, fluid milk. So-called low-fat milks are 2% butterfat; whole milk ranges from 3.5% to 4%, according to local regulations and individual dairy standards. To produce lower fat milks, part of the butterfat is removed from whole milk, and dried milk solids are added. Low-fat (2%) milk contains 135 kcal/cup (8 oz). Whole milk, 4%, contains 170 kcal/cup, 3.5%, 150 kcal/cup. Nonfat milk contains 80 kcal/cup.

2. Nonfat dried milk is the best bargain of all forms. Reconstituted with water it provides a fluid nonfat milk at less than half the cost of fresh form. It can also be used in innumerable ways in cooking to add valuable nutrition.

3. If the family size warrants it, buy milk in large containers. Fluid milk sometimes costs less in the half-gallon or the large bulk containers than in the quart container.

4. If cheese is used often, buy it in bulk, It costs less and keeps better.

5. Cottage cheese is an unripened, soft curd (80% moisture) and hence a rapidly perishable item. Buy it only as you use it to avoid waste resulting from spoilage.

Poultry Buy poultry as the whole bird. Usually the larger, more mature birds cost less than the young broilers and fryers and can be made equally tender with longer, moist, cooking methods such as braising, stewing or pressure cooking.

Organ meats Liver, kidney, heart are nutritious bargains; use them often. A good cookbook will have appetizing ways of preparing them for family acceptance.

Fish This is usually a good buy, since it is sold in cuts that contain little or no waste. Shellfish is more costly. Fresh fish in season is usually less expensive. Less expensive packed styles of canned fish should be used. For example, tuna is packed according to sizes of pieces. Fancy or solid pack (large pieces) is most expensive. Chunk style is made up of moderate-sized pieces and is moderate in price. Flake or grated style consists of smaller pieces and is cheapest in price.

Red meats Since meat is commonly one of the most costly food items, learn how it is graded, cut, processed, and marketed. Excellent educational material is available through the local county home advisor, a USDA extension service. Avoid cuts with large amounts of gristle, bone, and fat. The lower grades provide good quality, less fat, and cost less.

Additional Resources
Farmers' Markets

In farmers' markets local produce is made available directly to consumers. This produce has the advantage of being fresh at prices lower than that found in the supermarket. It also offers opportunities for socializing experiences between grower and consumers and gives a sense of community cohesion.

Consumer Cooperatives

Consumer cooperatives focus on the economics of food marketing as well as on the issue of nutrition and ecology. The newer food cooperatives customarily deal in bulk sales of whole and minimally processed foods. Belonging to a food cooperative increases personal responsibility and individual choice, and brings food issues more under the control of the consumer.[5,6] Many of these food cooperatives stress the purchase of locally grown foods, thus strengthening the local farmers while providing fresh foods for consumers.

Home Gardens

With a little effort any extra yard space may be turned into a home garden. Many persons are now turning to their backyards, alloted community spaces, window boxes, planter boxes on porches, and indoor potted plots to grow at least a portion of their own produce.

To Sum Up

A major role of health care professionals is to translate the large amount of nutrition information available so that it can meet the needs of clients and families. They must present it in such a way that it is easily understood, is retained and applied by the learner, and can be evaluated to improve its effectiveness and ability to meet continuing care needs. Valid health and nutrition education must focus on the needs of the learner. Goals for planning counseling and educational activities and the methods for meeting these goals must be based on identifiable client and family needs.

Families under economic stress need counseling concerning financial assistance. Various U.S. food assistance programs operate to help families in need. Referrals to appropriate agencies may be made. The nutrition counselor may also need to assist the family in planning the most economic and nutritious meals possible within their limited circumstances. The family may need help in learning good shopping and food handling practices—planning ahead, buying wisely, storing safely, and cooking appropriately to preserve nutritional values.

Questions for Review

1. Identify and describe the skills necessary for an effective nutrition counseling session.
2. Identify the basic principles of learning and describe how they may be used in planning nutrition education for one of your clients and family.
3. What government food assistance programs are available to help low-income families? What other local food resources are available in your community?
4. List and discuss the "best food buys" described in this chapter. How many of the recommended practices do you follow in selecting, storing, and preparing foods?

References

1. Report: Profile of the federal food programs, Washington, D.C., 1982, Food Research and Action Center.
2. Longen, K.: Domestic food programs: an overview, USDA Economical, Statistical, and Cooperative Services, Pub. No. ESCS-81, 1981.
3. Cleveland, L.E., and Peterkin, B.B.: USDA 1983 family food plans, Fam. Economics Rev. **2**:12, 1983.
4. Field, C.R., and others: Nutrition knowledge and preferences of food-cooperative shoppers, J. Am. Diet. Assoc. **82**(4):389, 1983.
5. Ehlers, K.M., and Fox, H.: Food-cooperative shoppers: nutrition knowledge, attitudes, and concerns, J. Am. Diet. Assoc. **80**(2):160, 1982.

Further Readings

Black, H., ed.: The Berkeley co-op food book: eat better and spend less, Palo Alto, Calif. 1980, Bull Publishing Co.

  A helpful guide for price-conscious families who want to become informed consumers.

Briley, M.E., and others: Validation and application of nutrition education objectives, J. Am. Diet. Assoc. **82**(4):385, 1983.

  A good study reporting a comprehensive list of learning objectives under seven concepts that can provide useful reference for planning nutrition education.

Diaz-Duque, O.F.: Advice from an interpreter, Am. J. Nursing **82**:1380, 1982.

  Good article concerning folk jargon and the "nodding" syndrome—the quick nod by patients to questions not really understood—which can lead to a language barrier, sometimes with dire results.

Lauer, P., Murphy, S.P., and Powers, M.J., Learning needs of cancer patients: a comparison of nurse and patient perceptions, Nurs. Res. **31**(1):11, 1982.

  Study revealing patients' and their nurses' differing views on patients' needs in areas of disease process, diagnosis, views of treatment, and nutrition.

USDA Food and Nutrition Service, Building a better diet, Program Aid No. 1241, 1979.

USDA Food and Nutrition Service, Eating for better health, Program Aid No. 1290, 1981.

USDA Human Nutrition Information Service, Your money's worth in foods, Home and Garden Bulletin #183, 1982.

  Practical booklets filled with information on meal planning, food shopping and preparation—a counseling aid for families who want to economize on food; prepared especially to help persons on a food stamp budget eat healthy foods.

Issues and Answers

Person-Centered Diabetes Education

A recent investigation of national patient education programs indicated that many of them provided information and skills training without incorporating learning theories in the design of the program. They also lacked a systematic way of assessing and influencing learner attitudes.

Learning theories are usually based on the psychosocial as well as educational needs of the persons involved. This relationship has an extremely important role to play in diabetes education. Since approximately 75% of all treated persons with diabetes fail to follow their prescribed diets, we should start to examine what we are doing in designing instruction for persons with diabetes. Ask yourself these questions:

Is the Teaching Process Effective?
Does it take into account the following:

- How people learn?
- What is worth learning?
- Who really is responsible for a person's health?
- What responsibilities for learning lie with the learner vs. the instructor?

Is the Learning Process Effective?
Does it consider the following:

- How significant the condition is to the person at that point in his/her life?
- How the person's sense of "psychological safety" is affected? (i.e., does the person feel accepted well enough to discuss diabetes control problems openly and honestly?)
- How the instructor will know if the person's attitude has changed toward receiving or using new information?

When you are planning a diabetes education program, these questions will remind you of important factors that influence learning behavior. While these questions seem to be immediately beyond the realm of nutrition, they are extremely important in any aspect of the care plan and learning process because *diabetes control lies primarily in the hands of the person with the diabetes.* No matter how much information is provided, it is ultimately up to the individual person to decide what foods will be selected, how much will be eaten, and when it will be eaten.

Diabetes educators often fail to consider major aspects of the person's individual and personal life that may influence these decisions: family, finances, work situation, or social activities. They also may fail to recognize the effect these activities have on the individual's sense of personal responsibility for health. These considerations may influence the type of instruction provided or even the decision to provide instruction at that time at all.

Issues and Answers—cont'd

The educator must be able to assess the person's sense of responsibility for continuing self-care and use this information to develop or revise instruction and counseling that will lead to positive behavior. Health workers may benefit from the systematic methods of assessment that have already been developed in the field of clinical psychology. Therapists have identified five levels of responsibility and client characteristics, with possible intervention methods for each level:

Levels of personal Responsibility	Client Characteristics	Intervention Method
Being diabetic is a disaster	Feels hopeless, helpless, defeated; self-care may be impossible	Educate family member or other caregiver
Being diabetic is a burden	Blames problem on others; expects others to feel sorry for him; feels angry, threatened	Provide emotional support; help client accept anger in order to move on
Being diabetic is a problem	Blames self as often as others; personal growth is possible	Reinforce attitudes that reflect sense of responsibility; examine nonresponsibility; examine nonresponsibility; examine nonresponsible attitudes in nonjudgmental way
Being diabetic is a challenge	Rarely blames others for problem; recognizes responsibility but does not act on it; good self-care expected	Point out discrepancies between stated need and actual behavior
Being diabetic is an opportunity	Takes total responsibility for the problem; acts positively on decisions; optimal self-care is expected	Provide tools required for good self-care

Such a system of assessing client attitudes has specific benefits:
1. It recognizes—and reinforces in the instructor—the fact that the client is ultimately responsible for his/her own health.
2. It gives the instructor an objective, measurable way of assessing client attitudes so that these can be compared and evaluated for indications of progress.
3. It serves as a basis for selecting appropriate teaching methods or counseling techniques, which can then be changed to match the client's current level of responsibility.

References
Anderson, R.M., Genthner, R.W., and Alogna, M.: Diabetes patient education: from philosophy to delivery, Diabetes Educator 8:33, 1982.
Surwit, R.S., Scovern, A.W., and Feinglos, M.N.: The role of behavior in diabetes care, Diabetes Care 5(3):337, 1982.

Chapter 11
Nutrition During Pregnancy and Lactation

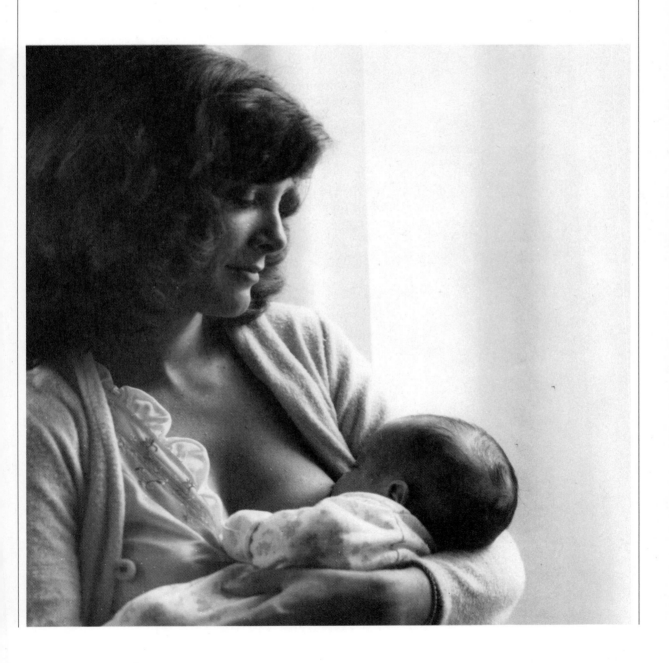

Preview

Human reproduction involves complex processes of rapid, specialized growth. Given a positive environment, including sufficient nutritional support, both mother and child possess tremendous powers of adaptation that enable them to meet these demands. We have seen in the previous chapters of our study that healthy body tissues depend directly on certain essential nutrients in food. Here we see that the infant's development relates directly to the diet of the mother.

In this chapter we start our journey through human needs during the life cycle. Here we look at the beginnings of life. We will explore the nutritional needs of pregnancy and the vital role this basic support plays in its successful outcome.

Chapter Objectives

After study of this chapter, the student should be able to:

1. Relate the mother's specific increased nutritional demands during her pregnancy to her changed physiology.

2. Plan realistic food patterns to meet these increased maternal nutritional needs.

3. Identify functional problems sometimes encountered during pregnancy and make general dietary suggestions for their control.

4. Identify possible complications of pregnancy and related dietary management.

5. Develop food plans to meet the nutritional needs of breast-feeding mothers.

Maternal Nutrition and the Outcome of Pregnancy

Background for Change

Early Practices: False Assumptions and Folklore

For centuries, in all cultures, a great body of folklore has grown up around pregnancy. Traditional practices and diet have been followed, many of which have had little basis in fact. Early obstetricians even developed the notion that semistarvation of the mother during pregnancy was really a blessing in disguise because it produced a small, lightweight baby, easy to deliver. To this end they used diet restricted in kilocalories, protein, water, and salt. Incredible as it now seems—despite the lack of any scientific evidence to support such ideas—this general view became planted in obstetric textbooks and practice and for some time was passed on from one generation of physicians to the next. Two assumptions grew and governed practice: (1) *the parasite theory:* whatever the fetus needs it will draw from the stores of the mother despite the maternal diet, and (2) *the maternal instinct theory:* whatever the fetus needs, the mother will instinctively crave and consume. Both of these theories are false. On the contrary, the current weight of scientific evidence underscores meeting increased nutritional needs for a successful pregnancy.

Current Practice: Positive Physiologic Demands

Clinical observations and developing science in both nutrition and medicine have refuted these prior false ideas and laid a sound base for positive nutrition in current obstetric practice. The benchmark report of the National Research Council, *Maternal Nutrition and the Course of Human Pregnancy,*[1] provided clear direction for a new positive approach to the nutritional management of pregnancy. Continuing research has reinforced this positive direction, guides for nutritional care of pregnant women have been issued by both the American College of Obstetrics and Gynecology and the American Dietetic Association. These guides, as outlined here, provide physicians, nutritionists, dietitians, and nurses with fundamental principles of nutrition for prenatal care. A child is nutritionally 9 months old at birth, even older when one considers the significance of the mother's preconception nutritional status. Ancient Chinese wisdom has long assigned the counting of age at birth as 1 year.

Factors Determining Nutritional Needs

Increased knowledge and the wide experience of many practitioners clearly demonstrate that maternal nutrition is critically important to both mother and child. It lays the fundamental foundation for the successful outcome of pregnancy—a healthy and happy mother and child (Figure 11-1). Several vital considerations emerge as factors governing nutritional requirements during pregnancy.

Age and Parity of the Mother

The teenage mother adds her own growth needs to those imposed by her pregnancy.[2] At the other end of the reproductive cycle, hazards increase with age. The number of pregnancies—**parity**—and the intervals between them also influence the needs of the mother and the outcome of the pregnancy.

Parity The number of children born alive.

Figure 11-1
A healthy child and mother—
happy participants in the
WIC Program.

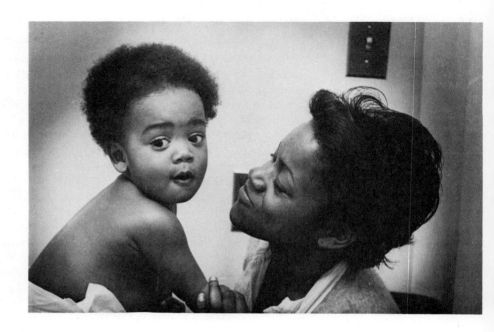

Placenta Tissue that
becomes active during
pregnancy, providing a
selective exchange of soluble
particles in the blood to and
from the fetus.

Preconception Nutrition

The mother brings to her pregnancy all of her previous life experiences, including her diet. Her general health and fitness and her state of nutrition at the time of her infant's conception are products of her lifelong dietary habits and genetic heritage.

Complex Metabolic Interactions of Gestation

Three distinct biologic entities are involved in pregnancy: the mother, the fetus, and the **placenta**. Together they form a unique biologic whole. Constant metabolic interactions go on among them. Their functions, while unique, are at the same time interdependent.

Basic Concepts Involved

As a result of our increased knowledge of pregnancy and nutrition, we can provide better nutritional guidance. Three basic concepts form a fundamental framework for assessing maternal nutrition needs and for planning supportive prenatal care for both parents.

Perinatal Concept

The prefix *peri-* comes from the Greek root meaning *around, about,* or *surrounding.* As knowledge and understanding increase, we see that the whole of the mother's life experiences surrounding her pregnancy must be considered. Cultural and social influences have shaped beliefs and values of both parents about pregnancy. Previous years of living and food habits have determined the mother's current nutritional status and nutrient reserves for the present pregnancy. All these influences are important.

Synergism Concept

Synergism is a term used to describe biologic systems in which the cooperative action of two or more factors produces a total effect greater than and different from the mere sum of their parts. In short, a new whole is created by the unified, joint effort of blending of parts in which each part influences the action of the other. Of the many biologic and physiologic interactions providing examples of synergism, pregnancy is a prime example. Maternal organism, fetus, and placenta combine to create a new whole, not existing before, and producing a total effect greater than and different from the sum of their parts. This collaborative effort exists for the sole purpose of sustaining and nurturing the pregnancy and its offspring. Physiologic measures change. Blood volume increases, cardiac output increases, and ventilation rate and tidal volume increase. The physiologic norms of the nonpregnant woman do not apply. The normal physiologic adjustments of pregnancy cannot be viewed as pathologic with application of treatment procedures for that same type of response in an abnormal state. For example, a normal physiologic generalized edema of pregnancy is a protective response. It reflects the normal increase in total body water necessary to support the increased metabolic work of pregnancy and is associated with enhanced reproductive performance.

Life Continuum Concept

Each child becomes a part of the ongoing family and continuum of life. Through the food each mother eats, she gives to her unborn child the nourishment required to begin and sustain fetal growth. Both parents carry over their nutritional beliefs and habits in their feeding and teaching of their growing child. These attitudes and values are internalized and passed on to future generations of children. Parenting includes both mother and father.

Positive Nutritional Demands of Pregnancy

The period of **gestation** is an exceedingly rapid growth period.[3] The human life grows from a single fertilized egg cell (ovum) to a fully developed infant weighing about 3 kg (7 lbs). What nutrients must the mother's diet supply to meet the nutritional demands of the fetus and of her own chaning body during this critical period of human growth and development? Throughout the pregnancy there is an increased need for all the basic nutrients (Table 11-1). Individual variations such as body size, activity, and multiple pregnancy need to be considered. Also quantitative need for nourishment of pregnant adolescents must be noted.[4] We use the Recommended Dietary Allowances (RDA) nutrient standards wisely when we view them as guidelines not requirements because they are not intended to represent merely literal (minimal) requirements of average individuals, but to cover substantially the individual variations in the requirements of healthy people.[5] In considering the needs of the healthy pregnant woman, we will review here the nutrient elements in terms of (1) the general amount of increased intake indicated, (2) why this increase is recommended, and (3) how it can be obtained in basic foods.

Energy

Kilocalories must be sufficient to (1) supply the increased energy demanded by the increased metabolic workload and (2) spare protein for

Table 11-1

Recommended Daily Dietary Allowances of Some Selected Nutrients for Pregnancy and Lactation (National Research Council, 1980 revision)

Nutrients	Nonpregnant girl		Nonpregnant women	Pregnancy				Lactation (850 ml daily)			
					Girl				Girl		
	12-14 yr 47 kg (103 lb)	14-18 yr 55 kg (120 lb)	25 yr 58 kg (128 lb)	Added Need	12-14 yr	14-18 yr	Woman 25 yr	Added Need	12-14 yr	14-18 yr	Woman 25 yr
Kilocalories	2200	2100	2000	300	2500	2400	2300	500	2700	2600	2500
Protein (g)	48	48	44	30	76	76	74	20	66	68	64
Calcium (g)	1.2	1.2	0.8	0.4	1.6	1.6	1.2	0.4	1.6	1.6	1.2
Iron (mg)	18	18	18	‡	18+	18+	18+	‡	18+	18+	18+
Vitamin A (RE)*	800	800	800	200	1000	1000	1000	400	1200	1200	1200
Thiamin (mg)	1.1	1.1	1.0	0.4	1.5	1.5	1.4	0.5	1.6	1.6	1.5
Riboflavin (mg)	1.3	1.3	1.2	0.3	1.6	1.6	1.5	0.5	1.8	1.8	1.7
Niacin equivalent and tryptophan (mg)	15	14	13	2	17	16	15	5	20	19	18
Ascorbic acid (mg)	50	60	60	20	70	80	80	40	90	100	100
Vitamin D (μg)†	10	10	5	5	15	15	10	5	15	15	10

*Retinol equivalents.
†Cholecalciferol; 10μg equals 400 IU vitamin D.
‡Required iron supplement 30-60 mg.

tissue-building. A minimum of about 36 kcal/kg is required for efficient use of protein during pregnancy. The RDA standard recommends an additional amount of energy—300 kcal, a 10% to 15% increase over the previous prepregnant standard or about 2200 kcal. This amount may be insufficient for an active, large, or nutritionally deficient woman, who may need as much as 2500 to 3000 kcal. Remember that a minimum of 1800 kcal is required just to avoid negative nitrogen balance, to say nothing of the added pregnancy and activity needs. This primary emphasis on sufficient kilocalories is critical to the support of the pregnancy and necessary to ensure nutrient and energy needs. Appropriate weight gain during the pregnancy will indicate whether sufficient kilocalories are provided.

Protein

Since protein is the essential growth element of the body, there is an increased essential requirement.

Amount of Increase

An additional daily allowance of 30 g of protein is recommended throughout the pregnancy. This added amount raises the 44 g required by the normal nonpregnant woman to at least 74 g daily. This represents an increase of about 66%.

Reasons for Increased Requirement

Protein, with its essential constituent nitrogen, is the nutrient basic to growth. Nitrogen balance studies give some indication of the large amount of nitrogen used by the mother and the child during pregnancy. More protein is essential to meet tissue demands posed by:

Rapid growth of the fetus A study of fetal tissue composition indicates the amount of nitrogen stored by the embryo rises from 0.9 g at conception to 55.9 g at delivery. The mere increases in size of the infant from one cell to multiple cells in a 3.5 kg (7 lb) child indicates how much protein is required for such rapid growth.

Development of the placenta The mature placenta at term has stored about 17 g of nitrogen. Sufficient protein is required for its complete development during pregnancy as a vital organ to sustain, support, and nourish the fetus.

Enlargement of maternal tissues Increased development of breast and uterine tissue is required to support the pregnancy. An estimated 17 g of nitrogen is incorporated into the developing maternal breast tissue and nearly 40 g into the increased uterine tissue. In addition, a general maternal reserve tissue is required. About 200 to 350 g of nitrogen is stored for the approaching losses during labor and delivery. For example, 300 to 500 ml or more of blood (protein tissue) may be lost during delivery. Also, the increased tissue is required in preparation for the physiologic demands of lactation to follow.

Increased maternal circulating blood volume A particular increase of protein is demanded by the increase in the mother's circulating blood volume of 20% to 50% or more above her normal volume. With this increase comes need for increased synthesis of the constituents of blood, especially hemoglobin and plasma protein, both of which are proteins vital to the support of the pregnancy. Increased hemoglobin is required to supply oxygen to the growing cells. Increased plasma protein (albumin) is required to keep the increased blood volume circulating by maintaining normal colloidal osmotic pressure and operation of the capillary fluid shift mechanism. This mechanism prevents accumulation of abnormal amounts of water in the tissues.

Formation of amniotic fluid The fluid surrounding the fetus is designed to protect it from shock or trauma. The fluid contains protein, hence its formation requires still more protein.

Storage reserves Increased storage reserves are required in maternal tissue to prepare for labor, delivery, the immediate postpartum period, and lactation. About 200 to 350 g of nitrogen is stored, thus, as a maternal reserve.

Food Sources

Milk, meat, egg, and cheese are complete protein foods of high biologic value. Protein-rich foods also contribute other nutrients such as calcium, iron, and B vitamins. The amounts of these foods that will supply the quantities of protein needed are indicated in the recommended daily food

Table 11-2
Core Food Plan for Daily Intake During Pregnancy and Lactation*

Food	Nonpregnant Woman	Pregnancy	Lactation
Milk, cheese, ice cream, skimmed or buttermilk (food made with milk can supply part of requirement	2 cups	3-4 cups	4-5 cups
Meat (lean meat, fish, poultry, cheese, occasional dried beans or peas	1 serving (3-4 oz)	2 servings (6-8 oz); include liver frequently	2½ servings (8 oz)
Eggs	1	1-2	1-2
Vegetable† (dark green or deep yellow)	1 serving	1 serving	1-2 servings
Vitamin C–rich food† Good source: citrus fruit, berries, cantaloupe Fair source: tomatoes, cabbage, greens, potatoes in skin	1 good source or 2 fair sources	1 good source and 1 fair source or 2 good sources	1 good source and 1 fair source or 2 good sources
Other vegetables, fruits, juices	2 servings	4-6 servings	4-6 servings
Bread‡ and cereals (enriched or whole grain)	6 servings	10 servings	10 servings
Butter or fortified margarine	Moderate amount	Moderate amount	Moderate amount

*Meets nutrient needs; add additional foods as needed for energy (kilocalorie) demands.
†Use some raw daily.
‡One slice of bread or ½ cup starch (grains or vegetables) equals 1 serving.

plan (Table 11-2). Additional protein may be obtained from legumes and whole grains while lesser amounts are available in nuts and seeds.

Minerals

The increased need for calcium and iron should be particularly emphasized throughout pregnancy.

Calcium

The pregnant woman should increase her daily calcium intake by 400 mg. Since the suggested intake for the nonpregnant woman is 800 mg, the total daily intake during pregnancy should be 1200 mg, about a 50% increase.

Reasons for increased requirements The size of the recommended increase indicates the importance of calcium to the mother and fetus. Calcium is the essential element for the construction and maintenance of bones and teeth. It is also an important constituent of the blood-clotting mechanism and is used in normal muscle action and other essential metabolic activities. The rapid fetal mineralization of skeletal tissue during the final period of growth demands more calcium.

Food sources Dairy products are a primary source of calcium. Some increase in milk or equivalent milk foods, such as cheese, ice cream, skim milk powder used in cooking, is recommended. Additional calcium is obtained in whole or enriched cereal grain and in green, leafy vegetables.

Iron

A woman should maintain a daily intake of 18 mg of iron throughout her childbearing years. This amount is necessary to replenish menstrual losses and to restore tissue and liver reserves after each pregnancy. To meet the iron needs of pregnancy, however, iron supplements in addition to dietary sources are usually recommended because the "iron cost" of a pregnancy is high. With increased demands of iron, often insufficient maternal stores, and inadequate provision through the usual diet, a regular daily supplement of 30 to 60 mg of iron is recommended for healthy women. If the woman is anemic at conception, a larger therapeutic amount, 120 to 200 mg iron, is recommended.

Reasons for increased requirement Increased iron is necessary to (1) maintain the mother's hemoglobin level given the increased blood volume; (2) provide for fetal development, especially a reserve in the fetal liver to last about 6 months after birth, since the boby's first food—milk—lacks iron; and (3) provide maternal iron stores to fortify the mother against blood losses at delivery.

Iron supplements The needed amount of iron can be obtained by checking the percentage of elemental iron in the iron preparation being used. For example, the commonly used compound *ferrous sulfate* is a hydrated salt $(FeSO_4) \cdot 7\ H_2O$, which contains 20% iron. It is usually dispensed as tablets containing 195, 300, or 325 mg of the ferrous sulfate compound. Each tablet, then, would contain 39, 60, or 65 mg of iron, respectively. Thus to supply a regular daily supplement of 60 mg of iron, one 300 mg tablet of ferrous sulfate should be used and, for a therapeutic dose of 120 mg iron, two tablets.

Increased blood circulation During pregnancy, the maternal circulating blood volume increases from 40% to 50% and more for multiple births. An adequate supply of iron prevents physiologic "dilution" anemia by providing for the increased hemoglobin demand.

Food sources Liver contains far more iron than any other food. You may encourage its use by suggesting appetizing ways of serving it. Other meat, dried beans, dried fruit, green vegetables, eggs, and enriched cereals provide additional sources of iron.

Vitamins

Increased amounts of vitamin A, B complex, C, and D are needed during pregnancy.

Vitamin A

A daily increase of 200 μg retinol equivalents (RE) is recommended for pregnancy. This is about a 25% increase over the usual adult intake. Vitamin A is an essential factor in cell development, maintenance of the integrity of epithelial tissue, tooth formation, and normal bone growth. Liver is an excellent food source. Other good sources include egg yolk, butter or fortified margarine, dark green and yellow vegetables, and fruits.

B Vitamins

There is a special need for B vitamins during pregnancy. These are usually supplied by a well-balanced diet that is increased in quantity and quality to supply all of the needed vitamins. The B vitamins are important as coenzyme factors in a number of metabolic activities related to energy production, tissue protein synthesis, and functions of muscle and nerve tissue. They play key roles in the increased metabolic activities of pregnancy.

There is an increased metabolic demand for folic acid during pregnancy. Folic acid deficiency usually occurs in conditions of general malnutrition. This makes the pregnant woman in a high-risk, low-socioeconomic situation especially vulnerable. A specific type of megaloblastic anemia caused by maternal folate deficiency sometimes occurs and warrants supplementation of the diet with folic acid. This added amount is particularly needed where such demands are greater, as in a multiple pregnancy. The RDA standard recommends a daily supplement of 400 μg of folic acid to prevent such deficiencies (see p. 259).

Vitamin C

Special emphasis must be given to the pregnant woman's need for ascorbic acid. This vitamin is essential to the formation of intercellular cement substance in developing connective tissue and vascular systems. It also increases the absorption of the iron needed for increasing quantities of hemoglobin. A daily increase of 20 mg is recommended. Added to the adult recommendation of 60 mg, this makes a recommended daily total of 80 mg during pregnancy or a 25% increase. Additional food sources such as citrus fruit and other fruits and vegetables should be included in the mother's diet to meet these increased needs.

Vitamin D

Adults who lead active lives with adequate exposure to sunlight probably need little additional source of vitamin D. During pregnancy, however, the increased need for calcium and phosphorus presented by the developing fetal skeletal tissue necessitates additional vitamin D to promote the absorption and use of these minerals. The recommended amount for pregnancy is 400 IU (15 μg calciferol) daily. Frequently supplementary vitamin D may be used. Food sources include fortified milk, butter, liver, egg yolk, and fortified margarine.

Dietary Patterns: General and Alternative
General Daily Food Pattern

A variety of familiar foods can usually supply the mother's need for added nutrients and make eating a pleasure. The increased quantities of essential nutrients needed during pregnancy may be met in many ways by planning around a daily food pattern and using key types of suggested foods. A general daily food pattern, which meets basic nutrient needs but not necessarily sufficient kilocalories, is suggested in Table 11-2. It may be used as a guide, with additional food added according to energy and nutrient needs, as well as personal desires. This pattern represents the "orthodox middle-class American diet." It has been labeled the "biomedically recommended prenatal diet," which is generally used by most health professionals in industrialized affluent countries worldwide.[6]

Alternative Food Patterns

It is always important to use the patient's own personal food patterns in diet counseling. Sometimes we rigidly adhere to the "orthodox biomedical" pattern above as *the only* pattern for all pregnant women. However, it is but one alternative diet pattern among many others from different countries, belief systems, and lifestyles. An extremist, unquestioning pursuit of "science as magic" may well lead us to label in turn *any* alternative practice as unscientific and reasonable and to close our minds to some possibly fruitful avenues of scientific exploration. *Specific nutrients*, not specific foods, are required for a successful pregnancy. These nutrients are found in a wide variety of food choices. If we are wise, we will encourage our clients to use foods that serve their nutritional needs, *whatever* those foods might be. A number of resources have been developed to serve as guides for a variety of alternative food patterns, ethnic and vegetarian.[7] In essence, two important principles govern the diet: (1) that the pregnant woman eat a sufficient quantity of food and (2) that she eat regularly, avoiding any habit of fasting or skipping meals, especially breakfast.

General Dietary Problems

Functional Gastrointestinal Problems

During pregnancy, the mother may encounter several general functional gastrointestinal difficulties. These are highly individual in form and extent and require individual counseling or control. Usually the complaints are short-term and relatively minor. However, if they persist or become extreme, they will need special attention.

Nausea and Vomiting

These symptoms, or so-called "morning sickness" of early pregnancy, are usually mild and transitory. A number of factors may contribute to the conditions. Some are physiologic and traceable to the hormonal changes that occur in early pregnancy. These changes are probably increased in some patients by psychologic factors, various situational tensions, or anxieties concerning the pregnancy itself. Simple treatment usually improves food toleration. For example, small frequent meals, fairly dry, and consisting chiefly of easily digested energy foods such as carbohydrates are more readily tolerated. Liquids may best be taken between meals instead of with food. If the condition develops to **hyperemesis gravidarum**—a severe, prolonged, persistent vomiting that can be life threatening—the mother is hospitalized and receives peripheral parenteral nutrition (see p. 520) and careful oral refeeding.[8]

Hyperemesis gravidarum
Severe vomiting that is potentially fatal.

Constipation

This complaint is seldom more than minor. Two factors during the latter part of pregnancy may make elimination somewhat difficult: (1) the pressure of the enlarging uterus on the lower portion of the intestine and (2) the added effect of the hormonal muscle-relaxant action of placental hormones on the gastrointestinal tract. In addition to adequate exercise, increased fluid intake and use of naturally laxative foods such as whole grains, dried fruits (especially prunes and figs), and other fruits and juices usually induces regularity. Laxatives should be avoided.

Weight Gain During Pregnancy

Amount of Weight Gain

Optimal weight gain of the mother during pregnancy is an important reflection of good nutritional status and contributes to a successful course and outcome. It should not become a problem. Usually the amount gained is about 11 to 13 kg (25 to 30 lb) as indicated in Table 11-3. The concept previously held by some practitioners of kilocalorie restrictions to avoid large total weight gains and thereby to avoid toxemia is without foundation. Evidence is mounting from a number of sources that women produce healthy babies within a wide range of total weight gain. For example, comprehensive data gathered over a number of years of study indicate that the range of weight gain in healthy pregnancies with normal outcomes varies widely according to individual need and situation. Indeed, the fulfillment of energy needs during pregnancy is a most critical demand for a successful outcome. Problems such as high-risk low-birth-weight babies are associated with inadequate maternal weight gain during the pregnancy (see p. 258).

Table 11-3
Approximate Weight of Products of a Normal Pregnancy

Products	Weight
Fetus	3400 g (7.5 lb)
Placenta	450 g (1 lb)
Amniotic fluid	900 g (2 lb)
Uterus (weight increase)	1100 g (2.5 lb)
Breast tissue (weight increase)	1400 g (3 lb)
Blood volume (weight increase)	1800 g (4 lb) (1500 ml)
Maternal stores	1800-3600 g (4-8 lb)
TOTAL	11000-13000 g (11-13 kg; 24 to 28 lb)

Quality of Weight Gain

The important consideration lies not so much in the quantity of weight gain but in the *quality* of the gain and the foods consumed to bring it about, rather than on a restriction on the amount of weight gained. Some practitioners have failed to distinguish between weight gained as result of edema and that due to deposition of fat—maternal stores laid down for energy to sustain fetal growth during the latter part of pregnancy and energy for lactation to follow.[9] Analysis of the total tissue gained in an average pregnancy shows that the largest component, about 62%, is water. Fat accounts for 31% and protein 7%. Water is also the most variable component of the tissue gained, accounting for a range of 8 kg (18 lb) to as much as 11 kg (24 lb). Of the 8 kg of water usually gained, about 5.5

kg (12 lb) is associated with fetal tissue and other tissues gained in pregnancy. The remaining 2.5 kg (6 lb) accumulates in the maternal interstitial tissues. Gravity causes the maternal tissue fluids to pool more in the lower extremities, leading to general swelling of the ankles. This condition is seen routinely in pregnant women. This fluid retention during pregnancy is a normal adaptive phenomenon designed to support the pregnancy and extert a postive effect on fetal growth. During pregnancy the connective tissue becomes more **hygroscopic** as a result of estrogen-induced changes in the ground substance of the tissue. The connective tissue thus becomes softer and more easily distended to facilitate delivery through the cervix and vaginal canal. Also, increased tissue fluid during pregnancy provides a means for handling the increased metabolic work and circulation of numerous metabolites necessary for fetal growth. Clearly, severe caloric restriction is unphysiologic and potentially harmful to the developing fetus and the mother. Such restriction inevitably is accompanied by restriction of vitally needed nutrients essential to the growth process. Thus *weight reduction should never be undertaken during pregnancy*. On the contrary, sufficient weight gain, more for the underweight woman than for the overweight woman, should be encouraged with the use of a nourishing diet as outlined.

Hygroscopic Taking up and retaining moisture readily.

Rate of Weight Gain

About 900 to 1800 g (2 to 4 lb) is an average gain during the first trimester. Thereafter, about 450 g (1 lb a week during the remainder of the pregnancy is usual. The individual woman who needs to gain more should not have unrealistic "grid patterns" imposed on her. It is only unusual patterns of gain—such as a sudden sharp increase in weight after the 20th week of pregnancy—which may indicate excessive, abnormal water retention, that should be watched.

Sodium

Sometimes in relation to weight gain, questions are raised about the use of salt during pregnancy. A regular moderate amount of dietary sodium is needed, about 2 to 3 g daily. This can be achieved through general use of salt in cooking and seasoning but limiting extra use at the table (see p. 259). Any routine restriction of sodium beyond this general use is unphysiologic and unfounded. Maintenance of the increased circulating blood volume, which is normal during pregnancy to support the increased metabolic work, requires adequate amounts of both sodium and protein. The National Research Council and both the professional nutrition and obstetrics guidelines have labeled routine use of salt-free diets and diuretics as potentially dangerous.

High-Risk Mothers and Infants
Identify Risk Factors Involved

To avoid the consequences of poor nutrition during pregnancy, mothers at risk should be identified as soon as possible. Risk factors that identify women with special nutritional needs during pregnancy are given in Table 11-4. These nutrition-related factors are based on clinical evidence of inadequate nutrition. However, rather than waiting for clinical symptoms of

Table 11-4
Nutritional Risk Factors in
Pregnancy

Risk Factors Presented at the Onset of Pregnancy	Risk Factors Occurring During Pregnancy

Age
  15 years or younger
  35 years or older
	Low hemoglobin and/or hematocrit
	  Hemoglobin less than 12.0 g
	  Hematocrit less than 35.0 mg/dl

Frequent pregnancies: three or more during a 2-year period	Inadequate weight gain
	  Any weight loss
	  Weight gain of less than 2 lb per month after the 1st trimester

Poor obstetric history or poor fetal performance	Excessive weight gain: greater than kg (2 lb) per week after the first trimester
Poverty	
Bizarre or faddist food habits	
Abuse of nicotine, alcohol, or drugs	
Therapeutic diet required for a chronic disorder	

Inadequate weight
  Less than 85% of standard weight
  More than 120% of standard weight	

poor nutrition to appear, a better approach would be to identify poor food patterns that will bring on nutritional problems and prevent these problems from developing. Look for three types of dietary patterns that will not support optimal maternal and fetal nutrition: (1) insufficient food intake, (2) poor food selection, and (3) poor food distribution throughout the day.[9] These patterns, added to the list of risk factors in Table 11-4, would provide a much more sensitive measure of nutritional risk.

Plan Personal Care

On the basis of such early assessment, practitioners can then give more careful attention to women identified as having higher risks in their pregnancies. By working closely with each woman and her own personal patterns of food intake and living situation, a food plan can be developed to ensure an adequate intake of all the nutrient increases demanded for support of the pregnancy and its successful outcome.

Recognize Special Counseling Needs

In addition to avoiding dangerous practices—such as diet fads, macrobiotics or fruitarianism (see p. 102), and **pica**—several special needs require sensitive counseling:

Pica Perverted appetite or craving for unnatural foods, such as chalk or clay, sometimes seen in pregnancy or in malnourished children.

Nulligravida A woman who has never been pregnant.

Primigravida A woman pregnant for the first time.

Age and parity Pregnancies at either age extreme of the reproduction cycle pose special problems. The adolescent pregnancy carries many social and nutrition-related risks. Imposed on a still-growing teenaged body are the additional demands of the pregnancy. **Nulligravidas** 15 years old and younger are especially at risk, since their own growth is incomplete. Sensitive counseling provides both information and emotional support. It should involve family or other persons significant to the young mother. On the other hand, the older **primigravida** (over 35 years of age) also requires special attention. She may be more at risk for hypertension, either preexisting or induced by the pregnancy, and may need more attention given to rate of weight gain and amount of sodium used. In addition, several pregnancies within a limited number of years leave a mother drained of nutritional resources and entering each successive pregnancy at a higher risk. Counseling may well include discussions of acceptable means of contraception and nutrition information and support.

Social habits: alcohol, cigarettes, and drugs These three personal habits are contraindicated during pregnancy. Studies with test animals have indicated that even small amounts of alcohol, especially during critical early weeks of cell differentiation and organ development, can cause tissue damage. Extensive or habitual alcohol use leads to the well-described *fetal alcohol syndrome.*[10,11] Cigarette smoking during pregnancy poses special problems, and the counseling of such mothers should certainly stress these. Smoking results in placental abnormalities and fetal damage including prematurity and low birthweight[12] (see box, p. 258). Drug use, both recreational and medicinal, also poses numerous problems. Self-medication with over-the-counter drugs has numerous adverse effects. The use of "street drugs" poses special hazards, resulting not only from the effect of the drug itself but also from the various impurities it contains. Also, megadosing with basic nutrients during pregnancy is contraindicated.

Socioeconomic problems Special counseling is required for women and young girls living in low-income situations or extreme poverty. Numerous studies and clinical observations indicate that lack of prenatal care, often associated with racial prejudices and fears as well as poverty, places the expectant mother in grave difficulty. Special counseling is required, especially sensitivity to personal needs, to help plan any needed resources for financial assistance. Resources include programs such as the special Supplemental Food Program For Women, Infants, and Children (WIC) (Figure 11-1) and the Commodity Distribution program (see p. 232).

Complications of Pregnancy

Anemia

Anemia is common during pregnancy. About 10% of the patients in large prenatal clinics in the United States have hemoglobin concentrations of less than 10 g/dl and a hematocrit reading below 32. Anemia is far more prevalent among the poor, many of whom live on diets barely adequate for subsistence. However, anemia is by no means restricted to the lower economic groups.

Nutritional Anemia

Two kinds of nutritional anemia may be encountered in pregnancy:

Iron deficiency Anemia due to iron deficiency is by far the most common cause of anemia in pregnancy. The cost of a single normal pregnancy in iron stores is large—about 500 to 800 mg. Of this amount nearly 300 mg is used by the fetus. The remainder is used in the expanded maternal blood volume and its increased red blood cells and hemoglobin mass. This iron requirement exceeds the available reserves in the average woman. Thus, in addition to including iron-rich foods in the diet, a daily iron supplement of 30 to 60 mg is recommended for all pregnant women. Treatment of highly deficient states requires more, daily therapeutic doses

Clinical Application

Who will have the Low Birthweight Baby?

The number of babies weighing less than 2500 g at birth is on the rise. Perinatal nutritionists are well aware of dietary factors that may influence this increase, especially poor weight gain during pregnancy. The prevalence of that turn-of-the-century adage to "grow the baby to fit the pelvis" continues to influence some physicians, nurses, and expectant mothers alike to limit prenatal weight gain to 20 lbs or less to avoid obstetrical problems, especially at delivery. This practice is harmful and is refuted by recent evidence that a gain of 25 to 35 lbs is strongly correlated with birthweights of greater than 2500 g.

The obsession with weight control during pregnancy can lead to harmful restrictions of vital energy and nutrients. Weight reduction should NEVER be attempted during pregnancy. Such regimens are extremely dangerous to the fetus. Even the common practice of skipping breakfast, especially late in pregnancy, may potentially impair intellectual development (as seen in studies with rats) by inducing a ketotic, pseudo-starvation state very quickly. Increased ketosis from fat breakdown can cause neurologic damage to the fetus.

Nondietary factors influencing this growing trend toward more low birthweight (LBW) babies were identified in a Baltimore study:

- Rise in number of older primigravidas (i.e., over 35 years of age)
- Rise in number of teenage pregnancies
- Previous induced abortions
- Single marital status (often an indicator of low economic status)
- Technologic advances in neonatal care, which keep premature infants alive longer
- Race: nonwhites continue to have higher rates of LBW infants than whites do

To reduce the risk of LBW infants in populations being served by your facility, you may want to:

- Explain the rationale for gaining approximately 25-30 lbs during pregnancy
- Discourage the use of cigarettes and alcohol
- Monitor excessive weight gain and sodium intake in older primigravidas, who are often at risk for prenatal essential hypertension and obesity
- Explore eating habits of adolescents in the local community, working with the girl and her "significant others" to incorporate nutrient-dense foods into her meal and snack selections
- Keep abreast of federal, state, and local supplemental foods programs (e.g., WIC) available to low-income women to ensure an adequate intake of nutrients and kilocalories
- Encourage regular eating patterns throughout pregnancy

References

Metzger, B.E., and others: "Accelerated starvation" and skipped breakfast in late normal pregnancy, Lancet **2**(8272):588, 1982.

Pomerance, J., and others: Attitudes toward weight gain in pregnancy, West. J. Med. **133**(4):289, 1980.

Strobino, D.M.: Trends in low birthweight infants and changes in Baltimore's childbearing population, 1972-1977, Pub. Health Reports **97**(3):273, 1982.

Weigley, E.S.: Nutrition and the older primigravida, J. Am. Diet. Assoc. **82**(5):529, 1983.

Megaloblastic anemia
Reduction in the number of red blood cells associated with the presence of large, premature cells in the bone marrow. Caused by a folic acid deficiency.

of 120 to 200 mg, which is usually continued for 3 to 6 months after the anemia has been corrected in order to replenish the depleted stores.

Folate deficiency A less common **megaloblastic anemia** of pregnancy results from folic acid deficiency. During pregnancy, the fetus is sensitive to folic acid inhibitors and therefore has increased metabolic requirements for folic acid and its derivatives. To prevent this anemia, the RDA standard recommends a preventive supplement for all pregnant women of 400 µg of folic acid daily.

Hemorrhagic Anemia

Anemia caused by blood loss is more likely to occur during labor and delivery rather than during pregnancy. Blood loss may occur earlier, as a result of abortion or ruptured tubular pregnancy. Most patients undergoing these physiologic problems receive blood by transfusion, and iron therapy may be indicated for adequate replacement hemoglobin formation.

Toxemia Formerly used term (current official term of American College of Obstetricians and Gynecologists is *pregnancy-induced hypertension—PIH*); a metabolic disturbance that usually manifests itself in the third trimester with symptoms of hypertension, abnormal edema, and albuminemia. if uncontrolled, it can lead to coma or convulsions.

Pregnancy-Induced Hypertension (PIH)
Relation to Nutrition

Clinical and laboratory evidence indicates that pregnancy-induced hypertension (PIH), formerly labeled **toxemia,** is a disease of malnutrition, especially related to diets poor in protein, kilocalories, calcium, and salt. Such malnutrition affects the liver and its metabolic activities. Classically, it is associated with poverty and found most often in women subsisting on inadequate diets with little or no prenatal care. Much of the PIH problem could be prevented by good prenatal care, which inherently includes attention to sound nutrition. A woman's fitness during pregnancy is a direct function of her past nutrition and her optimal nutrition throughout pregnancy.

Clinical Symptoms

PIH is generally defined according to its manifestations, which usually occur in the third trimester toward term. These symptoms are hypertension, abnormal and excessive edema, albuminuria, and in severe cases, convulsions or coma **(eclampsia).**

Eclampsia Advanced pregnancy-induced hypertension (PIH) manifested by convulsions.

Treatment

Specific treatment varies according to the individual patient's symptoms and needs. Optimal nutrition is a fundamental aspect of therapy in any case. Emphasis is placed on adequate dietary protein and increased kilocalories for energy requirements to protect protein for tissue-building needs. Correction of plasma protein deficits stimulates normal circulation of fluid tissue, with subsequent correction of the **hypovolemia** (see p. 172). In addition, adequate salt and sources of vitamins and minerals are needed for correction and maintenance of metabolic balance.

Hypovolemia Abnormal reduction in volume of circulatory plasma.

Clinical Conditions

Clinical conditions complicating pregnancy are managed according to the general principles of care related to pregnancy and to the particular disease involved. Examples of three such conditions are given here.

Table 11-5
Risk Factors in Pregnancy-Induced Hypertension

Fetal hydrops Extensive edema of the entire fetus associated with severe anemia.

Hydramnios An excess of amniotic fluid.

Hydatidiform mole An abnormal pregnancy resulting in a cystic mass resembling a bunch of grapes, formed by a pathologic ovum in the uterus; a molar pregnancy.

Before Pregnancy	During Pregnancy
Nulligravida	Primigravida
Diabetes mellitus	Large fetus
Preexisting condition (hypertension, renal or vascular disease)	Glomerulonephritis
Family history of hypertension or vascular disease	**Fetal hydrops**
Diagnosis of pregnancy-induced hypertension in a previous pregnancy	**Hydramnios**
Dietary deficiencies	Multiple gestation
Age extremes 20 years or younger 35 years or older	**Hydatidiform mole**

Hypertension

Problems associated with hypertension in pregnancy can be prevented by initial and continuing screening and monitoring by the prenatal nurse with referral to the clinical nutritionist for a plan of care.[13] Risk factors for hypertension before and during pregnancy are given in Table 11-5. Nutritional therapy should center on (1) prevention of weight extremes, such as underweight or obesity, (2) correction of any dietary deficiencies and maintenance of optimal nutritional status during pregnancy, and (3) management of any related preexisting disease such as diabetes mellitus. Sodium use may be moderate but should not be unduly restricted because of its relation to fluid and electrolyte balances during pregnancy. Initial and continuing client education and a close relationship between the client and the nurse-nutritionist care team contribute to successful management of the hypertension and prevent problems that may occur.

Diabetes Mellitus

The management of diabetes in pregnancy presents special problems. Therefore routine screening is necessary to detect gestational diabetes—which is related only to the pregnancy itself—and those women having a family history of diabetes. Team management is required for preexisting type I, insulin-dependent diabetes mellitus.[14] Refer to Chapter 18 for a detailed discussion of diabetes care.

Phenylketonuria (PKU)

Successful management of PKU babies and children has ensured their normal growth and development to adulthood. Now young women with childhood PKU are having children of their own. Maternal PKU presents potential fetal hazards. If it is untreated it can be associated with increased spontaneous abortions and stillbirths and congenital anomalies often causing death. Postnatal growth and development retardation is evident in surviving infants.[15] Careful management of the mother's low phenylalanine diet before conception, with a planned pregnancy, and continuing close follow-up throughout the pregnancy itself can improve the outcome

Table 11-6
Nutritional Components of
Human Milk (per 100 ml)

Milk Component	Colostrum	Transitional	Mature	Cow's Milk
Kilocalories	57.0	63.0	65.0	65.0
Vitamins, fat-soluble:				
A (µg)	151.0	88.0	75.0	41.0
D (IU)	—	—	5.0	2.5
E (mg)	1.5	0.9	0.25	0.07
K (µg)	—	—	1.5	6.0
Vitamins, water-soluble:				
Thiamin (µg)	1.9	5.9	14.0	43.0
Riboflavin (µg)	30.0	37.0	40.0	145.0
Niacin (µg)	75.0	175.0	160.0	82.0
Panthothenic acid (µg)	183.0	288.0	246.0	340.0
Biotin (µg)	0.06	0.35	0.6	2.8
Vitamin B_{12} (µg)	0.05	0.04	0.1	0.6
Vitamin C (mg)	5.9	7.1	5.0	1.1

of these pregnancies and avoid much of the risk. Such a diet is carefully constructed by a specialized clinical nutritionist and monitored for adjustment according to need throughout the pregnancy.

Nutrition During Lactation

Trends in Breast-Feeding

An increasing number of mothers in America and other developed countries are choosing breast-feeding for their infants (see Issues and Answers, p. 266-267). Several factors have contributed to this choice: (1) more mothers are informed about the benefits of breast-feeding, (2) practitioners recognize the ability of human milk to meet infant needs (Table 11-6), (3) maternity wards and alternative birth centers are being modified to facilitate successful lactation, and (4) community support is more available, even in work places. Exclusive breast-feeding by well-nourished mothers can be adequate for periods varying from 2 to 15 months. Solid foods are usually added to the baby's diet at about 6 months of age.

Nutritional Needs

A prenatal nutrient supplement may wisely be continued by the mother during her breast-feeding period. Basic dietary nutritional requirements for lactation include the following additions to the mother's prepregnant needs.

Energy

The recommended caloric increase is 500 kcal more than the usual adult allowance. This makes a daily total of about 2500 kcal. This additional energy recommendation for the overall total lactation process is based on three factors:

1. **Milk content** An average daily milk production for lactating women is 850 ml (30 oz). Human milk has a kcal range of 20 to 70 kcal/oz or an average of 24 kcal/oz. Thus 30 oz of milk has a value of about 700 kcal.

2. **Milk production** The metabolic work involved in producing this amount of milk requires from 400 to 450 kcal.
3. **Maternal adipose tissue storage** The additional energy needs during lactation are drawn from maternal adipose tissue stores laid down during pregnancy in normal preparation for lactation to follow in the maternal cycle. Depending on the adequacy of these stores, additional energy input may be needed in the lactating woman's daily diet.

Protein

An increase of 20 g over the quantity recommended for the nonpregnant woman is needed during lactation. This makes a total daily protein allowance of about 70 g.

Minerals

The quantities of calcium and iron required by the lactating mother are not greater than those needed during pregnancy. The increased amount of calcium that was required during gestation for mineralization of the fetal skeleton is now diverted into the mother's milk production. Iron, since it is not a principal mineral component of milk, need not be increased for milk production.

Vitamins

An increased quantity of vitamin C above that recommended for the prepregnant woman is recommended for the lactating mother. An increase of 40 mg over the nonpregnancy woman's need is necessary, making the total ascorbic acid requirement 100 mg daily. Increases over the mother's prenatal intake are recommended also for vitamin A and the B complex vitamins involved as coenzyme factors in energy metabolism. The quantities needed of these vitamins, therefore, always increase as kilocalorie intake increases.

Fluids

An increased intake of fluids is necessary for adequate milk production, since milk is a fluid tissue. Water and beverages such as juices, tea, coffee, and milk (not necessarily beer, as some have thought) all add to the fluid necessary to produce milk.

Rest and relaxation

In addition to the increased diet, the mother who wants to breast-feed her baby requires rest, moderate exercise, and relaxation. Often the nurse and the nutritionist may help the mother by counseling her about her new family situation. Together they may develop plans to accommodate these personal needs.

To Sum Up

Pregnancy involves synergistic interactions among three distinct biologic entities: the fetus, the placenta, and the mother. Maternal needs reflect the increasing nutritional needs of the fetus and the placenta, as well as the need to meet maternal needs and to prepare for lactation. An optimal weight gain of about 11 kg (25 lb), or more as needed, is recommended during pregnancy to accommodate the rapid growth taking place. Even more significant than the actual weight gain is the nutritional quality of the diet.

Common problems occurring during pregnancy include nausea and vomiting, heartburn, or constipation. In most cases they are easily relieved without medication by simple, often temporary changes in the diet. Unusual or erratic eating habits, age, parity, prepartum weight status, and low income are among the many related conditions that also place the woman at risk for complications.

The ultimate goal of prenatal care is a healthy infant and a mother physically capable of breast-feeding her child, should she choose to do so. Human milk provides essential nutrients in quantities required for optimal infant growth and development.

Questions for Review

1. List and discuss five factors that influence the nutritional needs of the woman during pregnancy. Which factors would place a woman in a high-risk category? Why?
2. List six nutrients that are required in larger amounts during pregnancy. Describe their special role and identify four food sources of each.
3. Identify two common problems associated with pregnancy and describe the dietary management of each.
4. List and discuss five major nutritional factors of lactation.

References

1. Food and Nutrition Board, Committee on Maternal Nutrition, National Research Council: Maternal nutrition and the course of human pregnancy, Washington, D.C., 1970, National Academy of Sciences.

2. Blume, R., and Goldhagen, J.: Teenage pregnancy in perspective, Clin. Pediatr. **20**:335, 1981.

3. Miller, J.A.: Finding factors for fast fetal growth, Science News **124**(1):12, 1983.

4. Worthington-Roberts, B.S.: Nutritional needs of the pregnant adolescent. In Worthington-Roberts, B.S., Vermeersch, J., and Williams, S.R., editors: Nutrition in pregnancy and lactation, ed. 3, St. Louis, 1985, The C.V. Mosby Co.

5. National Research Council: Recommended dietary allowances, ed. 10, Washington, D.C., 1985, National Academy of Sciences.

6. Cassidy, C.M.: Subcultural prenatal diets of Americans. In Alternative dietary practices and nutritional abuses in pregnancy, Committee on Nutrition of the Mother and Preschool Child, Food and Nutrition Board, National Research Council, National Academy of Sciences, Washington, D.C., 1982, The Academy Press.

7. Dwyer, J.T.: Vegetarian diets in pregnancy. In Alternative dietary practices and nutritional abuses in pregnancy, Committee on Nutrition of the Mother and Preschool Child, Food and Nutrition Board, National Research Council, National Academy of Sciences, Washington, D.C., 1982, The Academy Press.

8. Schulman, P.K.: Hyperemesis gravidarum: an approach to the nutritional aspects of care, J. Am. Diet. Assoc. **80**(6):577, 1982.

9. King, J.C.: Dietary risk patterns during pregnancy. Nutr. Update **1**:206, 1983.

10. Iber, F.L.: Fetal alcohol syndrome, Nutr. Today **15**(5):4, 1980.

11. Beagle, W.S.: Fetal alcohol syndrome: a review, J. Am. Diet. Assoc. **79**:274, 1981.

12. Luke, B., Hawkins, M.M., and Petrie, R.H.: Influence of smoking, weight gain, and pregravid weight for height on intrauterine growth, Am. J. Clin. Nutr. **34**:1410, 1981.

13. Willis, S.E., and Sharp, E.S.: Hypertension in pregnancy: I. Pathophysiology, II. Prenatal detection and management, Am. J. Nurs. **82**:792, 1982.

14. Williams, S.R.: Nutritional therapy in special conditions of pregnancy. In Worthington-Roberts, B.S., Vermeersch, J., and Williams, S.R., editors: Nutrition in pregnancy and lactation, ed. 3, St. Louis, 1985, The C.V. Mosby Co.

15. Acosta, P.B., and others: Nutrition in pregnancy of women with hyperphenylalaninemia, J. Am. Diet. Assoc. **80**(5):443, 1982.

Further Readings

Hales, D., and Creasy, R.K.: New hope for problem pregnancies, New York, 1982, Harper & Row, Publishers Inc.

A readable reference written in popular style. Directed toward parents experiencing problem pregnancies who need sound information presented in a supportive manner.

Worthington-Roberts, B.S., Vermeersch, J., and Williams, S.R.: Nutrition in pregnancy and lactation, ed. 3, St. Louis, 1985, The C.V. Mosby Co.

A comprehensive and popular reference for health care professionals in prenatal care. Contains background research, practical guides, and discussions of such wide-ranging areas of concern as the pregnant adolescent and the woman with diabetes or phenylketonuria.

Gormican, A., Valentine, J., and Satter, E.: Relationships of maternal weight gain, prepregnancy weight, and infant birthweight, J. Am. Diet. Assoc. **77**(6):662, 1980.

A clear presentation of a study exploring two philosophies regarding optimal weight gain in pregnant women in relation to the mother's prepregnant weight and the infant's birthweight.

Brown. J.E.: Nutrition for your pregnancy, Minneapolis, 1983, University of Minnesota Press.

An excellent resource written in an interesting popular style. Contains many references and tools. A good reference for parents.

Issues and Answers

**The Dynamic
Nature of Human
Milk**

Mother Nature is determined to give every breastfed infant all the
nutrients he/she needs, no matter *when* the child is born or *how*.

Mothers and physicians alike have been reluctant to consider
breast-feeding for babies born prematurely or delivered by cesarean
section, for fear that there may be some negative effect on the
quantity or quality of human milk. Uncertainty about the nutritional
quality of mother's milk has also led them to encourage adding
formula and/or solid foods to the diet to make sure the baby is "well-
fed." These practices are usually unnecessary. In some cases, they
may contribute to obesity, allergies, and digestive problems because of
the extra stress placed on an immature gut.

Breast Milk for the Preterm Infant
Levels of nutrients in mother's milk shift according to the gestational
age of the infant at birth. The preterm infant is often "spared" its
mother's milk by some hospital workers because they think of it as
"mature" milk having too little protein and too much lactose to meet
the nutritional and digestive needs of the child. An analysis of the
nutritional quality of preterm milk, however, revealed different
nutrient levels: energy and fat concentrations that were 20 to 30%
higher, protein levels 15 to 20% *higher,* and lactose levels 10% *lower*
than those found in mature milk. Thus premature milk can meet the
extra energy and protein needs of the rapidly developing preterm
infant.

Breast Milk During Weaning
Nutrient levels continue to change with time to match changing
growth patterns and developing digestive abilities. Despite its thin
watery appearance, mother's milk does provide sufficient kilocalories
and nutrients to keep babies well-fed without supplemental formula
and food. Even when the infant is being weaned, Mother Nature steps
in to ensure adequate levels of nutrients, just in case the new, solid-
food diet cannot meet the child's needs. In a study in which human
milk was collected during gradual weaning, it was found that the milk
had higher concentrations of protein, sodium, and iron. Lactose levels
fell, possibly so that higher amounts of kilocalories could be supplied
by fats—a more concentrated source—in case the new diet could not
provide enough.

Breast Milk and the Cesarean-Section Infant
The quality of human milk is not influenced by the way in which
babies come into the world, either. Many women fear that a baby
born by cesarean section cannot be nursed, mainly because of a fear
that this method delays or prevents the production of "mature" milk.
Milk production, however, is stimulated by the release of the
placenta, and this always occurs whether the delivery is vaginal or
not. A recent study of 19 women confirmed this when the workers

Issues and Answers—cont'd

found *no* significant difference in the length of time it took mature milk to "come in" after vaginal vs. cesarean deliveries.

Thus, premature or cesarean deliveries should not stop the woman who wants to breast-feed from doing so. In fact, breast-feeding may be encouraged to ensure the infant of an adequate supply of easily digestible nutrients and other factors designed to meet his/her nutritional and immunologic needs. In addition, mothers should not underestimate the nutritive quality of their milk simply because it does not appear as "rich" and thick as cow's milk. In nutritional and immunologic terms, breast milk remains the best milk for baby.

References

Anderson, G.H., Atkinson, S.A., and Bryan, M.H.: Energy and macronutrient content of human milk during early lactation from mothers giving birth prematurely and at term, Am. J. Clin. Nutr. **34**:258, 1981.

Garza, C., and others: Changes in the nutrient composition of human milk during gradual weaning, Am. J. Clin Nutr. **37**(1):61, 1983.

Kulski, J.K., Smither, M., and Hartmann, P.E.: Normal and cesarian section delivery and the initiation of lactation in women, Austr. J. Exp. Bil. Med. Sci. **59**(4):405, 1981.

Chapter 12
Nutrition for Growth and Development

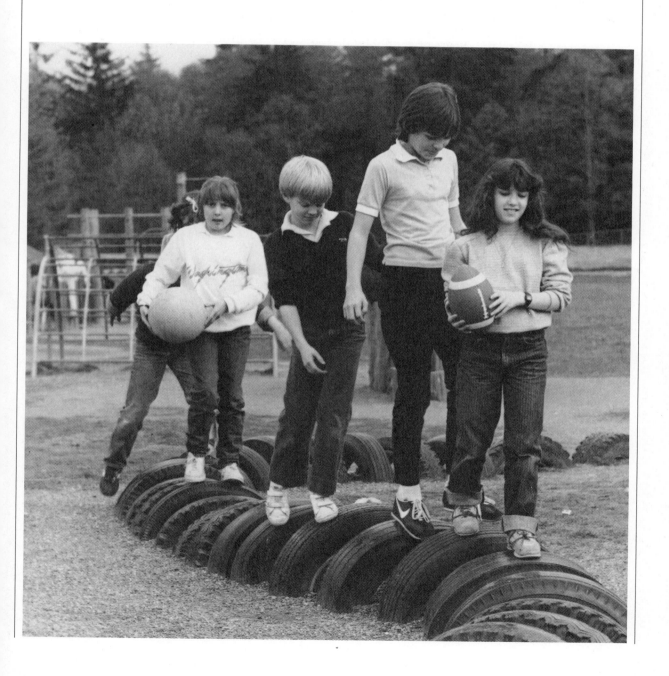

Preview

Human growth and development involves far more than physical processes alone. It encompasses social and psychologic influences and relationships—the entire environment and culture that nutures individual growth potential. Food and feeding during these highly significant years of childhood do not and cannot exist apart from this broader overall growth and development process. The *whole* process produces the *whole* person. In this chapter, therefore, we will consider food and feeding as a part of the whole development of the child. We will relate age-group nutritional needs and food habits to individual psychosocial development as well as to physical maturation normally achieved at each age level.

Chapter Objectives

After study of this chapter, the student should be able to:

1. Describe the normal physical growth pattern during the life cycle.

2. Identify ways of measuring childhood growth.

3. Relate basic nutrients to the growth process and identify nutritional needs for normal growth and development of children at each age level.

4. Relate food choices and feeding practices to basic physical and psychosocial development at each age period.

Growth and Development

Growth may be defined as an increase in size. Biologic growth of an organism occurs through cell multiplication. Development is the associated process in which growing tissues and organs take on increased complexity of function. Both of these processes are part of one whole, forming a unified concept of growth and development. Through these changes a small dependent newborn is transformed into a fully functioning independent adult. Throughout your study, however, remember that although we speak of general needs at a given age level, wide individual variations exist within normal ranges. In your care of children, then, never lose sight of each individual child's unique needs and growth potential.

Normal Life-Cycle Growth Pattern

The normal human life-cycle follows four general phases of overall growth.

Infancy

The infant grows rapidly during the first year of life, with the rate tapering off somewhat in the latter half of the year. At age 6 months an infant will probably have doubled the birth weight and at 1 year may have tripled it.

Childhood

The latent period of childhood between infancy and adolescence reflects a slowed and erratic growth rate. At some periods there are plateaus; at others small spurts of growth occur. The overall variable rate affects appetite accordingly. At times children will have little or no appetite, and at other times they will eat voraciously. Parents who know that this is a normal pattern will relax and not make eating a battleground with their children.

Adolescence

With the beginning of puberty the second rapid growth spurt occurs. Because of the hormonal influences involved, multiple body changes occur. These changes include the growth of long bones, the development of sex characteristics, and the development of fat and muscle mass.

Adulthood

In the final phase of a normal life cycle, growth levels off on the adult plateau. Then it gradually declines during old age.

Measuring Childhood Growth

Children grow at widely varying rates. Thus the wisest counsel that can be given to parents is that children are *individuals*. Parents can wisely avoid comparing one child with another and assuming that inadequate growth is taking place when the rate does not parallel that of another child. General measures of growth in children, however, relate to physical, mental, emotional, and social and cultural growth.

Physical Growth

Contemporary growth charts, developed by the National Center for Health Statistics (NCHS), reflect a broad base for growth patterns in children today. These charts are based on data from large numbers of a national representative sample of children. In clinical practice these charts are used as guides in assessing an individual child's pattern of growth in comparison with the percentile growth curves on these charts derived from measurement of numbers of children throughout the growth years. Several methods are used in practice for measuring physical growth of children:

Weight and height These common general measures of physical growth form a crude index without giving finer details of individual variations. They are used to look for patterns of growth over time, since an individual child's pattern is plotted on the related age group graph. As the child grows, weight and height can then be compared to averages on the growth charts (Figure 12-1).

Body measurements These measurements provide other helpful indications of growth. They include the length of the infant and standing height of the growing child, head circumference, mid-upper arm circumference and derived muscle circumference, measures of chest, abdomen, leg at the calf, pelvic breadth, skinfold thicknesses, and similar measures.

Clinical signs A general observation of vitality, a sense of well-being, good posture, healthy condition of gums and teeth, skin, hair, and eyes, muscle development, and nervous control all contribute measurably to a state of health, well-being, and optimum growth. Compare the signs of nutritional status as given in Table 1-1, p. 13.

Figure 12-1
Growth and developmental study being conducted at the University of California in Berkeley. Here weight of twins in the study is being recorded. Many other measures are taken, some by use of calipers.

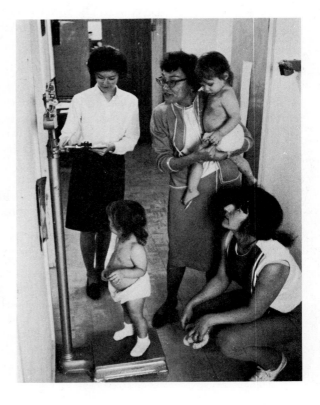

Laboratory tests In addition, other measures of growth can be obtained by various laboratory tests. These may include studies of blood and urine to determine levels of hemoglobin and vitamins. Radiographs of the hand and wrist may also be taken to indicate degree of bone development.

Nutritional analysis Measure of the growth of a child may be based on a nutritional analysis of general eating habits. This will give some measure of the adequacy of the diet to meet growth needs. The guides given in Chapter 10 (p. 223) may be used for such a diet history and analysis. Results of this analysis may then be used as a basis for diet counseling with the parents.

Mental Growth

Measurement of mental growth usually involves the testing of abilities in speech and other forms of communication, as well as the ability to handle abstract and symbolic material in thinking. Children originally think literally. As mental capacity develops, they can increasingly handle more than single ideas and develop constructive concepts.

Emotional Growth

Measurement of emotional growth reflects the capacity for love and affection and the ability to handle frustration and its anxieties. It also involves the child's ability to control aggressive impulses and to channel hostility from destructive to constructive activities.

Social and Cultural Growth

Social development of a child is measured in terms of the ability to relate to others and to participate in group living in a cultural setting. These social and cultural behaviors are first learned through relationships with parents and family, all of which have much influence on food habits and feeding patterns. As horizons broaden, the child develops relationships with others outside the family—with friends and persons in the community. For this reason, a child's play in the early years is a highly purposeful activity.

Nutritional Requirements for Growth

Energy Needs

During childhood the demand for kilocalories is relatively large. However, there is much variation in need with age and condition. For example, the total daily caloric intake of a 5-year-old child is spent in the following way: (1) about 55% supplies *basal metabolic requirements,* 5% of which is involved in the *specific dynamic effect* of food—especially protein—in generally stimulating metabolism, (2) various *physical activities* require about 25%, (3) 12% is needed for *tissue growth,* and (4) about 8% is represented in *fecal loss.* Of these kilocalories, carbohydrate is the main energy source and is also important as a protein-sparer to ensure that protein vital for growth will not be diverted for energy needs. Fat kilocalories are important to ensure certain fatty acids that are essential fro growth, especially linoleic acid; however an excess of fat, especially from animal sources, should be avoided.

Protein Needs

Protein is the *growth element* of the body. It supplies the essential building materials for tissue growth—amino acids. These building materials are necessary for formation and maintenance of muscle and nerve tissue, bone matrix, and fluid tissues and secretions. As a child grows, the protein requirements per unit of body weight gradually decrease. For example, for the first 6 months of life an infant requires 2.2 g/kg of body weight. This amount gradually decreases until adulthood, when protein needs are only 0.8 g/kg. Usually a healthy, active, growing child will consume the necessary amount of kilocalories and protein in the variety of foods provided.

Water Requirements

Water is essential to life, second only to oxygen. The infant's need for water is even greater than that of an adult for two reasons: (1) a greater percentage of total body weight is made up of water and (2) a larger proportion of total body water is outside the cells and hence is more easily available for loss. Generally an infant consumes daily an amount of water equivalent to 10% to 15% of body weight, compared with adult daily consumption of water equivalent to 2% to 4% of body weight. A summary of approximate daily fluid needs during the growth years is given in Table 12-1.

Table 12-1
Approximate Daily Fluid
Needs During Growth Years

Age	ml/kg
0-3 months	120
3-6 months	115
6-12 months	100
1-4 years	100
4-7 years	95
7-11 years	90
11-19 years	50
> 19 years	30

Minerals and Vitamins

In your previous study of minerals and vitamins you learned of their essential roles in tissue growth and maintenance and in overall energy metabolism. Positive childhood growth and development depends on an adequate amount of these essential substances. For example, calcium is necessary for rapid bone mineralization that takes place during growth. It is also needed for developing teeth, muscle contraction, nerve irritability, blood coagulation, and the action of the heart muscle. Another mineral of concern is iron, essential for hemoglobin formation. The infant's fetal store is diminished in 4 to 6 months after birth and the first infant food—milk—lacks iron. Thus the infant needs solid food additions at about 4 to

6 months of age to help supply iron. Such initial foods as enriched cereal, egg, and, later, meat supply this need.

A summary of the nutritional needs for growth, as recommended by the National Research Council, is given in Table 12-2.

Hypervitaminosis

Excess amounts of two vitamins, A and D, are of concern in feeding children. Excess intake of these vitamins may occur over prolonged periods because of misunderstanding, ignorance, or carelessness. Parents must be instructed to use only the amount directed and no more. These excesses bring clear toxic symptoms:

Vitamin A Symptoms of toxicity from excess vitamin A include lack of appetite, slow growth, drying and cracking of the skin, enlargement of the liver and spleen, swelling and pain of long bones, and bone fragility.

Vitamin D Symptoms of toxicity from excess vitamin D include nausea, diarrhea, weight loss, excess urination especially at night, and eventual calcification of soft tissues, including those of renal tubules, blood vessels, bronchi, stomach, and heart.

Age Group Needs

Stages of Human Growth

Throughout the human life-cycle, food and feeding not only serve to meet nutritional requirements for growth and maintenance but they also relate intimately to personal psychosocial development. The nutritional age group needs of children cannot be understood apart from the child's overall maturation as a *person*.

Psychosocial Development

The eight stages of human growth as developed by Erikson provide a helpful framework for study.[1,2] At each stage the child struggles between a positive ego value and its conflicting negative aspect. Given favorable circumstances, a growing child develops the positive aspect of the developmental problem at each life stage and builds increasing strength to meet the next life crisis. Erikson's eight stages of growth and development point us to areas of need:

1. **Infancy**—trust vs. distrust
2. **Toddler**—autonomy vs. shame and doubt
3. **Preschooler**—initiative vs. guilt
4. **School-age child**—industry vs. inferiority
5. **Adolescent**—identity vs. role confusion
6. **Young adult**—intimacy vs. isolation
7. **Adult**—generativity vs. stagnation
8. **Older adult**—ego integrity vs. despair

Given favorable circumstances, a growing child develops through each of these life stages, building inner resources. The struggle at any age, however, is not forever won at that point. A residue of the negative remains, and in periods of stress, such as illness, regression in some degree usually occurs. As the child gains mastery at each stage of development, however, assisted in significant positive relationships of support, integration of self-control takes place. Various related developmental tasks sur-

Table 12-2
Recommended Daily Dietary Allowances for Growth (National Research Council 1980 version)

	Age (yr)	Weight kg	Weight lb	Height cm	Height In	Energy (kcal)	Protein (g)	Vit. A µg RE	Vit. A IU	Vit. D (µg*)	Vit. E (mg αTE)
Infants	Birth-0.5	6	13	60	24	kg × 115	kg × 2.2	420	1400	10	3
	0.5-1	9	20	71	28	kg × 105	kg × 2.0	500	2000	10	4
Children	1-3	13	29	90	35	1300	23	400	2000	10	5
	4-6	20	44	112	44	1700	30	500	2500	10	6
	7-10	28	62	132	52	2400	34	700	3300	10	7
Males	11-14	45	99	157	62	2700	45	1000	5000	10	8
	15-18	66	145	176	69	2800	56	1000	5000	10	10
Females	11-14	46	101	157	62	2200	46	800	4000	10	8
	15-18	55	120	163	64	2100	46	800	4000	10	8

*As cholecalciferol; 10 µg cholecalciferol equals 400 IU vitamin D

round each of these stages. These are skills that, when accomplished, contribute to successful resolution of the core problem.

Physical Growth

These developmental tasks are integrated and associated with normal physical maturation at each point of growth. Various neuromuscular motor skills enable the child to accomplish related physical activities.

Food and Feeding Practices

In each of these stages of childhood, food choices and feeding practices are intimately related. Food habits do not develop in a vacuum. They are an integral part of both physical and psychosocial development. Here we will relate these two influences to the general age-group developmental characteristics.

Infancy (Birth to 1 Year)
The Premature Infant

Special care is crucial for these tiny, immature babies.

Physical characteristics Premature infants vary in weight and development. They are usually considered premature if they are born at fewer than 270 days of gestation or weigh less than 2500 g (5.5 lb). Similar infants who are *small for gestational age (SGA)* have suffered some degree of intrauterine growth failure and also have low birth weights and general growth retardation.[3] All of these infants have problems catching up with growth and nutrition. Because they are immature, their body composition differs from that of full-term infants: (1) they have much more water and less protein and minerals per kilogram of body weight, (2) there is little subcutaneous fat, (3) bones are poorly calcified, (4) the neuromuscular system is incompletely developed, making normal sucking reflexes weak, (5) digestive-absorptive ability and renal function are limited, and (6) the immature liver lacks developed enzyme systems or adequate iron stores.

	Water-soluble Vitamins							Minerals				
Vit. C (mg)	Fola-cin (μg)	Via-cin (mg)	Ribo-flavin (mg	Thia-min (mg)	Vit. B₆ (mg)	Vit. B₁₂ (μg)	Cal-cium (mg)	Phos-phorus (mg)	Iodine (μg)	Iron (mg)	Mag-nesium (mg)	Zinc (mg)
35	30	6	0.4	0.3	0.3	0.5	360	240	40	10	50	3
35	45	8	0.6	0.5	0.6	1.5	540	360	50	15	70	5
45	100	9	0.8	0.7	0.9	2.0	800	800	70	15	150	10
45	200	11	1.0	0.9	1.3	2.5	800	800	90	10	200	10
45	300	16	1.4	1.2	1.6	3.0	800	800	120	10	250	10
50	400	18	1.6	1.4	1.8	3.0	1200	1200	150	18	350	15
60	400	18	1.7	1.4	2.0	3.0	1200	1200	150	18	400	15
50	400	15	1.3	1.1	1.8	3.0	1200	1200	150	18	300	15
60	400	14	1.3	1.1	2.0	3.0	1200	1200	150	18	300	15

Food and feeding If these "tinest babies" are to survive, they require special feeding. Special consideration has to be given to the type of milk used and methods of feeding.

Type of milk Controversy continues regarding the relative merits of breast milk and special formulas for premature infants. Nonetheless, premature infants have done well on both forms of feeding.[4,5] There is some indication that milk produced by mothers of premature infants may be especially suited to the needs of the preterm infant, since in comparison to milk from mothers of full-term infants, it has a higher protein and mineral content and its fat is more digestible. For a number of reasons, however, the majority of preterm infants are fed special formulas at some stage. Several newer commercial preterm infant formulas have been developed. Table 12-3 shows a comparison of these special formulas with standard full-term infant formulas and with human milk.

Methods of feeding Tube feeding has been used for premature infants but it is hazardous and usually avoided. Long-term peripheral vein feeding is difficult in tiny infants and may become complicated by sepsis and jaundice. For most of these infants, bottle-feeding can successfully be instituted with care and support, using one of the newer special formulas.

The Full-Term Infant

Physical characteristics The growth rate during infancy is rapid. Consequently energy requirements are high. The full-term infant has the ability to digest and absorb protein, a moderate amount of fat, and simple carbohydrates. There is some difficulty with starch, since amylase, the starch-splitting enzyme, is not being produced at first. However, as starch is introduced, this enzyme begins to function. The renal system functions well, but more water relative to size is needed than in an adult to manage urinary excretion. Since teeth do not erupt until about the 4th month, the initial food must be liquid or semiliquid. The infant has limited nutritional

Table 12-3
Nutritional Value of Special Formulas and Human Milk for the Preterm Infant

Nutritional Component	Advisable Intake Birth Weight 1.0 kg (2.2 lb)	1.5 kg (3.3 lb)	Human Milk Content Preterm	Mature	Standard Formulas Enfamil* Similac† SMA‡	Special Premature Formulas Enfamil Premature with Whey*	Similac Special Care†	"Preemie" SMA‡
Kilocalories/deciliter			73	73	67	81	81	81
Protein (g/100 kcal)	3.1	2.7	2.3§	1.5	2.2	3.0	2.7	2.5
Vitamins, fat-soluble								
D (IU/120 kcal/kg/day)	600	600	—	4.0	70-75	75	180	76
E (IU/120 kcal/kg/day)	30	30	—	0.3	2-3	2	4	2
Vitamins, water-soluble								
Folic acid (µg/120 kcal/ kg/day)	60	60	—	8.0	9-19	36	45	14
Vitamin C (mg/120 kcal/kg/day)	60	60	—	7.0	10	10	45	10
Minerals								
Calcium (mg/100 kcal)	160	140	40.0	43.0	66-78	117	178	92
Phosphorus (mg/100 kcal)	108	95	18.0	20.0	49-66	58	89	49
Sodium (mEq/100 kcal)	2.7	2.3	1.5‖	0.8	1.0-1.8	1.7	1.9	1.7

*Mead Johnson Nutritional Division, Evansville, Ind.
†Ross Laboratories, Columbus, Ohio.
‡Wyeth Laboratories, Philadelphia.
§Range: 1.9-2.8 g/100 kcal.
‖Range: 0.9-2.3 mEq/100 kcal.

Beikost Solid and semisolid baby foods.

stores remaining from fetal development, especially in iron, so that supplements of vitamins and minerals are needed. These are first given in concentrated drops and later in **beikost**—solid food additions to milk. The newborn's *rooting reflex* and somewhat recessed lower jaw are natural adaptations for feeding at the breast.

Psychosocial development The core psychosocial problem during infancy is the development of *trust vs. distrust*. Feeding is the infant's main means of establishing human relationships. The close mother-infant relationship in the feeding process fills the basic need to build trust. The need for sucking and the development of oral organs—lips and mouth—as sensory organs represent adaptations to ensure an adequate early food intake for survival. As a result, food becomes the infant's general means of exploring the environment and is one of the main early means of communication. As muscular coordination involving the tongue and the swallowing reflex develops, the infant will accept solid foods when such foods are started at about 6 months of age. As physical and motor maturation develop, the infant will want to help in the feeding process. When these stages of development occur, the exploration of new powers should be

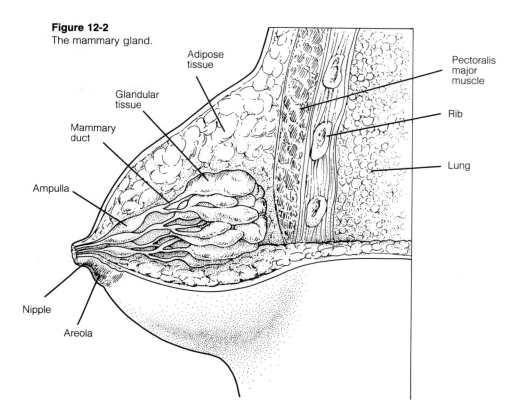

Figure 12-2
The mammary gland.

encouraged. If the needs for food and love are fulfilled in this early relationship with the mother or other feeding adult, and in broadening relationships with other family members, trust is developed. The infant shows this trust by an increasing capacity to wait for feedings while they are being prepared.

Food and feeding Certain considerations and choices are important in feeding full-term infants.

Breast-feeding The ideal food for the human infant is human milk. It has specific characteristics that match the infant's nutritional requirements during the first year of life. The process of breast-feeding today, as in the past, is successfully initiated and maintained by most women who try. The female's breasts, or mammary glands, are highly specialized secretory organs (Figure 12-2). They are composed of glandular tissue, fat, and connective tissue. The secreting glandular tissue has 15 to 20 lobes, each containing many smaller units called *lobules*. In the lobules secretory cells called *alveoli* or *acini* form milk from the nutrient material supplied to them by a rich capillary system in the connective tissue. During pregnancy the breast is prepared for lactation. The alveoli enlarge and multiply and toward the end of the prenatal period secrete a thin, yellowish fluid called *colostrum*. As the infant grows, the breast milk develops, adapting in composition to the needs of the developing child.

Breast milk is produced under the stimulating hormone *prolactin*, produced by the anterior pituitary gland. After the milk is formed in the

Figure 12-3
Breast-feeding the newborn
infant. Note that the nurse, in
assisting the mother, avoids
touching the infant's outer
cheek so as not to counteract
his natural rooting reflex at
the touch of the breast.

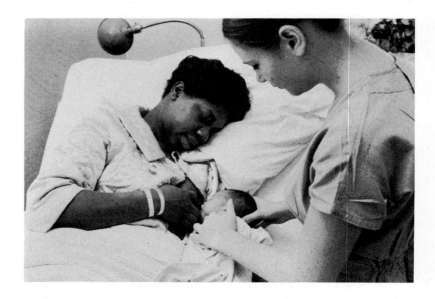

mammary lobules by the clusters of secretory cells (alveoli or acini), it is
carried through converging branches of the *lactiferous ducts* to reservoir
spaces under the *areola,* the pigmented area of skin surrounding the nipple. These reservoir spaces under the areola are called *ampullae.* From 15
to 20 excretory lactiferous ducts carry the milk from the ampullae out to
the surface of the nipple. Two other pituitary hormones, principally *oxy-
tocin* and to a lesser extent *vasopressin* (antidiuretic hormone or ADH),
stimulate the ejection of the milk from the alveoli to the ducts, releasing
it so that the baby can obtain it. This is commonly called the *let down reflex.*
It causes a tingling sensation in the breast and the flow of milk. The initial
sucking of the baby stimulates this reflex. The newborn rooting reflex,
oral needs for sucking, and the basic hunger drive usually make breast-
feeding simple for the healthy, relaxed mother (Figure 12-3). A nutritionally adequate diet will support ample milk production (see p. 250).

Bottle-feeding Formula feeding by bottle may be preferred by some
mothers. If the mother does not choose breast-feeding or stops early, bottle feeding of an appropriate formula is an acceptable alternative. Both
breast milk and formula have approximately the same energy value—20
kcal/oz. About 90% of these mothers use a commercial formula. A variety
of these formulas that approximate the composition of human milk are
available. Commercial infant formulas are based on several types of constituent proteins: cow's milk, soy protein, protein hydrolysate, or meat
base. A description of these major types of standard commercial formulas
for full-term infants is given in Table 12-4. Some of the milk-based formulas are whey-adjusted to more nearly approximate the protein ratio in
human milk. The standards for levels of nutrients required in infant formulas are set by the Infant Formula Act of 1980, P.L. 97-359, which is
based on recommendations from the American Academy of Pediatrics.[6]
These standards are given in Table 12-5 and can be compared to the
standards recommended by the National Research Council for infants

Table 12-4

A Comparison of Types of Formulas Manufactured for Full-Term Infants

Type of Formula/Use		Protein Content	Fat Content	Carbohydrate Content
Milk-based routine	Source:	Nonfat cow's milk	Vegetable oils	Lactose
	G/100 kcal:	2.2-2.3	5.4-5.5	10.5-10.8
	% Kcal:	9	48-50	41-43
Whey-adjusted routine	Source:	Nonfat cow's milk plus demineralized whey	Vegetable and oleo oils	Lactose
	G/100 kcal:	2.2	5.4	10.8
	% Kcal:	9	48	43
Soy isolate/cow's milk sensitivity	Source:	Soy isolate	Vegetable oils	Corn syrup solids and/or sucrose
	G/100 kcal:	2.7-3.2	5.1-5.6	9.9-10.2
	% Kcal:	12-13	45-51	39-40
Casein hydrolysate/ protein sensitivity, galactosemia	Source:	Casein hydrolysate	Corn oil or corn oil and MCT*	Tapioca starch and glucose, sucrose, or corn syrup solids
	G/100 kcal:	2.8-3.3	3.9-4.0	13.1-13.6
	% Kcal:	11-13	35	52-54
Meat-based cow's milk sensitivity, galactosemia	Source:	Beef hearts	Sesame oil and beef heart fat	Tapioca starch and sucrose
	G/100 kcal:	4.0	4.8	9
	% Kcal:	16	47	37

*Medium-chain triglycerides.

from birth to 6 months. When bottle formula is used and the infant is obviously satisfied, extra milk should not be forced, regardless of the amount remaining in the bottle. Any remaining formula should be thrown away and not refrigerated for use again. A healthy infant will take the amount of formula needed. Today most infants are fed on a so-called demand schedule, according to individual need, about every 3 to 4 hours. A healthy infant will soon establish an individual pattern according to growth requirements.

Cow's milk Regular unmodified cow's milk is not suitable for infants. It may cause gastrointestinal bleeding; also its solute load is too heavy for the infant's renal system to handle. Also, infants should *not* use milks of reduced fat content, such as skim or 2% milk, for two reasons: (1) *insufficient energy* is provided to support maintenance requirements, causing the use of body fat to make up the deficit, and (2) *linoleic acid* in the fat portion of milk is an essential fatty acid needed for growth and development of body tissues. A specific form of eczema has been observed in infants deficient in linoleic acid. To meet special infant needs, the American Academy of Pediatrics recommends breast milk or formulas up to 1 year of age, with a gradual addition of appropriate foods beginning at 6 months.

Table 12-5
Nutrient Standards for
Formulas Manufactured for
Healthy, Full-Term Infants

Nutrient	RDA (1980) (up to age 6 months)	Nutrient Requirements of the Infant Formula Act of 1980	
		Minimum	Maximum
Energy (kcal)	570-870	670	
Protein (g)	13.2	12.1	30.2
Essential fatty acids			
Linoleate, % kcal	3.0	2.7	
Vitamins, fat-soluble			
A (IU)	1400 (420 μg)	1675 (503 μg)	5025 (1508 μg)
D (IU)	400 (10 μg)	268	670
E (IU)	4.5	4.7	
K(μg)	12.0*	27.0	
Vitamins, water-soluble			
C (mg)	35.0	54.0	
B_1 (thiamin) (μg)	300.0	268.0	
B_2 (riboflavin) (μg)	400.0	402.0	
B_6 (pyridoxine) (μg)	300.0	235.0	
B_{12} (μg)	0.5	1.0	
Niacin	6.0 mEq	1.68 mg	
Folacin (μg)	30.0	27.0	
Pantothenic acid (mg)	2.0*	2.0	
Biotin (μg)	35.0	10.0	
Choline (mg)		47.0	
Inositol (mg)		27.0	
Minerals			
Calcium (mg)	360.0	335.0	
Phosphorus (mg)	240.0	168.0	
Magnesium (mg)	50.0	40.0	
Iron (mg)	10.0	1.0†	
Iodine (μg)	40.0	34.0	
Zinc (mg)	3.0	3.4	
Copper (μg)	500-700*	402.0	
Manganese (μg)	500-700*	34.0	
Sodium (mg)	115-350*	134.0	402.0
Potassium (mg)	350-925*	536.0	1340.0
Chloride (mg)	275-700*	369	1005.0
Fluoride (μg)	100-500*		
Chromium (μg)	10-40*		
Selenium (μg)	10-40*		
Molybdenum (μg)	30-60*		

*Based on estimated safe and adequate daily dietary intakes. Some figures are given in ranges because of a lack of information on which to base allowances.

†Based on iron content of nonfortified infant formula (0.15 mg/100 kcal). The Committee on Nutrition recommends that infants receive 1.0 mg/100 kcal formula.

Beikost (solid food additions) There is no nutritional need for introducing solid foods to infants before 6 months of age. Earlier use may contribute to allergies or overweight. Nutritional and medical authorities agree that for the first 6 months of life the optimal single food for the infant is human milk, or alternative formula feeding when necessary. Until that time the infant does not need any additional foods and is not able to fully

Table 12-6
Guideline for Adding of Solid
Foods to Infant's Diet During
the First Year*

When to start	Foods added	Feeding
Sixth month	Cereal and strained cooked fruit	10 AM and 6 PM
	Egg yolk (at first, hard boiled and sieved, soft boiled or poached later)	
	Strained cooked vegetable and strained meat	2 PM
	Zweiback or hard toast	At any feeding
Seventh to ninth month	Meat: beef, lamb, or liver (broiled or baked and finely chopped)	10 AM to 6 PM
	Potato: baked or boiled and mashed or sieved	
Suggested meal plan for age 8 months to 1 year or older		
7 AM	Milk	240 ml (8 oz)
	Cereal	2-3 tbsp
	Strained fruit	2-3 tbsp
	Zweiback or dry toast	
12 NOON	Milk	240 ml (8 oz)
	Vegetables	2-3 tbsp
	Chopped meat or one whole egg	
	Puddings or cooked fruit	2-3 tbsp
3 PM	Milk	120 ml (4 oz)
	Toast, zweiback, or crackers	
6 PM	Milk	240 ml (8 oz)
	Whole egg or chopped meat	2 tbsp
	Potato: baked or mashed	2-3 tbsp
	Pudding or cooked fruit	
	Zweiback or toast	

*Semisolid foods should be given immediately before milk feeding. One or two teaspoons should be given at first. If food is accepted and tolerated well, the amount should be increased to 1 to 2 tbsp per feeding.

NOTE: Banana or cottage cheese may be used as substitution for any meal.

handle them. There is no one specific sequence of food additions that must be followed. A general guide is given in Table 12-6. Individual responses and needs may be a basis for choices. Single foods are introduced first, one at a time in small amounts, so that if there is an adverse reaction, the offending food can be identified. The traditional transition food is cereal—*iron-fortified infant cereal*—with a little milk or formula, then fruits, vegetables, egg, potato, and finally meat. Small amounts are given initially, usually before the milk feeding. Over time the child will be introduced to a wide variety of foods and come to enjoy many of them. A variety of commercial baby foods are available, prepared today without the formerly used ingredients of sugar, salt, or monosodium glutamate. Some mothers prefer preparing their own baby food. This can easily be done by cooking and straining vegetables and fruits, freezing a batch at a time in ice cube trays, then storing the cubes in plastic bags in the freezer. Then a single cube can be reheated conveniently for use at a feeding.

Two basic factors should guide the feeding process: (1) *necessary nutrients* are needed, not any specific food and (2) food is a basis of *learning*. Food serves not only for physical sustenance but also supplies other personal and cultural needs. Good food habits begin early in life and continue as the child grows older. By the time infants are approximately 8 or 9 months old, they should be able to eat so-called family foods—chopped, cooked foods, simply seasoned—without needing special infant foods. Throughout the first year of life the infant's needs for physical growth and psychosocial development will be met by breast milk or formula, a variety of solid food additions, and a loving, trusting relationship between parents and child (Figure 12-4).

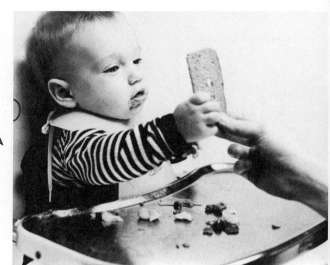
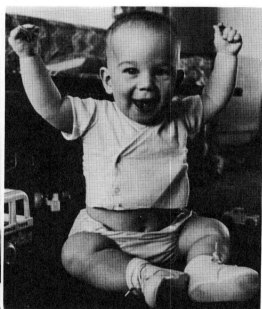

Figure 12-4
A, This 6-month-old boy is taking a variety of solid food additions and is developing wide tastes. Here feeding has become a bond of relationship between mother and child and is serving as a source not only of physical growth but also of psychosocial development. **B,** Optimum physical development and security are evident, the result of sound nutrition and loving care.

Childhood (1-12 Years)
Toddler (1-3 Years)

Physical characteristics and growth After the rapid growth of the first year, the parents may be concerned when they observe the toddler eating less food and at times having little appetite. Beginning with the second year and through the latent years of childhood, the rate of gain is less and the pattern of growth changes. The legs become longer, and the child begins losing baby fat. There is less body water and more water inside the cells. The young child begins to look and feel less like a baby and more like a child. Important muscle development takes place as the child begins to walk. The big muscles of the back, buttocks, and thighs need to be strengthened for erect posture and walking. Bones begin to lengthen, although the overall rate of skeletal growth slows. There is more deposit of mineral for strengthening the bones to support the increasing weight than in great lengthening of the bones. The child needs fewer kilocalories (less total quantity of food) but more protein and mineral matter for growth. The child has about 6 or 8 teeth at the beginning of the toddler period. Most of the deciduous "baby" teeth have erupted by the end of the third year.

Psychosocial development The core psychosocial problem toddlers struggle with is the conflict between *autonomy vs. shame and doubt.* There is an increasing sense of self, or "I," of being a person, distinct and individual, apart from the mother and not just an extention of her. The very fact of beginning to walk gives an increasing sense of independence. A growing curiosity leads to much exploration of the environment, and increasingly the mouth is used as a means of exploring. Touch is important, providing the means of learning what objects are like. Often the constant use of "no" is not perverse negativism as much as it is the struggle with ego needs in conflict with the parents' efforts to maintain control. The child wants to be more autonomous, but the attention span is fairly short because of an increasing diversion of interest to other things in the environment. Often the struggle for autonomy or selfhood takes the form of wanting to do things before being able to do them completely.

Food and feeding Both physical growth and psychosocial development during this period influence nutrient needs and food patterns (see box, p. 286). Energy (kilocalories) needs are not high during the toddler period, and they increase slowly and in spurts. The greater emphasis is on key nutrients such as proteins, minerals and vitamins to maintain the growth pattern. The bones are strengthening to keep pace with muscle development and increasing activity. To meet these needs, only two and sometimes three cups of milk are sufficient. Sometimes excess milk intake, a habit carried over from infancy, excludes some solid food from the diet. As a result, the child may be lacking iron and develop a "milk anemia." On the other hand, a child may dislike milk or begin to refuse it. In this case other milk products such as yogurt and cheese may be used instead. Also, milk solids can be used in soups, custards, or puddings, and dry milk can be used in cooked cereals, mashed potatoes, meatloaf, and other dishes. Giving the child an increasing variety of foods will help to develop good food habits. Studies indicate that food preferences of young children grow directly from frequency of exposure and thus increased opportunity to develop a familiarity with a number of foods. An emphasis on refined sweets is best avoided, reserving them for special occasions, not for habitual use or bribes to get a child to eat.

Clinical Application

Toddler-Feeding Made Simple

Parents waste a lot of time coaxing, arguing, begging, even threatening their 2- to 5-year-olds to eat more than 1½ green peas at dinnertime. You can help them save time by developing child-feeding strategies based on the developmental needs of their little ones.

The first step is to remind them that:

Their children are not growing as fast as they did during the first year of life. Consequently, they need less food.

A child's energy needs are sporadic. Just watch their activity level. Food should be provided to help their bodies keep up with the myriad of activities they have "planned" each day.

Next, offer a few suggestions that make child-feeding easier:

Serve small portions. Do not give much more than a baby food jar could hold. Let them ask for seconds if they're still hungry.

Guide them in serving themselves small amounts. This takes awhile because, like adults, children's eyes tend to be bigger than their stomachs. Constant gentle reminders will eventually help them learn when to stop.

Keep "quick-fix" nutritious foods around for "off-hour" meals. The term "snack" isn't appropriate for the amount of food some youngsters put away between meals. To keep from turning into a permanent short-order chef, the parent should consider keeping foods such as fruit, cheese, peanut butter to serve between meals and provide essential nutrients.

Don't put away the main meal before serving dessert. Amazing but true: some children will ask for main meal foods *after* finishing dessert, if they are still hungry!

Avoid overseasoning. If it's too spicy, no amount of screaming and cajoling will make them eat it.

Don't force foods that the child dislikes. Individual food dislikes usually don't last very long. If the child shuns one food, offer a similar one—If it's available at that meal (e.g., a fruit if the child shuns vegetables). If not, ignore it. And don't worry about malnutrition. At this rate, there's little chance of deficiency signs cropping up anytime soon.

Enroll the child in nursery school. Since food is not always available in the classroom, little students learn to eat at regular times. They also tend to try foods that are abhorred at home, probably because of peer pressure or a desire to impress a new authority figure—the teacher.

Be patient. While adults are discussing world events over broccoli, toddlers are learning how to pick it up with their forks.

They might take longer. They might not eat. But with flexibility, time, patience, and a sense of humor, most parents find they can get enough nutrients into their children to keep them alive and happy throughout the preschool years.

References
Mayer, J.: Eat! Health **11**(1):46, 1979.

Summary principles Two principles are important for parents to know, understand, and practice during this period:

1. The child needs fewer kilocalories but relatively more protein and mineral matter for physical growth. Therefore a variety of foods should be offered in smaller amounts to provide key nutrients.
2. The child is struggling for autonomy. This struggle often takes the form of refusal of food and a desire to do things before being fully able to do them completely. Again, if parents offer a variety of foods in small amounts and support and encourage some degree of food choice and self-feeding in the child's own ceremonial manner, then eating can be a pleasant, positive means of development. It can help fulfill the growing need for independence and the desire for ritual. Parents need to maintain a calm, relaxed attitude of sympathetic interest to understand this struggle and to give help where needed while avoiding both overprotection and excessive rigidity.

Preschooler (3-6 Years)

Physical characteristics and growth Physical growth continues in spurts. On occasion the child bounds with energy. Play is hard play—running, jumping, and testing new physical resources. At other times the child will sit for increasing periods of time engrossed in passive types of activities. Mental capacities are developing and the environment is being explored. Specific nutrients need emphasis. Protein requirements continue to be relatively high. The child continues to need calcium and iron for storage. Since vitamins A and C may be lacking in the diets of preschool and growing children, a variety of fruits and vegetables should be provided.

Psychosocial development Each age period builds on the previous one. The toddler whose physical and psychosocial needs have been fulfilled by understanding and able parents has a foundation on which the preschool period builds. The child is continuing to form life patterns in attitudes and basic eating habits as a result of social and emotional experiences. The two-fold guiding principle for parents remains the same—(1) to provide a variety of key foods to meet physical needs and (2) to provide climate that promotes and supports social and emotional growth.

The core psychosocial problem preschool children struggle with is that of *initiative vs. guilt.* The superego (conscience) is beginning to develop. As powers of locomotion increase, so do imagination and curiosity. This very capacity often leads to troubled feelings about changing attitudes, especially towards parents. This is a period of increasing imitation and of sex identification. The little boy will imitate the father; the little girl will imitate the mother. In their play, much of this becomes evident in the use of grown-up clothes and role playing in domestic situations. Wise parents will avoid sex-stereotyping responses, especially during this formative period. Eating assumes greater social significance. The family mealtime is an important means of socialization and sex identification. The children imitate their parents and others at the table. Depending on the examples set for them here, this may be negative rather than positive training.

"Food jags" Colloquial expression referring to repeated use of single foods over a brief period of time.

Food and feeding Because of developing social and emotional needs, the preschool child frequently follows **"food jags"** that may last for several days. However, they are usually short-lived and of no major concern. Again, the key is food variety. The child usually prefers single foods to combination dishes such as casseroles or stews. With mental development and the learning of language, the child prefers a single food that is easily identified and named because it has retained its characteristic texture, color, and form. The child likes foods that can be eaten with the fingers. Often raw fruit and raw vegetables cut in finger-sized pieces and offered to a child for selection help to meet these needs.

Allow the child to set goals in quantity of food. The portions need to be relatively small. Often if the child can pour milk from a small pitcher into a little glass, a greater amount may be consumed. The quantity of milk consumed usually declines during the preschool years. The child will consume two and sometimes three cups of milk during the day. Smaller children like their milk more lukewarm, not icy cold. Also, they prefer it in a small glass that will hold about a half to three fourths of a cup, rather than a large, adult-size glass. As the child begins to eat increasingly away from home, group eating becomes significant as a means of socialization. The child learns food patterns both at the family table and in group situations away from home. The child may be involved in a nursery or preschool situation in which group eating occurs. Food habits of preschoolers are greatly affected by the group, and food preferences grow according to what the group is eating. In such situations the child learns a widening variety of family food habits and forms new social relationships.

Young school-age child (6-12 Years)

Physical characteristics and growth The school-age period has been called the latent period of growth. The rate of growth slows and body changes occur gradually. However, resources are being laid down for the rapid adolescent growth ahead. Sometimes this period has been called the lull before the storm. By now the body type has been established, and growth rates vary widely. Girls usually outdistance boys in the latter part of this period.

Psychosocial development The core problem children struggle with during these early school years is the tension between *industry vs. inferiority.* With the stimulus of school and a variety of learning activities come increasing mental development, ability to work out problems, and competitive activities. The child begins moving from a dependence on parental standards to the standards of peers, in preparation for coming maturity. Pressures are generated for self-control of the growing body. There is a temporary disorganization of previous learning and developed personality. It is a kind of loosening up of the personality pattern for the inevitable changes ahead in adolescence. It is a diffuse period of gangs, cliques, hero worship, pensive daydreaming, emotional stresses, and learning to get along with other children.

Food and feeding The slowed rate of growth during this latent period results in a general decline in the food requirement per unit of body weight. This decline continues up to the latter part of the period just before approaching adolescence. Likes and dislikes are a product of earlier years. Family attitudes are imitated. As horizons widen, increasing interests and participation in other activities compete with mealtime, and often family conflict ensues. The important relationship of sound nutrition and learning has long been established. Breakfast is particularly important for a school child. It breaks the fast of the sleep hours and prepares a child for problem-solving while increasing memory span in the learning period at school. The school lunch program (see p. 231) provides a nourishing noon meal for many children who would not otherwise have one. Here a child can observe different food attitudes and taste new foods that he/she may not normally accept otherwise. Some favorite foods of American children are listed in Table 12-7. The school-age child is also increasingly exposed to new stimuli that influence food habits. Television becomes a strong source of food selection. There are positive learning opportunities in the classroom, particularly when parents provide support at home, and nutrition is integrated in other activities. Other school programs involve overweight children in a weight-management group situation involving behavior modification, nutrition education, and physical activity.

Table 12-7
Favorite Food Choices of American Children (listed in order of priority)*

Breakfast	Lunch or Dinner	Vegetables	Fruit	Beverage	Desserts	Sandwiches
Cereal	Steak or roast beef	Corn	Apple	Cola or soda	Ice cream	Peanut butter and jelly
Pancakes or waffles	Pizza	Carrots	Orange	Milk	Cake	Meat or cold cuts
Eggs	Spaghetti	Beans	Peach	Fruit punch	Pie	
French toast	Chicken	Tomatoes	Grape	Root beer	Pudding	Ham
Toast	Hamburger	Peas	Banana	Juices (other than orange)	Gelatin dessert	Tuna fish
Sweet rolls	Fish	Greens, collards or spinach	Watermelon		Banana split	Cheese
Doughnuts	Macaroni and cheese	Potatoes	Pear	Orange juice	Brownie	Bacon, lettuce, and tomato
				Lemonade		Roast beef

*Adapted from survey data of Lamme, A.J., and Lamme, L.L. Children's food preferences, J. Sch. Health **50**(7):397, 1980.

Adolescence (12-18 Years)

Physical characteristics and growth During the adolescent period, with the onset of puberty, the final growth spurt of childhood occurs. Maturation during this period varies so widely that chronologic age as a reference point for discussing growth ceases to be useful, if indeed it ever was. *Physiologic age* becomes more important in dealing with individual boys and girls. It accounts for wide fluctuations in metabolic rates, food requirements, scholastic capacity, and even illness.

Body changes in the adolescent period result from hormonal influences regulating the development of sex characteristics. The rate at which these changes occur varies widely and is particularly distinct in growth patterns that emerge between the sexes. For girls there is an increasing amount of subcutaneous fat deposit, particularly in the abdominal area. The hip breadth increases, and the bony pelvis widens in preparation for reproduction. A pelvic girdle of subcutaneous fat results. This is often a source of anxiety to many figure-conscious young girls. In boys physical growth is manifested more by an increased muscle mass and long-bone growth. A boy's growth spurt is slower than that of the girl, but he soon passes her in weight and height.

Food and feeding With the profound growth of adolescence comes increased demands for energy, protein, minerals, and vitamins. Caloric needs increase with the metabolic demands of growth and energy expenditure. Although individual needs vary, girls consume less food than boys do. Sometimes the increased appetite characteristic of this growth period leads adolescents to satisfy their hunger with snack foods that are high in sugar and fat and have very little essential protein content. Adolescent growth needs for protein are great, especially during the pubertal changes in both sexes and for the developing muscle mass in boys. Calcium and iron are particularly needed minerals. Bone growth demands calcium. Menstrual iron losses in adolescent girls predispose them to simple iron-deficiency anemia. The B vitamins are needed in increased amounts, especially by boys, to meet the extra demands of energy metabolism and muscle tissue development. Intake of needed vitamins A and C may be low because of erratic food intake.

Eating habits Physical and psychosocial pressures influence adolescent eating habits (see Issues and Answers, p. 293-294). Usually boys fare better than girls; their large appetite and the sheer volume of food it leads them to consume usually ensure an adequate intake of nutrients. Adolescent girls, however, may be less fortunate. Two factors combine to place them under pressure concerning body weight:

1. Because of physiologic sex differences associated with fat deposit during this period and a comparative lack of physical activity, adolescent girls may gain excess weight easily.
2. Social pressure and personal tensions concerning figure control will sometimes cause adolescent girls to follow unwise, self-imposed crash diets for weight loss. In some cases self-starvation diets may be followed, which result in complex and far-reaching eating disorders such as **anorexia nervosa** and **bulimia.** Usually these problems, which can assume severe proportions, involve a distorted body-image and a morbid, irrational pursuit of thinness. In one high school survey of 1268 adolescent girls aged 13-19,[7] 36% said that they were currently "dieting" to lose weight, 69% had been dieting at some time before the survey, 52% had begun dieting before age 14, and 14% were "chronic dieters." Despite their average weight being below age norms, all of the subjects perceived themselves as overweight. As a result of such malnourishment of varying degrees at the very time in life when the body is laying down reserves for approaching reproduction, many teenaged girls may suffer malnutrition. The hazards of such eating habits to the future course during potential pregnancies is clearly indicated in the studies relating preconception nutritional status to the outcome of gestation (see pp. 246, 256, and 334).

Anorexia nervosa Psychological condition manifested by a refusal to eat in order to achieve a thin, usually abnormally thin, appearance.

Bulimia Practice of bingeing on food, then inducing vomiting to prevent weight gain.

To Sum Up

Growth and development depend on nutrition to support physiologic and metabolic processes. Nutrition, in turn, depends on a multitude of social, psychologic, cultural, and environmental influences that affect individual growth potential throughout the life cycle. Four types of growth are usually measured during each phase of development: physical, mental, emotional, and sociocultural. Each type of growth is evaluated in assessing the child's nutritional status and planning an effective counseling approach.

Nutritional needs change with each growth period. *Infants* experience rapid growth. Breast-feeding is preferred during the first 6 months of life. The start of solid foods is delayed until 4 to 6 months of age to allow the infant's metabolic processes to mature. *Toddlers, preschoolers,* and *school-age children* experience a slowed and erratic latent growth in childhood. Their energy requirements per unit of body weight are not as great as the infant's. Their nutritional needs center on protein for growth with attendant minerals and vitamins. Social and cultural factors influence the development of food habits. *Adolescents* experience a second large growth spurt before reaching adulthood. This rapid growth is accompanied by sexual maturation as well as physical growth. Increased caloric and nutrient needs on the average are easier to achieve in boys than they are in girls, who more frequently feel social and peer pressure to restrict food intake for weight control. This pressure may inhibit their ability to acquire the nutritional reserves necessary for later reproduction.

Questions for Review

1. How is physical growth measured? What signs are used to measure mental, emotional, and sociocultural growth?
2. What factors are responsible for the major differences in nutritional and feeding needs of the preterm and full-term infant?
3. Why is breast-feeding the preferred method for feeding infants? What types of commercial formulas are available for bottle-fed babies?
4. Outline a general schedule for a new mother to use as a guide for adding solid foods to her infant's diet during the first year of life.
5. What changes in physical growth and psychosocial development influence eating habits in the toddler, preschool child, and school-age child? How do these factors influence the nutritional needs of each age group?
6. What factors influence the changing nutritional needs of adolescents? Who is usually at greater nutritional risk during this phase—boys or girls? Why? What nutritional deficiencies are associated with this more vulnerable age?

References

1. Erikson, E.: Childhood and society, New York, 1963, W.W. Norton & Co. Inc.
2. Hall, E.: A conversation with Erik Erikson, Psychology Today **17**(6):22, 1983.
3. Miller, J.A.: The littlest babies, Science News **124**(16):250, 1983.
4. Brooke, O.G.: Nutrition in the preterm infant, Lancet **1**(8323):514, 1983.
5. Brady, M.S., and others: Formulas and human milk for premature infants: a review and update, J. Am. Diet. Assoc. **81**(5):547, 1982.
6. Anderson, S.A., Chinn, H.I., and Fisher, K.D.: History and current status of infant formulas, Am. J. Clin. Nutr. **35**:381, 1982.
7. Johnson, C.L., and others: A descriptive survey of dieting and bulimic behavior in a female high school population. In Understanding anorexia nervosa and bulimia, Columbus, Ohio, 1983, Ross Laboratories.

Further Readings

Anderson, S.A., Chenin, H.I., and Fisher, K.D.: History and current status of infant formulas, Am. J. Clin. Nutr. **35**:381, 1982.

A comprehensive review of the history and development, types and uses, nutrition concerns and problems, current legislation and regulations, and research needs of infant formulas.

Owen, G.M.: Measurement, recording, and assessment of skinfold thickness in childhood and adolescence, Am. J. Clin. Nutr. **35**(3):629, 1982.

A good discussion that outlines techniques for measuring skinfold thickness. Reports percentiles that may be used as reference data but should not be considered as "norms," "standards" or "ideals." Presents problems in the use of these standards as a routine screening measurement in well-child care.

Shinwell, E.D., and Gorodischer, R.: Totally vegetarian diets and infant nutrition, Pediatrics, **70**(4):582, 1982.

Reports on a study of the deleterious effects of a vegan diet in infancy and the unsuccessful attempts to find dietary modifications that would satisfy both the vegan philosophy and the recommended dietary allowances.

Issues and Answers

Food Habits of Adolescents

Teenagers have gained the reputation of having the worst eating habits in the world. Is this justified? Here's a closer look at the actual eating habits of American adolescents during the last 15 years:

Skipping Meals

A study of California teens revealed that lunch (not breakfast, as most people assume) was the meal most frequently skipped. Breakfast was most frequently skipped by obese children, however. In all cases, the frequency of regular meals increased with income and social status.

Snacking

Another study indicated that 12- to 16-year-olds met or exceeded their RDA per 100 kcals for protein, riboflavin, and vitamin C through between-meal foods. But vitamin A, calcium, and iron levels were low.

Fast Foods

Having a limited range of items, fast foods are more likely to be lacking one or more essential nutrients. They are generally considered to be inadequate in calcium and vitamin A, and too high in kcals, saturated fats, and sodium. Current marketing practices continue to attract the young, and fast food restaurants have become popular "hang-outs" to escape the demands of an ever-encroaching adult world. These places will influence the nutritional quality of adolescent meals for some time.

Unusual Food Choices

Teenagers are likely to eat any type of food at any time of the day. They are as likely to have barbecued chicken for breakfast as pancakes for dinner. These food choices are only unusual in terms of the time of day at which they are consumed and usually present no threat to health or nutritional status.

Alcohol Consumption

As adolescents approach the drinking age in their locale, alcohol begins to provide a more significant portion of their total caloric intake. Even a mild form of abuse coupled with the elevated nutritional demands of adolescence may comprise nutritional status, especially in terms of folic acid, which is "destroyed" by excessive amounts of alcohol. Damage to the intestinal mucosa caused by chronic alcohol use could also influence the absorption of other nutrients.

In general, the adolescent diet may be no worse than the average adult diet, although intake of calcium, vitamin A, iron, and ascorbic acid are usually seriously inadequate for the teen years, especially among girls. In addition, eating habits and social pressures have made this age group susceptible to at least two important nutritional problems: obesity and anorexia nervosa.

Continued.

Issues and Answers—cont'd

■ *Obesity* affects approximately 10% to 20% of the adolescent population. As in adults, an excessive intake of kcals is less often the cause than lack of exercise. Concern about personal appearance could make the adolescent more reluctant than an adult to participate in activities (e.g., team sports, dance classes) that are popular ways of controlling weight.

■ *Anorexia nervosa* is considered the flip side of the weight management coin. It usually affects achievement-oriented, affluent girls, (although the problem now crosses socioeconomic—and sexual—barriers. This self-induced starvation is often attributed to an obsession to attaining a slim figure—a desire that goes so far as to result in self-starvation, emaciation, and serious health problems, including amenorrhea.

In all, the food habits of adolescents reflect a reduced influence of parents on the child's eating habits, increased peer pressure or desire to conform, extra sensitivity to appearance, and elevated needs for energy.

References
Truswell, A.S., and Darnton-Hill, I.: Food habits of adolescents, Nutr. Rev. **39**(2):73, 1981.

Chapter 13
Nutrition for Adults: Aging and the Aged

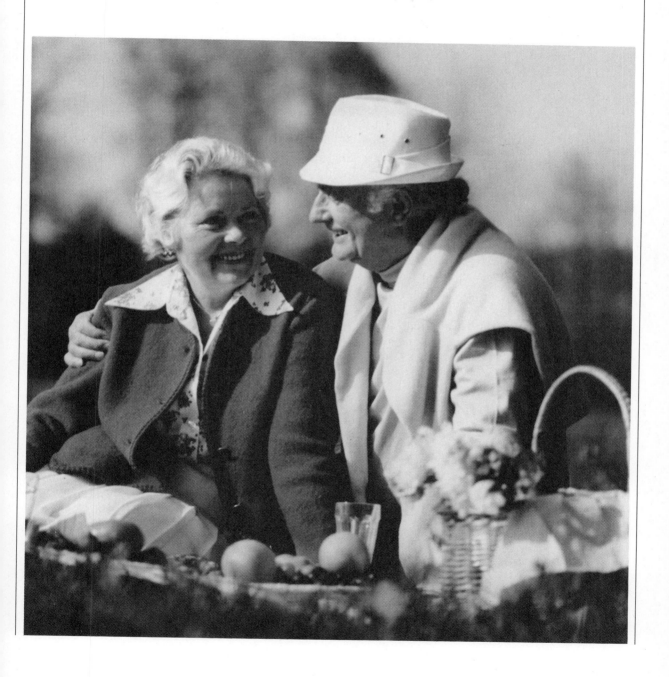

Preview

Following the tumultuous adolescent years come the challenges, problems, and opportunities of maturity. The cycle of human growth and development continues throughout the adult years.

Our population has been changing. There are more adults now and they are growing older. Thanks to the World War II "baby boom," the fastest growing group in America today is aged 35 to 44. This is an increase of almost 10% since the 1980 census, and this group now numbers about 28 million. Already there are 26.3 million Americans aged 65 and over, and the second fastest growing group is aged 85 and over. According to further census bureau projections, during the 1980s there will be a 15% increase in the 65- to 74-year-old population and a 33% increase in the 75-year-old and over group.

Behind all of these numbers are human beings—unique individuals experiencing the imprint of their life situation and facing problems, including health concerns. In our study, two important concepts govern our approach: (1) aging is an *individual* process and (2) aging is a part of a *total life* process—biologic, nutritional, socioeconomic, psychosocial, and spiritual.

Chapter Objectives

After study of this chapter, the student should be able to:

1. Identify social and economic problems of aging persons in American society today.

2. Define the role of nutrition in the aging process and the changes it brings in specific nutrient needs.

3. Identify nutrition-related clinical problems of aging.

4. Relate eating problems among aging clients to practical daily living situations and identify community resources to help meet these needs.

Aging in America

Aging is a positive concept. It encompasses the whole of life, and every period has its unique potential and fulfillment. The periods of adulthood—young, middle, and older—are no exception. Both psychosocial and physical development continue, although in changing patterns, as persons mature and grow older. The three adult stages of the human life span, as identified by Erikson (see p. 275), complete the whole of human development.

Psychosocial Development in Adulthood
Young Adulthood (18–40 Years)

In the years of young adulthood the individual has now become an autonomous person. Each individual must resolve the core problem of *intimacy vs. isolation.* The person who achieves the goal of intimacy is able to build intimate self-fulfilling relationships, either in marriage or in other personal relationships. Others who fail to do so become increasingly isolated from others. These are years of much stress but also much fulfillment. They are the years of career beginnings, of establishing one's own home, of parenthood, and of starting young children on their way through the same life stages. These are the years of early struggles to make one's way in the world, with their attendant joys and heartaches.

Middle Adulthood (40-60 Years)

Generativity Pertaining to the reproduction or continuance of the species.

In the years of middle adulthood the core problem the individual faces is **generativity** *vs. self-absorption.* Children have now grown and gone to make their own lives. For some these are the years of the "empty nest." For others it is an opportunity to expand personal growth—"it's my turn now." There is a coming-to-terms with what life is all about and a great opportunity of finding expression for stored learning in passing on life's teachings. It is a regeneration of one's life in the lives of young persons following the same way. To the degree that these inner struggles are not won, there is increasing self-absorption, a turning-in on oneself, and a withering rather than a regenerating spirit of life.

Older Adulthood (60-80 + Years)

In the last stage of life the final core problem is resolved between *integrity vs. despair.* Depending on a person's resources at this point, there is either a predominant sense of wholeness and completeness or a sense of bitterness and revulsion and of wondering what life was all about. If the outcome of life's basic experiences has been positive, the individual arrives at old age a rich person—rich in wisdom of the years. Building on each previous level, psychosocial growth has reached its individual, positive human resolution. But some of our elderly patients will not have resolved the core psychosocial conflicts. They still struggle with those that they have wrestled with in previous stages of life. Thus they arrive at middle and later years poorly equipped to deal with the adjustments of aging and health problems that may face them. On the other hand, many will have been enriched by life's experiences in their maturing process. In turn they will bring enrichment to our lives. The resulting relationship is a mutually rewarding one.

Socioeconomic and Psychologic Factors

Increasing industrialization and urbanization of American society, the complexity of the culture it is building, and the changes in age distribution in the population have all brought about changes in the lives of adults in the United States today.

Population Changes

Not only has the general population been increasing rapidly, but significant shifts have occurred in age distribution. More people are living longer. One out of every 7 Americans is now over the age of 60, and the number of older Americans has increased two and a half times as fast as the overall population. At age 65 the average life expectancy is 16 more years; at age 75, another 10. Recent surveys indicate that many adults are not only living longer but also living better.[1] Many older adults are active and able to take care of themselves for longer than the general American myth and stereotyping of **ageism** would picture them. But many persons are increasingly concerned about the "quality" of life, not merely its length. They are concerned about changing biologic, social, and environmental factors and their combined effect on the quality of lengthened life. Today our increased longevity has in general been influenced by two factors: medical care and living standards.

Ageism Discrimination on the basis of age, usually applying to older persons.

Medical care Great progress in care of infants and children has reduced infant mortality, controlled communicable diseases, and improved child care. The increased availability and quality of medical care during adult years is also a factor in health during maturing years. However, there has been relatively little progress in controlling chronic disease in old age or in relating general medical care practices to the needs of the aged.

Living standards General U.S. living standards are high, but many "new poor" have begun to suffer more since there is a sagging economy worldwide. In general more people have a better education, better housing, and improved nutrition through growth and early adult years, although in older age problems in socioeconomic status increase for many. The factors that have contributed to the increased number of older persons in the population have medical, social, and economic implications.

Social and Economic Factors

America's increasing industrialization and high technology, with subsequent changing social attitudes, have affected the position of older persons in American society. Economic insecurity creates pressures (Figure 13-1). A policy in industry of early retirement and employment difficulties with advancing age have created financial pressures. However, industry leaders are beginning to recognize that changes in the U.S. workforce, the economic status of the federal Social Security System, and the employability of older workers with much experience and skill are factors that will profoundly affect the composition of the workforce in the years ahead. In some instances changing social attitudes toward elderly persons and their capacities have increased institutional care and segregation in living situations. Many elderly persons, however, are able to live with extended families or in a variety of group or self-help situations. Only 1 of every 20

Figure 13-1
Elderly disabled man assisted by the Food Stamp Program to obtain needed food.

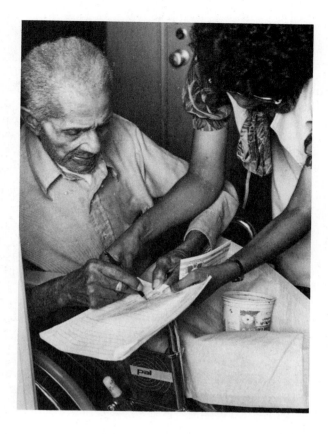

elderly persons is in a health care facility, and only 10% of those over 65 are confined in any serious way (see box, p. 300). Older persons are often removed from involvement in the activities of society, but they need such stimuli for as long as possible.

Psychologic Factors

Financial pressures and a decreasing sense of acceptance and accomplishment cause many elderly persons to suffer anxieties and loss of personal values. Many may feel inadequate. All persons need a sense of belonging, achievement, and self-esteem. Instead many elderly persons are often lonely, restless, unhappy, and uncertain. Primarily the greater part of the aging process in any area is culturally determined. Unfortunately in many instances our culture imposes a set of negative roles on persons as they reach older age.[2] Basic needs common to older persons include economic security, personal effectiveness, suitable housing, constructive and enjoyable leisure-time activities, satisfying social relationships, and spiritual values.

The Aging Process and Nutritional Needs

General Physiologic Changes

The general biologic process of growth and decline extends over the entire life span. It is conditioned by all previous life experiences and by the imprint of these experiences on individual genetic heritage.

Clinical Application

Improving the Nutritional Status of the Elderly in Long-term Care Facilities

The use of full-time nutritionists at long-term care facilities is a relatively new concept. A report of Canadian dietitians, employed by facilities that previously relied only on a food service supervisor, documents improvements in the nutritional status of residents as a result of professional nutrition services. They review various activities that help ensure optimal nutrition status of residents:

Administrative Duties
- Developing cyclic menus based on age group nutritional requirements
- Staff training to ensure proper food preparation, storage, and distribution
- In-service education for all health professionals and kitchen staff regarding the nutritional requirements of residents

Clinical Duties
- Making regularly scheduled nutritional assessments (weight, body composition, laboratory tests as needed [pp. 356-357])
- Conducting a baseline nutrition assessment of *every* resident at admission
- Making accurate calculations of diets as needed
- Discouraging abuse of alcohol, nicotine, laxatives, and other drugs
- Developing resident education programs such as weight and health management classes
- Encouraging eating by planning special events such as picnics and holiday meals that may include family members, creating a "homelike" atmosphere in the dining hall, preparing meals in general living areas to "entice" residents with food aromas, and encouraging residents to serve themselves.

References
Gardner, J., and Kelley, A.: Long-term care facilities: the benefits of having a dietitian, J. Can. Diet. Assoc. **44**(1):68, 1983.

Nature of Biologic Changes

During middle and older adulthood there are gradual cell losses and reduced cell metabolism, with a gradual reduction in the performance capacity of most organ systems. Radioisotope (potassium 40) estimations of lean body mass demonstrate a continuous age-related decline that accelerates in later life.[3] For example, by age 70 the kidneys and lungs lose about 10% of their weight in comparison with values in young adults, the liver loses 18% of its weight, and skeletal muscle diminishes by 40%. There is also an overall, gradual reduction in the body's reserve capacities. An important cause is the gradual reduction in cellular units. For example, functioning units of the kidney—nephrons—are lost as the "aging Western kidney" responds to our high-protein diet (see p. 485).

Effect of Changes on Food Patterns

Some physiologic factors may affect food patterns. For example, there is a diminished secretion of digestive juices and a decreased motility of the gastrointestinal tract. This causes decreased absorption and use of nutrients. Sensory perceptions, such as taste, smell, and vision, also diminish. These senses influence appetite and the amount of food consumed. Along with these biologic changes there often comes an increased concern about body functions, increasing social stress, personal losses, and diminished social opportunities to maintain self-esteem. All of these responses may affect food intake.

Individuality of the Aging Process

The biologic changes of aging are general. But in reality persons in the advancing years of life will display a wide variety of individual reactions. They simply get old at different rates. Each person bears the imprint of individual trauma and the accumulation of disease experience. This has a direct effect on individual aging. Thus specific needs of individuals must always be remembered and considered when caring for general aging and nutritional needs. The greatest influence of nutrition in the aging process takes place in earlier years. Nutrition's most effective role is in the growth and middle years. These years prepare the individual to meet the gradually declining metabolic processes of older age.

Nutritional Needs
Energy—Kilocalories

In adulthood the basal energy requirement is reduced by gradual losses in functioning protoplasm. This factor, together with the usual reduced physical activity, creates less demand for energy as age advances. Some studies with test animals indicate that the concept of a limited, less rich diet—undernutrition without malnutrition—may actually lengthen life.[4] The RDA standard is based on estimates of 5% decreased metabolic activity in middle and latter years. The average estimate of energy needed is an approximate caloric requirement of 1800 kcal. Men may require more—about 2200 kcal.

There are major gaps in our knowledge of energy and nutrient needs of the elderly. Some evidence indicates that nutrient uptake by cells declines with aging, so that older persons may need higher plasma levels of nutrients to maintain optimal tissue concentration. Living situations vary widely among older adults, so there is need for much more information on their daily life activities and the degree of energy that they may be capable of expending. Kilocalorie requirements are highly individual, according to activity. Primary consideration must be given to the living status of the person and the degree of activity in various phases of life. Perhaps the simplest basis for caloric intake is the maintenance of *normal* weight. But there is current rethinking of traditional standards of ideal weight based on weight-for-height tables (see p. 346). Recent reassessment of these and other data has raised the possibility that the greatest longevity is not associated with conventional "desirable" weights but with levels 10% to 25% greater.[3] In other words, very thin persons have a reduced life expectancy rather than a better outlook. This view has obvious nutritional implications in terms of optimal energy intake in adults of all ages.

Carbohydrates The optimal energy from carbohydrate intake is unknown, but it is usually recommended that about 50% of kilocalories in the diet come from carbohydrate foods, mostly complex carbohydrates such as starches. Easily absorbable sugars may also be used, and there is generally no disturbance in carbohydrate metabolism. The fasting blood sugar level is essentially normal in the aged. They can choose freely among carbohydrate foods, according to individual needs and desires and physical responses.

Fats Fats usually contribute about 30% of total kilocalories. They provide a source of energy, important fat-soluble vitamins, and essential fatty acids. A reasonable goal is to avoid large quantities of fat, with more emphasis on the quality of the fat consumed. Digestion and absorption of fats may be delayed in elderly persons, but these functions are not greatly disturbed with age. There is no need to be unduly restrictive. Sufficient fat for food palatability aids appetite. Excessive fat, however, should be avoided because of the delayed absorption capacity of elderly persons.

Protein There is a basic need for quality protein to meet the nutritional needs of the aging in our society.

Basic needs The RDA standard recommends a continuation of the daily protein intake for the aging individual at the same adult allowance given for age 25—0.8 g/kg of body weight. This amount provides an allowance for wide variation in individual needs. A recent study, however, of protein needs of elderly persons showed that a diet meeting the adult RDA for protein was inadequate to prevent loss of body protein.[3] It is possible that to maintain nitrogen balance, elderly persons may need relatively more protein as their energy intake is reduced. There is certainly an increased need for protein during illness, convalescence, or a wasting disease.

Protein quality Protein needs are influenced by two basic factors: (1) the biologic value of the protein—the quantity and ratio of its amino acids—and (2) adequate caloric value of the diet. It is estimated that 25% to 50% of the protein intake should come from animal sources, with the remainder from plant protein sources. Protein should supply from 15% to 20% of the day's total kilocalories. For healthy individuals there is usually no need for supplemental amino acid preparations. They are an expensive and inefficient source of available nitrogen.

Vitamins There is usually no requirement for additional vitamin intake in the healthy adult. There may be gradually decreasing tissue stores with normal aging but no difference in requirement from that for normal adults. Individual problems may stem from inadequate normal intake rather than from an increased need. A well-selected mixed diet with a variety of foods should supply vitamins in normally needed quantities. Increased therapeutic needs in illness should be evaluated on an individual basis.

Minerals There is usually no need for increased minerals in normal aging. The same adult allowances are sufficient if provided on a continuing basis and by a well-balanced diet. However, two essential minerals need emphasis and possible increase: calcium and iron. The adult RDA stan-

Osteoporosis Bone weakened by a loss of mineral content, mainly calcium.

dard for calcium intake is 800 mg/day. There has been some recent evidence that to prevent negative calcium balance, the level should be increased to at least 1200 mg in women over age 50 and in men over age 60 to prevent calcium loss from bone tissue and the development of **osteoporosis** (see p. 146).[3,5] Poor diets may also be deficient in iron, which is needed to prevent iron-deficiency anemia. Some individuals need increased attention and encouragement to ensure adequate dietary sources of these minerals among their daily food choices.

The Question of Nutrient Supplementation

There is no evidence that *healthy* adults in middle to older years require additional nutrient supplementation. The nutrition board of the National Research Council has stated that it is aware of no convincing evidence of unique health benefits accruing from consumption of a large excess of any one nutrient. Nonetheless the use of such supplements is widespread among older adults. There is some indication that nutrient supplementation might be a rational approach to improve cognitive function in disoriented elderly persons. In illness or debilitated states supplementation may well be needed to help restore tissue integrity and health (see Issues and Answers, pp. 309-311).

Clinical Needs

Chronic illness, such as heart disease (Chapter 20), often creates additional problems for aging persons. In addition, other environmental factors contribute to illness from malnutrition and produce clinical needs.

Malnutrition
Personal Food Habits

Generally poor dietary habits in young adulthood, as with any personal habit, tend to be set and accentuated in older age. Although surveys usually show adequate caloric intake on the average, there is frequent evidence of inadequate nutrient distribution in food choices. For example, there may be little use of animal protein, such as meat, egg, cheese, and milk. There may also be inadequate use of whole grains, fewer vegetables and fruits, and use of more sweets and desserts, even to the extent of about 20% of the day's kilocalories. Also, older persons are frequently prey to claims of food faddists concerning various restorative food products, tonics, or regulators.

Oral Problems

Peridontal disease Disease (inflammation) occurring in tissue surrounding the teeth; facilitates tooth loss.

Poor teeth, **peridontal disease**, or poorly fitting dentures make chewing difficult. A denture can only be as successful as the health of the tissue on which it rests. An analysis of the three stages of eating food—biting, chewing, and swallowing—will provide a basis for helping the person with new dentures adjust to using them. Poor appetite and limited financial means for adequate dental care discourage efforts to seek improvement in the situation. Also, mucosal changes in the mouth, as well as a decrease or change in the quality of salivary secretions, cause further difficulty in eating.

Gastrointestinal Problems

Diverticulitis Inflammation of "pockets" of tissue (diverticuli) in the lining of the mucous membrane in the colon.

Numerous gastrointestinal complaints vary from vague indigestion or "irritable colon" to specific diseases such as peptic ulcer (p. 425) or **divertic-**

ulitis (p. 426). Such problems generally reduce appetite and food intake. so the needed nutrients are not taken in. In other cases limited absorption of nutrients curtails nourishment still further.

Personal and Social Factors

Financial resources may be limited, and there may be little money available to purchase needed food. Persons may lack knowledge of the food needed for a well-balanced diet. Boredom, loneliness, anxiety, insecurity, and apathy compound the problem. Especially if an older person lives alone, the social value of eating is gone. They may also lack adequate cooking, refrigeration, or storage facilities. They may have no means of transportation to obtain food. A vicious cycle often ensues: funds are low, the person hesitates to spend, goes without, and suffers increasing weakness and **lethargy**. This state leads to still less interest and incentive. Finally, illness results.

Implications for Patient Care

The malnourished older person needs much personal care and support to build improved eating habits. Helpful attitudes and actions by practitioners are based on an understanding and realistic approach.

Analyze food habits carefully Learn the patient's personal attitudes, the precise situation, and its limiting factors. Nutritional needs can be meet with a variety of foods, so suggestions can be adapted to fit particular needs and personal situations and desires. Offer suggestions in a practical, realistic, and supportive manner.

Never moralize The statement, "Eat this because it's good for you," should be struck from everyone's vocabulary. It has little value for anyone, much less a person who is struggling to maintain personal integrity and self-esteem in a culture that largely alienates its aged.

Encourage food variety An unattractive bland diet is presumed by many to be necessary for all elderly persons. *It is not.* A variety of foods and adventures with new foods, tastes, and seasonings often prove to be the needed stimuli for poor appetite and lack of interest in eating. A decreased taste sensitivity in aging needs all the help it can get. Sometimes smaller amounts of foods and more frequent meals are helpful.

Weight Management

In a different sense, obesity may be considered a form of malnutrition. In middle and older adults it can be a potential health hazard in relation to diabetes and hypertension. Avoiding excessive weight in earlier growth years is a major nutritional measure for preventing problems in old age.

Causes of Overweight

Many of the same living situations and emotional factors that have been described here may also contribute to overweight. Such factors often lead to overeating as a compensation, and poor food choices result. Also physical activity is usually decreased and the caloric requirement lessened, but the same food habits continue.

Lethargy Drowsiness; indifference.

Individual Approach

Long-standing eating habits or excessive weight are difficult to change. Certainly a reasonable approach should be followed, avoiding drastic measures or diet and planning only for a slow gradual loss. Moderate physical activity should be encouraged whenever possible. Personal and realistic planning with every client or patient is mandatory because individual kilocalorie requirements vary widely and individual personalities and problems are unique. This initial approach should be followed by supportive guidance and encouragement. Such an individual program usually pays the greatest dividends.

**Community
Resources**

Government Programs for Older Americans
Older American Act—Title VII

In 1972, the Nutrition Program for Older Americans, Title VII of the Older Americans Act, was authorized by Public Law 92-258. The program was developed to meet both nutritional and social needs of persons 60 years of age and older who (1) cannot afford adequate diets, (2) are unable to prepare adequate meals at home, (3) have limited mobility, or (4) are isolated and lack incentive to prepare and eat food alone. The original program provided services such as outreach, escort and transportation, health services, information and referral, health and welfare counseling, nutrition and consumer education. In 1978 amendments to the Older Americans Act were authorized by Public Law 95-478, which coordinated nutrition services with other services for older people.[7] Under this amended act, Title III, the services founded after 1980 included the provision of meals, both congregate and home-delivered, and related nutrition services and education.

Congregate meals The program provides older Americans, particularly those with low incomes, with low-cost, nutritionally sound meals in senior centers and other public or private community facilities. In these settings older adults can gather for a hot noon meal and receive both food and social support.

Home-delivered meals For those persons who are ill or disabled and as a result unable to attend the congregate meals, meals are delivered by couriers to the home. This service provides both nutritional needs and human contact and support. Often the courier is the only person the homebound individual may contact during the day.

U.S. Department of Agriculture (USDA) Research Centers

A new $32.6 million Human Nutrition Research Center on Aging has been built by the USDA in cooperation with Tufts University in Boston. It is the largest research facility in the United States specifically authorized by Congress to study nutrition's role in aging. Current research investigations include protein needs in the aged, the nutritional status of elderly men and women, and the prevention and slowing of osteoporosis through nutritional support.[8]

USDA Extension Services

The USDA operates agricultural extension services in state universities. County home advisors aid communities with practical material and counsel for elderly persons and community workers.

Public Health Departments

Skilled health professionals work in the community through local and state public health departments. These resources are available to provide health guidance for elderly persons. The public health nutritionist is a significant member of the health care team and provides counseling and nutrition education services as well as community program planning. Counseling is also provided concerning the various food assistance programs available (see p. 233).

Professional Organizations and Resources

National Council on the Aging

This national organization was established in 1950 and is located in Washington, D.C. Its members include both professionals and volunteers who work on many fronts to improve the quality of life for older Americans. It provides a nonprofit, central national resource for research, planning, training, information, technical assistance, advocacy, program and standards development, and publications that relate to all aspects of aging, including nutrition.

American Geriatric Society

Geriatrics The study and treatment of diseases of old age; a branch of medicine concerned with medical problems associated with old age.

This professional organization of physicians engaged in medical care of elderly patients promotes research in **geriatrics** to advance scientific knowledge of the aging process and the treatment of its disease. A number of nurses and other health professionals are associate members. The society publishes the *American Journal of Geriatrics*.

The Gerontological Society

Gerontology The study of the aging process and its phenomena.

This society's membership includes a wide number of interested health professionals. Its committee on aging has stimulated increased interest among other related organizations and community and government agencies in **gerontology** and the problems of the aging person in our society. This organization publishes the *Journal of Gerontology*.

Community Groups

Local community groups representing health professions such as the medical society, nursing organizations, and dietetic associations sponsor a variety of programs to help meet the needs of elderly persons. In addition, there are qualified nutritionists and registered dietitians in private practice available in most communities for individual counseling and community program support. Senior citizen centers in local communities also provide a broad range of services and available nutrition counseling and education.

Volunteer Organizations

Many activities of volunteer health organizations such as the Heart Association and Diabetes Association relate to the needs of older persons.

To Sum Up

The challenge of meeting the nutritional needs of the older population is compounded by the lack of research in this area, the interaction of current and past social, economic, and psychologic factors, and the wide range of individual differences in the biologic process of aging. Nutritional requirements should, at least in part, be based on biologic changes caused by aging. However, standards are mainly based on data available for younger adult populations, as well as requirements to counteract disease processes prevalent in aging, such as cardiovascular disease.

Major illnesses found in elderly persons are associated with malnutrition and obesity. in counseling the older client, the nutritionist should analyze food habits carefully. Each client must be encouraged to make dietary changes at his/her own rate, with supportive guidance, encouragement, and patience.

Questions for Review

1. Identify three major biologic changes that occur with aging and give an example of each.
2. Identify and give examples of three major factors contributing to malnutrition in older adults. How do these factors influence the nutrition counseling process?
3. List and describe the purpose of several agencies providing nutrition-related services for elderly persons or for health professionals in geriatric practice.

References

1. Gelman, D.: Growing old, feeling young, Newsweek **C**(18):56, 1982.
2. Ferguson, T.: The prejudice against older people, Medical Self-Care **15**:10, Winter 1981.
3. Munro, H.N.:, Nutritional requirements in the elderly, Hosp. Pract. **10**:143, 1982.
4. Report: Limited food intake and longevity, Nutr. Rev. **40**(10):314, 1982.
5. Report: Osteoporosis and calcium balance, Nutr. Rev. **41**(3):83, 1983.
6. Raskind, M.: Nutrition and cognitive function in the elderly, J. Am. Med. Assoc. **249**(21):2939, 1983.
7. Greene, J.M.: Coordination of Older Americans Act programs, J. Am. Diet. Assoc. **79**(6):617, 1981.
8. Mathieu, M.: Nutrition and aging center, J. Am. Diet. Assoc. **82**(1):79, 1983.

Further Readings

Gelman, D., and others: Who's taking care of our parents? Newsweek **CV**(18):60, 1985.

An excellent review of the increasingly disturbing problem of quality of life in the care of America's aged. Because there is a growing number of older persons and complicated burdens borne by middle adults in caring for aging parents, we face a society in which the old will be looking after the very old.

Patten, S.E.: Nutrition and the elderly: a cultural perspective, Geriatrics **37**(5):141, 1982.

This book clearly states the relationship between social influences on eating behavior and successful resolution of nutritional problems in the elderly.

Young, E.A.: Nutrition, aging, and the aged, Med. Clin. North Am. **67**(2):295, 1983.

A thorough symposium report on concepts of aging, essential nutrients, nutritional assessment, factors influencing nutritional status, and selected nutrition-related problems in the elderly.

Report: Teaching hospitals? Why not "teaching nursing homes?" J. Am. Diet. Assoc. **80**(3):260, 1982.

An announcement of the plans of the National Institute on Aging (NIA) to set up research centers in nursing homes located near medical schools.

Issues and Answers

Can We Eat to Live Forever?

The world is getting older. Our lifespan has extended from age 45 at the turn of the century to 77 (74 in men) today. It is expected to climb even higher.

We owe today's longevity to the conquest of infectious disease, the provision of safer work environments, and the development of more effective medical technology. In short, we have largely conquered our external environment. The time has come to conquer our *inner* environment—through proper nutrition.

Scientists are beginning to consider the importance of nutrition in combating the physical deterioration that accompanies old age—a 10% loss of kidney and lung tissue, 18% of liver tissue, 40% of skeletal tissue, and as much as 25% (12% in men) of bone by the seventh decade of life. One would think that scientists could simply make biochemical calculations to find optimal blood levels for nutrients that could retard these losses and make recommendations for dietary intake. However, achieving an optimal diet among elderly persons is much more complex than that. Consider the following.

Sensory Deprivation

Elderly persons tend to live alone. Such physical and emotional isolation tends to diminish the desire to eat. When this is combined with the progressive deterioration in sight, smell, touch, and hearing, attempts to prepare meals are no longer merely frustrating—they become dangerous.

Taste and Smell

Oral infections, poor hygiene, and a reduced salivary flow rate contribute to the increased difficulty in taste and smell. To what extent does this affect the desire to eat? No one knows. Some scientists say very little, suspecting poor research techniques in studies of this problem. Other believe it is serious enough to warrant further research to arrest on-going losses.

Bone and Tooth Loss

Approximately one half of all adults have lost their teeth by age 65. The main culprit is **periodontal disease**. Researchers are beginning to look at this problem as a possible manifestation of osteoporosis. Therefore they are focusing study on calcium:

- **Calcium RDAs** Some suggest that 1000 to 1200 mg/day may be necessary to prevent calcium loss, rather than the current RDA of 800 mg.
- **Phosphate** Calcium and phosphorus maintain an inverse ratio in the blood (p. 144). Processed foods contribute heavily to phosphate levels in the American diet and are suspected of promoting calcium resorption from bone.
- **Megavitamins** One report associates excessive vitamin A levels with a greater loss of bone in elderly persons. Another study of 100 elderly subjects revealed that 60% took vitamin supplements,

Continued.

Issues and Answers—cont'd

with most taking three or more times the recommended daily allowance for vitamin A. This warrants further study.

■ **Protein** America's obsession with meat may harm aging bones, as a high protein intake results in increased loss of calcium in the urine.

Caloric Needs

It has repeatedly been reported that elderly persons fail to consume recommended amounts of kilocalories. Recent animal research indicates that they might have the right idea. Restricted kcal intake in rats has been associated with longevity and has retarded development of respiratory, cardiovascular, and renal disease, as well as cancer. This factor is still controversial. A recent reassessment of the effect of body weight suggests that we should all weigh 10% to 25% more than we do in order to live longer. As the reassessment does not associate body size with detrimental health habits, such as smoking, it, in turn, is itself controversial.

Gastrointestinal Problems

Peristalsis Wavelike motion of longitudinal and circular muscle fibers in the gastrointestinal tract that propels food along for variable distances.

Reduced production of digestive juices, less **peristalsis**, and reduced mucosal surface area all work to inhibit nutrient absorption and promote such digestive disorders as constipation.

Drugs

The high prevalence of chronic disease means a high prevalence of drug use, both prescription and over-the-counter use. Drugs, either individually or in combination, can alter taste, appetite, and other factors affecting nutritional status.

Poverty

Frequently many elderly persons either cannot work or are forced into retirement. For these reasons they tend to be among the poorest citizens. Even those individuals in good health often lack the money to shop, the transportation to reach shopping areas, or the means for adequate food preparation and/or storage equipment to maintain a reasonably healthful diet.

Based on the information available thus far, the most nutritionally supportive environment for elderly persons is one in which they

1. Have company for meals, congregate meal sites, family support, and friends
2. Have foods with pleasant but distinctive aromas and flavors
3. Consume meals that are lower in protein-rich and processed foods, higher in fiber-rich foods (complex carbohydrates and a variety of fresh fruits and vegetables) and calcium (from non-bovine as well as bovine sources, to avoid excessive protein levels), and meals that provide a moderate amount of kilocalories
4. Avoid excess supplements, especially of vitamin A

Issues and Answers—cont'd

5. Avoid unnecessary drugs and are informed of the action of each drug they do take
6. Are subsidized financially or live in situations such as senior centers, private homes, or with roommates that provide some financial, emotional, and nutritional support

These seem like reasonable recommendations for any age group. But nutrition in elderly persons presents such a myriad of long-standing compounding factors that a wide variety of services and professional assistance may be needed to avoid nutritional deficits. Thus counselors who hope to promote a nutritionally supportive environment for elderly clients must themselves maintain a network of professionals available for referrals and work together as a team to meet the unique needs of older persons.

References
Munro, H.N.: Nutritional requirements in the elderly, Hosp. Pract. 10:143, 1982.
Rivlin, R.S.: Nutrition and aging: some unanswered questions, Am. J. Med. 71:337, 1981.
Yearick, E.S., Wang, M.L., and Pisias, S.J.: Nutritional status of the elderly: dietary and biochemical findings, J. Gerontol. 35(5):661, 1980.

Chapter 14
Nutrition and Physical Fitness

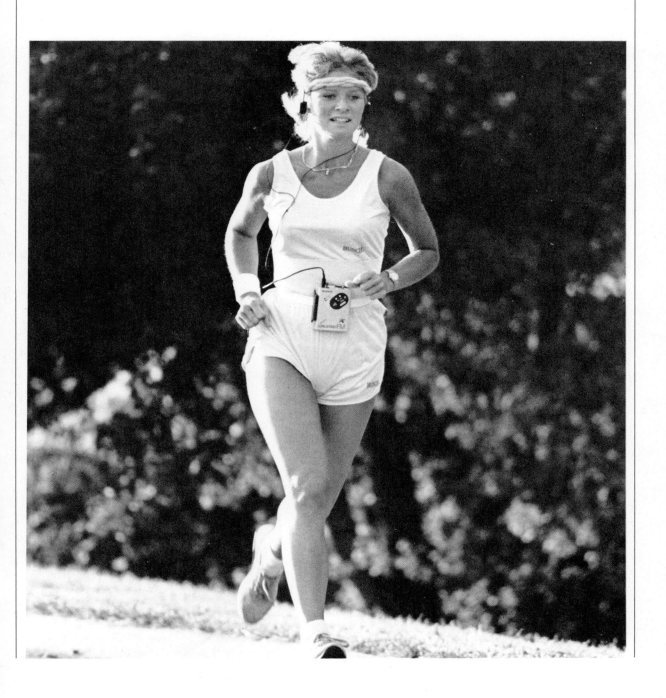

Recently there has been a growing interest in physical fitness. The modern approach of preventive medicine, as well as the necessity of dealing with demonstrated disease, calls for increased attention to the related roles of nutrition and physical fitness in health care. For both recreational desires and health imperatives, we need to provide our clients and patients with sound guidelines. We need to practice them ourselves.

After study of this chapter, the student should be able to:

1. Define physical fitness and describe how it is measured.

2. Identify sources of body fuel for different levels of physical activity.

3. Describe the nutritional needs of an active person.

4. Relate the degree of physical exercise to modern health problems.

5. Help individual clients develop realistic physical activity programs.

6. Describe an "optimal diet" for athletes.

Physical Activity and Energy Sources

Energy The capacity for work; power to affect changes in self and surroundings.

Kinetic Regarding or producing motion.

Substrate The substance that enzymes act on.

In Chapter 4 you learned that the term **energy** refers to the body's ability, or power, to do work. The energy required to do body work takes several different forms: mechanical, chemical, electric, light, radiant, and heat. Energy, like matter, can be neither created nor destroyed. Instead it is constantly being transformed or cycled from one form to another. We also speak of energy as being *potential* or **kinetic,** stored or active energy. Physical activity requires a base of sound nutrition to supply the **substrate** fuels, which along with oxygen and water meet widely varying levels of energy demand for muscle action.

Muscle Action: Fuels, Fluids, and Oxygen

The synchronized action of the millions of specialized cells and structures that make up our skeletal muscle mass make possible all forms of physical activity.

Muscle Structures

A finely coordinated series of small bundles within the muscle fibers (Figure 14-1) triggered by nerve endings produce a smooth symphony of action through simultaneous and alternating contraction and relaxation. These successively smaller muscle structures include:

1. **the particular muscle**—the large complete skeletal muscle
2. **the fascicules**—smaller bundles that make up muscle
3. **muscle fibers**—smaller muscle units that compose each fasciculus
4. **myobrils**—still smaller strands that compose each muscle fiber
5. **myofilaments**—the smallest of all the fiber bundles where muscle contraction occurs
6. **myosin** and **actin**—the contractile proteins within each myofilament that are the smallest moving parts of every muscle

Myofibril Slender thread of muscle; runs parallel to the muscle fiber's long axis.

Myosin A myofibril protein that acts in conjunction with actin to cause the contraction and relaxation of muscle.

Actin A myofibril protein that acts with myosin to cause the contraction and relaxation of muscle.

Muscle Action

Inside the cell membrane these contractile proteins, myosin and actin, are arranged in long parallel rows. These parallel rows slide together when the muscle contracts and pull apart when the muscle relaxes, allowing the muscle to shorten or lengthen as needed. The contraction of all of these muscle bundles occurs instantly and simultaneously when a specific motor nerve impulse excites these molecules of myosin and actin in the myofilaments to mesh together and thereby shorten the muscle. Periods of relaxation then occur between contractions. This alternating process continues until muscle fatigue builds up and the muscle can no longer respond. Muscle fatigue occurs for two reasons: (1) the supply of muscle **glycogen,** the immediate muscle fuel, is exhausted and therefore insufficient to sustain the required chemical reaction, and (2) **lactic acid,** the metabolic product of this chemical muscle reaction, accumulates during sustained high levels of exercise and cannot be removed fast enough.

Glycogen A polysaccharide, the main storage form of carbohydrate, largely stored in the liver and to a lesser extent in muscle tissue.

Lactic acid Produced by anaerobic glycolysis in muscles during exertion; can be converted to glucose by the liver.

Fuel Sources

Phosphate bonds form high-energy compounds in body metabolism (see Chapter 2). The main high-energy compound of the body cells is *adenosine triphosphate (ATP)*. It has rightly been called the "energy currency" of the cell (see p. 77). Various forms of energy are called on for successive energy needs.

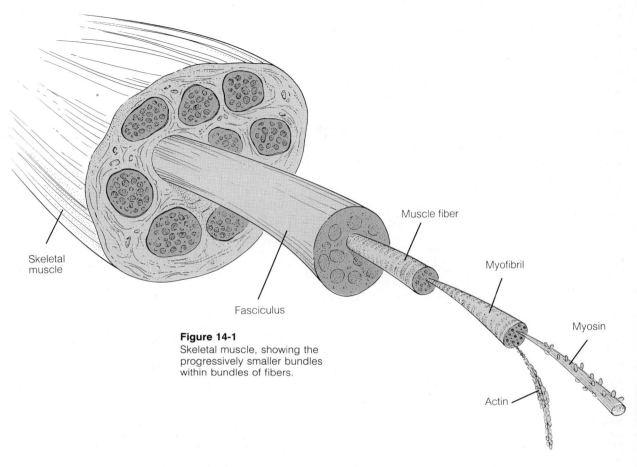

Figure 14-1
Skeletal muscle, showing the
progressively smaller bundles
within bundles of fibers.

Immediate energy High-power or immediate energy demands over a short time depend on ATP being readily available within the muscle tissue. This amount is used up rapidly and a backup compound, *creatine phosphate (CP)*, is made available. These high-energy phosphate compounds, however, will sustain all-out exercise only for about 5 to 8 seconds.

Short-term energy If an activity lasts longer than between 30 seconds and 2 minutes, *muscle glycogen* supplies the continuing need. Although the amount of available glycogen is small, it is an important rapid source of energy for brief muscular effort.

Long-term energy Exercise continuing more than 2 minutes requires an oxygen-dependent or **aerobic** energy system. A constant supply of oxygen in the blood is necessary for continued exercise. Special cell organelles, the **mitochondria,** which are located within each cell, produce large amounts of ATP. ATP is produced mainly from glucose and fatty acids and supplies continued energy needs (see p. 77).

Fluids and Nutrients

An increased intake of water is essential in the course of exercise. A deficiency can be dangerous and limits capacity greatly. As exercise continues,

Aerobic Requiring oxygen to proceed.

Mitochondrion The cell's "powerhouse;" a small, spherical to rod-shaped organelle located in the cell cytoplasm; principal site of energy generation (ATP synthesis); contains enzymes of Krebs cycle and cell respiration, as well as RNA and DNA for synthesis of some proteins.

the body temperature increases as part of the energy produced is released as heat. To control this temperature increase, the body shunts as much heat as possible to the skin, where it is released in sweat. Over time, and especially in hot weather, this excessive sweating can lead to **dehydration** (see p. 170). This is a serious complication.

Dehydration Excessive water loss from body tissues.

Nutrients also become depleted during continued exercise. As energy demands increase, the body burns blood glucose and muscle glycogen stores to provide energy. With prolonged exercise, the levels of these nutrients fall too low to sustain the body's continued demands. Fatigue follows and exhaustion threatens.

Oxygen and Aerobic Capacity

The most profound limit to exercise is the person's ability to deliver oxygen to the tissues and to use it for the production of energy. This vital ability depends on the fitness of the pulmonary and cardiovascular systems. In general a person's *aerobic capacity* depends on the degree of fitness and body composition.

Definition of Fitness Physical fitness may be defined in terms of aerobic capacity, which is the body's ability to deliver and use oxygen in sufficient quantities to meet the demands of increasing levels of exercise.[1,2] Aerobic capacity is expressed in terms of milliliters of oxygen consumed per kilogram of body weight per minute. This measurement allows for a more equal comparison of the aerobic capacity of individuals of differing sizes.

Body Composition Men have a higher aerobic capacity because of their difference in body composition. The tissues of the body that use more oxygen make up the **lean body mass,** the active metabolic body tissue. Men have a larger lean body mass than do women. When oxygen consumption is expressed only in terms of lean body mass instead of body weight, men and women have the same aerobic capacity. But women carry more body fat, which serves critical biologic functions and which is not as metabolically active as that of men. Since women must carry their entire body weight as part of their workload, their performance will be affected accordingly. It is evident that a person's aerobic capacity is affected by percentage of body fat and lean body mass—how much of the body's weight is active metabolizing tissue. Body composition is determined by the relative amounts of these two components of body weight.[3]

Lean body mass All component parts of the body, excluding neutral storage lipid; the entire fat-free mass.

Diet and Exercise

General Nutrient Needs

Our diet supplies the necessary fuel substrate for meeting our energy needs. We require carbohydrate and fat as basic fuels but have very little need for protein. General needs apply to all individuals, but there are special needs for the growing child.

Protein

Protein as fuel substrate Protein is usually discounted as a fuel substrate in energy production during exercise. Although some amino acids can feed into the cell's basic energy cycle, the extent of this input during exercise is minimal. There is evidence that some amino acid breakdown occurs during exercise and that nitrogen is lost in sweat. Authorities agree that protein makes an insignificant contribution to energy during exercise.[4]

Protein in the diet About 0.8 to 1.0 g/kg body weight is needed to meet general needs during exercise. This amounts to the usual adult RDA standard, which contributes about 10% to 12% of the kilocalories in the diet. Most Americans eat about twice this amount of protein, putting a taxing load on the kidneys (see p. 485) and on the liver over time. Nitrogen consumed in excess of need must be excreted. This requires an increase production of urea, which contributes to dehydration, a serious factor during strenuous exercise. High-protein diets can also lead to increased excretion of calcium in the urine.[5]

Fat

Fat as fuel substrate *(not directly dr. from diet but from bodyfatstores)* In the presence of oxygen, fatty acids provide energy. The rate at which this can take place is determined in part by the rate of mobilization of fatty acids from storage tissues. Free fatty acids are stored with glycerol as triglycerides in the body's adipose tissue. The enzyme *lipoprotein lipase* mobilizes these stores of fatty acids. This lipase is stimulated by exercise. Its activity is affected by levels of hormones also involved in exercise, especially growth hormone and epinephrine.

Fat in the diet It is important to recognize that fat as a fuel substrate is not drawn from the diet directly, but from body fat stores. Dietary fat is not necessary to maintain these body fat stores, since excess kilocalories in the diet will be stored as fat regardless of their dietary source. We do not need to eat in excess of our dietary needs to burn fat, and there is no danger of depleting our fat stores before exercise has proceeded to exhaustion.[1,2] Thus there is little basis for increased levels of fat in the diet. On the other hand, however, it is important to have some fat in the diet, especially as a source of the essential fatty acid, **linoleic acid.** In an apparent attempt to imitate the low-fat diet of the now famous runners, the Tarahumara Indians of the mountains of Mexico, some compulsive runners have virtually eliminated fat from their diets. This induces a linoleic acid deficiency. Since the heart muscle prefers fatty acids, especially linoleic acid, as an energy source, there have been reports of deaths resulting from cardiac arrest in some of these cases (see Issues and Answers, pp. 328-329). Although it is necessary to include some fat in the diet, the total amount should not exceed 25% to 30% of the total daily kilocalorie intake.

Carbohydrate

Carbohydrate as fuel substrate Although fat and protein have their specific roles to play in maintaining general health, the major nutrient for energy support in exercise is carbohydrate. Carbohydrates come from two sources, the circulating blood glucose and glycogen stored in muscle cells and the liver.

Carbohydrate in the diet Carbohydrate should contribute about 55% or more of the daily caloric intake.[5,6] Complex carbohydrates—starches—are preferable to simple ones—sugars. On the whole, the complex carbohydrates take longer to digest, provide a more sustained source of blood

Linoleic acid Essential fatty acid; preferred fuel for the heart muscle.

glucose, and are metabolized preferentially into glycogen. Simple sugars, on the other hand, are less efficient at maintaining the body's glycogen stores. They are mainly converted to fatty acids and stored as fat rather than as glycogen. Simple carbohydrates also provoke a sharper insulin response, contributing to the dangers of subsequent hypoglycemia. In addition, complex carbohydrates supply needed fiber, vitamins, and minerals. Studies have shown that during repeated bouts of intense exercise, low-carbohydrate diets were not able to restore tissue glycogen levels.[6] The low-carbohydrate diet resulted in decreased capacity for work, which intensified with each subsequent day on the diet. Conversely, high-carbohydrate diet restored glycogen levels nearly to their preexercise levels, but never completely. A day of rest was needed every week to accomplish this needed restoration of glycogen.

Numerous other studies have shown that low-carbohydrate diets inhibit exercise performance. Athletes, especially, experience fatigue, **ketoacidosis** (from excess **ketones**), dehydration, and hypoglycemia.[7] Well-conditioned athletes sometimes use a glycogen-loading procedure to buildup glycogen reserves for endurance events of 60 minutes or more. However, this diet manipulation carries dangers and should not be practiced often, certainly not without medical supervision.

Vitamins and Minerals

Vitamins and minerals as fuel substrate Vitamins and minerals cannot be used as fuel substrates. They are not oxidized or used up in the process of energy production. They are essential in the energy production process but only as cofactors in enzyme reactions.

Vitamins and Minerals in the Diet

Increased exercise levels are not correlated with increased dietary needs for vitamins or minerals, except with the possibility of riboflavin. Studies have shown that the standard RDA riboflavin recommendation may be low for very active women.[8] In general, exercise may well increase the body's efficient use of vitamins and minerals. Since athletes, for example, have an increased dietary need for energy, their larger caloric intake from good food sources would automatically increase their dietary intake of vitamins and minerals. Therapeutic iron supplements may be necessary for some athletes who experience "sports anemia" (see box, p. 320).

Exercise and Energy
Kilocalories

Physically active persons, especially athletes, need more fuel. Exercise raises the body's kilocalorie need. Also, exercise has the benefit of helping to regulate appetite to meet these needs. At mild to moderate levels of exercise, persons have actually been shown to eat less than inactive persons do. This may be related to an internal "set point" regulating the amount of body fat the person will carry. According to this theory (see p. 338), the set point is raised—that is, more body fat is stored—when the individual becomes inactive. In any case, when exercise levels rise above the mild or moderate to strenuous levels, caloric needs also rise.

Ketoacidosis Abnormally high concentration of ketone bodies (ketones) in body tissues and fluids; a complication of low-carbohydrate diets, diabetes mellitus, and starvation.

Ketone Intermediate fat metabolite; large class of organic compounds that contain the carbonyl group C=O, where the carbon atom is joined to two other carbon atoms.

Clinical Application

Sports Anemia

Some athletes experience periods of anemia with endurance exercise. Reduced hemoglobin in a runner's blood means reduced oxygen-carrying capacity, with obvious implications for aerobic capacity and ability to sustain an exercise workload.

The definition of anemia has been set at a hemoglobin (Hgb) value of less than 12 g% for women (normal 14) and less than 14 g% for men (normal 16). We know very little, however, about the relative influence on athletic performance of Hgb levels *within* the normal range. Some suggest that athletes' Hgb levels should be higher for optimal performance, although excessive concentrations of Hgb lead to increased blood viscosity and a decreased rate of flow. Maintenance of Hgb levels at least at the normal levels for women and men have been proposed.

Although frank anemia is rare among competitive athletes, low normal values are typical. Heavy exercise may induce transient anemia during the initial weeks of training, with Hgb stabilizing in the long run at the low end of normal. But strenuous continued exercise is also associated with low iron stores in athletes, which could pose long-term problems.

Possible causes of so-called "sports anemia" include: (1) a diet inadequate in iron, (2) decreased iron absorption, and (3) increased iron losses. Few studies have revealed a diet low in iron; decreased absorption and increased loss are more probable causes. Women athletes have cyclic menstrual loss of iron, unless they experience amenorrhea. Also, recent studies have shown significant amounts of iron lost in profuse sweating. Another possibility is occasional *intravascular hemolysis,* the rupture of red blood cells (RBC) as a result of the stresses of heavy exercise. This effect could be transient or chronic. It is manifested as free Hgb in the urine but has not been reported often.

Another factor in athletes' low-normal Hgb levels may be *hemodilution.* Strenuous training leads to an increase in both plasma volume and absolute quantity of Hgb, but the increases may not be proportional—plasma volume increases more than Hgb. Hemodilution with increased iron loss and increased red blood cell turnover could account for the prevalence of low-normal values among athletes. Obviously, this situation is complicated if the diet is inadequate in bioavailable iron.

References
Hunding, A., Jordal, R., and Paulev, P-E.: Runner's anemia and iron deficiency, Acta Med. Scand. **209**(4):315, 1981.
Pate, R.R.: Sports anemia and its impact on athletic performance. In Haskull, W., Scala, J., and Whittam, J., editors: Nutrition and athletic performance, Palo Alto, Calif., 1982, Bull Publishing Co.
Puhl, J.L., and others: Hematological and iron status of elite track and field women, Med. Sci. Sports Exerc. **14**(2):154, 1982.

Nutrient Fuels

Even for the athlete, there is no significantly greater need for protein or fat than for a nonactive person. Carbohydrate is the preferred fuel and critical foodstuff for the active person. These carbohydrates should be complex in form at an intake that will not only meet increased energy needs but also supply added vitamins and minerals. The following ratio is the approximate recommended dietary composition for support of physical activity:

Protein:	10% to 15% of total kilocalories (1.0 to 1.5 g/kg)
Fat:	30% of total kilocalories
Carbohydrate:	55% to 60% of total kilocalories (or remainder of kilocalories to meet energy needs)

Nutrition and Athletic Performance

Athletes and Coaches: A Vulnerable Group
Misinformation.

Athletes and their coaches are particularly suseptible to myths and magic claims about foods and dietive supplements. They search relentlessly for the competitive edge (see Issues and Answers, pp. 328-329). Knowing this, marketers unremittingly exploit this search, making this group particularly vulnerable. Manufacturers sometimes make distorted and false claims for products. Pangamic acid, for example, trade-named "vitamin B_{15}" but not a vitamin at all, has carried claims about its ability to enhance oxygen transport during exercise. Naturally, if such a compound were available, it would be of interest to athletes and their trainers. However, scientific research has exposed these claims as unfounded.

Myths

In addition to specific frauds, the world of athletics is beset with superstitions and misconceptions. Some of these myths include the following.

- Athletes need protein for extra energy
- Extra protein is needed to build bigger and stronger muscles
- Muscle tissue is broken down during exercise, and protein supplements are needed to replace this breakdown
- Vitamin supplements are important to enable the athlete to use more energy
- Vitamins and minerals are burned up in workouts and training sessions
- Electrolyte solutions are important during exercise to replace losses in sweat
- A pregame meal of steak and eggs ensures maximal performance
- Sugar is needed before and during performance to enhance energy-levels
- Drinking water during exercise will produce cramps

Pregame Meal

Steak and eggs have been the ritual precompetition meal. However, if such a meal is eaten less than 6 hours before the athletic event, it will still be in the stomach during the event. Protein and fat delay the emptying of the stomach and neither contributes to the glycogen stores needed during exercise. On the contrary, the ideal pregame meal is a light, low-fat, low-protein meal high in complex carbohydrate (starches), eaten 3 to 4 hours before competition. This allows the body time to digest, absorb, and transform it into stored glycogen.[6]

Hydration: Water and Electrolytes
Water—The Problem of Dehydration

Dehydration can be a serious problem for athletes. Its extent depends on the intensity and duration of the exercise, the surrounding temperature, the level of fitness, and the preexercise or pregame state of hydration. It is most severe in endurance events. For example, marathon runners sometimes collapse from dehydration. They may also have many other problems such as cramps, delirium, vomiting, hypothermia, or hyperthermia—all caused by dehydration.[9]

Cause About 60% of the energy from the breakdown of glucose is released as heat. In minimal physical exercise this heat production maintains desirable body temperature. But during exercise it exceeds the body's needs and sometimes its heat tolerance. Sweating is our main mechanism for dissipating body heat. The major source of fluid lost in sweat is plasma fluid. Endurance events can cause the loss of several liters of water as sweat, which is pulled from the plasma fluid to control body heat. Unless this amount is replaced, serious consequences can follow.

Prevention The thirst mechanism fails to keep pace with the body's increased need for fluid during exercise. The dehydrated person, therefore, must push fluids. To prevent dehydration, athletes are advised to drink more water than they think is needed, without dependence on the normal thirst mechanism. Cold water, about the temperature inside a refrigerator, is absorbed more quickly from the stomach. It is important to speed rehydration and to minimize the discomfort that a full stomach can give the athlete. Small cups of cold water should be drunk every 15 minutes during athletic events of long duraton. Until quite recently it was thought that drinking water immediately before or during an athletic event would cause cramps. There is no basis for this claim.

> Fluid replacement equivalent: 1 lb (2.2 kg) fluid weight = 500 ml.

Electrolytes

There is much ado focused—and money being made—on electrolytes. The marketing of **ergogenic** aids claims that the electrolytes lost in sweat must be replaced. This is true, but how? Sweat is more dilute than our internal fluids, and we thus lose proportionately, not just absolutely, much more water than anything else. Adding electrolytes and sugar to water simply delays its emptying from the stomach.[6] Water is the rehydration fluid of choice. Electrolytes will be replaced with the athlete's next meal.

> **Ergogenic** The tendency to increase work output.

Building a Personal Exercise Program

Health Benefits

In several other chapters we discuss physical activity in relation to various health problems. These chapters can be referred to for questions about particular conditions. Here we summarize health benefits of aerobic exercise for some of these conditions.

Treatment of Coronary Heart Disease

There are several benefits of exercise for those persons with coronary heart disease (see Chapter 20).

Cardiac output The volume of blood propelled from the heart with each contraction, also called *stroke volume*.

1. Aerobic exercise increases heart size and strength.[1]
2. The heart's stroke volume is also increased.[1] The heart then needs to pump fewer times per minute to circulate the same amount of blood. This represents a long-term reduction in the heart's workload.
3. Exercise raises blood levels of high-density lipoproteins (HDL), creating a more favorable ratio of high-density lipoproteins to low-density lipoproteins (LDL). This effect is more marked in men, although exercise will have the same effect in women if it is of high intensity.
4. Exercise enhances the circulatory system by increasing the oxygen-carrying capacity of the blood and increasing the blood volume.

↓ in total & LDL c.

Diabetes Management

Exercise helps control diabetes by enhancing the action of insulin through an increase in the number of insulin receptor sites[10] (see Chapter 18). This effect is particularly useful in the management of Type II diabetes in obese individuals. In the management of Type I diabetes, or insulin-dependent diabetes, the nature and scheduling of physical activity must be balanced with food and insulin to prevent hypoglycemic reactions. Such management can be done.

Weight Management

Exercise is extremely beneficial in weight management because it (1) helps to regulate appetite, (2) increases the basal metabolic rate, and (3) reduces the fat deposit "set point" level (see Chapter 15). Exercise also helps to reduce stress-related eating, since it provides a physical outlet for working off the hormonal physiologic events produced by stress in the body.

Bone Disease

Exercise increases bone mineralization, thus reducing the risk of bone weakness and of potential osteoporosis.[11]

Mental Health

Exercise stimulates the production of brain opiates, associated with a decreased susceptibility to pain, as well as an improved mood, including an exhilaration or kind of "high." It has also been found to be beneficial in the treatment of schizophrenia.[12]

Assessing Personal Condition and Exercise Needs

There are different kinds of exercise. Choosing those kinds that are best depends on individual health and personal needs, the aerobic benefits involved, and personal enjoyment.

Health and Personal Needs

In planning an exercise program, it is important to assess individual health status, personal needs, present level of fitness, and resources required. What do you want to gain from your exercise? How much time

Table 14-1

Target Zone Heart Rate According to Age to Achieve Aerobic Physical Effect of Exercise

Age	Maximal Attainable Heart Rate (pulse: 220 minus age)	Target Zone	
		70% Maximal Rate	85% Maximal Rate
20	200	140	170
25	195	136	166
30	190	133	161
35	185	129	157
40	180	126	153
45	175	122	149
50	170	119	144
55	165	115	140
60	160	112	136
65	155	108	132
70	150	105	127
75	145	101	124

can you commit to it? How much, if anything, does it cost? Perhaps it is even more important to ask yourself what you really like to do. If the exercise you choose isn't fun, you will soon stop doing it and it will benefit no one. Also, it is wise to start slowly and build gradually rather than risk injury and discouragement. *Moderation* and *regularity* are key guides in developing a physical activity program.

Beneficial Level of Exercise

Cardiac rate Number of heart beats per minute; pulse rate.

To build aerobic capacity, the level of exercise must raise the pulse to within 70% of maximal heart rate. Unless you have had an exercise tolerance or stress test and know precisely what your maximal exercising heart rate is, the rule of thumb is to determine your **cardiac rate** by subtracting your age from 220 (Table 14-1). This calculation estimates your maximal heart rate. About 70% of this figure tells you the rate to which you want to raise your pulse in the course of exercise. This rate should then be maintained for an uninterrupted period of at least 20 minutes and be practiced at least 3 times a week to have aerobic benefits.[13] Check your resting pulse before starting the exercise period, then again during and immediately afterward. Monitor your progress in developing your maximal exercising heartrate and aerobic capacity.

Types of Physical Activity
General Exercise

There are many exercises from which you may choose. Many of them are enjoyable but do not reach aerobic levels. For example, golf is a passion for many, but it is far too slow and sporadic to be aerobic. Also, most sports in the hands of amateurs, rather than those with fast-paced extraor-

Table 14-2
Aerobic Exercises for
Physical Fitness (maintained
at aerobic level for at least 30
minutes)

Type of Exercise	Aerobic Forms
Ballplaying	Handball Raquetball Squash
Bicycling	Stationary Touring
Dancing	Aerobic routines Ballet Disco
Jumping rope	Brisk pace
Running/jogging	Brisk pace
Skating	Ice skating Roller skating
Skiing	Cross country
Swimming	Steady pace
Walking	Brisk pace

dinary skill to provide sustained exercise, are too slow-paced to be aerobic. These include tennis, football, baseball, and basketball. Weight-lifting develops and strengthens muscles but is not a form of aerobic exercise.

Aerobic Exercise

Forms of exercise that can be sustained at a necessary level of intensity to provide aerobic benefits include swimming, running, jogging, bicycling, and the recently popular aerobic dancing routines and workouts (Table 14-2). However, perhaps the simplest and most popular form of stimulating exercise is *walking*. If the pace is fast enough to elevate your pulse and if it is maintained for the requisite 20 minutes, walking can be an excellent form of aerobic exercise. It is convenient and requires no equipment other than good walking shoes. It is also emotionally satisfying to many people for whom running, swimming, cycling, and dancing may be inappropriate.

Preparation for Exercise

Once you have chosen a sport or exercise, adequate preparation is essential, and safety precautions must be observed. Runners and joggers need appropriate shoes of good quality. Cyclists need good helmets. Whatever the form of exercise, before beginning stretch the muscles to prevent stress and injury. Also take time after completing the exercise to cool down. Many exercise-related injuries, such as pulled muscles and stress fractures, are connected to inadequate preparation.[13] It is also possible to exercise beyond the limits of tolerance. Incidences of injuries related to running begin to rise dramatically at the 25-miles-per-week mark. Also, endurance exercise and low body fat are associated with amenorrhea in women.[14,15] Some recent studies have compared the personality profiles of compulsive runners with those of anorexic persons.[16] Certainly any level of compulsion that comes to dominate one's life is *unhealthy*. Listen to your own body. When you are tired, rest. When you hurt, stop. When the level of exercise you do is no longer a challenge and you want to increase it, do so—but only then.

To Sum Up

Anaerobic Not requiring oxygen to function.

Glycolysis Anaerobic enzymatic conversion of glucose to simpler compounds of lactate or pyruvate; results in stored energy in the form of ATP in muscles; differs from respiration in that organic substances, rather than oxygen, are used as electron receptors.

The energy "currency" of the body is ATP. The cell's storehouse of energy is creatine phosphate. These two high-energy phosphate compounds are in limited supply. They can provide energy only for a few seconds and need to be replenished for exercise to continue. This added supply is made available by **anaerobic** glycolysis, with added energy made available after 3 to 4 minutes of continued exercise by the body's aerobic system of energy production. **Glycolysis** metabolizes only carbohydrate substrate, furnished either by blood glucose or stored glycogen. Dietary carbohydrate is necessary to replenish these fuel sources. Protein contributes little to total energy production for exercise, whereas the body's ability to burn fat as fuel depends on the level of fitness. The higher the body's efficiency in using oxygen, the more fatty acids will contribute to the energy supply. Even in the best-trained athletes, fatty acid oxidation must be accompanied by glucose metabolism.

The protein needs of the diet are not increased by exercise, contrary to popular belief, and neither is the body's need for vitamins or minerals. Exercise does increase the body's need for kilocalories and water. Cold water taken in small, frequent amounts is the best way to prevent dehydration. Electrolytes lost in sweat are replaced by a diet of adequate quality and quantity. Adding electrolytes or sugar to water delays its emptying from the stomach and thus delays rehydration.

The optimal diet for the athlete is 10% to 15% of the kilocalories from protein, 30% or less from fat, and 55% to 60% from carbohydrate. The pregame meal should be small, requiring little or no protein and relying mainly on complex carbohydrate (starches).

The health benefits of general and aerobic exercise are many and increase with practice. A minimal level of aerobic exercise need for cardiovascular fitness is achieved by elevating the heart rate to 70% of maximum for a sustained period of at least 20 minutes at least three times a week. Excellent aerobic exercises include sustained fast walking, swimming, jogging, running, and aerobic dancing or workouts.

Questions for Review

1. What are the component muscle structures and how do they produce muscle action?
2. What type of substrate fuel does the body use for immediate energy needs? Short-term needs? Long-term needs?
3. Outline the nutrition and physical fitness principles you would discuss with a client who is an athlete. Plan a diet for this client that would meet nutrient and energy needs.
4. Why is fluid balance vital during exercise periods? How is water and electrolyte balance achieved?
5. How would you conduct a counseling session for a patient with coronary disease about the role of exercise in cardiovascular health? With an overweight client with Type II diabetes?

References

1. Katch, F.I., and McArdle, W.D.: Nutrition, weight control, and exercise, Philadelphia, 1983, Lea & Febiger.
2. Coleman, E.: Eating for endurance, Riverside, Calif., 1980, Rubidoux Printing Co.
3. Wilmore, J.H.: Body composition in sport and exercise: directions for future research, Med. Sci. Sports Exer. **15**(1):21, 1983.
4. Evans, W.J., and others: Protein metabolism and endurance exercise, The Physician Sports Med. **11**(7):63, 1983.
5. Butterfield, G.E.: Fats, carbohydrates, and proteins: why we need them, and how they are obtained. In Haskell, W., Scala, J., and Whittam, J., editors.: Nutrition and athletic performance, Palo Alto, Calif., 1982, Bull Publishing Co.
6. Costill, D.L., and Miller, J.M.: Nutrition for endurance sport: carbohydrate and fluid balance, Int. J. Sports Med. **1**:2, 1980.
7. Felig, P., and others: Hypoglycemia during prolonged exercise in normal man, N. Engl. J. Med. **306**(15):895, 1982.
8. Belko, A.Z., and others: Effects of exercise on riboflavin requirements of young women, Am. J. Clin. Nutr. **37**(4):509, 1983.
9. Moore, M.: Boston Marathon medical coverage: the road racer's safety net, Physician Sports Med. **11**(6):168, 1983.
10. Holloway, J.F., Lewis, S.B., and Dohrmann, M.L.: The role of exercise in the retardation of glucose intolerance and coronary risk factors in diabetics, Med. Sci. Sports Exerc. **15**(2):91, 1983.
11. Stillman, R.J., and others: The relationship of bone mineral content and physiological activity in women over the age of thirty, Med. Sci. Sports Exer. **15**(2):149, 1983.
12. Levin, S.J., and Gimino, F.A.: Psychological effects of aerobic exercise in schizophrenic patients, Med. Sci. Sports Exerc. **14**(2):116, 1982.
13. Hales, D., and Hales, R.E.: How much is enough? Am. Health 37, July/Aug., 1983.
14. Schwartz, B., and others: Exercise-associated amenorrhea: a distinct entity? Am. J. Obstet. Gynecol. **141**(6):662, 1981.
15. Spiak, D.L., and Katch, F.I.: Relative body fat and menstrual function in athletes and non-athletes, Med. Sci. Sports Exerc. **15**(2):174, 1983.
16. Yates, A., Leehey, K., and Shisslak, C.M.: Running—an analogue of anorexia? N. Engl. J. Med. **308**(5):251, 1983.

Further Readings

ADA Report: Nutrition and physical fitness, J. Am. Diet. Assoc. **76**(5):437, 1980.

This paper presents ADA's position on nutrition and physical fitness in two parts. Part I suggests recommendations for the general public. Part II covers recommendations for athletes involved in training or competition.

Cooper, K.H.: The aerobics program for total well-being, New York, 1982, M. Evans and Co.

An expanded reference by the early developer of aerobic exercise programs; provides useful material for planning an individual exercise regimen as part of overall health care.

Report: How exercise protects the heart, Sci. News **121**(1):171, 1982.

A summary of research that concludes that moderate regular exercise may prevent or retard coronary heart disease in primates and suggests that such exercise this should begin in childhood and continue into adulthood.

Issues and Answers

The Winning Edge—or Over the Edge?

Athletes, their coaches, and indeed our entire culture have become increasingly aware that the percentage of body fat vs. the percentage of lean body mass can be a major influence on athletic performance. Each extra pound of body fat an athlete carries into competition is extra, nonproductive weight. Muscles, the lean body mass, provide the strength, agility, and endurance required to win.

Athletes, therefore, strive to achieve as low a percentage of body fat as possible while still maintaining good health. In reaching for such a goal, however, many young athletes develop an abhorence of body fat, resulting in food aversion and the undertaking of excessive weight loss regimens. These self-generated excesses are commonly reinforced by people surrounding the young athletes: coaches, teammates, and perhaps most demanding of all—parents. A fear of failure—failure to make the team, failure in competition, failure to live up to others' expectations—pushes the young person in his/her campaign to best this "opponent—their level of body fat—and to win this particular contest by a large, decisive amount. Such an all-consuming focus can result in compulsive behavior that leads the young person to set unrealistic goals resulting in abusive weight loss.

Fortunately, the reasons prompting such excessive voluntary weight loss in these young athletes are not the result of chronic emotional problems. Instead, they are superficial, resulting from an accumulation of immediate, short-term goals and concerns. These athletes usually respond to counseling in an excellent manner, reversing the excessive behavior, particularly with the support of concerned friends and teammates.

Yet for some individuals, excessive, compulsive fixation on lean body mass and the loss of body fat can become obsessive and enduring. For example, a compulsive runner's ideal of 5% body fat is found only in ballet dancers, gymnasts, models, and victims of anorexia nervosa. Our culture reinforces this "positive" attribute of beauty—slimness in women, physical prowess in men. But when a susceptible individual enters a time of stress or a search for a firm identity, he/she may see our cultural sterotypes as providing this self-concept. For women, this stress is usually encountered in adolescence, when physical attraction becomes important. For men, their sense of self is more closely tied to vocational and sexual effectiveness, both of which can be related to physical abilities. A man's abilities are tested more often in adulthood, resulting in a preoccupation with physical fitness as a way to deny any decline in strength or ability. This may be why the majority of compulsive runners—those who feel they must run despite everything, including injury or ill health—are men.

While our culture views compulsive dieting—anorexia nervosa—as a serious emotional disorder, compulsive training is seen as a positive personality trait showing dedication. In reality, both are symptomatic

Issues and Answers—cont'd

of an unstable self-concept and attempt to establish a firm sense of identity. They are perceptual disorders: whereas the anorexia victim sees herself as fat, the compulsive runner sees himself as out-of-shape. No goal, once attained, is sufficiently satisfying. If 5% body fat is achieved, 4% is strived for. Ignoring the physical indications against it, such striving has resulted in persons suffering permanent disabilities and even death, sometimes from cardiac arrest caused by linoleic acid deficiency. These driven individuals have a spartan attitude, unable to enjoy any of life's more passive, receptive pleasures.

While physical fitness and athletic accomplishments may be admirable goals, for a small percentage of participants the "thrill of victory" may be a hollow one if the victory is at the expense of their health and peace of mind. The ability to slow down, stop and "smell the roses," and enjoy life may mean more to the quality and quantity of a person's lifespan than the color of a coveted ribbon or medal.

References

Herbert, W.: Runners and anorexics: an ascetic disorder? Sci. News **123**(7):102, 1983.

Smith, N.J.: Excessive weight loss and food aversion in athletes simulating anorexia nervosa, Pediatrics **66**(1):139, 1980.

Yates, A., Leehey, K., and Shisslak, C.M.: Running—an analogue of anorexia? N. Engl. J. Med. **308**(5):251, 1983.

Chapter 15
Nutrition and Weight Management

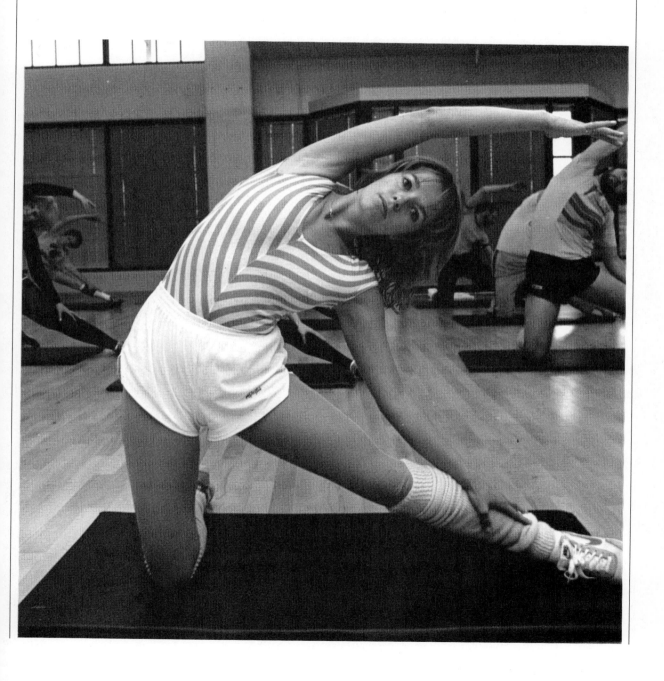

Preview

Even as you read these lines, one out of every four Americans is on some kind of a weight-reduction diet. Use of these "diets" is increasing daily, with a bewildering array of them constantly appearing in the public press. Even in light of such an obsession with weight loss, however, we as a people are getting heavier. The average American has gained about 2.25 kg (5 lb) since the mid-1960s. A large part of the answer lies in our becoming less and less physically active since our growing technology is producing a sedentary society.

But the sad fact is that all of these reducing "diets" have one thing in common: the weight, once lost, is almost always put back on again. Only about 5% of these "dieters" manage to maintain their weight at the new lower level after such a "diet." Perhaps this result points to the failure of the traditional "medical (or illness) model" of obesity and the need for a more realistic "health model." In this chapter we will try and move toward such a positive health model. We want to help our clients and patients feel better about themselves, whatever their weight, and to help those with related problems such as diabetes and hypertension plan more realistic and effective personal weight-management programs.

Chapter Objectives

After study of this chapter, the student should be able to:

1. Identify social and physiologic costs of America's obsession with weight and thinness.

2. Identify causes of obesity and describe current related social trends.

3. Relate overweight to health.

4. Plan weight management programs for clients based on a "health model."

Body Composition: Fatness and Leanness

Obesity Excessive adipose fat tissue, more than is required for optimal body function.

Meanings and Methods
Body Weight vs. Body Fat

Sometimes the common terms *obesity* and *overweight* are used without a necessary attention to body composition.

Obesity As it is used in the traditional medical model, the word "**obesity**" is a clinical term for excess body weight. It is generally applied to a person who is 15% to 20% or more above the "ideal" weight. The problem, however, lies in defining the word "ideal." It is usually defined in reference to average weight according to height and frame. But an "average" person doesn't really exist. Every person is individual, and *normal* values in healthy persons vary over a wide range. Also, until recently, *age* has been overlooked as an important variable in setting a reasonable or ideal body weight.[1] There is no one best or ideal weight associated with longevity in adults aged 25 to 59. In terms of minimal mortality, body weight is lower in young adults than in middle-aged adults.[2-4]

Overweight We often use the term *overweight* as a synonym for obesity. But these two terms are not interchangeable and the distinction is important. For example, a football player in peak condition can be markedly "overweight," according to standard weight-height charts. That is, he can weight considerably more than the average man of the same height, and much of this weight may not be fat at all.

Body composition A determination of how much of the body weight is fat and how much is lean body mass.

Body composition What is critical in determining a reasonable body weight is **body composition**. This refers to how much of the body weight comes from fat and how much is from lean body tissue or lean body mass. This lean tissue mass consists of muscles, bones, connective tissue, and so on. Thus it would be more correct to talk in terms of *fatness* and *leanness* than overweight. When we speak of weight, we need to ask for whom, under what circumstances, and by what measures. In practice, various measures of body size, contours, or skinfold thicknesses, are used to measure the layer of subcutaneous fat and help determine body composition. In research, more specific methods are used such as weighing a person under water and determining the amount of water displacement as a means of learning total fat content of the body. Given this way of determining fat content, obesity occurs when the percentage of body fat is more than 20% for men and more than 30% for women.

Standard Weight-For-Height Measures

Two basic approaches have been used to calculate reasonable weights: a general guide and standard weight tables:

General guide In common usage, a general rule of thumb has been passed along to determine proper weight:
1. For men, 106 lb (47.7 kg) for the first 5 ft (150 cm), then add 6 lb/in (2.7 kg/2.5 cm), plus or minus 10 lb (4.5 kg)
2. For women, 100 lb (45 kg) for the first 5 ft, then add 5 lb/in (2.25 kg/2.5 cm), plus or minus 10 lb

For many persons, however, especially women, unrealistically low figures are produced by this method, and it is seldom used in practice.

Weight-height tables Most of the standard tables are based on the Metropolitan Life Insurance Company's "ideal" weight-for-height charts. However, these charts have been derived from life expectancy data gathered by the company since the 1930s. There are problems with the data these tables have been based on and how representative they may be of our total current population[5] (see Issues and Answers, pp. 346-349). Also, a number of studies have found that health risks are as great, if not greater, in the very thin, low-weight range as for the extremely obese group. Within each age group, extremely thin as well as extremely fat persons have higher mortality rates. The message seems to be that persons should strive to be neither excessively overweight nor excessively underweight and that the multitude of health problems attributed to *moderate* amounts of overweight are unfounded.

Ideal Weight

Why is the term *ideal weight* difficult to define? Several factors may help to indicate why this is not a useful concept, and why some body fat is essential to health.

Individual variation The basic problem with the idea of ideal weight is that it really doesn't exist. A person's ideal body weight depends on many different factors, including age, body shape, metabolic rate, genetic makeup, sex, extent of physical activity, and many other factors. Persons need varying amounts of weight and can carry different amounts of weight in good health.

Menarche Onset of menstruation.

Necessity of body fat It is important to remember that some body fat is essential to survival. This has been demonstrated in times of human starvation. Such victims die of fat loss, not protein depletion. For mere survival men require 3% body fat; women require 12%. Especially for reproductive health, women require about 20% body fat.[6] Menstruation (**menarche**) begins when the female body reaches a certain size or, more precisely, when the young girl's body fat reaches this critical proportion of body weight, about 20%—the amount needed for ovulation and thus for any eventual pregnancy.

Obesity and Health

Many common beliefs about the relation of obesity and health conflict with data available from scientific studies.

Common Beliefs

Common folk knowledge holds that being fat is "bad for you." Also, traditional medical opinion has contended for years that obesity of any amount contributes to a wide number of health problems, including hyperlipidemia, carbohydrate intolerance, surgical risk, anesthesia risk, pulmonary and renal problems, pregnancy complications, diabetes, and hypertension.

Conflicting Data

Often in such broad statements a distinction is not made between moderate overweight states and massive or "morbid" obesity, which poses a different problem entirely. Both extremes of weight variance—fatness and thinness—pose medical problems, but the major issue affecting most Americans is a degree of general overweight in the population that requires closer study. Careful examination of the data collected in recent years reveals that there are only two health problems that have valid relationships to weight—hypertension and diabetes.[2] Clearly, there are health risks in *extreme* obesity, but unless a person is at least 30% *overfat*, there is questionable relationship of weight to mortality.[7]

Specific Relationships

These data, however, might obscure other important implications of obesity. Obesity is related to type II diabetes and to hypertension, which in turn contribute to coronary heart disease. Losing weight is associated with improvement of hypertension and diabetes. In obese persons with type II diabetes or with hypertension, a weight loss can induce significant reductions in elevated blood sugar or blood pressure.

Social Images: Fear of Fatness

Recently, a model of thinness, especially for women, has developed in American society with social blame placed upon fatness.

The Thinness Model

Fueled by capital investment in Madison Avenue advertising, a successful attempt has been made to use an exaggerated image of thinness for marketing many products. The "ideal" woman has been remade in the eyes of America. The gaunt, almost cadaverous models adorning the covers of many glamour magazines seem to mock most women's attempts to feel good about themselves and their bodies. This extreme degree of thinness now popular in America, however, goes against body wisdom and often contributes to marginal health or reproductive capacity.

The Fatness Blame

Overweight persons, especially women, don't conform to these social norms and are somehow blamed for their condition. Many people still hold to our popular mythology that fat people are (1) *gluttonous*—they eat much more than they should, (2) *lazy*—if they wanted to, they would lose weight, (3) *neurotic*—they have an oral fixation caused by arrested development during childhood, or (4) *unhappy*—they eat because they are depressed. However, studies of comparative behavior have shown no evidence for any of these superstitious beliefs about overweight persons.[6]

Effects of the Thin-Fat Images

Anorexia nervosa Extreme psychophysiologic aversion to food, resulting in life-threatening weight loss.

Bulimia Morbidly increased appetite, often alternating with periods of anorexia or purging.

Many Americans *are* unhappy. They can never live up to the thinness ideal. This national obsession has devoured the creative energies of many people. Unfortunately this obsession with thinness has resulted in two serious eating disorders: (1) **anorexia nervosa**, a form of self-induced starvation that has reached alarming proportions among adolescent girls, and (2) **bulimia**, a gorging-purging syndrome that creates both emotional and physical problems. Also, many of the fad weight-loss diets produce nutrient deficiencies. When they are practiced apart from a wise exercise program, the caloric intake is usually too low—less than 1200 kcal/day for women—to provide enough vitamins and minerals. In general there is a problem of iron intake for American women.

Physical Fitness: a New Health Image

Fortunately another "ideal type" is receiving more attention in America today. We seem to have "discovered" a physical fitness model. However, this too can be taken to extremes. In general, though, it seems to be a healthy direction and can provide at least part of the answer to the problem of weight management.

Problem of Weight Management

How would a person go about losing excess weight? Simple, you say—just reverse the process by which you gained it. When energy intake does not equal energy expended, the difference is reflected in weight either stored or lost. About 3500 kcal is the equivalent of 0.45 kg (1 lb) of body fat (Table 15-1). Well, that's part of the answer, but it isn't altogether quite that simple. There are many individual differences that often lead to extreme practices, and there are both physical and psychosocial factors involved.

Individual Differences and Extreme Practices
Valid Factors in Energy Balance

A number of real factors influence an individual's point of energy balance. Keeping a weight balance score in purely arithmetic terms is not that easy. First, it's difficult to know *precisely* just how many kilocalories are in the food you are eating. Second, it's even more difficult to know how many kilocalories you are actually burning up. This depends particularly on your basal metabolic rate (BMR), body size, amount of lean body mass, age, sex, and physical activity, among other things. Third, it is true that some persons do have more metabolic efficiency. Recent work indicates that some people do "burn" food more easily than others (see p. 85).

Extreme Practices

Individual differences in energy needs, combined with social pressures, lead many obese individuals to use various approaches to weight loss, which often create problems:

Fad diets The constant array of various weight-loss diets, to the extent that they work at all, are based on the arithmetic of energy balance. Many, however, are nutritionally inadequate. Without close medical supervision, the extreme, very low-calorie diets can be dangerous.

Fasting This drastic approach is dangerous also. Its effects are those of starvation: acidosis, postural hypotension, an increase in urinary loss of important electrolytes, an increase in serum uric acid, constipation, and a decrease in **basal metabolic rate (BMR)**. Sometimes there is sufficient loss of heart muscle to cause death.[8]

Basal metabolic rate (BMR) Rate of internal chemical activity in resting tissue.

Clothing and body wraps Special "sauna suits" are claimed to help weight loss in specific spots of the body or to help clear up so-called "cellulite" tissue. To the scientific community "spot reduction" is a fabrication as is "cellulite." This word was coined some years ago in Europe by a "beauty operator" and has no factual basis. This mummylike body wrap-

Figure 15-1
Gastroplasty is a type of restrictive gastric surgical procedure used for treatment of severe obesity.

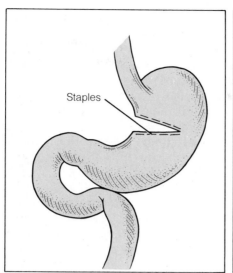
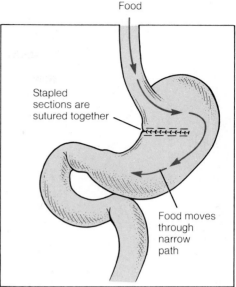

ping is endured by some persons in an attempt to reduce body size. What small weight loss may result is usually caused by temporary water loss. The only way to lose weight is to burn up more kilocalories than are consumed.

Drugs Amphetamines, commonly called "speed," were once popular in the treatment of obesity. However, they are no longer used because of their danger to health. Common over-the-counter drugs in use now include *phenylpropylamine (PPA),* a stimulant similar to amphetamine. PPA has been linked to increased blood pressure and damage to the blood vessels in the brain, leading to central nervous system disorders such as confusion, hallucination, stroke, and psychotic behavior.[6]

Surgery Surgical techniques are usually reserved for medical treatment of extreme, or "morbid," obesity. These procedures include various gastric stapling procedures (Figure 15-1) and wiring the jaws shut. These techniques, however, involve considerable risk and sometimes result in the development of other health problems as side effects.

Causes of Obesity
Genetic Factors

Genetic inheritance probably influences a person's chance of becoming fat more than any other factor. A genetic base regulates differences in body fat and sexual differences in weight. Within families, if one parent is obese, a child has a 40% chance of becoming obese. This chance is 80% if both parents are obese and only 7% if neither parent is obese.[9] Families also exert social pressure and teach children habits and attitudes toward food.

Psychologic Factors

Fat persons are seen as having less control over their appetites and as being more responsive to external cues than to internal ones. Therefore, some people believe that obese persons eat: (1) when it is mealtime or when they are surrounded by food, instead of when they are hungry, (2) when they are unhappy, or (3) because as children they associated food with maternal love. Studies have shown, however, that these factors cannot be applied to fat persons as a group.[9] They have no more tendency to these actions and feelings than anyone else. But there is no question about the role that psychology must play in any weight-maintenance program. Our cultural "ideal" thin-body type and resulting social discrimination against obese persons have created psychologic problems in many individuals. Social support, in the form of counseling, support groups, friends, or family, is critical for a successful weight-maintenance program.

Social Factors

Class values of different social groups also influence obesity. As a person moves upward in social class, there is a tendency to be more highly motivated to maintain a moderate to "normal" body weight. In lower socioeconomic status groups obesity is fairly common and considered normal. In higher-level groups greater social value is usually placed on the thinner state. The length of exposure to these values and their pressure on individuals in any social class determines reaction to them.

Physiologic Factors

The normal physiology of growth and development during the life cycle contributes to accumulation of fat tissue deposits. There are critical periods for the development of obesity: early childhood, early stages of puberty, and adulthood as persons grow older with no diet adjustment for their decreased physical exercise. For women other times may be during pregnancy and after menopause, since hormonal factors are involved. Two theories of physiologic factors contributing to weight management problems have developed:

Fat cell theory This theory holds that the percentage of body fat an individual carries is determined by the number of fat cells in the body, which is partly determined by inheritance and partly by eating patterns developed in early childhood. Once the body has added fat cells to accommodate extra fuel storage, these cells remain and can store varying amounts of fat.

Set-point theory Several investigators have proposed a completely new way of looking at obesity.[6,10] This view maintains that an internal mechanism, a so-called *set-point*, regulates the amount of body fat an individual carries. This theory places obesity on a physiologic basis and is in direct distinction from those claims that it is a purely psychologic problem and that obese persons are at fault.[1,7,11] The theory provides a possible basis for understanding why it is so difficult for some obese persons to lose weight and maintain weight loss. The idea of set-point in the human body is that the individual will eat to regain whatever amount of fat the body is "set," or genetically "programmed for," and will similarly lose weight gained in excess of this internally regulated point. Apparently the major way of manipulating this set-point is by increasing physical exercise. To date this is the only known way to lower the set-point, to raise the BMR, and to "program" the body to store less fat than it did before. Thus increased levels of physical activity, especially aerobic exercise, will help the body regulate itself at a lower level of body fat. In combination with a well-balanced diet that moderately restricted in energy value, increased exercise offers the main support for gradual and sustained weight loss.

The Health Model: A Positive Personal Approach

General Components

In common practice the general approach to management of simple obesity is based on underlying energy balance and the client's personal situational needs. The two main aspects of the approach are (1) motivation and support and (2) a personalized program.

Motivation and Support

Motivation is a prime factor. A nutrition counselor, through initial interviews, determines individual needs, attitudes toward food, and the meaning food has for the client. The nutritionist recognizes emotional factors involved and provides support to meet the client's particular needs.

A Personal Program

To be successful, a weight-management program must meet personal needs. Such a program should emphasize some of the following factors:

Food behaviors Note the usual quantity of food served and consumed. Then use smaller portions, attractively served. Take time to eat *slowly* and savor food taste and texture. Reduce hidden factors added in food preparation such as fat, sugar, and salt. Increase fiber content. Choose a variety of foods from a basic food guide, such as an exchange system (see p. 342), which can serve as a focus for sound nutrition education. Emphasize whole primary foods and minimal use of processed foods. Plan a fairly even food distribution throughout the day.

Exercise behaviors Plan a regular daily exercise schedule. Start with simple walking, building to a brisk pace, for about a half hour a day. Add some form of aerobic exercise, such as swimming, or develop a set of body exercises, including stretching exercises, body and muscle development, an aerobic goal, and a cool-down period (see box, p. 340). Set occasional goals and note progress. Above all, use a variety of activities and enjoy them.

Relaxation exercises Practice progressive muscle relaxation and stress-reduction exercises. Learn a simple pattern as a guide, using imagery as a focusing device. Use background tapes or environmental records if they are helpful. Select a suitable time and stay with it for daily practice. Start with a brief 10-minute period, then increase as desired.

Personal interest areas Develop some creative interest area for intellectual stimulation, personal enjoyment, and fulfillment. Explore various community resources to support such activities.

Follow-up program The nutrition counselor and the client should develop a follow-up schedule of appointments. On subsequent visits, progress should be noted, problems discussed, and solutions mutually explored.

Clinical Application

Benefits of Aerobic Exercise in Weight Management Programs

The goal of weight management is to reduce adipose tissue and, in most cases, to build *lean body mass (LBM)*. However, both tissues are lost when a person tries to reach a weight goal by reducing food intake alone.

Optimal body composition can be achieved by combining food restriction with aerobic exercise. This type of exercise consists of activities that are sustained long enough to draw on the body's fat reserves for fuel while increasing oxygen intake (thus, the name "aerobic"). Lean body tissue burns fats in the presence of oxygen. Thus aerobic activity is best suited for achieving the ideal high LBM/low fatty tissue balance in the body.

The benefits of aerobic exercise to the overweight person in a weight management program include:
- Lowering of set-point
- Suppressed appetite
- Reduced body fat
- Higher basal metabolic rate
- Increased energy expenditure
- Retention or building of LBM levels

Sometimes clients complain of difficulty or disappointment in a slow rate of weight loss, difficulty in controlling appetite, consistent "flabbiness" despite continuing diet management. These persons may welcome the suggestion of aerobic activity to help meet these needs. You may want to recommend a brisk daily walk, jumping rope, swimming, bicycling, jogging, running, or some other activity that can be sustained long enough for it to have an aerobic effect (p. 324). Note carefully the physical stress this activity may place on individuals who have not exercised for some time or who have medical prolems related to exertion. Advise these clients to have a physical check-up before beginning such a program on their own or joining a local gymnasium or other community fitness center.

Continuing support should be provided. Practical suggestions for dealing with such things as realistic goals, food binges, weight plateaus, meals away from home, and other special situations need to be discussed. These may help the client anticipate needs, avoid pitfalls, and sustain motivation.

Behavioral aspects Practioners in a health care setting recognize the need for supportive therapies for weight management that focus on the behavioral aspects of the problem. Food behavior is rooted in many human experiences and varying life situations. These experiences often produce addictive forms of eating response or conditioning. Behavior-oriented therapies help the obese person change such inappropriate food and eating patterns through increased insight and understanding, motivation, and reconditioning.[11]

Principles of a Sound Food Plan

On the basis of careful interviewing, the nutrition counselor assesses nutritional status, food habits, and situational factors. A sound food plan is developed with the client based on the following dietary components:

Energy Balance

The energy intake level (kilocalories) is adjusted to meet individual weight-reduction requirements. A decrease of 1000 kilocalories daily is the necessary adjustment to lose about 900 g (2 lb) a week; 500 kcal is needed to lose 450 g (1 lb) a week (Table 15-1). An average sound diet prescription for energy balance for women is about 1200 kcal/day. For larger women and for men the prescription would be about 1500 to 1800 kcal/ day. Some persons may wish to determine what their total energy needs are as a basis for planning a reduced energy intake for their weight-management program (Table 15-2).

Nutrient Balance

Basic energy nutrients are outlined in the diet prescription to achieve the following nutrient balance:

1. **Carbohydrate** About 50% of total kilocalories, with emphasis on complex forms such as starch with fiber, and a limit on simple sugars.
2. **Protein** Approximately 20% of total kilocalories, with emphasis on lean food and small portions.
3. **Fat** About 30% of total kilocalories, with emphasis on low animal fats, scant use, and alternate seasonings.

Table 15-1
Kilocalorie Adjustment
Required for Weight Loss

To lose 454 g (1 lb) a week—500 fewer kcal daily

Basis of estimation	
1 lb body fat	= 454 g
1 g pure fat	= 9 kcal
1 g body fat	= 7.7 kcal (some water in fat cells)
454 g × 9 kcal/g	= 4086 kcal/454 g fat (pure fat)
454 g × 7.7 kcal/g	= 3496 kcal/454 g body fat (or 3500 kcal)
500 kcal × 7 days	= 3500 kcal = 454 g body fat

Table 15-2
General Approximations for
Daily Adult Basal and Activity
Energy Needs

Basal Energy Needs (avg. 1 kcal/kg/hr)		Male (70 kg) kcal 70 × 24 = 1680	Female (58 kg) kcal 58 × 24 = 1392
Activity energy needs			
Very sedentary	+20% basal	1680 + 336 = 2016	1392 + 278 = 1670
Sedentary	+30% basal	1680 + 504 = 2484	1392 + 418 = 1810
Moderately active	+40% basal	1680 + 672 = 2352	1392 + 557 = 1949
Very active	+50% basal	1680 + 840 = 2520	1392 + 696 = 2088

In general this nutrient balance approximates the recommendations of the U.S. Dietary Goals (see pp. 69-71). This can serve as a good basic guide.

Distribution Balance

Spread food evenly through the day to meet energy needs. Consider any daily "problem times" and use simple, planned snacks as needed for such periods.

Food Guide

Use some type of general food list, such as those in the food exchange system (see Appendix H). Some examples of general food plans using this system are given in Table 15-3. This sytem provides a good general ref-

Table 15-3
Weight Reduction Food Plans Using the Exchange System of Dietary Control* (Total Kilocalorie Distribution: 50% Carbohydrate, 20% Protein, 30% Fat)

Food Exchange Groups	1000 kcal	1200 kcal	1500 kcal	1800 kcal
Total Number Exchanges/day				
Milk (nonfat)	2	2	2	2
Vegetable	3	3	4	4
Fruit	3	3	4	4
Bread	4	5	7	9
Meat	3	4	5	7
Fat	4	4	5	5
Meal Pattern of Food Exchanges				
Breakfast				
Fruit	1	1	1	1
Meat			1	1
Bread	1	1	2	2
Fat	1	1	1	1
Milk	½	½	½	½
Lunch/Supper				
Meat	1	1	1	2
Vegetable	1	1	2	2
Bread	1	2	2	3
Fat	1	1	2	2
Fruit	1	1	1	1
Milk	½	½	½	½
Dinner				
Meat	2	2	2	3
Vegetable	2	2	2	2
Bread	1	1	2	3
Fat	2	2	2	2
Fruit			1	1
Milk	½	½	½	½
Snack (afternoon or evening)				
Milk	½	½	½	½
Meat		1	1	1
Bread	1	1	1	1
Fruit	1	1	1	1

*See food exchange lists, Appendix H.

erence guide for comparative values and portions, variety in food choices, and basic meal planning. Food items should be combined into desired dishes. Use alternate seasonings, such as herbs and spices, onion, garlic, lemon juice, vinegar, wine, broth (fat-free), mustard, and other condiments.

Personal Needs
Individual Adaptations

Throughout the planning remember to focus on the individual client and his/her personal needs. If the plan is unrealistic it will not be followed. Some persons find that keeping a daily journal is helpful. This should include notes of food intake, environmental food cues, feelings, physical symptoms, and any stress factors related to food behavior. It may also include notes about other activities such as physical exercise or stress-reduction practice. A review of such notes may help in making general observations, determining problem areas, monitoring progress, and gaining insights for setting personal goals to achieve desired behavior changes.

Treatment Choices

What is a reasonable classification of weight levels that practitioners can use to help plan the best approach to weight management for the client? A simple classification used in general practice is based on degree of overweight:[12]

1. **Mild**—20% to 40% overweight (about 91% of all obese women). Only a moderate caloric restriction is indicated, along with nutrition education, behavior therapy, and increased physical exercise. Such a program is best provided by nonphysician health professionals or community groups.
2. **Moderate**—41% to 100% (9% of all obese women). Special programs, sometimes including very low-kilocalorie diets, may be indicated.[7]
3. **Severe**—greater than 100% (0.5% of all obese women). Only surgical treatment using gastric restrictive procedures appears to have any measure of success.

Essential parts of all programs are nutrition counseling and education, behavior therapy, and increased physical activity. Working with persons in the latter two groups above requires medical supervision. It is best accomplished through a team of health professionals.

Preventive Approach

In the last analysis, it would seem that the most constructive work with weight management would be aimed at *prevention*.[13] Support for young mothers and children before the obese condition develops will help prevent many problems later in adulthood. This support should include early nutrition counseling and education, with positive food behavior and habit formation.

To Sum Up

Body weight has traditionally been used as an indicator of obesity, which may raise the risk of health problems. New methods of determining body weight reveal that the underlying *composition* of that weight, the lean vs. fat tissue, is its most important aspect. Weight-management programs have traditionally been designed for obese persons. However, a recent growing obsession with thinness has created a "new" weight-management problem—eating disorders that result in self-starvation. These disorders are strongly associated with societal pressures and psychologic counseling is an important part of therapy. Problems involved in planning a weight-management program, either for the obese or malnourished person, include the metabolic and energy needs of the individual, personal food choices and habits, and variations in needs for fatty tissue during different stages of the life cycle.

The health model is based on personal motivation and support for the individual. Aspects of such a program include changing food behaviors, increasing physical activity, practicing relaxation techniques, and developing personal interests. Behavior modification techniques help the individual examine the effect of life situations on eating habits and change those situations that encourage overeating. A sound weight-management plan is based on an adjusted kilocalorie level that allows for (1) a moderate rate of weight loss (1 to 2 lb/week), (2) nutrient levels based on the requirements of growth as well as the U.S. Dietary Goals with meals distributed throughout the day, and (3) ongoing monitoring of other food-related behaviors (environmental cues, stress, physical activity) to help the individual achieve personal goals. The ideal weight-management plan begins with prevention, stressing positive food habit formation in early childhood to prevent major problems later in life.

Questions for Review

1. What is meant by "ideal weight"? Explain the variables involved in determining this factor. What role does it play in weight-management?
2. Describe two major eating disorders associated with America's growing obsession with thinness. What social factors contribute to this obsession? Compare how these factors contribute to the growing tendency toward overweight.
3. What is the "set-point" theory? What implications does it present for the future of weight-management methods?
4. Describe five components of the "health model" for weight-management. How does it differ from the traditional medical model?
5. What are the basic principles of a sound food plan for weight-management programs?

References

1. Stern, J.S.: Obesity treatment, J. Am. Diet. Assoc. **84**(4):405, 1984.
2. Andres, R.: Effect of obesity on total mortality, Int. J. Obesity **4**:381, 1980.
3. Gurin, J.: What's your natural weight? Am. Health **3**(3):43, 1984.
4. Rhoads, G.G., and Kagan, A.: The relation of coronary disease, stroke, and mortality to weight in youth and in middle age, Lancet **1**:492, 1983.
5. Weigley, E.S.: Average? Ideal? Desirable? A brief overview of height-weight tables in the United States, J. Am. Diet. Assoc. **84**(4):417, 1984.
6. Bennett, W., and Gurin, J.: The dieter's dilemma, New York, 1982, Basic Books, Inc.
7. Brownell, K.D.: The psychology and physiology of obesity: implications for screening and treatment, J. Am. Diet. Assoc. **84**(4):406, 1984.
8. Report: Survey of very-low-calorie weight reduction diets, Arch. Intern. Med. **143**(7):1423, 1983.
9. Foreman, L.: The fat fallacy, Health **15**(9):23, 1983.
10. Keesey, R.E., and Corbett, S.W.: Metabolic defense of the body weight set-point. In Stunkard, A.J., and Stellar, E., editors: Eating and its disorders, New York, 1984, Raven Press.
11. Atkinson, R.L. and others: A comprehensive approach to outpatient obesity management, J. Am. Diet. Assoc. **84**(4):439, 1984.
12. Stunkard, A.J.: The current status of treatment for obesity in adults. In Stunkard, A.J., and Stellar, E., editors Eating and its disorders New York, 1984, Raven Press.
13. Edelman, B.: Developmental differences in the conceptualization of obesity, J. Am. Diet. Assoc. **80**(2):122, 1982.

Further Readings

Bray, G.A.: "Brown" tissue and metabolic obesity, Nutrition today **17**(1):23, 1982.
    Good explanation with many illustrations of the nature and function of "brown fat" and its possible relationships to obesity by a leading researcher in the field.

Huse, D.M., and Lucas, A.R.: Dietary treatment of anorexia nervosa, J. Am. Diet. Assoc. **83**(6):687, 1983.

Mayer, A.: The gorge-purge syndrome, Health **14**(7):50, 1982
    Two articles providing increased understanding of the personal pain involved in these extreme eating disorders and possible approaches to treatment and care. mayer describes the experience of a young nurse with bulimia. Huse and Lucas, a dietitian-physician team, outline the details of their program of care for young persons with anorexia nervosa at the Mayo Clinic.

Levine, A.S., and Morley, J.E.: The shortening pathways to appetite control, Nutri. Today **18**(1):6, 1983.
    Readable, informative article updating research progress in identifying mechanisms of appetite control. Good review of agents involved, centering on the function of the hypothalamus, with discussion of a sliding set-point and numerous diverse substances that act as chemical messengers. Many illustrations and extensive references.

Stunkard, A.J., and Stellar, E., editors: Eating and its disorders, New York, 1984, Raven Press.
    In various chapters, experts discuss topics such as fat cells and body weight, dietary obesity, metabolic defense of body weight set-point, physical exercise, behavior therapy, current treatment status, etc.

Issues and Answers

The Use and Abuse of Height-Weight Tables

On March 1, 1983, with considerable media coverage, the Metropolitan Life Insurance Company (MLI) issued its "new" weight-height tables. These charts list recommended weigh ranges for women and men of varying body frames at different heights. The last time they were revised was in 1959. Now, after analyzing mortality data on 4.2 million people for 22 years, the company statisticians have determined that Americans can weigh from 2 to 13 lbs more than they do now and expect to live longer than their leaner counterparts.

The public may welcome this news, as expressed in the public press with statements such as, "Now it's OK to weigh more." On the other hand, various investigators and practitioners in medicine and nutrition are raising more serious questions about the uses and abuses of these tables over the years. There is evidence from many sides that we are rethinking the relationship of overweight, health, and longevity. Questions are being raised not only about the difference in the two most recent tables, the 1959 and 1983 versions, but also, and more significantly, the conceptual basis of their construction in the first place. Which table is best? Is either one valid as a health standard for clinical practice? How can we deal with weight management issues related both to health dictates and to social demands? A better understanding of how these tables came to be and what current research teaches us concerning their appropriate use in practice will help us use them in a broader and more appropriate manner in our own practice.

Development of Standard Height-Weight Tables

The earliest weight tables appeared in Europe in 1836, simply based on the weights of "a moderate number of Belgians." Through the intervening years, the development of weight-height tables as we have come to know them has been dominated mainly by the insurance industry and used by insurance companies as a guide for evaluating life insurance applicants. Early industry leaders candidly admitted that weight-height concerns had no commercial significance until life insurance came into being. Standards were set by the industry on the assumption that overweight people were bad insurance risks and higher premiums were set for these persons, if they were accepted at all.

Over the last few decades, a leader in the insurance industry, the Metropolitan Life Insurance Company, has taken the lead in revision of earlier tables. In 1942 and 1943, MLI challenged the previous tables' use of only average weights as standard. Instead, they sought to relate weight to disease and mortality. They also introduced the idea of bodyframe size as a factor in appropriate weight but gave no guildelines for determining body type. Their data base for analysis came from a sampling of their policyholders. The weight statistically

Issues and Answers—cont'd

associated with longevity they called "ideal weight" and so titled their 1942-1943 table. In 1959, they issued a revision of the table, based again on data from policyholders, this time including persons insured by 26 life insurance companies in the United States and Canada— The Build and Blood Pressure Study, 1959. They concluded that the lowest mortality rates were associated with below-average weight and thus used the term "desirable weight" in the title of their 1959 table revision.

Currently, with their new 1983 revision based on data from 25 insurance companies and over 4 million policyholders, MLI statisticians have dropped both terms—"desirable" and "ideal." Instead the new table is simply titled with the date of issue and includes a footnote that weights of persons at ages 25 to 59 are based on lowest mortality. Weights are again given in terms of body-frame size, with the same three designations. Instructions are included this time for finding your frame size by measuring your elbow bones with fingers and a ruler—not exactly an easy procedure. The designated weights are only slightly higher than those in the 1959 tables, the greatest increases being for shorter men and women.

Changing Concepts
Over the past few years, the data and philosophy behind the 1959 tables and, currently, the 1983 revisions have been increasingly questioned by researchers and practitioners. These concerned leaders include such persons from medicine as Reuben Andres, clinical director of the Gerontology Research Center at the National Institute on Aging, and Ancel Keys, a pioneer researcher in the field of nutrition and medicine. Their questions have focused mainly on limitations built into the tables by the nature of their population database and the factors of age and frame used in the tables' analysis and construction.

Limitations of Population Base
Many persons, even including MLI actuaries and statisticians themselves, have pointed out that insurance policyholders are not representative of the population at large. Three reasons have been cited: (1) They are persons valuing insurance and able to afford it— largely white, middle-class, adult males. (2) Underwriting practices vary widely from strict to lenient, with weight measurements and health data inaccurate or falsely self-reported—unsuitable for medical or public health purposes. (3) The population of American policyholders does not reflect the general population incidence of chronic disease or acute illnesses because such persons usually do not apply for insurance or may be rejected if they do. Moreover, overweight persons charged higher rates may have been motivated to purchase insurance by fear of a hidden health problem that could lead to an early death.

Continued.

Issues and Answers—cont'd

Age Factor

Andres was among the first to voice concerns about the dangers of thinness and to question the risk of being moderately overweight. He has since analyzed the data himself and found that the new MLI tables were "too liberal for young adults and too restrictive for older people." He has constructed a new table, using the insurance data, that gives safe ranges of weight for different heights *and ages*. Based on his research, he offers a simple formula for finding your own "safe" weight range. Pull out your pocket calculator and find your own best weight:

- Measure your height without shoes, in inches, and divide that figure by 66
- Multiply this result by itself
- Multiply that result by your age plus 100

This final number is the middle of your "safe weight range," which is within about 15 pounds on either side, unless you have hypertension or diabetes.

The biologic fact is that most persons get fatter as they get older. Thus, according to Andres, the "safe" range of weight raises with age. Adults who gain about 8 to 10 lbs a decade may actually be helping themselves to keep healthy. Both Andres and Keys conclude that unless an individual has hypertension or diabetes, overweight does not increase mortality or the development of coronary heart disease.

Body Frame

The concept of body frame as used in these tables is without scientific foundation. Keys has stated that these frame types were created simply by dividing the weight distribution of the data into thirds and labeling those thirds as "small," "medium," and "large." In fact, Andres calls such distinction of frame size a "fiction." The American Medical Association has also pointed out the difficulties of scientifically determining frame size.

What is the Answer?

So the question remains: Which weight-height standard do we use—1959 or 1983? The answer is *neither*. These tables may be useful as guides but should not be used as standards for determining "ideal" body weight. How can they? Ideal weight is based primarily on the amount of lean body tissue. Health professionals cannot tell the percent body fat, or lean tissue, from a table. They *might* be able to estimate it, by measuring subcutaneous fat with calipers at designated spots on the body or by submerging the individual in a water tank and gauging the percent fat by the amount of water that is displaced. If they do, they may find that some of their "overweight" clients are, in fact, very lean, with well-developed musculature contributing to excess weight. Conversely, some of their "ideal weight" clients may, in fact, be obese in the true sense of the word—having too much

Issues and Answers—cont'd

body fat. Worst of all, they might find out that some of their formerly undernourished patients who start to gain weight "quite nicely" are, in fact, edematous and in dire need of nutritional intervention.

It is unfortunate that the medical community and the public have taken these guidelines so seriously for so long. Perhaps the time has come to alleviate the anxiety surrounding weight by taking these charts down from their traditional havens over our scales and placing them in their rightful place on the desk or in the drawer as one of our reference guides. Perhaps then both patient and counselor will be released from "the numbers game." We can then delve further into the physiologic, cultural, economic, and social factors that *really* count in the process of weight management. With this tool in proper perspective, we can focus our clinical concerns on those with "dangerous" weights—the very thin and the extremely obese—and give primary attention from a health care standpoint to those middle-weight persons who have weight-related disease such as diabetes and hypertension.

As for the social issues involved, our weights and our looks remain intensely personal. But many moderately overweight middle adults, unhappy for years with their bodies, will escape from the tyranny of the tables and feel better about themselves. Ultimately, all our ideas about what looks good may gradually change, and we'll discover that we're in better shape than we thought.

References
Andres, R.: Effect of obesity on total mortality, Int. J. Obesity **4**:381, 1980.
Gurin, J.: What's your natural weight? Am. Health **3**(3):43, 1984.
Keys, A.: Overweight, obesity, coronary heart disease, and mortality, Nutr. Rev. **38**:297, 1980.
Seltzer, F.: The Metropolitan Life Insurance Company's height-weight tables, Diet. Currents **10**(4):1, 1983.
Weigley, E.S.: Average? Ideal? Desirable? A brief overview of height-weight tables in the United States, J. Am. Diet. Assoc. **84**(4):417, 1984.

Part Three

Introduction to Diet Therapy

Chapter 16

Nutritional Assessment and Therapy in Patient Care

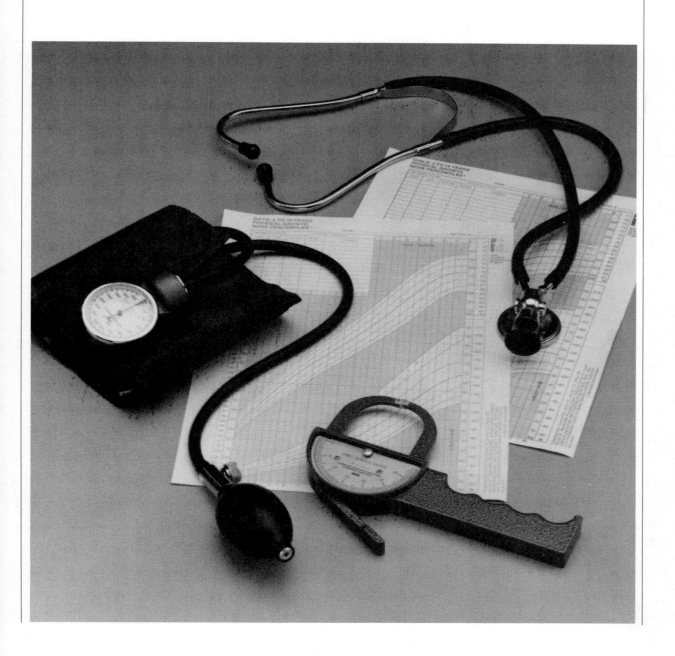

Preview

Persons face acute illness or chronic disease and its treatment in a variety of settings: the acute care hospital, the long-term rehabilitation center, the extended care facility, the clinic, the private office, and the home. In all instances nutritional care is fundamental. It is a vital support for any medical treatment being given. Frequently it is the primary therapy in itself. Comprehensive nutritional assessment provides the necessary data for appropriate nutritional therapy based on identified patient needs. Clinical nutritionists and dietitians with sound clinical judgment and expertise work with an effective clinical care team. Together these professionals provide an essential component for successful medical treatment. They assist the patient in recovery from illness or injury, help the person maintain follow-up care to promote health, and also help control costs.

In this chapter we focus on the comprehensive care of the patient's nutritional needs. Wherever the place of care and whatever the need, the health care practitioners, the patient, and the family work together to support the healing process and promote health.

Chapter Objectives

After study of this chapter, the student should be able to:

1. Recognize the aspects of our modern health care system that can create problems in patient care and plan ways of minimizing their effects.

2. Identify and describe the components of the therapeutic process in patient care.

3. Relate methods of basic nutritional assessment to planning sound nutritional care.

4. Plan and carry out quality standards of nutritional care for all patients.

Hospitalized Patients: The Therapeutic Process

Setting and Focus of Care
Hospital Setting and Health Care Team

In the modern hospital setting, the therapeutic encounter between health care providers and their patients occurs under stressful conditions at best. Each injured or ill patient is a unique person, requiring special treatment and care. At the same time, a confusing array of health care providers seeks to determine needs and implement what they perceive to be appropriate care. It's small wonder that the course does not always run smoothly. Sometimes our complex system and highly specialized technology get in the way and we lose sight of our reason for being—fulfilling individual human needs and personal care. Constant open and validating commincation is essential, both among the health team members and between the health care provider and the patient and family. In this team effort to provide quality nutritional care, the clinical dietitian—who is a clinical nutrition specialist—together with the physician, carries the primary responsibility. The nurse and other primary care practitioners provide essential support. In the setting of the individual medical center, then, with its strengths and shortcomings and within the essential team care provided, the clinical nutritionist or dietitian must care for the patient's nutritional needs in close relationship to the medical and nursing care. Determining these needs is a primary concern.

Patient-Centered Care

The primary principle of nutritional practice, too often overlooked in many routine procedures, should be evident: to be valid, nutritional care must be *person-centered*. It must be based on identified needs and updated constantly with the patient. A second fundamental fact also needs emphasis: despite all methods, tools, and technologies described here or elsewhere, *the most therapeutic tool you will ever use is yourself*. It is to this seemingly simple yet profound healing encounter that you must bring yourself.

Phases of the Care Process
Assessment: Data Base

Nutritional status Condition or situation related to degree of body nourishment.

A broad base of relative information about the patient's **nutritional status**, food habits, and life situation is necessary for making accurate initial assessments. Useful background information may come from a variety of sources such as the patient, the patient's chart, family or other relatives and friends, oral or written communication with other hospital personnel or staff, and related research.

Analysis: Problem List

A careful analysis of all data collected determines specific patient needs. Some needs will be immediately evident. Others will develop as the situation unfolds. On the basis of this analysis, a list of problems may be formed to guide continuing care activities.

Planning Care: Needs and Goals

Valid care is planned on identified problems. The plan must always be based on personal needs and goals of the individual patient, as well as the identified medical care requirements.

Implementing Care: Actions

The patient care plan is put into action according to realistic and appropriate activities within each situation. For example, nutritional care and education will involve decisions and actions concerning an appropriate food plan and mode of feeding, as well as the training and education needs of the patient, staff, and family who will carry it out.

Evaluating and Recording Care: Results

As every care activity is carried out, results are carefully checked to see if the identified needs have been met. Appropriate revisions of the care plan can be made as needed for continuing care. These results are carefully recorded in the patient's medical record. Clear documentation of all activities is essential.

Nutritional Assessment and Analysis

Nutritional assessment To judge or evaluate by measurement of values involved. Evaluation of nutritional status by broad study of nutrition-related measures and values involved—physical, physiologic, psychosocial, personal, cultural, medical, and dietary—and environmental influences affecting them, for the purpose of maintaining health or treating disease.

The fundamental purpose of **nutritional assessment** in general clinical practice is to determine the overall nutritional status of the patient, current health care needs, both physiologic and psychosocial as well as personal, and related factors influencing these needs in the person's current situation. A clinical nutritionist, with the help of other health team members as needed, uses several basic types of activities for nutritional assessment of patients' needs. These include anthropometric measures, biochemical tests, clinical observations and physical examination, and dietary evaluations based on careful personal history, including diet-drug interactions and social, family, and medical histories. The patient's full history is a fundamental tool for planning health care; history-taking is a primary skill for all health professionals (see p. 217). Also, a broad number of tests may be used for research purposes in a large facility with an access to highly sophisticated equipment. However, the procedures outlined here provide a good base in general clinical practice.

Gathering Nutritional Data
Anthropometric Measures

Skill gained through careful practice is necessary to minimize the margin of error in making body measurements. Selection and maintenance of proper equipment and attention to careful technique are essential in securing accurate data.

Weight Hospitalized patients should be weighed at consistent times—for example, before breakfast after the bladder has been emptied. Clinic patients should be weighed without shoes in light, indoor clothing or an examining gown. For accuracy, using regular clinic beam scales with nondetachable weights is necessary. An additional weight attachment is available for use with very obese persons. Metric scales with readings to the nearest 20 g provide specific data. However, the standard clinic scale is satisfactory. All scales should be checked frequently and calibrated every 3 to 4 months for continued accuracy.

After carefully reading and recording the patient's weight, ask about the usual body weight and compare it with standard height-weight tables[1,2] (see Issues and Answers, pp. 369-370). Interpret present weight in terms of percentage of usual and standard body weight for height. Check for any significant weight loss: 1% to 2% in the past week, 5% over the past month, 7.5% during the previous 3 months, or 10% in the last 6 months. These amounts of weight loss are significant. More than this rate can be severe. Values charted in the patient's record should indicate percentage of weight change.

Height If possible use a fixed measuring stick or tape on a true vertical flat surface. If such is not available, the moveable measuring rod on the platform clinic scales may be used with reasonable accuracy. Have the patient stand as straight as possible, without shoes or cap, heels together, and looking straight ahead. The heels, buttocks, shoulders, and head should be touching the wall or vertical surface of the measuring rod. Read the measure carefully and compare it with previous recordings. Note the growth of children or the diminishing height of adults. Metric measure of height in centimeters provide accurate data. A satisfactory substitute, more easily obtained in the bedfast patient, is a measure of arm length.[3] This is a measure of the total arm length, from the tip of the acromial process of the scapula to the end of the styloid process of the ulna. This is a useful alternative to full body-height measure, especially in older patients. In these older adults, a general thinning of weight-bearing cartilages—the "bent-knee gait"—and a possible **kyphosis** of the spine may make height measurement inaccurate.

Kyphosis An increased, abnormal convexity of the upper part of the spine; hunchback.

Body Measures In general clinical practice, the clinical nutritionist uses two basic body measurements—the mid-upper–arm circumference and the triceps skinfold thickness—and from these calculates a third measure, the mid-upper–arm muscle circumference. First, using a centimeter tape made of nonstretchable material, the midpoint of the upper arm is located on the nondominant arm, unless it is affected by edema. The circumference is measured at this midpoint, securing the tape snugly but not so tightly as to make an indentation. The measure is read accurately to the nearest tenth of a centimeter and recorded. The resulting measure is compared with previous measurements to note possible changes. Next, using a standard millimeter skinfold caliper, a measure is taken of the triceps skinfold thickness at this same midpoint of the upper arm. This measure provides an estimate of subcutaneous fat reserves. Together with the mid-arm circumference at the same spot, it enables the practitioner to make a good estimate of general skeletal muscle mass, an indicator of body composition. Then, using these two measures in a standard formula developed by research, the practitioner can calculate the mid-upper–arm muscle circumference. This derived value gives an indirect measure of the body's skeletal muscle mass. Finally, to interpret the patient's measurements for monitoring nutritional status, these values are compared as percentages of standards provided in reference tables.

Biochemical tests

A number of laboratory tests are available for studying nutritional status. In general clinical nutrition practice, the tests most commonly used for assessing and monitoring nutritional status and planning nutritional care are listed here. General ranges for normal values are given in standard texts.

Measures of plasma protein Basic measures include serum albumin, hemoglobin, and hematocrit. Additional ones may include serum transferrin or total iron-binding capacity (TIBC) and ferritin (see p. 523).

Creatinine Byproduct of creatine metabolism; levels in the urine indicate the amount of lean body mass.

Measures of protein metabolism Basic 24-hour urine tests are used to measure urinary **creatinine** and *urea nitrogen* levels. These materials are products of protein metabolism. The patient's 24-hour excretion of creatinine is interpreted in terms of ideal creatinine excretion for height—the creatinine-height index (CHI). Comparison is made with standard values for this index. The patient's 24-hour nitrogen excretion is used with calculated dietary nitrogen over the same 24-hour period to determine nitrogen balance.

Measures of immune system integrity (anergy) Basic measures are made of lymphocyte count. Additional measures may be made by skin testing, observing delayed sensitivity to common recall antigens such as mumps or purified protein derivative of tuberculin (PPD). Skin tests are read at 24 and 48 hours, with greater than 5 mm considered positive and the presence of one positive test indicating intact immunity.

Clinical Observations

Keen observation is made of possible malnutrition signs as well as those evident through vital signs and physical examination.

Clinical signs of malnutrition Careful attention to physical signs of possible malnutrition provides an added dimension to the overall assessment of general nutritional status. A guide for a general examination of such signs is given in Table 16-1. The practitioner should make a careful descriptive record of any such observations in the patient's medical record.

Vital signs and physical examination Other physical data may include pulse rate, respiration, temperature, and blood pressure. A study of the common procedures of a normal physical examination will provide useful background orientation. An interesting and sound popular version of such a guide has been provided by a New York cardiologist,[4] who translates medical jargon into plain English with both humor and compassion.

Diet Evaluation

A careful nutrition history, including nutritional information related to living situation and other personal, psychosocial, and economic problems, is a fundamental part of nutritional assessment. But obtaining accurate information about basic food patterns and dietary intake is not a simple matter. We need methods that simplify data collection and analyses and provide accurate information on the intake of individuals.[5] However, a sensitive practitioner may obtain some useful information by using one or more of the basic tools described here.

Diet history In clinical practice, we need general knowledge of the patient's basic eating habits to determine any possible nutritional deficiencies. In conjunction with the patient's usual living situation and related food attitudes and behaviors, social and family history, and medical history with current status and treatment, the nutrition interview[6] provides an essential base for further personal nutrition counseling and planning

Table 16-1
Clinical Signs of Nutritional Status

Body Area	Signs of Good Nutrition	Signs of Poor Nutrition
General appearance	Alert, responsive	Listless, apathetic, cachexic
Weight	Normal for height, age, body build	Overweight or underweight (special concern for underweight)
Posture	Erect, arms and legs straight	Sagging shoulders, sunken chest, humped back
Muscles	Well developed; firm, good tone; some fat under skin	Flaccid, poor tone; undeveloped; tender, "wasted" appearance; cannot walk properly
Nervous control	Good attention span; not irritable or restless; normal reflexes; psychological stability	Inattentive, irritable, confused; burning and tingling of hands and feet (paresthesia); loss of position and vibratory sense; weakness and tenderness of muscles (may result in inability to walk); decrease or loss of ankle and knee reflexes
Gastrointestinal function	Good appetite and digestion, normal regular elimination, no palpable (perceptible to touch) organs or masses	Anorexia, indigestion, constipation or diarrhea, liver or spleen enlargement
Cardiovascular function	Normal heart rate and rhythm, no murmurs, normal blood pressure for age	Rapid heart rate (above 100 beats/minute tachycardia), enlarged heart, abnormal rhythm, elevated blood pressure
General vitality	Endurance, energetic, sleeps well, vigorous	Easily fatigued, no energy, falls asleep easily, looks tired, apathetic
Hair	Shiny, lustrous, firm, not easily plucked, healthy scalp	Stringy, dull, brittle, dry, thin and sparse; depigmented; can be easily plucked
Skin (general)	Smooth, slightly moist, good color	Rough, dry, scaly, pale, pigmented, irritated; bruises; petechiae
Face and neck	Skin color uniform, smooth, pink, healthy appearance, not swollen	Greasy, discolored, scaly, swollen; skin dark over cheeks and under eyes; lumpiness or flakiness of skin around nose and mouth
Lips	Smooth, good color, moist, not chapped or swollen	Dry, scaly, swollen, redness and swelling (chelosis), or angular lesions at corners of the mouth or fissures or scars (stomatitis)
Mouth, oral membranes	Reddish pink mucous membranes in oral cavity	Swollen, boggy oral mucous membranes
Gums	Good pink color, healthy, red, no swelling or bleeding	Spongy, bleed easily, marginal redness, inflamed, gums receding
Tongue	Good pink color or deep reddish in appearance, not swollen or smooth, surface papillae present, no lesion	Swelling, scarlet and raw, magenta color, beefy (glossitis), hyperemic and hypertrophic papillae, atrophic papillae
Teeth	No cavities, no pain, bright, straight, no crowding, well-shaped jaw, clean, no discoloration	Unfilled caries, absent teeth, worn surfaces, mottled (fluorosis), malpositioned
Eyes	Bright, clear, shiny; no sores at corner of eyelids; membranes moist and healthy pink color, no prominent blood vessels or mount of tissue or sclera; no fatigue circles beneath	Eye membranes pale (pale conjunctivas), redness of membrane (conjunctival injection), dryness, signs of infection; Bitot's spots, redness and fissuring of eyelid corners (angular palpebritis), dryness of eye membrane (conjunctival xerosis), dull appearance of cornea (corneal xerosis), soft cornea (keratomalacia)
Neck (glands)	No enlargement	Thyroid enlarged
Nails	Firm, pink	Spoon shaped (koilonychia), brittle, ridged
Legs, feet	No tenderness, weakness, or swelling, good color	Edema, tender calf, tingling weakness
Skeleton	No malformations	Bowlegs, knock-knees, chest deformity at diaphragm, beaded ribs, prominent scapulas

Williams, S.R.: Nutritional guidance in prenatal care. In Worthington-Roberts, B.S., Vermeersch, J., and Williams, S.R., editors: Nutrition in pregnancy and lactation, St. Louis, 1985, The C.V. Mosby Co.

Figure 16-1
Interviewing of patient to plan
personal care.

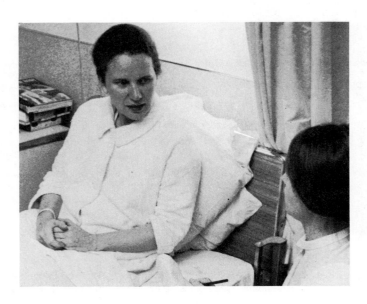

of care (Figure 16-1). For example, an activity-associated day's food intake pattern, using a tool such as the one discussed, may guide you in obtaining a fairly valid picture of food habits and eating behaviors (see box, p. 361). In addition to food and nutrition information, drug therapy data must be obtained from the medical record and the patient or family to determine any possible drug-nutrient interactions involved or any teaching needed by the patient (see Chapter 17). Research carefully *all* prescription and over-the-counter drugs your patient is taking.

Food record For measures such as the creatinine and urea nitrogen excretion tests, a specific 24-hour period of urine collection is required. During this same period a specific and detailed record of all food intake is essential for determining total protein and energy values of the diet. The protein value is used for calculation of nitrogen balance. A careful and simple explanation for your patients should be provided concerning the use of the record in calculating this nitrogen balance—an important measure of nutritional status. The caloric value will indicate how well the patient is meeting goals for energy input. These goals are based on the energy expenditure demands of the patient's illness or health maintenance requirements. At times a longer food record is needed for full analysis of all nutrient values. This analysis is usually done by computer (see p. 566).

$$\text{N balance} = \frac{\text{total protein}}{6.25}$$

Analyzing Nutritional Data

Valid patient care planning requires analysis of all nutritional data collected. On this basis problems requiring solutions can be identified.

Data Analysis

A detailed analysis of the nutritional information collected is necessary for determining nutritional diagnosis, any primary or secondary nutritional disease, as well as underlying nutrition-related conditions.

Clinical Application

**Nutrition History:
Activity-Associated
General Day's
Food Pattern**

Name _____ Date _____
  Height _____ Weight (lb) _____ (kg) _____ Age _____
                                      Ideal weight _____

Referral
Diagnosis
Diet order
Members of household
Occupation
Recreation, physical activity

Present food intake

	Place	Hour	Frequency, form, and amount checklist
Breakfast			Milk
			Cheese
			Meat
			Fish
			Poultry
Noon meal			Eggs
			Cream
			Butter, margarine
			Other fats
Evening meal			Vegetables, green
			Vegetables, other
			Fruits (citrus)
			Legumes
Extra meals			Potato
			Bread—kind
			Sugar
			Desserts
			Beverages
Summary			Alcohol
			Vitamins
			Candy

Nutritional diagnosis All the various nutritional data for each individual patient, collected by the clinical nutritionist and other team members through the broad assessment activities just described, must be carefully analyzed to reach a valid nutritional diagnosis and plan of care. The nutritional diagnosis will require information about all aspects related to the individual patient's needs: nutrient deficiencies, underlying disease requiring a modified nutrient or food plan, any personal cultural and ethnic needs, or economic needs as well as mode of feeding and dietary management.

Primary and secondary nutritional disease The nutritionist coordinates these nutrition activities and carries a major responsibility on the health care team for interpreting nutrition-related data and making decisions and recommendations concerning any primary or secondary nutritional states. Any nutritional deficiency disease—which may underlie or contribute to overall illness—may be classified as primary or secondary, depending on the cause. *Primary* deficiency disease results from a lack of an essential nutrient in the diet, for whatever reason. *Secondary* nutrition deficiency disease results from one or more barriers to the use of the nutrient substances after they are consumed. This inability to use a given nutrient may stem from digestive or malabsorption problems. Such problems may be caused by lactose intolerance, celiac disease, **chemotherapy** or radiation treatments, or cell metabolism problems in genetic disease.

Chemotherapy Treatment of disease with chemicals that destroy unhealthy tissue (see Chapter 23).

Nutrition-related conditions Related problems with nutritional involvement will also be considered. These include such conditions as heart disease, hypertension, cancer, liver and renal disease, and surgery. Any quantifiable data collected can be analyzed by computer (see Chapter 24). Laboratory data may be handled in a similar manner, with general patterns of change monitored over time. Careful appraisal of medical and personal data from histories, records, reports, and interviews will help focus on various needs and problems and provide a realistic picture of nutritional and eating difficulties.

Problem list On the basis of this careful analysis, a problem list is usually developed. Around such a list realistic and relevant care may be planned. Every aspect of the patient's needs is considered. In conference with the health care team, the patient, family, or any significant others, personal goals are determined for care. These goals help establish priorities for immediate care as well as long-term care.

Planning and Implementing Nutritional Care

Basic Concepts of Diet Therapy
Normal Nutrition Base

The primary concept of diet therapy is that such treatment is based on normal nutritional requirements of the patient. This is an important initial fact to grasp and to impart to the patient. For example, it is a great source of encouragement to the parents of a newly diagnosed diabetic child that the diet plan will be based on normal growth and developmental needs and will use regular foods. A therapeutic diet is but a modification of normal nutritional needs, modified only in so far as the specific disease in the specific individual necessitates.

Disease Application

The principles of a specific therapeutic diet will be based on modifications of the nutritional component of the normal diet. These changes may include one or more of the following types of modification:

1. **Nutrients** Modifications in one or more of the basic nutrients such as protein, carbohydrates, fat, minerals, and vitamins

2. **Energy** Modification in energy value as expressed in kilocalories
3. **Texture** Modification in texture or seasoning, such as liquid or low residue

Background Information Needed

Four areas of knowledge, therefore, are needed to plan and carry out valid nutritional care in therapeutic diets:

1. **Personal needs** What personal desires, concerns, or life situation needs must be met?
2. **Disease** How does this disease affect the body and its normal metabolic function?
3. **Nutritional therapy** How and why does the diet need to be modified in terms of its nutritional components to meet the needs created by this particular disease?
4. **Food plan guidelines** How do these necessary nutritional modifications affect daily food choices?

Individual Patient Adaptation

A workable plan for a specific person must be based on individual food habits within the specific personal life situation. This can be achieved only through careful planning *with the patient,* based on an initial interview to obtain a diet history and knowledge of personal food habits, living conditions, and related factors. In this way, diet principles can be understood and motivation secured to follow through. Whatever the problems, nutritional care is valid only to the extent that it involves this kind of knowledge, skills, and insights. Individual adaptations of the diet to meet individual needs are imperative for successful therapy.

Routine House Diets

A schedule of routine "house" diets, based on some type of cycle menu, is usually followed in hospitals for those patients not requiring a special diet modification. According to general patient need and tolerance, the diet ordered may be liquid (clear liquid or full liquid with milk used on the full liquid diet), soft (no raw foods, except lettuce in some instances, and generally bland in seasoning), and regular (a full, normal-forage diet). Occasionally an interval step between a soft and regular diet may be used—the light diet. Sample menus from hospital staff dietitians may be compared to note differences.

Managing the Mode of Feeding

Depending on the patient's condition, the clinical nutritionist may manage the diet by using any one of four feeding modes:

Enteral: Oral Diet

As long as possible, of course, regular oral feedings are preferred. Supplements are added if needed. According to the patient's condition, there may also be need for assistance in eating (Figure 16-2).

Enteral: Tube Feeding

If a patient is unable to eat but the gastrointestinal tract can be used, tube feeding may provide needed nutritional support. A number of commer-

Figure 16-2
Child with fractured arm is
assisted in eating by student
nurse.

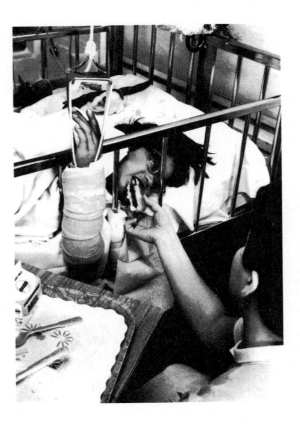

cial formulas are available or a blended formula may be calculated and
prepared.

Parenteral: Peripheral Vein Feeding

If the patient cannot take in food or formula via the gastrointestinal tract,
intravenous (IV) feeding will be needed. Solutions of dextrose, amino acids, vitamins, and minerals, with intermittent lipid formula, can be fed
through peripheral veins when the need is not extensive or long term.

Parenteral: Total Parenteral Nutrition (TPN)

If the patient's nutritional need is great and support therapy may be required for a longer time, feeding through a larger central vein is needed.
This is a special surgical procedure. It requires special nutrient solutions
determined and monitored by clinical nutritionist and physician, prepared
by trained pharmacists, and administered by specially trained nurses. This
skilled nutritional support team is essential for successful therapy. Details
of all these various modes of feeding are given in later chapters, as they
apply to various conditions.

Evaluation: Quality Patient Care

General Considerations

When the nutritional care plan is carried out, patient care activities need
to be considered in terms of the nutritional diagnosis and treatment objectives. The extent to which each of the care activities helps to meet the

particular goals of the patient and the family are evaluated. This evaluation is both continuous and terminal. It seeks to validate care while it is being given as well as to determine the effectiveness of a particular course of care. Various areas need to be questioned and investigated:

Estimate the Achievement of Nutritional Therapy Goals

What is the effect of the diet or mode of feeding on the illness or the patient's situation? Is there need for any change in the nutrient ratios of the diet as a originally calculated, in the meal-distribution pattern, or in the feeding mode?

Judge the Accuracy of Intervention Actions

Is there need to change any of the nutritional care plan components? For example, is there need for a change in type of food or feeding equipment, environment for meals, procedures for counseling, or types of learning activities for nutrition education?

Determine Patient Ability to Follow Prescribed Nutritional Therapy

Are there any hinderances or disabilities that prevent the patient from following the treatment plan? What is the impact of nutritional therapy on the patient, the family, or the staff? Were the necessary nutritional assessment procedures for collecting nutrition data carried out correctly? Do the patient and the family understand the information given for self-care? Have any community resources required by the patient and family been available or convenient for use? Has any needed food assistance program been sufficient to meet needs for the patient's care?

Quality Patient Care
PSROs

Since the establishment of Professional Standards Review Organizations (PSROs) in 1972, there has been an increased emphasis on the setting of practice standards to ensure the delivery of quality patient care. In addition, at present, an increased focus on cost control in health care settings requires that mechanisms be developed for effectively evaluating patient care programs on the basis of (1) cost effectiveness and (2) provision of nutritional services by the most qualified personnel.

Quality Care Models

Within dietetics, standards for both professional and support level staff have been developed in a number of medical care settings.[7] These models of quality care have established specific standards for (1) identifying patients who require increased nutritional support or nutrition education, (2) determining patient care priorities and spelling out the degree of care required, and (3) defining role responsibilities for carrying out each part of the care plan. These models for quality care have been applied to specific patient care needs, such as a standard of practice for quality assurance in nutritional care for patients with cancer.[8]

Role of the Nurse

The nurse works closely with the clinical dietitian or nutritionist in supporting the nutritional care planned and carried out by the clinical dietitian for all patients. Thus skills in consultation and referral are essential. At varying times, depending on need, the nurse may serve as coordinator, interpreter, or teacher.

Coordinator

Because of their close relationship with patients and their more constant attendance, nurses are best able to coordinate any special services or treatments required by the patient. The nurse may help schedule activities to prevent conflicts or secure needed consultation for the patient with a social worker, dietitian, or other health team member. Sometimes hospital-induced malnutrition exists in a patient because meals are interrupted by various procedures. For example, an audit in one hospital revealed that in 1 week 5% of the patient trays were not served at all, 24% were held back for patients having medical procedures done at mealtime, and 15% were accepted but uneaten because of poor patient appetite.[9]

Interpreter

Since the nurse works closely with the patient, she/he can help reduce tension by careful, brief, easily understood explanations concerning various treatments and plans of care. This will include basic interpretation of the therapeutic diet from the clinical nutritionist or the physician and of the resulting food selections on the tray. The nurse may sometimes assist the patient in making appropriate selections from menus provided.

Teacher or Counselor

One of the nurse's most significant roles in nutritional care is that of basic health teaching and counseling. There are innumerable informal opportunities during daily nursing care for planned conversation about sound nutrition principles, which will reinforce the counseling of the clinical nutritionist. In addition, according to patient situation, nurses may work with the clinical nutritionist or dietitian during periods of instruction to provide the patient with information concerning principles of the patient's modified diet integrated with general health teaching about the disease process. They can help coordinate medical and nutritional management of the patient's illness by the physician and clinical dietitian into overall nursing care and patient education. The clinical dietitians are also excellent resources for teaching materials and needed nutrition information.

Clearly, learning about the patient's nutritional needs is a continuing activity beginning with hospital admission. It should follow through and include plans for continuing application in the home environment. Follow-up care may be provided by the hospital's clinical dietitian, by consultation with clinical nutritionists or dietitians in community private practice, by public health nutritionists or nurses, or by referrals to community resources.

To Sum Up

The basis for an accurate assessment of the patient's nutritional needs begins with the individual patient and family. Physical as well as psychologic, social, economic, and cultural factors in and out of the clinical setting all play a role in estimating the patient's health status and any possible problems with adherence to a nutritional care plan.

Nutritional assessment is based on a broad foundation of pertinent data: physiologic, psychosocial, medical, and personal data, including food and drug uses and values. The effectiveness of an assessment based on analysis of these data depends in turn on effective communication with the patient, family members, or "significant others" in the development of an appropriate care plan, as well as with other members of the health care team. The patient's medical record is a basic means of communication among health care team members.

Nutritional therapy, based on a combination of the personal and physiologic needs of the patient, requires a close working relationship among nutrition, medical, and nursing staff in the health care facility. The nurse's schedule offers many opportunities to reinforce the nutritional principles of the diet. Nutritional therapy doesn't end with the patient's discharge. Outpatient nutrition services, appropriate social services, and food resources in the community help meet continuing needs of patients and their families.

Questions for Review

1. Identify and discuss the possible effects of various psychologic factors on the outcome of nutritional therapy.
2. Outline a procedure for assessing the nutritional needs and building a care plan for a 65-year-old widower hospitalized with coronary heart disease (refer to Chapter 20, if necessary). Include community agencies the patient could be referred to for follow-up care, services, and information.
3. List and describe five commonly used anthropometric measures, five serum and two urinary products tested for nutritional information, and six clinical signs used to assess nutritional status.
4. Describe the nature and purpose of quality assurance plans for standards of nutritional care.

References

1. Weigley, E.S.: Average? Ideal? Desirable? A brief overview of height-weight tables in the United States, J. Am. Diet. Assoc. **84**(4):417, 1984.
2. Gurin, J.: What's your natural weight? Am. Health **3**(3):43, 1984.
3. Mitchell, C.O., and Lipschitz, D.A.: Arm-length measurement as an alternative to height in nutritional assessment of the elderly, J. Parent. Enter. Nutr. **6**(3):226, 1982.
4. Rosenfeld, I.: The complete medical exam, New York, 1978, Simon and Schuster.
5. Striff, J.L., and others: A comparison of dietary methods in nutritional studies, Am. J. Clin. Nutr. **37**:300, 1983.
6. Swan, E., and Rohrback, C.: Nutritional assessment—an investigative interview, Nutr. Support Serv. **1**(5):14, 1982.
7. Ometer, J.L., and Oberfell, M.S.: Quality assurance, I. A levels of care model, J. Am. Diet. Assoc. **81**(2):129, 1982.
8. Oberfell, M.S., and Ometer, J.L.: Quality assurance, II. Application of oncology standards against a levels of care model, J. Am. Diet. Assoc. **81**(2):132, 1982.
9. Kared, F.A., Becker, D.S., and Finkelstein, G.: Unreceived meals source of malnourishment, Hospitals **56**:47, 1982.

Further Readings

Freed, B.A., Chase, G., and Kaminski, M.V., Jr.: Initiation of an admission nutritional screening program in an urban community hospital, Nutr. Support Serv. **2**(8):19, 1982.

Winborn, A.L., and others: A protocol for nutritional assessment in a community hospital, J. Am. Diet. Assoc. **78**:129, 1981.

Weissberger, L.E., Sowa, D., and Weddle, D.: Clinical nutritional assessment: a two-month evaluation, J. Am. Diet. Assoc. **81**(1):58, 1982.

These three articles provide guidance, from the experiences of two Chicago nutrition support teams, for beginning and evaluating hospital-wide admission nutritional screening programs and determining the most effective procedures to use. Many charts and references.

Wright, R.A., Nutritional assessment, J. Am. Med. Assoc. **355**:559, 1980.

A good summary review of investigations showing effect of nutrition status on the course of disease and the outcome of surgery and the effectiveness of chemotherapy.

Issues and Answers

**"How Much
Should I
Weigh?"—Methods
of Measuring Body
Fat**

When a client asks you this question, you could simply weigh the person on a scale and compare the resulting figure with a standard weight/height table. This will only tell you the total weight, however, and not the amount of *fat*, which is a true indicator of obesity.

Several methods of estimating body fat are available, though none are perfect. Some have the advantage of being simple to perform, are inexpensive, and are convenient for use in most clinical settings:

Skinfold Thickness

This method involves the use of calipers (or **ultrasound**) to measure the amount of fat lying underneath the skin at specific body sites: biceps, triceps, and subscapular and suprailiac areas. This method has its drawbacks in use with the individual client because it fails to account for differences in age, the compressibility of fat in each area, skin thickness, and the fact that fat-free mass (FFM) may not be constant in all individuals. However, it is a cheap assessment method and tends to work well in epidemiologic studies and in clinical work—if done accurately.

Ultrasound Sound waves at a frequency above that which can be heard by the human ear (20 kilocycles/second); in controlled doses, can be used as a therapeutic or diagnostic tool (e.g., to determine skinfold thickness).

Muscle Metabolites

Levels of two metabolites in the urine are measured to estimate tissue: creatinine and 3-methyl histidine. The latter may be a more accurate indicator of fat-free weight, though its use is limited in a disease state because of a higher turnover rate in its levels in muscular tissue. creatinine is easier to measure. However, urine levels fluctuate with mestruation, age, infection, fever, trauma, and disease.

Body Density

Another method of estimating body fat is growing in popularity, despite its inconvenience and expense. Body density measurement involves underwater weighing in a closed container to estimate body fat by the amount of water such fat displaces. Two methods are used: (1) total immersion, in which results can be affected by residual air in the gut (calculations account for residual air in the lungs) and (2) use of the plethysmograph, a vessel that requires the subject to stand in water only up to the neck, with the air in the lungs, gut, and surrounding spaces measured by a special pump. The latter method tends to be the more accurate of the two.

Other more exotic methods involve the use of traceable radioactive or nonradioactive **isotopes** of natural elements, which diffuse throughout the body:

Total Body Water

Isotope An element that has the same number of protons (atomic number) as another element but which has a different number of neutrons (atomic number).

This method involves giving a dose of a special **isotope** of water and measures the amount of isotope given off after it has reached an equilibrium with regular body water, a process that takes only 3 to 4 hours. This test assumes that the water content of nonadipose tissue— or fat-free mass (FFM)—remains constant. If this is true, the amount of FFM could be subtracted from the entire body weight to estimate

Continued.

Issues and Answers—cont'd

Cachexia General poor health and malnutrition, usually indicated by an emaciated appearance.

the amount of body fat. This assumption fails, however, in light of the fact that (1) water levels rise when muscle-wasting occurs, and (2) adipose tissue itself contains water, which is not accounted for in this test. Both facts indicate that this test will underestimate the amount of water in the body.

Total Body Potassium

This method uses a naturally occurring isotope of potassium, ^{40}K, to measure lean body tissue. Results match those of other tests very closely for healthy, non-obese subjects 20 to 29 years of age. However, this test overestimates the amount of fat in patients suffering from **cachexia** and underestimates the amount of lean in obese subjects. The lean tissue of obese persons apparently has less potassium, and their excess adipose tissue may inhibit the measurement of ^{40}K in lean tissue.

Total Body Nitrogen

This measure reflects total body protein in muscle and nonmuscle lean tissue. Estimating fatty tissue is simply a matter of subtracting this amount from the total body weight. Because it measures more than muscle, it is less likely to underestimate lean body mass in individuals with muscle-wasting conditions (e.g., cancer). The main drawback, however, is cost of the test and accessibility of equipment.

Fat-Soluble Gases

Another method based on diffusion, but not using radioactive elements, uses fat-soluble gases, such as those used in anesthesia. These gases should be good indicators of body fat when they are absorbed into it. Unfortunately, they take a long time to be absorbed and are not absorbed evenly throughout all body fat.

Whole Body Conductivity

This new technique takes advantage of the fact that lean tissue conducts electricity better than fat. Tests based on this theory have worked well on farm animals. It is believed that they will work equally well on humans.

Perhaps in the near future, technology will have developed a simple, inexpensive, and accurate method of measuring body fat. The nutrition counselor could then at long last answer more accurately the most frequently asked question and work with the client to develop a truly effective strategy for weight reduction.

References

Cohn, S.H., and others: Comparison of methods of estimating body fat in normal subjects and cancer patients, Am. J. Clin. Nutr. **34**(12):2839, 1981.

Garrow, J.S.: New approaches to body composition, Am. J. Clin. Nutr. **35**:1152, 1982.

Heymsfield, S.B., and others: Measurement of muscle mass in humans: validity of the 24-hour urinary creatinine method, Am. J. Clin. Nutr. **37**(3):478, 1983.

Chapter 17
Drug-Nutrient Interaction

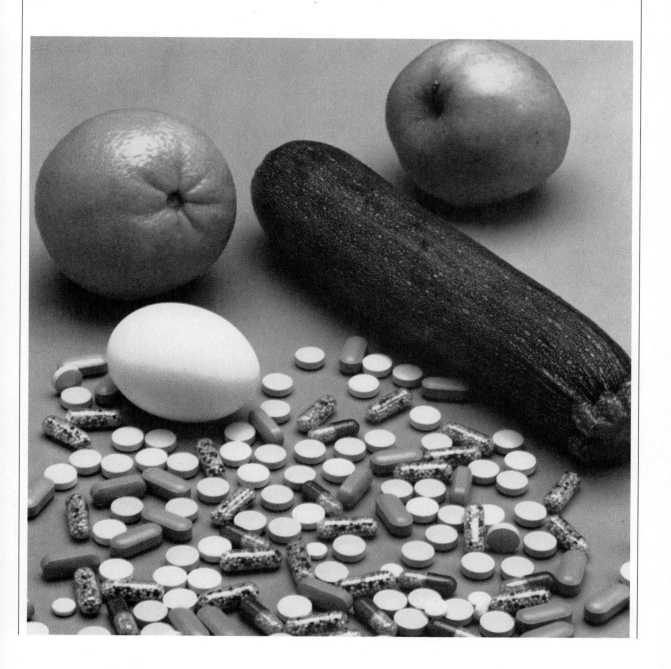

Preview

Consumers today have general information about drug misuse. However, many are dangerously uninformed or misinformed about the specific drugs they may be taking, especially in relation to the food they eat.

The influence of food and dietary patterns on drug absorption and bioavailability is complex. All members of the health care team must have basic knowledge of both drug action and nutrition to make the wisest and most effective use of drug and nutritional therapy. In this chapter we look briefly at some major effects of combining food and nutrients with drugs. We will see how these interactions affect nutritional therapy and education for our clients and patients.

Chapter Objectives

After study of this chapter, the student should be able to:

1. Describe ways in which food and its nutrients affect the use of drugs in the body.

2. Identify effects of drugs on appetite, nutrient absorption, vitamins, and minerals.

3. Identify effects of food nutrients and cooking methods on drug distribution and metabolism in the body.

4. Identify points along the gastrointestinal tract where foods just consumed might affect the efficiency of drug action.

5. Relate food intake to whether it either helps or hinders the body's use of drugs.

Drug-Nutrient Problems in Modern Medicine

Our Medicated Society
Extent of the Problem

The field of nutrient-drug interaction is both complex and confusing. We face a drug-oriented medical environment and a bewildering array of drug items. Every year American physicians prescribe and pharmacists dispense a total amount of drugs sufficient to provide seven individual medications for each woman, man, and child in the United States. To this amount we can then add the large volume of nonprescription drugs that Americans purchase over the counter. Some concerned persons have come to view our overmedicated society with alarm. Knowledgeable and concerned pharmacologists indicate that outside of extremely serious illness, most general medical problems can be treated with less than 25 drugs.[1] The World Health Organization (WHO) has estimated that only some 150 to 200 drugs are actually needed to take care of almost all ordinary illnesses around the world. Yet on our American market there are 54,000 drugs, many of them only slight variations of other drugs, the so-called "me too" drugs.

Possible Cause and Effect

The modern medical world is increasing in complexity and specialization because of advancing technology. Specialty areas or disciplines can easily become isolated from many other important interacting factors when the care of clients and patients falls outside their primary area of expertise. Physicians who prescribe medications, pharmacists who fill these prescriptions, or nurses who administer them may not be fully aware of a particular drug's impact on an individual patient's nutritional state. They may also be unaware of the patient's diet and how it may influence the effects of medication. Similarly a clinical nutritionist/dietitian may provide a diet prescription and food plan yet not be fully aware of the client's medication program and its implications for sound nutritional care.

Drug Use and Nutritional Status
Elderly Persons at Risk

All of us, at any age, risk harmful drug or drug-nutrient interactions. However, elderly persons are particularly vulnerable. Several things contribute to this increased risk among the elderly: (1) they are likely to be taking more drugs for longer periods of time to control chronic diseases, and (2) illness, mental confusion, or lack of drug information may increase errors in self-care. As a result, concerned physicians, nutritionists, pharmacists, and nurses are working more and more together as a team to provide drug and nutritional education and therapy on a sounder basis. A number of drug-nutrient interactions demand this type of team work in patient care.

General Hospital Malnutrition

Studies on hospital malnutrition indicate that there are a number of possible mechanisms of nutrient-drug interaction. The results of these studies give us information on the contributing causes to general malnutrition. Such causes are especially prevalent in hospitalized patients and require informed therapy. These nutrient-drug mechanisms that can affect nutrition include the following drug actions, which are responsible for:

1. Decreased intestinal absorption
2. Increased renal excretion
3. Direct competition or displacement of nutrients from carrier protein sites
4. Interference with synthesis of necessary enzyme, coenzyme, or carrier
5. Hormonal effects on genetic systems
6. The drug delivery system
7. Components in drug formulation

In this chapter we will review briefly various effects of drugs on food and nutrients and vice versa, with some examples in each case.

Effects of Drugs on Food and Nutrients

Drug Effects on Food Intake
Increased Appetite

A number of drugs have the effect of increasing appetite.[2] These drugs include the following:

Antihistamines These drugs can lead to marked increase in appetite and subsequent weight gain. One of these agents, both an antihistamine and a serotonin antagonist, is cyproheptadine hydrochloride (Periactin).

Psychotropic drugs Some of the tranquilizers may lead to **hyperphagia** (the opposite of **hypophagia**) (see Issues and Answers, pp. 386-387). Tranquilizers that lead to weight gain when given to psychotic patients may have the opposite effect on geriatric patients. Some of these drugs include chlordiazepoxide hydrochloride (Librium), diazepam (Valium), chlorpromazine hydrochloride (Thorazine), and meprobamate (Equanil). As with the tranquilizers, other types of antidepressant drugs such as amitriptyline hydrochloride (Elavil) may promote appetite and lead to marked weight gain.

Steroids Anabolic steroids, including testosterone, promote nitrogen retention, increased lean body mass, and subsequent weight gain. Glucocorticoids may also increase appetite, leading to weight gain.

Decreased appetite A number of drugs have the opposite effect of depressing the appetite.[2] Some examples of these drugs include:

Insulin A rapid drop in blood sugar, *hypoglycemia,* can be induced by insulin. This effect is not marked by hunger but often causes nausea, weakness, and aversion to foods. The hypoglycemic reaction is distinct from the effect of general insulin use in the management of diabetes, which may bring a feeling of hunger as nutrient metabolism is improved.

Alcohol Abuse of alcohol can lead to loss of appetite, reduced food intake, and malnutrition. This *anorexia*—loss of appetite—can stem from various effects of alcoholism, such as gastritis, lactose intolerance, hepatitis, cirrhosis, ketoacidosis, pancreatitis, alcoholic brain syndrome, drunkenness, and withdrawal symptoms. The resulting reduced food intake can then lead to malnutrition, which further complicates the anorexia by causing deficiencies of thiamin, zinc, or protein.

Hyperphagia Eating or ingesting more food than necessary for optimal body function.

Hypophagia Eating less than necessary for optimal health.

Clinical Application

The Proof of the Pudding . . .

The senses of taste and smell greatly affect our responses to various foods. The loss of these senses can drive persons to constantly seek elusive satisfaction by overeating, or it may stop them from eating entirely. In either case, the pleasure of eating has gone and nutritional status suffers. Patients on drugs that affect taste and smell need counseling concerning food choices, combinations, and seasonings that can help overcome this difficulty. Some of these drugs include the following:

- **Anesthetics, local** Benzocaine, cocaine, procaine
- **Antibiotics** Amphotericin B, ampicillin, griseofulvin, lineomycin, streptomycin, tetracyclines
- **Anticoagulants** Phenindione
- **Antihistamines** Chlorpheniramine maleate
- **Antihypertensive agents** Captopril, diazide, ethacrynic acid
- **Anti-infectious agents** Metronidazole
- **Cholesterol-lowering agents** Clofibrate
- **Hypoglycemic agents** Glipizide
- **Psychoactive agents** Carbamazepine, lithium carbonate, phenytoin, and amphetamines
- **Toothpaste ingredients** Sodium lauryl sulfate

Indeed, the proof of the pudding . . . *is* **in the taste thereof!**

References
Barley, B.: Taste killers, Am. Health, **3**(1):22, 1984.

Amphetamines These drugs act as stimulants to the central nervous system and have the effect of depressing the desire for food and can lead to marked loss of weight. For this reason they have been used as appetite-depressant drugs in the treatment of obesity. However, long-term use of these drugs in such treatment has caused problems, since appetite may not be the primary causative factor in the excess weight status. For this reason, amphetamines are rarely used now in the treatment of obesity.

Dysgeusia Altered sense of taste.

Chelating agent Substance that combines with a metal, firmly binding it; chemotherapeutic use for metal poisoning.

Taste changes A loss of taste, **dysgeusia**, may be caused by a number of drugs. For example, the **chelating agent** D-penicillamine is used in the treatment of conditions such as heavy metal poisoning, rheumatoid arthritis, or cystinuria.[2] The taste loss in this case is presumably caused by a drug-induced zinc deficiency. Other drugs affecting taste acuity include diuretics, anticancer agents such as methotrexate, doxorubicin hydrochloride (Adriamycin), and agents used to treat Parkinson's disease. Even a 1-g dose of aspirin can increase perception of a bitter taste. Sodium lauryl sulfate, a substance often used in toothpaste to make it clean teeth better, can make orange juice taste bitter.[3] A number of other drugs affect taste and smell (see box above).

Nausea Many drugs have the effect of decreasing appetite because they contribute to nausea and vomiting. For example, cardiac glycosides, digitalis, and related drugs can produce nausea if used in relatively large amounts. A number of drugs used in cancer chemotherapy have similar effects and also contribute to malnutrition and weight loss.

Bulking effects Various agents such as methyl cellulose and other dietary fiber products interfere with absorption of nutrients and contribute to their loss. These bulking agents can also contribute to decreased intake of food by creating a sense of fullness and lack of desire for food intake. For this reason they have been used as adjunct therapy in weight management.

Drug Effects on Nutrient Absorption and Metabolism

Increased Nutrient Absorption

A number of drugs can benefit nutritional status by increasing nutrient absorption. For example, cimetidine (Tagamet), a gastric antisecretory agent, has helped patients with many different gastrointestinal problems. The drug reduces gastric acid and volume output, lowers duodenal acid load and volume, reduces jejunal flow, maintains pH, decreases fecal fat, nitrogen, and volume and thus improves absorption of protein and carbohydrate.[2] This drug is helpful in the treatment of numerous disorders,

Table 17-1
Drugs Causing Primary Nutrient Malabsorption*

Drug	Use	Nutrients Lost	Action
Cholestyramine	Holds bile acid; hypo-cholesterolemic agent	Fat; fat-soluble vitamins A, D, and K; vitamin B_{12}; iron	Binding agent for bile salts and nutrients
Colchicine	Antigout agent	Fat; vitamin B_{12}, provitamin A (carotene); lactose; sodium, potassium	Enzyme damage; inhibits cell division; structural defect
Methyldopa	Antihypertensive agent	Vitamin B_{12}, folic acid; iron	Unclear; possible autoimmune action
Mineral oil	Laxative	Fat-soluble vitamins A, D, and K; provitamin A (carotene)	Nutrients dissolve in oil and are lost in feces
Neomycin	Antibiotic	Fat; vitamin B_{12}; nitrogen; lactose, sucrose; sodium, potassium, iron, calcium	Binds bile salts; lowers pancreatic lipase; structural defect
Para-aminosalicylic acid	Antituberculosis agent	Fat; folic acid, vitamin B_{12}	Blocks mucosal uptake of vitamin B_{12}
Phenolphthalein	Laxative	Calcium, potassium; vitamin D	Rapid intestinal transit; loss of structural tissue integrity
Potassium chloride	Potassium replacement	Vitamin B_{12}	Lowered ileal pH
Salicylazosulfapyridine (Azulfidine)	Antiinflammatory agent (ulcerative colitis)	Folic acid	Blocks mucosal uptake of folic acid

*Adapted from Roe, D.A.: Interactions between drugs and nutrients, Med. Clin. North Am. **63**(5):985, 1979.

including peptic ulcer disease and bowel resection. It has become one of the leading agents in current drug sales.

Decreased Nutrient Absorption

A number of drugs contribute to both primary and secondary malabsorption:

Primary malabsorption Colchicine, a drug used in the treatment of gout, can lead to vitamin B_{12} deficiency, causing megaloblastic anemia. Alcohol abuse can provoke malabsorption of thiamin and folic acid, causing peripheral neuritis and anemia.[4] Laxatives can produce severe malabsorption, leading to conditions such as osteomalacia.

Secondary malabsorption Some drugs inhibit vitamin D absorption, leading to malabsorption and consequent deficiency of calcium. For example, the antibiotic neomycin causes tissue changes in the intestinal villi, which precipitate bile salts, prevent fat breakdown by inhibiting pancreatic lipase, and decrease bile acid absorption.[4] These effects lead to **steatorrhea** and failure to absorb fat-soluble vitamins A, D, E, and K. Malabsorption of vitamin D in turn leads to a calcium deficiency. Other drugs cause malabsorption of folic acid or impair its use, causing malabsorption of still other nutrients. Methotrexate, for example, is a folic acid antagonist and impairs the intestinal absorption of calcium. Summaries of the drugs causing primary and secondary nutrient malabsorption are given in Tables 17-1 and 17-2.

Mineral Depletion

Certain drugs lead to mineral depletion through induced gastrointestinal losses or increased renal excretion.

Diuretics Diuretic drugs are intentionally used to reduce levels of excess tissue water and sodium. But they may also result in loss of other minerals, such as magnesium, zinc, and potassium. Potassium deficiency is marked by weakness, anorexia, nausea, vomiting, listlessness, apprehen-

Steatorrhea Excessive fat amounts in the feces, often due to malabsorption syndromes.

Diuretic A substance that increases or promotes urine excretion.

Table 17-2
Drugs Causing Secondary Malabsorption of Calcium*

Drug	Use	Action
Diphenylhydantoin, phenobarbital, primidone	Anticonvulsant agents	Accelerated vitamin D metabolism
Diphosphonates	Paget's disease (increased bone resorption and deformity)	Vitamin D hormone [1,25,(OH)$_2$D$_2$] formation decreased
Glucocorticoids, such as prednisone	Collagen disease; allergies	Calcium transport decreased
Glutethimide	Sedative	Impaired calcium transport
Methotrexate	Leukemia	Folic acid antagonist—acute deficiency of the vitamin

*Adapted from Roe, D.A.: Interactions between drugs and nutrients, Med. Clin. North Am. **63**(5):985, 1979.

sion, and sometimes diffuse pain, drowsiness, stupor, and irrational behavior.

Chelating agents Penicillamine attaches to metals and can lead to deficiency of zinc and copper.

Alcohol The abuse of alcohol can lead to diminished levels of potassium, magnesium, and zinc.

Antacids These commonly used over-the-counter medications are of concern because they produce phosphate deficiency, with symptoms of anorexia, malaise, **paresthesia,** profound muscle weakness, and convulsions.[4]

Paresthesia Abnormal sensations, such as prickling, burning, "crawling" of skin, etc.

Aspirin Salicylates such as aspirin (acetylsalicylic acid—ASA) can induce iron deficiency by causing low-level blood loss from erosions in the stomach or intestinal tissue. Aspirin is a widely used analgesic agent for relief of common minor aches and pains. Its mechanism of action is through inhibition of certain *prostaglandins* (see p. 62). These hormonelike substances have profound influence on a wide number of physiologic functions, including blood clotting, blood pressure, the inflammatory process, contraction of voluntary muscles, and transmission of nerve impulses. But it is important to remember that aspirin is a *drug*. Since it is an irritant to the stomach and gut, its continuous use can erode mucosal tissue and cause chronic loss of iron, leading to iron-deficiency anemia.

Thus traditional practice in the past has advised taking aspirin with meals for maximum therapeutic effect and minimal irritation. However, current research does not support this practice.[2,4-7] Studies indicate that when aspirin is taken with food, only about half of the aspirin dose gets absorbed and at a slowed rate of time. In comparison, when aspirin is taken with a full glass (250 ml) of water, without food, the full dose is more completely and rapidly absorbed and without increased irritation. This positive effect is due to: (1) total gastric acid dilution by increased cold water, (2) increased dissolution of the drug by increased fluid, and (3) faster stomach emptying, which is delayed by food. Of course, persons with ulcers or bleeding disorders or scheduled for surgery, as well as those with kidney problems or gout, should not use aspirin at all without medical supervision. And it should never be taken with alcohol or vitamin C tablets because both will increase aspirin's irritating effect.

Therefore the best way to take aspirin for minimal irritation *and* maximum therapeutic effect, contrary to prior opinion, is on an empty stomach with a *full* glass of water.[4,5] This fact is important: the absorption of aspirin is facilitated by a large volume of water and inhibited by the presence of food. Taking aspirin—especially on an empty stomach—without a large fluid intake, invites irritative erosion of the stomach lining.

Vitamin Depletion

Certain drugs act as metabolic antagonists to certain vitamins and thus cause a deficiency of the vitamin involved.

Vitamin antagonists Various drugs have been used successfully to treat disease because they are antagonists of certain vitamins. For example, coumarin anticoagulants inhibit regeneration of vitamin K, which is necessary for blood clotting (see p. 115). Some cancer chemotherapy drugs such as

Table 17-3
Examples of Drugs that Act
as Vitamin Antagonists*

Target Vitamin	Drugs
Vitamin K	Coumarin anticoagulants
Folic acid	Methotrexate
	Pyrimethamine
	Triamterene
	Trimethoprin
Vitamin B_6	Cycloserine
	Hydralazine
	Isoniazid
	Levodopa

*Adapted from Roe, D.A.: Interactions between drugs and nutrients. Med. Clin. North Am. **63**(5):985, 1979.

methotrexate inhibit folacin metabolism and thus prevent synthesis of cell reproduction materials—DNA, RNA, and protein. In a similar manner, the anti-malaria drug, pyrimethamine, inhibits the action of folic acid in protein synthesis. A list of vitamin-antagonist drugs is given in Table 17-3.

Hypovitaminoses from use of oral contraceptives Users of oral contraceptive agents (OCA) have developed subclinical deficiencies of folic acid, riboflavin, and vitamins B_6, B_{12}, and C. OCAs induce a greater demand for these nutrients. Table 17-4 includes a list of some of these effects on nutritional status.

Table 17-4
Interactions between Oral
Contraceptive Agents (OCA)
and Vitamins and Minerals
Affecting Nutritional Status*

Nutrient Affected by OCA	Effect	Clinical Result
Vitamins		
Retinol (vitamin A)	Impairs liver storage; increases plasma binding	Unclear
Pyridoxine (vitamin B_6)	Alters metabolism of tryptophan and vitamin B_6	Abnormal protein metabolism; mood changes
Cobalamin (vitamin B_{12})	Reduces vitamin B_{12} serum levels	Unclear
Folic acid	Reduces red cell concentration; increases folate-binding protein	Megaloblastic anemia
Minerals		
Copper	Increases plasma levels of ceruloplasmin	Unclear
Iron	Increase serum levels of transferrin	Unclear
Zinc	Reduces serum levels of zinc	Unclear

*Data adapted from Butterworth, C.E., Jr., and Weinser, R.L.: Malnutrition in hospital patients: assessment and treatment. In Goodhart, R.S., and Shills, M.E., editors: Modern nutrition in health and disease, ed. 6, Philadelphia, 1980, Lea & Febiger.

Table 17-5
Adverse Drug Reactions Caused by Alcohol and Specific Foods

Type of Reaction	Drugs	Alcohol/Foods	Effects
Flushing	Chlorpropamide (diabetes) Griseofulvin Tetrachlorethylene	Alcohol	Dyspnea, head-ache, flushing
Disulifiram reaction	Aldehyde dehydrogenase inhibi-tors: Disulfiram (Antabuse) Calcium carbimide Metronidazole Nitrofurantoin Sulfonylureas	Alcohol Foods containing alcohol	Abdominal and chest pain, flush-ing, headache, nausea and vomit-ing
Hypoglycemia	Insulin-releasing agents: Oral hypoglycemic drugs	Alcohol Sugar, sweets	Mental confusion, weakness, irra-tional behavior, unconsciousness
Tyramine reaction	Monoamine oxidase inhibitors (MAOI): Antidepressants such as phe-nelzine Procarbazine Isoniazid (isonicotinic acid hy-drazide)	Foods containing large amounts of tyramine: Cheese Red wines Chicken liver Broad beans Yeast	Cerebrovascular accident (CVA), flushing, hyperten-sion

*Adapted from Roe, D.A.: Interactions between drugs and nutrients, Med. Clin. North Am. **63**(5):985, 1979.

Special Adverse Reactions

Several reactions are related to specific drug interactions with particular nutrients (Table 17-5).

Vasoactive Having an effect on the diameter of blood vessels.

Monoamine oxidase inhibitors (MAOIs) These antidepressant medica-tions increase the cardiovascular effect of simple **vasoactive** amines, such as tyramine and dopamine, in foods.[6] The resulting *tyramine syndrome* is marked by headache, pallor, nausea, and restlessness. With increased ab-sorption, symptoms may escalate to apprehension, sweating, palpatations, chest pain, fever, and increased blood pressure, at times to the extent of hypertensive crisis and stroke. A low-tyramine food list is given here (see p. 547) for use with any patient taking one of these antidepressant drugs.

Flushing reaction Short-term reaction resulting in redness of neck and face.

Dyspnea Labored, difficult breathing.

Flush reaction A number of drugs react with alcohol to produce a **flush-ing reaction** along with **dyspnea** and headache. Central nervous system depressants, including hypnotic sedatives, antihistamines, phenothiazines, and narcotic analgesics, may cause a loss of consciousness if taken in com-bination with alcohol.

Hypoglycemia Drugs such as chlorporpamide (Diabinese) and similar oral medications used to control Type II diabetes mellitus (see p. 401), are hypoglycemic agents. They precipitate a rapid release of insulin, which may provoke hypoglycemia. This response is increased when the drugs are used together with alcohol. The symptoms of hypoglycemia include weakness, mental confusion, and irrational behavior. If not treated, loss of consciousness can follow.

Disulfiram A white to off-white, crystalline powder antioxidant; inhibits oxidation of the acetaldehyde metabolized from alcohol.

Disulfiram reaction The drug, **disulfiram**, commonly called Antabuse, is used in the treatment of alcoholism. It combats alcohol consumption by producing extremely unpleasant side effect when taken with alcohol. Within 15 minutes flushing ensues, followed by headache, nausea, vomiting, and chest or abdominal pain.

Effects of Food and Nutrients on Drugs

Food Effects on Drug Absorption
Factors Affecting Drug Absorption

The absorption of drugs is a complex matter. Food can affect eventual drug absorption in a number of ways:

Solution Before an orally administered tablet or capsule can dissolve, it must first disintegrate. The drug's absorption from solution in acid gastric juice or in the more alkaline and bilary excretions of the intestine may be more or less complete. The drug then passes through the intestinal mucosa and liver circulation before entering systemic circulation. Here it may be subject to metabolism, deactivation, and elimination through the so-called "first-pass" mechanism. Food may affect eventual drug absorption at any of these points.

Stomach-emptying rate The composition of the diet affects the rate at which the food enters from the stomach. Fats, high temperatures, and solid meals prolong the amount of time food stays in the stomach. Food usually increases secretion of bile, acid, and gut enzymes. It also enhances intestinal motility and **splanchnic** blood flow. Drugs may adsorb to certain food particles.

Splanchnic Pertaining to the large interior organs of the body, especially those located in the abdomen.

Clinical Significance

Any clinical significance of these effects depends on the extent of the effect and the nature of the drug. A small change in absorption may be critical for a drug with a steep dose-response curve but unnoticable for a drug with a wide range of effective concentration. In general the amount of absorption is clinically more important than the rate, since it has more impact on the steady-state plasma concentration of the drug after multiple doses.[6] Table 17-6 gives some examples of drugs whose amount and rate of absorption is influenced by food.

Increased Drug Absorption

Various circumstances contribute to the increased absorption of a drug[2,6]:

Dissolving characteristics When a drug does not dissolve rapidly after it has been taken, the time it remains in the stomach with food is prolonged. This increased time in the stomach may increase its effectiveness and consequent absorption.

Gastric-emptying time Delayed emptying of food from the stomach can have the effect of doling out small portions of a drug, creating more optimal saturation rates on the absorptive sites in the small intestine.

Nutrients Some nutrients promote absorption of certain drugs. For example, high-fat diets increase absorption of the antifungal drug, griseofulvin. This drug is fat-soluble, and high-fat diets stimulate secretion of

Table 17-6
Food Effect on Drug
Absorption*

	Absorption Reduced by Food	Absorption Delayed by Food
	Amoxicillin	Acetaminophen
	Ampicillin	Amoxicillin
	Aspirin	Aspirin
	Demethyl chlortetracycline	Cephalexin
	Doxycycline	Cephradine
	Isoniazid	Digoxin
	Levodopa	Furosemide
	Methacycline	Potassium ion
	Oxytetracycline	Sulfadiazine
	Penicillin G, V(K)	Sulfamethoxine
	Phenethicillin	Sulfamethoxypyridazine
	Phenobarbital	Sulfanilamide
	Propantheline	Sulfasymazine
	Rifampicin	Sulfisoxazole
	Tetracycline	

*Adapted from Roe, D.A.: Interactions between drugs and nutrients, Med. Clin. North Am. **63**(5):985, 1979.

bile acids, which aid in the absorption of the drug. Vitamin C, as well as gastric acid, enhances iron absorption.

Blood flow Food intake increases splanchnic blood flow. This increased circulation increases absorption.

Nutritional status In addition to the presence of specific nutrients, nutritional status may also affect bioavailability of certain drugs. Chloramphenicol is absorbed more slowly in children with protein-energy malnutrition (PEM), but elimination of the drug is also slower in well-nourished children, resulting in a net increased bioavailability of the drug.[8]

Decreased Drug Absorption

The absorption of some drugs is delayed or reduced by the presence of food:

Aspirin The absorption of aspirin is reduced and delayed by food, so it should be taken on an empty stomach with ample water, preferably cold[4,5] (see p. 378).

Tetracycline Nutritional status may also have an impact on drug absorption. Tetracycline absorption is impaired in malnourished individuals.[9] Absorption of this commonly used antibiotic is also hindered when it is taken with milk, as well as with antacids or iron supplements. Tetracycline combines with these materials to form new insoluble compounds that the body cannot absorb.

Phenytoin The presence of protein inhibits the absorption of phenytoin. Carbohydrate increases its absorption, but fats have no impact.[10]

Food Effects on Drug Distribution and Metabolism
Carbohydrate and Fat

Dietary carbohydrate and fat, especially their relative quantities, influence liver enzymes that metabolize drugs. For instance, the presence of fats increases the activity of diazepam (Valium). Fat increases the concentration of the unbound active drug by displacing it from binding sites in plasma and tissue protein.

Indoles

Indole Compound produced in the intestines by the decomposition of tryptophan; obtained from indigo and coal tar.

The **indoles** in **cruciferous vegetables** (cabbage, brussel sprouts, broccoli, cauliflower) can speed up the rate of drug metabolism. They apparently induce mixed-function oxidase enzyme systems in the liver.[11,12]

Cooking Methods

Cruciferous vegetables Vegetables belonging to the botanical family *Cruciferae* or *Brassicaceae*, whose members have crosslike, four-petaled flowers; e.g., broccoli, cabbage, brussel sprouts, cauliflower.

The method of cooking foods may alter the rate of drug metabolism. Charcoal broiling, for example, increases hepatic drug metabolism through enzyme induction.[6,12-14]

Changes in Intestinal Microflora

Changes in intestinal microflora related to amount of dietary protein or fiber, for example, may influence intestinal drug metabolism.[2,13]

Vitamin Effects on Drug Action

Vitamins influence drug action in several ways:

Effects of vitamins on drug effectiveness Pharmacologic doses of vitamins can decrease blood levels of drugs when vitamins interact with drugs. For example, megadoses of folic acid or vitamin B_6 can reduce blood level and the efficacy of phenytoin (Dilantin) or phenobarbital for seizure control.[2]

Control of drug intoxication Riboflavin can be useful in treating boric acid poisoning.[2] Boric acid combines with the riboflavin and eliminates it in the urine. Also, vitamin E combats pulmonary oxygen toxicity. Premature human infants at risk for development of bronchopulmonary dysplasia by oxygen therapy have been protected by vitamin E administration during the acute phase of respiratory distress requiring oxygen treatment.

To Sum Up

The field of nutrient-drug interaction is in its infancy. More research is needed to sort out complicated relationships and possible effects. Drugs can have multiple effects on the body's absorption, metabolism, retention, and nutrient status. They can provoke adverse reactions in combination with certain foods and can influence appetite, either repressing it or artificially stimulating it. Drugs can either increase an individual's absorption of nutrients, or more commonly, decrease absorption, sometimes leading to clinical deficiencies. Drugs can also induce mineral and vitamin deficiencies by their mode of action.

Just as drugs affect our use of food, food affects our use of drugs. Food can affect the absorption of drugs in a variety of ways. Foods also have an effect on subsequent distribution and metabolism of drugs. Vitamins may interfere with drug effectiveness, especially if they are taken in large doses. On the other hand large doses of specific vitamins can be effective in countering certain drug toxicity conditions.

Questions for Review

1. Name four ways food may affect drug use and give examples of each.
2. If your patient were using a prescribed MAOI such as Parnate, what foods would you instruct him/her to avoid?
3. What is the most effective way to take aspirin, with what type of liquid, and with or without food? Why?
4. What foods would you suggest to a hypertensive patient on the diuretic drug hydrochlorothiazide as good sources of potassium replacement?
5. Outline suggestions you would discuss with a patient experiencing a drug-induced taste loss. How would you explain the taste loss?
6. How does cimetidine (Tagamet) help to improve the nutritional status of persons with gastrointestinal disease?

References

1. Napoli, M.: Prescription drugs, Health Facts **6**(26):1, 1981.
2. Roe, D.A.: Interactions between drugs and nutrients, Med. Clin. North Am. **63**(5):985, 1979.
3. Barley, B.: Drugs: taste killers, Am. Health **3**(1):22, 1984.
4. Koch, P.A., and others: Influence of food and fluid ingestion on aspirin bioavailability, J. Pharm. Sci. **67**(11):1533, 1978.
5. Toothaker, R.D., and Welling, P.G.: The effect of food on drug bioavailability, Ann. Rev. Pharmacol. Toxicol. **20**:173, 1980.
6. Rogers, H.J.: Food and medicine incompatibility, Royal Soc. Health **102**(1), 1982.
7. Ribakove, B.M.: Aspirin, Health, **14**(2):40, 1982.
8. Mehta, S.J., and others: Disposition of four drugs in malnourished children, Drug-Nutrient Interactions **1**(3):205, 1982.
9. Raghuram, T.C., and Krishnaswamy, K.: Tetracycline absorption in malnutrition, Drug-Nutrient Interactions **1**(1):23, 1981.
10. Johanson, O., and others: Opposite effects of carbohydrate and protein on phenytoin absorption in man, Drug-Nutrient Interactions **2**(2):139, 1983.
11. Pantuck, E.J., and others: Stimulatory effect of brussel sprouts and cabbage on human drug metabolism, Clin. Pharm. Ther. **25**(1):88, 1979.
12. Anderson, K.E., Conney, A.H., and Kappas, A.: Nutritional influences on chemical biotransformations in humans, Nutri. Rev. **40**(6):161, 1982.
13. Carr, C.J.: Food and drug interactions, Ann. Rev. Pharmacol. Toxicol. **22**:19, 1982.
14. Kappas, A., and others: Effect of charcoal-broiled beef on antipyrine and theophylline metabolism, Clin. Pharmacol. Ther. **23**(4):445, 1978.

Further Readings

Avorn, J.: Why Tums don't go with tetracycline, Am. Health **1**(2):74, 1982.

Report: Here are some things you should know about prescription drugs, FDA Consumer, Health and Human Services Pub. No. (FDA) 82-3124, Public Health Service, June, 1982.

Two sound, very readable articles from the public press providing consumers and professionals alike with much practical information about drug-nutrient actions. Good basis for patient education.

Moore, A.O., and Powers, D.E.: Food medication interactions, Tempe, Arizona, 1981, Ann O. Moore and Dorothy E. Powers, Publishers.

This small pocket size booklet provides a good review and ready reference for clinical work with patients.

Smith, C.H., and Bidlack, W.R.: Food and drug interactions, Food Technol. **36**:99, 1982.

Brief, excellent review with charts relating drug action to nutrient supplements and various foods and beverages.

Smith, C.H., and Bidlack, W.R.: Nutrition and the elderly: food and drug interactions, Nutrit. M.D. **8**(11):1, 1982.

This nutritionist-pharmacist team apply drug-nutrient interaction information to the special needs of elderly persons. They discuss such topics as heart disease, arthritis, gastrointestinal problems, diabetes, depression, and dietary habits.

Issues and Answers

The Calming of America?

American medicine has many names for the psychoactive drugs that act on the mind to dull its reactions. But all these drugs interact dangerously with alcohol and in some cases with commonly eaten foods. Perhaps the name that best fits the effect of these drugs is *tranquilizer*, from a Latin root meaning "calm, quiet, stillness." This meaning signifies the escape many persons seek from a turbulent, confusing world.

We live in an age of stress, often called the "era of anxiety." We also live in a culture committed to "instant" cures and the avoidance of discomfort. Often, instead of probing the causes of our problems and striving to alter the conditions that produce them, we feel somehow that we must never feel uncomfortable. And if we do, we take something for it. We seek the "magic potion" to ease the pain and often the symptoms.

To what extent do we actually use such antianxiety drugs in our search for relief? According to the National Academy of Sciences, some 8.5 million Americans take prescription sleeping pills at least once a year. Two million take them every night for periods of at least 2 months at a time. A study conducted by the National Institute on Drug Abuse indicated that 17 million Americans have used stimulants, 28 million have taken sedatives, and 51 million—nearly 1 out of every 4 Americans—have taken tranquilizers.

America's single most widely prescribed tranquilizer drug is *diazepam (Valium)*. For example, in one recent year, 3.2 billion pills were sold legally, up 50% from the year before, enough to provide every man, woman, and child in the United States with 145 pills a year. Today Valium remains the country's most widely prescribed drug, although a similar antianxiety agent, *lorazepam (Ativan)*, is close on its heels. It is difficult to explain just why Valium is the most frequently prescribed psychoactive drug in the United States. Certainly from a scientific or a pharmacologic viewpoint, no superior effectiveness has been proved. Its popularity may be explained by an aggressive marketing program, leading more physicians to prescribe it, and increased quantities of the drug that are being manufactured. In turn, the increased availability of the drug has lead to increased black market exposure and easy street usage. Also, probably the pale blue Valium tablets were more appealing than the dark green capsules or yellow tablets of some of its competitors.

Valium belongs to a group of psychoactive drugs, first introduced in 1960, called *benzodiazepines*. These antianxiety drugs bind to specific receptor sites in the brain. Their clinical effects are mediated through the central nervous system. For some time scientists have sought the identity of the body's natural compound that occupies these receptor sites in the brain. Now pharmacologists report purification of this natural substance. Paradoxically, they have discovered that this new 104-amino acid brain peptide not only blocks

Issues and Answers—cont'd

the receptor-binding action of the antianxiety drugs but also appears to induce anxiety, indicating that it is not a natural tranquilizer, but has just the opposite effect. Thus this newly identified compound has been named *diazepam-binding inhibitor (DBI)* peptide. These scientists suggest that the naturally occurring DBI acts to trigger anxiety-associated behavior. Apparently, then, drugs such as Valium achieve their antianxiety effect by getting in the way of this naturally occurring anxiety-producing brain peptide.

Along with its desired effect, a drug usually causes some unwanted side effects. In the case of antianxiety drugs such as Valium, several interactions and side effects relate to nutrition counseling needs:

■ **Alcohol.** Tranquilizers and alcohol do not mix. These drugs enhance the effects of alcohol and other central nervous system (CNS) depressant drugs that slow down the nervous sytem. In addition to alcohol, other CNS depressant drugs include over-the-counter antihistamines or medicine for hay fever, other allergies, or colds, as well as prescribed anticonvulsants (e.g., Dilantin), pain medications, or narcotics. Long-term use of alcohol also induces liver enzyme changes leading to more rapid metabolism, reducing the effect of drugs that are detoxified by the liver. Thus in the alcoholic, benzodiazepines may be metabolized more rapidly and the person may use larger and larger doses to achieve the desired effect.

■ **Weight gain.** Persons on these antianxiety drugs often experience a marked increase in appetite with subsequent weight gain. This may bring added concern and require general weight management counseling.

■ **Gastrointestinal problems.** Some general side effects interfere with food intake and use. These problems range from heartburn, nausea and vomiting, to constipation or diarrhea. Individual counseling relating to food choices, combinations, and forms may be needed.

■ **Pregnancy and lactation.** Some cases of birth defects from benzodiazepine use during the first 3 months of pregnancy have been reported. In addition, continued use during pregnancy may cause fetal dependency with withdrawal side effects after birth. During lactation these drugs may pass into the breast milk and cause unwanted effects in the infant.

Such widespread use—and abuse—of transquilizers means that we will frequently encounter them in clinical practice. Nutrition counseling must involve assessment of all possible food, drug, and alcohol interactions, with related guidance concerning dietary management.

References
Hughes, R., and Brewin, R.: The daze of our lives, Family Health **11**(10):28, 1979.
Miller, J.A.: Brain peptides in a chemistry of anxiety, Science News **123**(5):388, 1983.
U.S. Pharmacopeial Convention, The physicians' and pharmacists' guide to your medicines, New York, 1981, Ballantine Books.

Chapter 18
Diabetes Mellitus

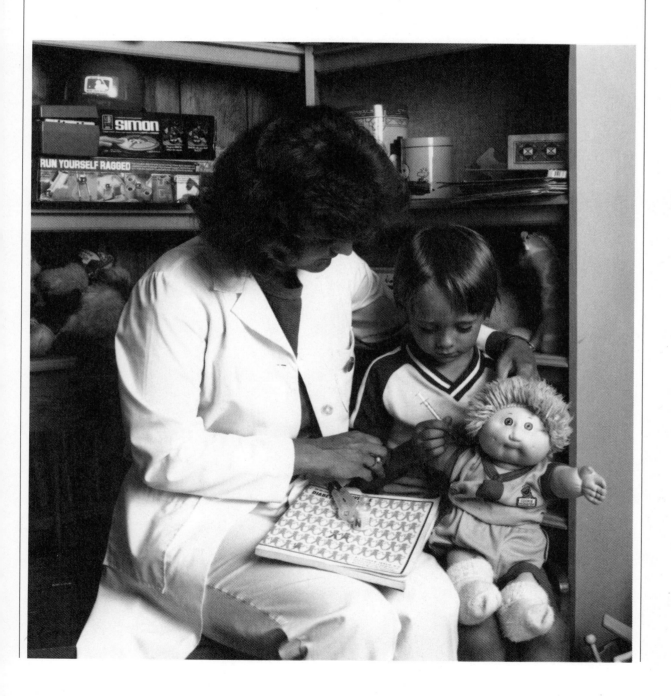

Preview

Nearly 11 million Americans have diabetes. One in twenty will be afflicted with the disorder. Of this total, 15% are insulin-dependent and 85% are non-insulin-dependent. In the North American population, diabetes complications have become the fifth-ranking cause of death from disease.

Diabetes is a disease with both ancient roots and a rapidly expanding modern research base. Many current studies are helping to explain early observations of its nature and the development of better means of care. During the past few years newer information about diabetes indicates that the disease has multiple causes. The current concept held by investigators is that diabetes is not a single disease but a syndrome consisting of many disorders characterized by hyperglycemia and, in a large number of persons, various complications. Sound nutritional therapy remains the fundamental base of management for all persons with diabetes. Newer forms of insulin and self-monitoring of blood glucose have become indispensible tools of control for many.

Chapter Objectives

After study of this chapter, the student should be able to:

1. Describe the nature and extent of diabetes mellitus in the population according to type and identify contributing causes and symptoms.

2. Identify the basic goals of current diabetes management and describe the forms of treatment necessary to achieve these goals.

3. Help persons with diabetes plan and maintain good self-care with sound management and practical tools and resources.

The Nature of Diabetes

Contributing Causes
Insulin Activity

For some time, insulin assay tests that were developed to measure the level of insulin activity in the blood have found insulin-like activity levels in early diabetes to be two or three times the normal insulin levels. Investigators postulated that the insulin was present but bound with a protein, making it unavailable. It is now evident that diabetes is a condition with multiple forms, resulting from: (1) lack of insulin, as in type I, insulin-dependent, diabetes mellitus or from (2) insulin resistance as in type II, non-insulin-dependent, diabetes mellitus.

Weight

Diabetes has long been associated with weight. Early clinicians observed that diabetes improved in overweight patients who lost weight. One investigator described two kinds of diabetes: "fat diabetes" and "thin diabetes."[1] All of these observations preceded any knowledge about insulin or a relationship between the pancreas and diabetes. Current research has reinforced the relationship between the overweight state and type II, or non-insulin-dependent, diabetes.

Heredity

Diabetes has usually been defined in terms of heredity. However, increasing evidence from many research centers indicates that there is considerable *genetic variation* between type I and type II diabetes. Environmental factors, in particular, play a role in revealing an underlying diabetes genotype in type II, non-insulin-dependent diabetes. This relationship with heredity has been based on the so-called "thrifty gene" hypothesis.[2] This theory is founded on the belief that in the past diabetes was a saving, or "thrifty," trait that provided better storage and metabolism of food during times when our ancestors lived under more primitive and difficult survival conditions. Then as food supplies became plentiful, the negative aspects of the diabetic trait began to appear. This state is clearly illustrated with the experience of the Pima Indians of Arizona. In earlier times they ate a limited diet mainly of carbohydrates harvested by heavy physical labor from a primitive agriculture. Now, however, with the "progress" of civilization, the Pimas are less active, have become obese, and *half* of the adults have type II diabetes. This is the highest reported prevalence of this type of diabetes in the world. This same pattern is seen among populations of urbanized Pacific Islanders as well as migrant Asian Indians. The evidence indicates that these groups have a genetic susceptibility (diabetic genotype) to type II diabetes and that the disease is triggered by environmental factors, including obesity.

Classification

Increasing evidence indicates differences between insulin-dependent and non-insulin-dependent diabetes, and epidemiologic studies have provided newer clinical and pathogenetic information. Based on this growing evidence, an international work group of the National Institutes of Health has provided an improved classification for the diabetes syndrome.[1] This classification, though still indicating the two main types, provides a basis for further analysis of subtypes within the two broad classes.

Type I, Insulin-Dependent, Diabetes Mellitus

In its insulin-dependent form, diabetes develops very rapidly and is more severe and unstable. This form occurs more frequently in children, and the child is usually underweight. Acidosis is fairly common.

Type II, Non-Insulin-Dependent, Diabetes Mellitus

In this non-insulin-dependent form, diabetes develops more slowly and is usually milder and more stable. This form occurs mainly in adults, and the person is usually overweight. Acidosis is infrequent. The majority of patients improve with weight loss and are maintained on diet therapy alone. Sometimes there is a need for an oral hypoglycemic medication.

Symptoms
Initial Observations

Early signs of diabetes include the following: (1) increased thirst (polydipsia), (2) increased urination (polyuria), (3) increased hunger (polyphagia), and (4) weight loss (type I) or obesity (type II).

Laboratory Test Data

Various clinical laboratory tests taken at this time reveal the following results: (1) glycosuria (sugar in the urine), (2) hyperglycemia, and (3) abnormal glucose tolerance tests.

Other Possible Symptoms

Additional signs that may appear are (1) blurred vision, (2) skin irritation or infection, and (3) weakness and loss of strength.

Results of Uncontrolled Diabetes

Continued symptoms that can occur as the uncontrolled condition becomes more serious are (1) fluid and electrolyte imbalance, (2) acidosis (ketosis), and (3) coma.

The Metabolic Pattern of Diabetes

Because the initial apparent symptoms, glycosuria and hypoglycemia, are related to excess glucose, diabetes has been called a disease of carbohydrate metabolism. However, as more becomes known about the intimate interrelationship of carbohydrate metabolism with fat and protein metabolism, diabetes is being increasingly viewed as a general metabolic disorder resulting from a lack of insulin (absolute, partial, or unavailable) affecting more or less each of the basic nutrients. It is especially related to the metabolism of the two fuels—carbohydrate and fat—in the body's energy system.

Normal Blood Sugar Controls

Control of blood sugar within its normal range of 70 to 120 mg/dl is vital to life. A knowledge of these controls in maintaining a normal blood sugar level is essential to understanding the impairment of these controls in diabetes (see Chapter 2). These normal balancing controls are reviewed in Figure 18-1.

Figure 18-1

Sources of blood glucose (food and stored glycogen) and normal routes of control.

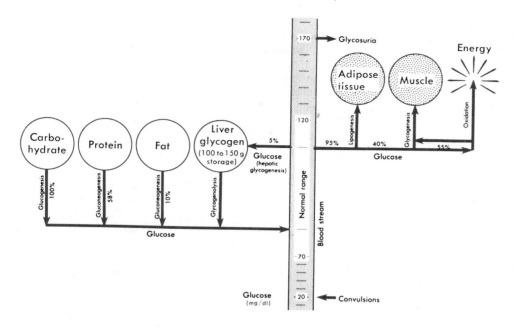

Glycogen A long, branched chain of glucose units that serves as the storage form of glucose in animals.

Glycogenolysis Breakdown of stored glycogen to yield glucose.

Glycogenesis Formation of *glycogen,* the storage form of carbohydrates in animals.

Lipogenesis Conversion of carbohydrates and protein into body fat.

Glycolysis Breakdown of glucose to pyruvate and lactate by enzymes.

Sources of Blood Glucose

To ensure a constant supply of the body's primary fuel, there are two sources of blood glucose: (1) *diet*—the energy nutrients in our food, dietary carbohydrate, protein, and fat, and (2) **glycogen**—the backup source from constant turnover of "stored" liver glycogen by a process called **glycogenolysis.**

Uses of Blood Glucose

To prevent a continued rise of blood sugar above 120 mg/dl, there are several basic uses for blood glucose constantly available according to need. These include (1) **glycogenesis**—conversion of glucose to glycogen for "storage" in the liver and muscle, (2) **lipogenesis**—conversion of glucose to fat and storage in adipose tissue, and (3) **glycolysis**—cell oxidation of glucose for energy.

Pancreatic Hormonal Controls

Three types of islet cells scattered in clusters throughout the pancreas (Islets of Langerhans) provide hormones closely interbalanced in regulating blood glucose level. This specific arrangement of human islet cells is illustrated in Figure 18-2. The largest portion of the islets is occupied by *B cells* filling the central zone or about 60% of the gland. These B cells synthesize insulin. Arranged around the outer rim of the islets are the *A cells,* one to two cells thick, making up about 30% of the total cells. These A cells synthesize glucagon. Interspersed between A and B cells, or occasionally between A cells alone, are the *D cells,* the remaining 10% of the total cells. These D cells synthesize somatostatin. Juncture points of the three types of cells act as sensors of the blood glucose concentration and its rate of change. They constantly adjust and balance the rate of secretion of

Figure 18-2
Islets of Langerhans, located
in the pancreas.

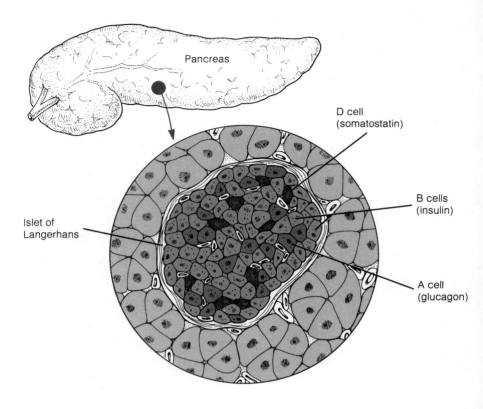

glucagon, insulin, and somatostatin to match whatever conditions prevail
at any time. These three hormones have specific interbalanced functions:

Insulin Although the precise mechanisms are not entirely clear, **insulin**
has a profound effect on these glucose-control mechanisms. It functions
in several ways: 1. It facilitates the transport of glucose through cell membranes by way of specialized insulin receptors. The cells of obese individuals with diabetes have fewer than the normal number of insulin receptors. As weight loss occurs, these receptors increase in number. They are
also increased by physical exercise. 2. It aids in the conversion of glucose
to glycogen with its consequent storage in the liver (glycogenesis). 3. It
stimulates the conversion of glucose to fat for storage as adipose tissue
(lipogenesis). 4. It inhibits fat breakdown (lipolysis) and the breakdown of
protein. 5. It promotes the uptake of amino acids by skeletal muscles and
increases protein synthesis. 6. It influences glucose oxidation through the
main glycolytic pathway.

Glucagon This hormone secreted by the A cells in the Islets of Langerhans functions as a coordinating antagonist to insulin. It rapidly breaks
down liver glycogen and, to a lesser extent, fatty acids from adipose tissue
to serve as body fuel. This action raises blood glucose levels in order to
protect the brain and other tissues. Thus it helps maintain normal blood
sugar levels during fasting and sleep hours. A lowering of the blood glu-

Insulin Hormone formed in
the beta cells of the
pancreas. It is secreted when
blood glucose and amino
acid levels rise and assists
their entry into the cells.

Glucagon Hormone
produced by the alpha cells
in the Islets of Langerhans
and secreted when blood
sugar levels are low or in
response to growth hormone.

Figure 18-3
Abnormal metabolism in uncontrolled diabetes.
From Harper, H.A.: Review of physiological chemistry, ed. 10, Los Altos, Calif., 1963, Lange Medical Publications.

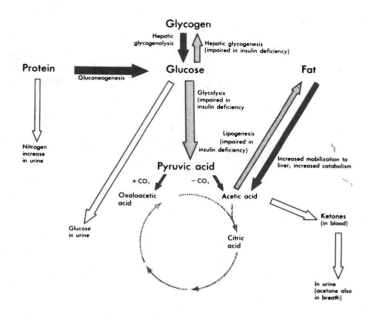

Somatostatin Hormone produced by the delta cells of the islets of Langerhans and the hypothalamus.

cose concentration, increased amino acid concentration, or sympathetic nervous system stimulation triggers the secretion of glucagon.

Somatostatin The pancreatic islet D cells are the major source of somatostatin, although this hormone is also synthesized and secreted in different regions of the body, including the hypothalamus. This hormone acts in concord with insulin and glucose to inhibit their reactions as needed to maintain normal blood glucose levels. It also helps regulate blood glucose levels by inhibiting the release of a number of other hormones as needed.

Metabolic Changes in Diabetes

In uncontrolled diabetes, insulin is lacking to facilitate the operation of normal controls on blood sugar level. Abnormal metabolic changes occur, as illustrated in Figure 18-3:

1. **Glucose** cannot be oxidized properly through the main glycolytic pathway in the cell to furnish energy. Therefore it builds up in the blood (hyperglycemia).

2. **Fat** formation (lipogenesis) is curtailed, and fat breakdown (lipolysis) increases. This leads to excess ketone formation and accumulation (ketoacidosis). The appearance of one of these ketones, **acetone**, in the urine indicates the development of ketoacidosis.

3. **Protein** tissues are also broken down in an effort to secure energy. This causes weight loss and nitrogen excretion in the urine.

Acetone Byproduct of the breakdown of fats for energy.

General Management of Diabetes

Diagnosis
Glucose-Tolerance Testing

The guiding principles for treating diabetes are early detection and prevention of complications. Current research and expert committees of both the National Institutes of Health (NIH) and World Health Organization

(WHO) have brought about a change in the conventional oral glucose tolerance test for diagnosing diabetes.[3] The new procedure uses a 75-g dose of glucose and only two blood glucose tests: (1) fasting and a (2) 2-hour plasma glucose test. A 2-hour plasma glucose level of 200 mg/dl or above indicates diabetes, while 140 mg/dl is the upper limit of normal. Those values falling between 140 and 200 mg/dl are labeled *impaired glucose tolerance*. Clinical experience indicates that persons in this latter group tend to develop overt diabetes at a rate of about four times that of normal persons. Thus, those diagnosed as diabetic and those with impaired glucose tolerance should have follow-up diet therapy and monitoring for glucose management. These diagnostic and follow-up procedures are now usually followed in general clinical practice.

Glycosylated Hemoglobin A_1c

This is an additional blood test used for diabetes screening and monitoring.[4] Glycohemoglobins are relatively stable molecules within the red blood cell. During the life of the cell (about 120 days), glucose molecules attach themselves to the hemoglobin. This irreversible glycosylation of hemoglobin depends on the concentration of blood glucose. The higher the level of circulating glucose over the life of the red blood cells, the higher the concentration of glycohemoglobin. Thus the measurement of hemoglobin A_1c relates to the level of blood glucose over a long period of time. It provides an effective tool for evaluating long-term management of diabetes and degree of control.

Treatment Goals
Basic Objectives

A health team should be guided by three basic objectives in the care of the person with diabetes:

Maintenance of optimal nutrition The first objective is to fulfill the basic requirement for general health, adequate growth and development, and the maintenance of a desirable lean weight.

Avoidance of symptoms This objective is designed to keep the person relatively free of symptoms, such as hyperglycemia and glycosuria.

Retinopathy Noninflammatory disease of the retina. In diabetes, it is characterized by small hemorrhages from broken arteries, yellow, waxy discharge, and retinal detachment.

Neuropathy Two kinds: (1) presence of disease and/or change in function of the peripheral nervous system, (2) noninflammatory injury to the peripheral nervous system; a complication of diabetes.

Nephropathy Disease of the nephrons in the kidneys; a complication of diabetes.

Prevention of complications The third objective recognizes the increased risk a person with diabetes faces for developing problems in tissues such as the eye **(retinopathy),** in nerve tissues **(neuropathy),** and renal tissues **(nephropathy).** In addition, coronary artery disease occurs in persons with diabetes about four times as often as in the general population. Peripheral vascular disease occurs about 40 times as often. There is some evidence that good care and control may reduce these chronic manifestations.[5]

Self-Care Role of Client

To accomplish these objectives, the person with diabetes must be given a central control position. Daily self-discipline and informed self-care are required for sound diabetes management because ultimately all persons with diabetes must treat themselves. Currently, more emphasis is being placed on comprehensive diabetes education programs that encourage self-monitoring and self-care responsibility.

Principles of Nutritional Therapy: The Balance Concept

The core problem in diabetes is energy balance, the regulation of the body's primary fuel—blood glucose. Based on this concept of balance, three main principles of nutritional therapy emerge: (1) total energy balance, (2) nutrient balance, and (3) food distribution balance. However, the fundamental underlying principle of care for all persons with diabetes may be stated very simply—*the diet for any person with diabetes is always based on the normal nutritional needs of that individual.* Personal diet is expressed in terms of (1) total requirement of kilocalories for energy, (2) a ratio of these kilocalories in relative amounts of carbohydrate, protein, and fat, and (3) a food distribution pattern for the day.

Total Energy Balance

Weight Management

Since type I diabetes usually begins during childhood (average age is 11), the weight-height measure for children is an index to adequate growth. In their adult years, the maintenance of a lean weight is a continuing objective of care (see Chapter 15). Since type II diabetes usually occurs in overweight adults, the major objective of care is weight reduction.

Kilocalories

The energy value of a diabetic diet should be expressed in kilocalories sufficient to meet individual needs for normal growth and development, physical activity, and maintenance of a desirable lean weight.

Nutrient Balance

The ratio of carbohydrate, protein, and fat in the diet is based on current recommendations for ideal glucose regulation and lower fat intake to reduce risks of cardiovascular complication (Table 18-1).

Carbohydrate

A more liberal use of carbohydrates, mainly in complex forms, is needed for smoother blood sugar control. About 50% to 55% of the total kilocalories of the diabetic diet is assigned to carbohydrates.

Complex carbohydrates The majority of the carbohydrate kilocalories, about 40% of the total kilocalories, should be consumed as complex car-

Table 18-1
Distribution of Major Nutrients in Normal and Diabetic Diets (as percentages of total calories)

	Starch and Other Polysaccharides* (%)	Sugars† and Dextrins (%)	Fat (%)	Protein (%)	Alcohol (%)
Typical American diet	25-35	20-30	35-45 ⅔ saturated	12-19	0-10
Traditional diabetic diets	25-30	10-15‡	40-45	16-21	0
Newer diabetic diets: current therapy	30-45	5-15‡	25-35 less than ½ saturated	12-24	0-6

*A substantial majority of these calories are starch, but complex carbohydrates also include cellulose, hemicellulose, pentosans, and pectin.
†Monosaccharides and disaccharides, mainly sucrose, but also included are fructose, glucose, lactose, and maltose.
‡Almost exclusively natural sugars, mainly in fruit and milk (lactose).

bohydrates (starches). In most cases these complex carbohydrates break down more slowly than simple sugars and release their available glucose over time.

Glycemic index Modification of carbohydrate food use will eventually have to take into account the varying glycemic index (effect on blood glucose level) of single foods and food combinations. Research in this area is in its early stages but may influence the groupings and selection of foods for improved dietary management in the future.[6,7]

Fiber The degree to which fiber is present in foods such as grains, vegetables, and other starches will influence the rate of absorption of the starch component and alter the effect of complex carbohydrates on the blood sugar level. An increased fiber content in the diet is an important aspect of regulating blood glucose levels.[8]

Simple carbohydrates The remainder of the carbohydrate kilocalories can be used as simple carbohydrates. In general, simple carbohydrates and single or double sugars found in fruits and milk as well as sucrose-sweetened food items should be controlled. They are readily absorbed and have a more immediate effect on the blood sugar level. Research on the glycemic index of various foods, however, has indicated that a small amount of sucrose or fructose is not necessarily detrimental, but it needs to be carefully controlled and used in mixed forms with other foods. Honey is a form of sugar (mainly fructose) and is *not* a sugar substitute, as some persons may believe.

Sugar substitute sweeteners The most commonly used non-nutritive sweetener has been saccharin, although there is still debate about its continued use. Aspartame, a recently marketed agent also known as Nutrasweet or Equal is made from two amino acids, phenylalanine and aspartic acid, and is metabolized as such. A summary of dietary sweeteners is given in Table 18-2.

Protein

Normal age requirements for protein govern the amount indicated for persons with diabetes. About 15% to 20% of the total kilocalories are assigned to protein to meet growth and development needs in children and to maintain tissue integrity. Lean food forms are used to help control fat.

Fat

Fat should always be used in moderation with greater attention given to the control of saturated (animal) fats. No more than 25% to 30% of the total kilocalories should be assigned to fat, with less than half of the total fat allowance used as saturated fats. The recommendation for control of fat, especially saturated fat, is based on the general indication of a relationship between saturated fats and coronary artery disease (see p. 455) and the greater risk factor for such disease in persons with diabetes.

Food Distribution Balance
General Rule

In general, fairly even amounts of food should be eaten throughout the day, adjusted to blood glucose self-monitoring. This will help avoid exces-

Table 18-2

A Summary of Dietary Sweeteners

Sweetener	Commercial Use	Comparative Sweetness*	Effectiveness in Carbohydrate Metabolism and Diabetes Control	Problems
Nutritive Sweeteners (provide 4 kcal/g)				
Aspartame Combination of two amino acids: aspartic acid and a methyl ester of phenylalanine	Soft drinks Chewing gum Powdered beverages Whipped toppings Puddings Gelatin Tabletop sweetener	180-200	Does not contribute significant amount of kilocalories or carbohydrates	Possibly tumerogenic† Possible source of excess phenylalanine for PKU children

Fructose
  Naturally occurring monosaccharide found in honey, fruits, and high-fructose corn syrup
	Baked products
	Frosting mixes
	Tabletop sweetener
	Home food preparation
		1.4
		
		Enhanced by
		  Use in liquids
		  Low temperature
		  Acidity
		  Dilution
			Absorbed more slowly than sucrose
			
			Does not require insulin for entry into cells
			
			Achieves similar level of sweetness with smaller amounts
			
			Contributes moderate amounts of calories and carbohydrates to prevent hypoglycemia
			
			Should not be used by poorly controlled, obese diabetics
				Caloric, carbohydrate values must be considered in calculating diets and recipes
				
				Intake of more than 75 g/day increases risk of hyperglycemia

Sorbitol
  Sugar alcohol naturally occurring in fruits and vegetables
	Baked products
	Sugar-free gum
		0.67	Not generally recommended for diabetes control because
			  Large amounts are needed to sweeten foods
			  Lack of insulin results in increased conversion to glucose‡
				Doses of more than 50-60 g/day result in diarrhea

Xylitol "Wood sugar" found in straw, fruits, corncobs	Banned for commercial use in the United States in 1982	1.22		Tumerogenic
L-Glucose, L-fructose: (Mirror images [isomers] of D-glucose and D-fructose)	Currently under study for possible commercial use	Same as D-glucose (0.72) and D-fructose (1.4)	Contributes no calories or carbohydrates because isomeric configuration prevents absorption	
Nonnutritive Sweeteners (noncaloric)				
Saccharin	Baked products Soft drinks Tabletop sweetener	300-600	Contributes no calories or carbohydrates to the diet	Bladder cancer in test animals§
Cyclamate	Banned for commercial use in the United States in 1970			Bladder cancer in test animals

*The sweetness of sucrose is assigned the value of 1.0.

†A breakdown product of aspartame, diketopiperazine, is considered tumerogenic by some researchers.

‡Sorbitol is metabolized to fructose, then glucose.

§FDA plan to ban saccharin in 1977 failed because of saccharin's popularity.

sive intakes at some points with longer fasting periods between, eliminating the "peaks and valleys" in food intake and consequent blood sugar swings. For persons with type I diabetes, a *regular* schedule of meals at fairly consistent times throughout the day with interval snacks as needed between meals and at bedtime is a basic pattern to build on. For persons with type II diabetes, a consistent meal schedule is not as important but is an aid in general weight management (see Chapter 15).

Daily Activity Schedule

Food distribution needs to be planned ahead and adjusted according to each day's scheduled activities. Practical consideration should be given to work, social events, and stress periods.

Exercise

For persons with type I diabetes, it is especially important that any exercise period or additional physical activity of any kind be accommodated in the food distribution plan. For persons with type II diabetes, exercise is an essential part of a successful weight management program.

Drug Therapy

The food distribution pattern will also be influenced by any form of drug therapy required for control.

Types of insulin Most persons with type I diabetes use a form of medium-acting insulin such as neutral protamine Hagedorn (NPH), lente, or globin. These insulins are compounded forms designed to last over a 24-hour cycle. They are usually given in the morning about a half hour before breakfast, reach their peak of activity in 8 to 10 hours (about mid-afternoon), and last from 20 to 24 hours. The meal distribution to balance with the insulin activity would then be a regular three-meal pattern, with allocations for between-meal and evening snacks as needed. Sometimes the medium-acting insulin is combined with short-acting regular insulin to provide for additional coverage through the first part of the day. Regular crystalline or semilente forms cover about a 4-hour period of time. Thus they affect only the one meal following their use. For control of more labile or **"brittle"** forms of type I diabetes, regular short-acting insulin may be used before each meal, the dose adjusted according to blood glucose self-monitoring (see p. 409). Several special refined insulins are used where allergies or other reactions have been encountered. More recently human insulins have been developed through adaptation of pig insulin, synthesis of human insulin, and genetic engineering. Smaller doses of the human insulin may meet most needs.

Insulin and exercise balance Exercise increases insulin efficiency by increasing the number of insulin receptors on muscle cells. Thus exercise is a useful addition to diet and insulin therapy. However, physical activity must be regular to be effective. A detailed history of personal activity and physical exercise habits provides the information needed as a basis for planning a wise program of *regular* moderate exercise. Guidelines for extra food to cover periods of heavier exercise, or athletic practice and competition, can be included (see p. 405). In general, exercise programs make

"Brittle" diabetes Form of Type I diabetes, difficult to control; sensitive to hypoglycemia and to acidosis.

persons feel better both physically and psychologically. Also, blood glucose self-monitoring (see p. 409) is a simple procedure and can be a helpful means of determining the balance needed at any point in time between exercise, insulin, and food.

Oral agents For some persons with type II diabetes, an oral hypoglycemic agent may be used. The use of an oral hypoglycemic agent (which has the effect of inducing hypoglycemia, a lowering of elevated blood sugar) has been curtailed currently, although it is still used in some cases. Such drugs belong to a group of compounds called sulfonylureas and include agents such as tolbutamide.

A third type of diabetes, although it combines the effects of both types I and II, usually requires no drug therapy. This type is currently referred to as *maturity-onset diabetes of the young (MODY)*.[9] This type of diabetes is characterized by asymptomatic hyperglycemia and patients have a family history suggestive of an autosomal dominant trait. It appears in children, adolescents, and young adults with or without obesity. Diet therapy alone has been shown to control the hyperglycemia of this combination type of diabetes.

Diet Management

Many of the basic therapy principles carry over for both type I and type II diabetes. For example, the nutrient ratios for both types are approximately the same. However, energy balance needs will vary widely. The growing child with type I diabetes will require an increased intake of kilocalories to accommodate rapid growth periods, but the major focus in type II diabetes is determining kilocalorie requirements for weight reduction in obese adults. Also, since type II diabetes is non-insulin-dependent, there is no need for snacks between meals to balance with peaks of insulin activity, nor is the timing of meals as crucial as with type I diabetes. A summary of the comparative nutrient ratios and dietary strategies for type I and type II diabetes is provided in Tables 18-1 and 18-3.

Table 18-3
Dietary Strategies for the Two Main Types of Diabetes Mellitus

Dietary Strategy	Type I (nonobese)	Type II (usually obese)
Decrease energy intake (kilocalories)	No	Yes
Increase frequency and number of feedings	Yes	Usually no
Have regular daily intake of kilocalories of carbohydrate, protein, and fat	Very important	Not important if average caloric intake remains in low range
Plan consistent daily ratio of protein, carbohydrate, and fat for each feeding	Desirable	Not necessary
Use extra or planned-ahead food to treat or prevent hypoglycemia	Very important	Not necessary
Plan regular times for meals/snacks	Very important	Not important
Use extra food for unusual exercise	Yes	Usually not necessary
During illness, use small, frequent feedings of carbohydrate to prevent starvation ketosis	Important	Usually not necessary because of resistance to ketosis

Individual Needs

First the practitioner seeks to discover as much as possible about each client's needs through a comprehensive history (see p. 361). A wide range of areas should be included in the discussion, such as personal and family needs, psychosocial development, social activities, work and school commitments, a typical day's routine, and description food habits. Also, a full medical history should be reviewed with particular reference to the diabetes, its course, and the client's personal experience with it. Pertinent medical and nutritional status data include laboratory tests and anthropometric measures of weight, height, and body composition (see p. 356). Then, based on information gathered through the comprehensive nutrition history, the clinical nutritionist determines the appropriate diet prescription for the patient and calculates the nutritional needs according to the balance concept of nutritional therapy described previously.

The Food Exchange Systems

In most health care centers, the Food Exchange System for planning diabetic diets is commonly used. This system of control, based on the concept of food equivalents, has been developed jointly by the American Diabetes Association and the American Dietetic Association. The system has some limitations and is not appropriate for all persons with diabetes; in such cases the clinical nutritionist devises other guidelines to meet individual needs. However, in most cases, with initial instruction and continued counseling by a professional diet counselor—usually a registered dietitian

Table 18-4
Food Exchange Groups

Food Group	Unit of Exchange	Composition Carbohydrate (g)	Protein (g)	Fat (g)	Calories	Characteristic Items
Milk	1 cup					
Skim		12	8	—	80	Equivalents to 1 cup whole
Low fat		12	8	5	120	milk listed; 1 cup skin + 2 fat
Whole		12	8	10	170	exchanges = whole milk
Vegetables	½ cup	5	2	—	35	Medium carbohydrate
Fruit	Varies	10	—	—	40	Portion size varies with carbohydrate value of item; all portions equaled at 10% carbohydrate
Bread	Varies; 1 slice bread	15	2	—	70	Variety of starch items, breads, cereals, vegetables; portions equal in carbohydrate value to 1 slice bread
Meat	28 g (1 oz)	—				Protein foods; exchange units
Lean		—	7	2.5	50.5	equal to protein value of 28 g
Medium fat		—	7	5	75	lean meal (cheese, egg, seafood)
Higher fat		—	7	7.5	95.5	
Fat	1 tsp					Fat food items equal to 1 tsp
Polyunsaturated		—	—	5	45	margarine (oil, mayonnaise, olives, avocados)
Monounsaturated		—	—	5	45	
Saturated		—	—	5	45	

with extensive clinical experience—the person with diabetes will find the diet a helpful tool for planning meals and snacks. It can be a sound means of dietary regulation that is flexible enough to meet a wide variety of living situations. Six food groups are listed in the Food Exchange System: milk, vegetables, fruit, bread, meat, and fat. The revised food lists incorporate the low saturated fat modification in subgroups. These complete food lists are given in Appendix H. A general description according to composition and characteristics is given in Table 18-4. In using the food groups as a guide, food items within any one group may be freely exchanged, since all foods in that group, in portions indicated, are of approximately the same food value. These food groups form the basis for calculating diet needs (Table 18-5) and helping clients learn to make wide food selections and substitutions.

Personal Food Plan

On the basis of the individual's calculated diet pattern, the nutritionist and the client work out a personal food plan. The client learns how to plan a menu by using the meal/snack food distribution pattern. A variety of foods from the Food Exchange system are chosen in the amounts indicated to meet the overall food plan. A sample menu based on a 2200-kcal diet as calculated in Table 18-5 is given on p. 404.

Special Concerns

In the course of daily living, a number of special concerns arise and become part of on-going diet counseling.

Special diet items There is little use for special "dietetic" or "diabetic" foods in the diet of a person with diabetes. Usually these products are more expensive than their regular counterparts, and the diet of the person with diabetes can be planned using regular foods. Also, in the case of sugar substitutes, there is still some question concerning the use of more than only moderate amounts of the two products approved, saccharin and aspartame[10] so that excess of either are unwise (see Table 18-2).

Alcohol Occasional use of alcohol in the diet of persons with diabetes can be planned, but caution must be used. Occasional use is defined as mod-

Table 18-5

Calculation of Diabetic Diet: Short Method Using Exchange System (2200 kcal)

Food Group	Total Day's Exchanges	Carbohydrate: 27 g (50% kcal)	Protein: 110 g (20% kcal)	Fat: 75 g (30% kcal)	Breakfast	Lunch	Dinner	Snacks PM	HS
Milk (low fat)	2	24	16	10	1				1
Vegetable	3	15	6			1	2		
Fruit	4	40			1	1		1	1
		79							
Bread	13	195	26		3	3	3	2	2
		274	48						
Meat	9		63	45	1	2	4	1	1
			111	55					
Fat (polyunsaturated)	4			20	1	1	2		
				75					

Sample Menu Prescription:
2200 kcal—275 g carbohydrate
(50% kcal) + 110 g protein
(20% kcal) + 75 g fat (30% kcal)

Breakfast	1 medium, sliced fresh peach	
	Shredded Wheat cereal	
	1 poached egg on whole-grain toast	
	1 bran muffin	
	1 tsp margarine	
	1 cup low-fat milk	
	Coffee or tea	
Lunch	Vegetable soup with wheat crackers	**Afternoon Snack**
	Tuna sandwich on whole-wheat	10 crackers with 2 tbsp peanut butter
	bread	Orange
	Filling: Tuna (drained ½ cup)	
	Mayonnaise (2 tsp)	
	Chopped dill pickle	
	Chopped celery	
	Fresh pear	
Dinner	Pan-broiled pork chop (trimmed well)	**Evening Snack**
	1 cup brown rice	3 cups popped, plain popcorn
	½-1 cup green beans	1 oz cheese
	Tossed green salad	1 cup low-fat milk
	Italian dressing (1-2 tbsp)	
	½ cup applesauce	
	1 bran muffin	

erate intake (less than 6% of the total kilocalories on a given day) not more than once or twice a day (see Issues and Answers, pp. 413-414). With type II, weight management is a primary concern. Since alcohol is metabolized like fat, the appropriate caloric substitution in the diet should be a reduction in fat intake. The alcohol kilocalories would then be accounted for by substitution for equal caloric value in fat exchanges. However, the situation is different in type I diabetes. Here the main concern is control of blood glucose levels, which may fluctuate widely. In these situations, alcohol-induced hypoglycemia can develop within 6 to 36 hours after alcohol ingestion in individuals whose food intake has been markedly restricted.[11] Thus when a person with type I diabetes chooses to use alcohol, it must be in small occasional amounts and should *not* be adjusted with substitution of food exchanges because of the possibility of hypoglycemic reactions. In either case, alcohol used in cooking does not have to be accounted for in the diet because the alcohol ingredient vaporizes in the cooking process and is not present in the finished product.

Physical activity For any unusual physical activity, the person with type I diabetes needs to make special plans ahead. This is particularly true of a young person with "brittle" diabetes engaging in strenuous athletic competition or practice (see p. 405). (You will find a discussion of the energy demands of exercise in Chapter 14.)

Illness When general illness occurs, food and insulin need to be adjusted accordingly. As needed, the texture of the food can be modified to incorporate easily digested and absorbed liquid foods while still maintaining as

Meal-Planning Guide for
Active People with Type I
Diabetes Mellitus

Moderate Activity

Exchange Needs For	Sample Menus
30 minutes	
1 bread OR 1 fruit	1 bran muffin OR 1 small orange
1 hour	
2 bread + 1 meat OR 2 fruit + 1 milk	Tuna sandwich OR ½ cup fruit salad + 1 cup milk

Strenuous Activity

Exchange Needs For	Sample Menus
30 minutes	
2 fruit OR 1 bread + 1 fat	1 small banana OR ½ bagel + 1 tsp cream cheese
1 hour	
2 bread + 1 meat + 1 milk OR	Meat and cheese sandwich + 1 cup milk OR
2 bread + 2 meat + 2 fruit	Hamburger + 1 cup orange juice

much as possible the glucose equivalents of the usual food plan (see box, pp. 406-407). This same procedure may be followed for glucose equivalent replacement of meals not eaten, as shown below.

Travel When a trip is planned, the diet counselor and the client should confer to decide on food choices according to what will be available to the traveler (see box, pp. 406-407).

How to Modify a Diabetic
Meal Plan for Sick Days

Usual Food Intake	Exchange	Carbohydrate (g)
½ chicken breast, roasted	3 meat	0
1 tsp margarine	1 fat	0
½ cup rice	1 bread	15
Tossed green salad, lemon wedge	Free food	0
¾ cup strawberries	1 fruit	10
1 cup skim milk	1 milk	12
	TOTAL	37

Sick Day Intake*	Exchange	Carbohydrate (g)
2 cups broth	Free food	0
1 cup gelatin	2 fruit	20
1 cup ginger ale (regular)	2 fruit	20
2 cups herbal tea	Free food	0
	TOTAL	40

*OBJECTIVE: to provide required amounts of carbohydrate for times when the person with diabetes just doesn't feel like eating much.

Clinical Application

Travel and Illness: "Real-life" Diabetic Situations

Routine meal-planning tips are all well and good. But what do you do when your "real-life" client with diabetes wants to travel or catches a cold? In both cases, the client will have too many distractions to concentrate fully on planning the most ideal menu. The fact remains, however, that in both travel and illness, diabetes management relies heavily on the food plan and, in the case of Type I diabetes, on meal/snack flexibility to meet changing demands.

Travel

Promote confidence about meal-planning skills. Review the number and type of exchanges allowed at each meal; encourage the client to practice measuring portion sizes; review tips on eating out.

Learn about the foods that will be available. For a cruise, have the client get a copy of the menu in advance. For air travel, order diabetic meals in advance. If foreign travel is involved, have the client ask the travel agent for information about foods commonly served to tourists.

Select appropriate snacks. Remind the client to meet extra carbohydrate and caloric needs during extra physical activities, such as hiking, swimming, skiing, mountain climbing.

Plan for time. Have the client avoid extended driving time and plan to include 20 g of carbohydrate for every 2 hours of travel. For emergencies and unexpected delays, the client should plan to have on hand food for two meals and two snacks, including nonperishable items and liquids.

Plan for time zone changes. The schedule may need to be changed. If so, discuss any needed meal revisions with the client for balancing the insulin-activity pattern.

Prepare companions. Companions must recognize signs and symptoms of hypoglycemia and know its treatment. Remind the client to carry quick-acting carbohydrates at all times. To support the medical regimen of insulin-dependent clients, remind them to: (1) carry an ID bracelet, pendant, or card at all times, (2) ask their physicians for a letter explaining the need for syringes, and (3) take a prescription for insulin and learn brand names used for insulin in the country to which they are traveling.

Sick-Day Survival

Nausea and diarrhea. Remind the client that fluid and electrolyte replacement is crucial. To replace *sodium,* the client should use salted crackers, broth or soups, as tolerated. To replace *potassium,* Coca Cola (small amounts of high-sugar foods can be tolerated as replacement for short periods of time, as during illness), tea, broth, or orange juice can be used. To replace *liquids,* the client should drink *something* at least every 2 to 3 hours.

Gastrointestinal disturbances. Insulin dosage may need to be decreased. The client should try a *clear liquid diet,* including fruit

---

Clinical Application—cont'd

---

juices, fruit ices, and soups for adequate amounts of carbohydrate. *Protein supplementation* through elemental nutrition may be necessary if symptoms last longer than 72 hours. As food tolerance improves, progress to a *soft diet* that includes milk drinks, custards, and eggs.

Colds and fever. These conditions are often treated with aspirin, which tends to lower sugar level. Remind the client of two major guidelines:

- **Do not skip meals.** If necessary, subdivide regular meals into small, frequent snacks.
- **Do not omit insulin.** If totally unable to eat, contact the physician for advice regarding insulin dosage.

In summary, the person with diabetes who is ill should (1) maintain intake of food every day, (2) replace carbohydrate solid foods with equal liquid or soft foods, (3) monitor blood frequently for sugar, and (4) contact a physician if the illness lasts more than a day or so.

Eating out Similar guidelines and suggestions can be provided for various situations when the person with diabetes eats meals away from home. As a general rule, the plan should be made ahead of time so that accommodations for what is eaten at home before and after the meal away from home can reflect continuing balance needs for the day. Such planning is more crucial in the case of a person with type I insulin-dependent diabetes.

Stress Any form of physiologic or psychosocial stress will be reflected in variations of diabetes control. These variations are caused by hormonal responses antagonistic to insulin. Persons with diabetes, especially type I, should learn useful stress-reduction exercises and activities as part of their diabetes education program.

Diabetes Education Program

Goal: Person-Centered Self-Care
Changing Roles

In past years a traditional medical model has guided diabetes education in its methods, language, and respective roles assumed. The professionals viewed themselves as having major authoritative roles and assigned the more passive role of "patient" to the person with diabetes. With notable exceptions, this model has been followed in most cases. However, because of an increasing movement toward changing roles of practitioners and consumers in the health care system (see p. 9), persons with diabetes are assuming a more active voice in planning and conducting their own care. Barriers in our traditional system stem from three sources: (1) our culture, (2) our health care delivery system, and (3) our professional training and habits.

Communication Needs

Essentially, much of the core problem centers on communication.[12,13] For example, here is a list of words we too commonly use that are objectionable to persons with diabetes, along with some suggestions of preferred language we might use instead.

"Diabetic" used as a noun The word "diabetic" is an adjective and should not be used alone as a noun. Use instead the phrase "person with diabetes."

Compliance The word "compliance" raises red flags in the minds of those with diabetes. It is a purely medical term and connotes an authoritative physician position. Instead use the word "adherence." This word has been adopted recently by national committees and associations working in the field of diabetes. The word "adherence" indicates that the decision-making responsibility rests with the person who has diabetes to determine courses of action in varying situations.

Patient Use instead the phrase "person with diabetes." Persons with diabetes are patients *only* when they are in the hospital or seeing a physician for an illness.

Cheating A particularly abusive word in the minds of many persons with diabetes—especially parents of children and young people with diabetes—is the word "cheating." This flagrant language abuse suggests dishonesty or failure to live up to an external code. By and large, persons with diabetes do not "cheat." They may kid themselves or they may be inaccurate in their reporting, but they do not cheat. Use instead phrases such as "having difficulty" or "having a problem with."

Content: Tools for Self-Care

Necessary Skills

Guidelines developed by diabetes educators and the American Diabetes Association (based on learning needs) build on necessary skills and content areas required for self-care of diabetes.[14] The necessary skills a person with diabetes must have for the best possible control—as well as favorable surrounding factors related to life situations and psychosocial needs—include six basic content areas:

1. Fulfillment of basic needs in relation to diabetes
2. Having a sound nutrition and meal plan
3. Understanding insulin (or oral medication) effects and how to regulate them
4. Monitoring of both blood glucose and urine sugar and acetone
5. Hypoglycemia control
6. Learning how to deal with illness and other special needs of daily living.

These educational needs can be organized on three levels that have been discussed so far: (1) survival level, (2) home management level, and (3) lifestyle level. (Personal ID registration with Medic Alert is also important.)

Educational Materials: Person-Centered Standards

A confusing array of diabetes education materials are available. Some are excellent, but some should be discarded. We are wisely reminded, especially by parents of some of our young adolescent clients, that whatever we use should measure up to several basic person-centered requirements. As health care providers, we should:

1. Give the client credit for having intelligence and wanting new information.
2. Inform persons fully and completely of health care information, giving both sides of an issue when experts disagree—as surely they will on occasion.
3. Appeal to various levels of understanding, ranging from basic to sophisticated.
4. *Never* be patronizing, dehumanizing, or childish.

In the last analysis whatever methods or materials we use, one central fact must be remembered: the person who has diabetes is the most important and fully equal member of the diabetes care team. Approaches and strategies that involve this recognition can be fruitfully developed and are the most likely to succeed.

Future Trends in Diabetes Care

Education of the person with diabetes may also include information concerning developing trends in diabetes care. Some of these areas include:

New insulins With the development of a method for applying genetic engineering to the manufacture of insulin, a new human insulin is being marketed under the trade name *Humulin*. This new insulin is produced by rapidly reproducing bacteria that have been given the human gene that codes for the manufacture of insulin in the pancreas. An advantage of the new product is that persons with diabetes who are allergic to animal insulin will be able to use the human insulin. Novo industry, which dominates the European insulin market, also has introduced "humanized" insulin, in which pig insulin is chemically converted to match the human type.

Insulin delivery systems In an efort to control blood glucose fluctuations in more "brittle" forms of type I diabetes, a continuous subcutaneous insulin infusion method of delivering insulin has been developed. Already more than 6000 people with type I diabetes are wearing these infusion pumps that provide a steady supply of insulin through subcutaneous needles inserted into the abdomen. The pump is about the size of a small cassette player and is worn on a belt (Figure 18-4). Studies indicate that this system helps make the diabetes diet more manageable for the client and leaves him without short-term or long-term metabolic risk factors for cardiovascular complications. However, insulin pumps are not suited for all persons, and great care must be exercised in selecting clients for such intensive glycemic control. An implantable insulin delivery system is in the research stages using test animals, and future experiments in human beings are being planned. Still another line of research centers on the effort to develop a "sugar sensor," which would monitor levels of blood glucose as well as controlling hormones, through small coded wire sensors implanted in small veins or body tissue. This device would measure glucose concentration as it fluctuates in blood fluids.

Blood glucose self-monitoring A blood glucose self-monitoring technique in the management of diabetes is being rapidly developed. It is valuable for several reasons:

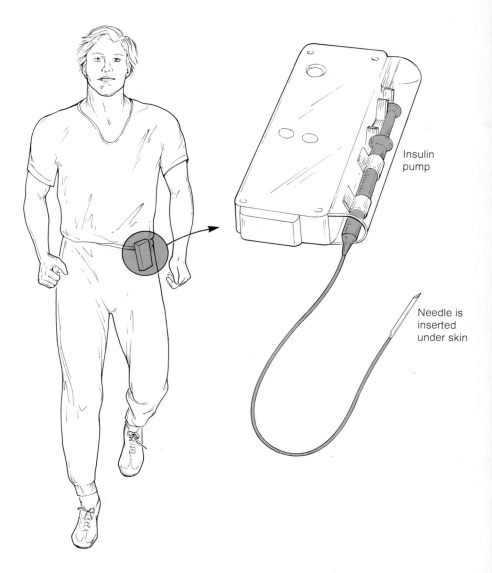

Figure 18-4
Use of an insulin pump with careful control by selected persons with diabetes allows them greater freedom of activity—including jogging.

Insulin pump

Needle is inserted under skin

1. It provides a means for closer control of blood glucose in variable day-to-day living situations and hence lessens the risk of a person developing vascular complications over time.
2. It offers a means, with reduced risk of complications in emergency situations, of controlling the economic cost of diabetes in lost work hours and health care expenses. Such costs have exceeded 10 billion dollars annually.[15]
3. It provides the only practical method for control of maternal glycemia in women with diabetes during pregnancy, consequently reducing infant mortality and morbidity in diabetic pregnancies.
4. It allows persons with unstable "brittle" type I diabetes to live a more normal life.

Although this technique is not for everyone, there are specific groups of diabetic persons who should be encouraged and given the opportunity to use it. These include: (1) women with preexisting diabetes during pregnancy, (2) persons with unstable type I diabetes, (3) persons with diabetes who have renal disease, (4) insulin infusion–pump users, and (5) persons with diabetes who are color-blind. Persons with type II diabetes may also find blood glucose self-monitoring a helpful means to control blood sugar since it increases motivation for closer dietary management. The success thus far of blood glucose self-monitoring indicates that this method is becoming the predominant means for daily personal diabetes management, with increased personal freedom and control.

To Sum Up

Diabetes mellitus is a syndrome composed of many metabolic disorders collectively characterized by hyperglycemia and other symptoms. The treatment relies heavily on a basic type of therapy—a carefully planned diet. Blood sugar levels are controlled primarily by the pancreatic hormones: *insulin,* which facilitates the passage of glucose through cell membranes via membrane receptors; *glucagon,* which ensures adequate levels of glucose to prevent hypoglycemia; and *somatostatin,* which controls the actions of insulin and glucagon to maintain normal blood glucose levels. The diabetic state results from inadequate insulin secretion or insulin resistance as a result of fewer receptor sites. Symptoms range from polydipsia, polyuria, polyphagia, and signs of abnormal carbohydrate metabolism to fluid and electrolyte imbalances, acidosis, and coma in seriously uncontrolled conditions.

Type I insulin-dependent diabetes mellitus affects approximately 15% of all persons with diabetes. It occurs more often in children and is more severe and unstable. Its treatment involves blood glucose self-monitoring, insulin administration, and scheduled meals and exercise to balance insulin activity.

Type II non-insulin-diabetes mellitus occurs mostly in adults, particularly those who are obese or overweight. Acidosis is rare. Its treatment consists of weight management through kilocalorie modification and exericse. The food plan should be rich in complex carbohydrates and fiber, low in simple sugars and fats (especially saturated fats), and moderate in protein. Moderate regular exercise increases the number of insulin receptor sites on cell membranes and aids in weight control.

Questions for Review

1. Describe the major characteristics of the two types of diabetes mellitus. Explain how these characteristics influence differences in nutritional therapy. List and describe medications used to control these conditions.
2. Identify and explain symptoms of uncontrolled diabetes mellitus.
3. Mr. Smith just found out that he has diabetes mellitus. He is a sedentary, 38-year-old man who is 170 cm (5 ft, 8 in) tall and weighs 94 kg (210 lb). No medications were prescribed. What is his desirable lean body weight? What would be an appropriate diet order in kilocalories and how should these kilocalories be distributed among the energy nutrients? If he decides to drink, how much alcohol could be allowed and how would it be fitted into his diet? Should he purchase sugar substitutes or diet foods? Defend your answer. What advice would you offer Mr. Smith to help his children reduce their chances of developing diabetes?

References

1. Whitehouse, F.W.: Classification and pathogenesis of the diabetes syndrome: a historical perspective, J. Am. Dietet. Assoc. **81**(3):243, 1982.

2. Mann, R.J., and Mann, F.D.: Professor Palmer's food-efficient rats, Nutri. Today **17**(5):21, 1982.

3. Ito, C., Mito, K., and Hara, H.: Review of criteria for diagnosis of diabetes mellitus based on results of follow-up studies, Diabetes **32**:343, 1983.

4. Verrillo, A., and others: The relationship between glycosylated haemoglobin levels and various degrees of glucose intolerance, Diabetologia **24**:391, 1983.

5. Bleicher, S.J., and others: Effect of blood glucose control on retinal vascular permeability in insulin-dependent diabetes mellitus, Diabetes Care **3**:184, 1980.

6. Crapo, P.A., and Olefsky, J.M.: Food fallacies and blood sugar, N. Engl. J. Med. **309**:44, 1983.

7. Jenkins, D.J.A.: Lente carbohydrate: a newer approach to the dietary management of diabetes, Diabetes Care **5**:634, 1982.

8. Burgess, B.E., Rationale for changes in the dietary management of diabetes, J. Am. Diet. Assoc. **81**:258, 1982.

9. Lawson, V.K., Young, R.T., and Kitabchi, A.E.: Maturity-onset diabetes of the young: an illustrative case for control of diabetes and hormonal normalization with dietary management, Diabetes Care **4**(1):108, 1981.

10. Horwitz, D.L., and Bauer-Nehrling, J.K.: Can aspartame meet our expectations? J. Am. Dietet. Assoc. **83**(2):142, 1983.

11. Franz, M.J.: Diabetes mellitus: considerations in the development of guidelines for the occasional use of alcohol, J. Am. Dietet. Assoc. **83**(2):147, 1983.

12. Hoover, J.: "Compliance" from a patient's perspective, The Diabetes Educator **6**:9, 1980.

13. Sims, D.F.: Barriers to adherence, Diabetes Care **2**:524, 1979.

14. Prater, B.: Education guidelines for self-care living with diabetes, J. Am. Dietet. Assoc. **82**(3):283, 1983.

15. McNeil, L.: Self blood glucose monitoring: an update, The Diabetes Educator **8**:15, 1983.

Further Readings

Anderson, J.W.: A diabetic in the family? Health **15**(7):48, 1983.

Monagan D.: Healing lifestyle, Am. Health **2**(5):29, 1982.

These two articles from the popular press provide good background for diabetes education and counseling based on experiences of persons with diabetes and professionals who work with them. Practical tools and information are given, showing the values of sound diet and exercise.

McNeil, L.: Self blood glucose monitoring: an update, Diabetes Educator, **8**:15, 1983.

Good review of current materials and products for monitoring, with a chart of standard blood sugar target levels and annual cost estimates for equipment. Useful for client counseling and education.

Poplin, L.E.: Diabetes that first occurs in older people, Nutri. Today **17**(5):4, 1982.

Readable review of the nature and treatment of Type II non-insulin-dependent diabetes. Excellent illustrations and charts.

Prater, B.: Education guidelines for self-care living with diabetes, J. Am. Diet. Assoc. **82**(3):283, 1983.

Wylie-Rosett, J.: Development of new educational strategies for the person with diabetes, J. Am. Diet. Assoc. **81**(3):268, 1982.

Two articles with helpful guidelines for developing a sound diabetes education program based on realistic needs and learning principles. Stresses important principles on self-care attitudes, knowledge, and skills.

Issues and Answers

Alcohol and Diabetes: Do They Mix?

Two shots of whiskey on an empty stomach can lower blood sugar dramatically. For this reason, among others, alcohol has been taboo for years for persons with diabetes. It definitely has some negative effects, since it:

- Interferes with the body's ability to regulate insulin-induced hypoglycemia. Persons in poor control are most susceptible to this effect.
- Increases serum cholesterol levels, though this effect is transient.
- Leads to hyperlipoproteinemia when used in excess by susceptible persons, including persons with diabetes.
- Leads to hyperglycemia when used in excess, though this is a transient effect usually lasting only a few hours.
- Induces a diabetic condition when used in excess by a prediabetic individual. In such persons, however, the blood sugar returns to normal following total abstinence, without having to resort to the use of insulin or other oral hypoglycemic agents.

For the person with diabetes, however, alcohol may not be quite as bad as most people think it is because it: (1) does not require insulin for its metabolism, (2) enhances the glucose-lowering effect of hypoglycemic agents, including insulin, when used in *moderate* amounts, and (3) raises HDL-cholesterol levels when used in *moderate* amounts, thus possibly providing some protection against cardiovascular disease.

In light of this information, it appears that diabetes and alcohol can mix—if shaken gently. For your clients who choose to use alcohol, you will want to suggest that they:

- Carry a personal diabetes ID at all times, in case of a hypoglycemic attack induced by alcohol
- Ask the physician if there are any contraindications to using alcohol (e.g., hypertriglycerides, gastritis, pancreatitis, some types of cardiac and renal disease) and any drug interactions (e.g., with the use of barbiturates or tranquilizers)
- Always sip alcoholic drinks slowly
- Never drink alcohol on an empty stomach
- Limit alcohol use to no more than one or two alcohol equivalents per day 2 or 3 days a week. Equivalents are:
  1½ oz (a shot glass) of distilled alcoholic beverage (whiskey, Scotch, rye, vodka, brandy, cognac, rum)
  4 oz dry wine
  2 oz dry sherry
  12 oz beer (preferably Light)
- Avoid sweet drinks: liquers, sweet wines, drinks mixed with tonic, soda, fruit juice, or other liquids that have a high concentration of sugar

Continued.

Issues and Answers—cont'd

In addition, warn clients taking oral hypoglycemic drugs of problems that may occur when they drink alcohol—e.g., nausea, deep flushing, tachycardia, and impaired speech. The effect begins 3 to 10 minutes after taking a drink and lasts an hour or longer.

Warn clients on insulin that they should not reduce their food intake. They should continue to eat their full diet as prescribed because of their susceptibility to hypoglycemia induced by the alcohol. Tell persons with non-insulin-dependent diabetes to consider the caloric value of the alcohol and omit two fat exchanges for each drink.

References

Feingold, K.R., and Siperstein, M.D.: Normalization of fasting blood glucose level in insulin-requiring diabetes: the role of ethanol abstention, Diab. Care, **6**(2):186, 1983.

Franz, M.J.: Diabetes mellitus: considerations in the development of guidelines for the occasional use of alcohol, J. Am. Dietetic Assoc. **83**(2):147, 1983.

Chapter 19
Gastrointestinal Problems

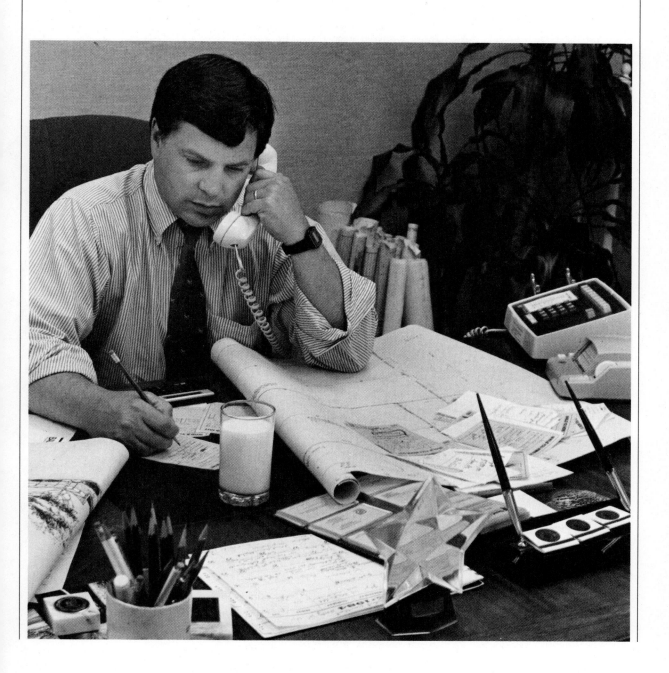

Preview

Surrounding every stomach there is a person. The gastrointestinal tract is a sensitive mirror of the individual human condition. Its physiologic function reflects both physical and psychologic conditioning. In adapting nutritional therapy to treat patients with gastrointestinal disorders, we deal not so much with a specific food item per se as with the state of the body that receives it.

Ingestion, digestion, and absorption of the food begins in the mouth and esophagus and ends in the remaining gastrointestinal tract. A series of intimately related secretory and neuromuscular mechanisms accomplish these vital tasks. It is on this highly individual but interrelated functional network of human life that we must base our nutritional therapy.

Chapter Objectives

After study of this chapter, the student should be able to:

1. Identify food-related problems that occur in the mouth and esophagus and describe the general nutritional therapy needed in each case.

2. Describe the current nutritional therapy for peptic ulcer disease and contrast it with previous traditional therapy.

3. Describe the rationale for current nutritional treatment of diverticulosis in contrast to former therapy.

4. Relate nutritional therapy for inflammatory bowel disease to the underlying problems involved and outline a specific patient's care plan.

5. Describe the food intolerance problem in phenylketonuria and its related nutritional therapy.

6. Compare the underlying problem in both galactosemia and lactose intolerance and compare the nutritional therapy in each case.

7. Identify basic food allergy or sensitivity problems and develop realistic plans for nutritional therapy.

8. Compare liver functions and nutritional problems in hepatitis, cirrhosis, and hepatic encephalopathy, relating the therapy in each case.

9. Relate gallbladder function to nutritional therapy in gallbladder disease.

Problems of the Mouth and Esophagus

Mouth Problems

Cleft Palate and Cleft Lip

Cleft palate in infants and younger children results from abnormalities in the structure of the mouth. When parts of the upper jaw anad palate separating the mouth and nasal cavity do not fuse properly during fetal development, the anatomic abnormality creates difficult feeding problems. The premaxillary and maxillary processes normally fuse early in gestation, between the fifth and eighth week of intrauterine life. Fusion of the palate is completed about 1 month later. If this fusion fails to occur, cleft lip (hairlip) or cleft palate results.

Feeding difficulties Since the infant with cleft palate or lip is unable to suck adequately, early feedings are tiring and lengthy. A softened nipple with an enlarged opening, through which the infant can obtain milk by a chewing motion, is helpful. In some instances a medicine dropper or gavage feedings may be used initially. The infant should be held in an upright position and fed slowly, in small amounts, to avoid aspiration. There should be brief rest periods and frequent burping to expel the large amount of air swallowed.

Surgical repair Corrective surgery of a cleft palate or lip is usually done at about 6 months of age. Follow-up work is done as needed depending on the extent of the deformity and the growth of the child. During the surgery period the child is usually cared for by a team of specialists. Preparation for surgery demands good nutritional status (see p. 509). Following surgery, special nutritional support and nursing care are essential. The infant or child is usually fed a fluid or semifluid diet by use of a syringe or large medicine dropper in the corner of the mouth. Great care must be exercised to protect the suture line and avoid any strain.

Dental Caries

Over the past 2 decades there has been a significant, if not surprising, decline in the caries rate. According to data from the recent National Caries Prevalence Survey (1979-1980) involving school children aged 5 to 17, there has been a 32% decline in caries incidence over the past 10 years.[1] Some of this decline is the result of increased use of fluoridated public water supplies and fluoridated toothpastes as well as better dental hygiene. However, during this same period the use of sugar in foods consumed by children did not decline. For example, from 1963 to 1980 there was a downward trend in the consumption of refined cane and beet sugar, but this was compensated for by an increase in corn sweeteners. The net result is that the use of sugars is relatively unchanged.[2] The large amount of dietary sugar consumed by children is still a nutritional concern.

Causes Three factors combine to produce tooth decay:

A susceptible host Differences in caries suseptibility vary widely among individual children. Some of these are hereditary differences in the anatomic characteristics of the tooth. But the ultimate form of the teeth is influenced by interrelationships between inherited characteristics and the environment that sustains tooth development. Since teeth once formed are stable structures, this positive nutritional influence can have an effect only during growth and development of the enamel-forming organ in the gums (see p. 110) and the tooth bud. Vitamins and minerals, especially vitamins A and D, calcium, and phosphorus play a large part.

Oral bacteria Streptococci comprise the highest number of bacteria in dental plaque, the gelatinous coating on the teeth. These organisms have a particular affinity for carbohydrates, acting on them rapidly, producing acids that lower the pH of the dental plaque and erode the enamel. But oral flora is complex. Bacterial effects can vary because of symbiosis between two or more microorganisms. However, it is their substrate—simple carbohydrates and sugars—that is mandatory for the metabolism of caries-producing organisms.

Diet As carbohydrate food accumulates in the mouth, it provides the necessary media for the normal growth of these acid-producing microorganisms that cause tooth decay. At sites on the tooth where shape contributes to retention of food particles—especially of sticky, gummy foods, which adhere and remain more readily on these tooth surfaces—the bacterial activity is greatest. Persistent and continuous snacking on such sticky carbohydrates, therefore, is a prime factor in tooth decay.

Dietary implications Although the problem of dental caries has decreased in recent years, it is by no means solved. Recent advances in the knowledge of nutrition and its relationship to caries has provided helpful steps in solving that problem. Two nutritional factors are apparent: 1. Adhesive simple carbohydrates, such as sweets, candy bars, caramels, consumed at frequent intervals do increase dental caries. However, simple carbohydrates in liquid form are less cariogenic than those in solid form. 2. Fluoridated public water supplies do decrease dental caries rates, although this practice still remains a source of some controversy in various communities.

Dentures

In some older persons, loss of teeth or ill-fitting dentures may cause problems with chewing and hence digestion of foods. The health of the gums on which the dentures rest is imperative for a successful fit and use. Vitamins A and C are particularly related to the integrity of gum tissue and may need special attention in the diet when healing or strengthening is necessary. When dental problems exist or when dentures are not available, a *mechanical soft* diet may be used. In this diet all foods are soft-cooked. Meats are ground and sometimes mixed with sauces or gravies, thus requiring less chewing to make eating easier.

Fractured Jaw

A fractured jaw or other surgical procedure on the mouth or neck can pose obvious eating problems. After the initial jaw injury has been corrected with surgical wiring, the resulting immobility prevents normal eating. A high-protein, high-caloric liquid diet is needed to provide healing nutrients. A straw should be used to drink the liquid formula. A typical formula is given in Table 19-1. As healing continues, soft foods requiring little effort in chewing can be introduced at first.

Table 19-1
High-Protein, High-Calorie Formula for Patient with Hepatitis

Ingredients	Amount	Approximate Food Value	
Milk	1 cup	Protein	40 g
Eggs	2	Fat	30 g
Skim milk powder	6 to 8 tbsp	Carbohydrate	70 g
or Casec	2 tbsp	Calories	710
Sugar	2 tbsp		
Ice cream	2.5 cm (1 in) slice or 1 scoop		
Cocoa or other flavoring	2 tbsp		
Vanilla	Few drops, as desired		

Esophageal Problems

After food is taken into the mouth, chewed and swallowed, it passes through the esophagus to the stomach aided by peristalsis and gravity. At the entry to the stomach, the *gastroesophageal sphincter muscle* forms a controlling valve. It relaxes to receive the food, then closes to hold each **bolus** for digestive action of enzymes in the gastric acid mix. A number of conditions may interfere with this normal food passage and create problems. These conditions vary widely from brief periods of functional discomfort—**dysphagia** ("indigestion")—to serious disease and complete obstruction. In any case, choice of food and feeding mode is adapted to the degree of dysfunction. Several types of esophageal problems encountered in general clinical practice are briefly described here.

Reflux Esophagitis

Regurgitation of the acid gastric contents into the lower part of the esophagus creates tissue irritation. The hydrochloric acid and pepsin cause tissue erosion, with symptoms of substernal burning, cramping, pressure sensation, or severe pain. These symptoms are aggravated by lying down or by any increase of abdominal pressure, such as that caused by tight clothing. This condition is related to (1) an incompetent gastroesophageal sphincter muscle, (2) frequency and duration of the acid reflux, and (3) the inability of the esophagus to produce normal secondary peristaltic waves to prevent prolonged contact of the esophageal mucosa with the acid and pepsin. A *hiatal hernia* may or may not be present. In addition, the acid reflux may be caused by pregnancy, obesity, pernicious vomiting, or nasogastric tubes. The most common symptom is **pyrosis.** It is frequently severe, occurring 30 to 60 minutes after eating. Sometimes pain radiates into the neck and jaw or down the arms. Other symptoms include iron-deficiency anemia, with chronic tissue bleeding, or aspiration, which may cause cough, dyspnea, or pneumonitis. The most common complications are **stenosis** and *esophageal ulcer.* Also, significant **gastritis** in the herniated portion of the stomach may cause occult bleeding and anemia. Treatment centers on the often associated or precipitating factor of obesity. Thus weight reduction is essential. The patient should avoid lying

Bolus A rounded mass of food that is ready to be swallowed.

Dysphagia Difficulty in swallowing.

Pyrosis Heartburn.

Stenosis Narrowing or closing of a canal or duct.

Gastritis Inflammation of the stomach.

down immediately after meals and should sleep with the head of the bed elevated. Frequent use of antacids helps control the symptoms. From 85% to 90% of persons with esophagitis respond to weight reduction and conservative measures.

Hiatal Hernia

Hiatus An opening or gap.

Normally the lower end of the esophagus enters the chest cavity at the **hiatus,** an opening in the diaphragmatic membrane, and immediately joins the upper portion of the stomach. A hiatal hernia occurs when a portion of the upper part of the stomach at this entry point of the esophagus protrudes through the hiatus alongside the lower portion of the esophagus (Figure 19-1). Food is easily held in this herniated area of the stomach and mixed with acid and pepsin. Then it is regurgitated back up into the lower portion of the esophagus. Gastritis can occur in this herniated portion of the stomach and cause bleeding and anemia. The reflux of acid gastric contents causes symptoms similar to those described above. Since obesity is frequently associated with hiatal hernia, weight reduction is a primary consideration. Avoiding tight clothing helps to relieve discomfort. Patients will need to avoid leaning over or lying down immediately after meals and should sleep with the head of the bed elevated. Antacids help to relieve the burning sensation. Large hiatal hernias or smaller sliding hernias may require surgical repair.

Diverticula

Small outpouchings in the gastrointestinal tract are called *diverticula.* These pouches may occur in the esophagus, as well as in the lower intes-

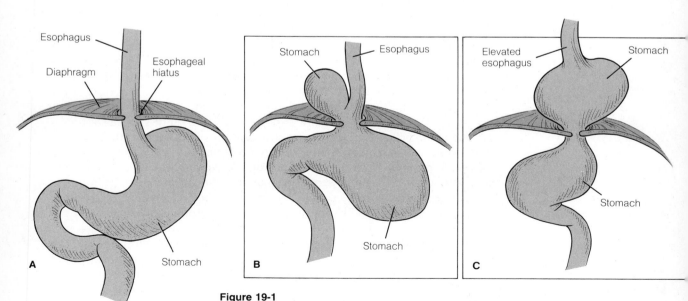

Figure 19-1
Hiatal hernia in comparison with normal stomach placement. **A,** Normal stomach. **B,** Paraesophageal hernia (esophagus in normal position). **C,** Esophageal hiatal hernia (elevated esophagus).

tine. Esophageal diverticula cause general dysphagia with regurgitation of undigested or partially digested food. If the diverticula are located in the upper part of the esophagus, the main symptoms are dysphagia, regurgitation, coughing, bad breath, and a foul taste in the mouth. Difficulty in swallowing increases, and eating becomes more difficult. Weight loss and impaired nutrition follow. If the diverticula are in the middle or lower portion of the esophagus, the symptoms are more delayed after beginning to eat. Ultimately, however, the condition produces dysphagia and pain. Nutritional therapy centers on selecting foods according to tolerance and helping patients develop habits of eating slowly and chewing food well. Surgical removal of large, symptom-producing diverticula may be indicated.

Peptic Ulcer Disease

Throughout the world peptic ulcer disease affects about 10% of the population. It is the subject of millions of dollars of research and causes the loss of many productive work hours as a result of illness. It can occur at any age, but the highest incidence is in middle adulthood, between ages 45 and 55. Gastric and duodenal ulcers, along with the complication of perforation, occur more often in men than in women, but related frequencies vary with the patient's age and the type of ulcer involved. Peptic ulcers may occur together with other diseases or with injuries such as burns—the so-called stress ulcer.

Causes

The exact cause of peptic ulcer is unclear. There is some evidence that a genetic factor may be involved, since close relatives of patients with ulcers have approximately three times as many ulcers as members of the general population. It is evident, however, that both physical and psychogenic factors are involved.

Physical Factors

Peptic ulcer is the general term given to an eroded mucosal lesion in the central portion of the gastrointestinal tract. Affected areas can include the lower portion of the esophagus, the stomach, and the first portion of the duodenum, the "duodenal bulb." Esophageal and gastric ulcers are less common. Most ulcers occur in the duodenal bulb, where gastric contents emptying into the duodenum through the pyloric valve are most concentrated. Gastric ulcers occur usually along the lesser curvature of the stomach. Peptic ulcer itself is a **benign** disease. Gastric ulcers, however, are more prone to develop into **malignant** disease. The underlying lesion results from an imbalance between the gastric acid and pepsin secretions and the degree of tissue resistance to these secretions.

Benign Not malignant or recurring.

Malignant Not improving, worsening; resulting in death.

Gastric acid and pepsin In ulcer formation, large amounts of hydrochloric acid and the gastric enzyme pepsin are secreted. Although much research is being conducted on this hypersecretion of acid, little is understood about its underlying causes.

Tissue resistance The balancing factor in the development of peptic ulcer disease is the degree of mucosal tissue resistance that can withstand the erosive and digestive action of these secretions. Several factors seem to influence the tissue's ability to withstand such destructive action: (1) the integrity of mucosal cells, (2) the ability of epithelial cells to regenerate themselves, (3) the mucosal barrier, and (4) the blood supply. Various topical irritants interfere with normal function of this tissue, including aspirin, alcohol, certain drugs, caffeine, or bile acids that may come in contact with the mucosa. Thus factors that contribute to weakened mucosa resistance in patients with gastric ulcer revolve around poor nutrition, diminished mucosal blood flow, and a defect in the inhibition of gastric acid and pepsin secretion. In the development of gastric ulcers, although the presence of acid is essential, the degree of tissue sensitivity seems to be the paramount factor. In the patient with duodenal ulcer, excess production of acid and pepsin is the primary factors. In either case, gastric hydrochloric acid is the necessary factor in the development and recurrence of peptic ulcer.

Psychogenic Factors

The influence of psychologic factors in the development of peptic ulcer is highly variable. Such stress factors may well play some role in the development of duodenal ulcer, but there is no distinct personality type that is free from the disease. Men are affected two to three times more frequently than are women, and the average age of incidence has increased. These are the adult years when career and personal strivings are at a peak. Also, stress ulcers occur in conjunction with emergency injuries such as burns or long-term rehabilitation processes.

Symptoms and General Management
Clinical Symptoms

Basic symptoms of peptic ulcer are increased gastric tone and painful hunger contractions when the stomach is empty. In duodenal ulcer, the amount and concentration of hydrochloric acid is increased; in gastric ulcer it may be normal. Nutritional deficiencies are evident in low plasma protein levels, anemia, and loss of weight. Hemorrhage may be the first sign in some patients. Diagnosis is based on clinical findings, x-ray tests, or visualization by gastroscopy.

General Medical Management

The prime objective in medical management is to provide psychologic rest and support tissue healing. Three factors form the basis of care:

1. **Drug therapy** Antacids buffer excess acid present; other drugs inhibit acid secretion. Currently the most commonly used drug to inhibit acid secretion is *cimetidine* (Tagamet). This drug is an antihistamine that acts as an antagonist to block histamine-stimulated gastric acid secretion. Routine use of anticholinergic agents has lessened, but they may sometimes be used together with cimetidine for additive effect.
2. **Rest** Both physical and mental rest are required for healing. This rest is aided as needed by sedative therapy and stress-reduction relaxation techniques.
3. **Diet** Nutritional therapy for peptic ulcer has changed considerably. Its basic objective is to support healing and prevent further tissue damage.

Dietary Management
Traditional "Bland" Diets

The so-called "bland" diets used in the past for treatment of peptic ulcer have proved to be unwarranted and ineffective. A more liberal individual approach prevails today in modern clinical practice.

Basis for Change

The development of more liberal approaches in the care of persons with peptic ulcer is based on recognition of individual need and use of a sound nutritional base for healing. Clinical experiences and experimental testing have refuted many past food dogmas.

Protein foods Milk and other protein foods have been considered effective buffering agents because of their amphoteric nature—acting as both acids and bases (see p. 89). However, although they do have some buffering effect, they also induce gastric secretions, as do all foods ingested. Volume of any food sufficient to exert antrum pressure against the stomach wall stimulates gastric secretion through the gastrin mechanism (see p. 29). Some investigators have questioned the effect of milk on gastric acid secretion, whereas opposing views have been expressed by others. Any form of fat tends to suppress gastric secretion and motility through the enterogastrone mechanism (see p. 29), accounting for some of the effect of whole milk. Also milk continues to be a source of needed nutrient factors for healing purposes.

Seasonings Other studies indicate that herbs and spices and other condiments have had little or no irritating effect on the majority of persons with ulcers. The sight, smell, and taste of most food normally initiates gastric secretion. But no significant change in gastric pH has been noted with the use of any particular items, except *alcohol, caffeine, black pepper,* and *meat extractives*. No food is sufficiently acid of itself to effect a significant pH change or cause direct irritation of an ulcer.

Food texture The routine omission of any fiber in the diet to treat ulcers seems to have no basis in fact. A regular diet, including good food sources of dietary fiber, has been found by investigators to be beneficial in the treatment of duodenal ulcer.[3]

Gas formers Routinely omitting a number of foods because of their reputation for being "gas formers" has also been questioned. Clinical observations show that tolerance for a variety of standard foods is highly individual. Patients with gastrointestinal disease have shown no greater intolerance for such foods than have patients with other conditions.

Current Liberal Management

Sound nutritional management is essential in the total medical care of the person with peptic ulcer disease. The patient is not "an ulcer;" he is a *person* with an ulcer. Therefore two basic principles should guide the current liberal approach:

1. **The individual must be treated as such** A careful initial history will give information about daily living situations, attitudes, food reactions, and tolerances. On the basis of such a detailed history, a rea-

sonable and adequate nutritional program *that can be followed* may be worked out.

2. **The activity of the patient's ulcer will influence dietary management** During acute periods of active ulceration more modified treatment may be needed to control acidity and initiate healing. However, when pain disappears, feedings can be liberalized according to individual tolerance and desire, using a variety of foods. Sound nutrition and improved emotional outlook hasten recovery. During quiet periods and for long-term prophylaxis when the patient is asymptomatic, a judicious choice from a wide range of foods and regular, unhurried eating habits provide the best course of action.

Principles of Nutritional Therapy for Peptic Ulcer

There are several current principles of nutritional therapy for ulcers that should be followed.

Sound total nutrition There must be optimal overall nutritional intake to support recovery and maintain healthy tissue, based on individual needs and food tolerances.

Protein Since protein provides the necessary amino acids for synthesis of tissue protein, there must be adequate dietary protein for tissue-healing needs. This means that adequate carbohydrate is needed to supply energy requirements to spare protein for necessary tissue healing.

Fat Moderate amounts of fat help to suppress gastric secretion and motility. If cardiovascular disease is a concern, reduction of saturated fat may be desired, with substitution of polyunsaturated fat (see p. 462).

Meal pattern Meals and snacks at regular intervals in small proportions will help maintain individual control of gastric secretions. These may be frequent, small feedings during more active stress periods. Regular meals, moderate in size and sufficient in number for individual need should be established as a regular habit.

Individual needs Positive individual needs and a flexible program should guide food planning. Individual counseling that meets personal needs should form the keystone of wise peptic ulcer therapy.

A general dietary guide incorporating nutritional therapy principles for a liberal approach to control of peptic ulcer disease in given in the box on p. 425.

Intestinal Diseases

General Functional Disorders
Irritable Bowel Syndrome

This general stress-related functional disorder of the intestine may occur at any age but is more frequent in women. It may be caused by irritation of the mucous membrane, with symptoms varying between spastic constipation and "nervous" diarrhea. These harried individuals develop patterns of irregular eating and bowel habits and often resort to excessive use of laxatives, cathartics, enemas, and a variety of other medications. General dietary measures are designed to provide optimal nutrition and regulate bowl motility. There should be additional amounts of bulk foods,

Liberal Food Guide for Peptic Ulcer

General Directions

- Respect individual responses or tolerances to specific foods experienced at any given time, remembering that the same food may evoke different responses at different times depending on the stress factor.
- Eat smaller meals more often, eat slowly, and savor your food in a calm environment as much as possible.
- Try to avoid caffeine beverages such as coffee, cola, and tea; also avoid alcohol.
- Cut down on or quit smoking cigarettes—not only to help the ulcer but also to help food taste better.
- Avoid excessive pepper on food or concentrated meat broths and extractives.
- Avoid frequent use of aspirin or other drugs that may damage the stomach lining.

Foods	Recommended Foods	Controlled Foods
Bread, cereals (at least 4 servings daily)	Any whole-grain or enriched bread, cereals, crackers, pasta	None
Vegetables (at least 2 servings daily)	Any vegetable, raw or cooked; vegetable juices	None
Potatoes, other starches	White potatoes, sweet potatoes, or yams; enriched rice, brown rice; corn, barley, millet, bulgur; pasta	Fried forms
Fruits (at least 2 servings daily)	Any fruit, raw or cooked; fruit juices	None
Milk, milk products (2 servings daily as desired)	Any form of milk or milk drink; yogurt; cheses	None
Meats or substitutes (2 servings daily)	Poultry, fish and shellfish, lean meats; eggs, cheeses; legumes—dried beans and peas, lentils, soybeans; smooth peanut buter	Fried forms or too highly seasoned or fatty
Soups, stews	Mildly seasoned, less concentrated meat stock base; any cream soups	More highly seasoned or concentrated base
Desserts	Any desserts tolerated	Items containing nuts or coconut; fried pastries
Beverages	Decaffeinated coffee, cocoa, fruit drinks, mineral waters, noncola soft drinks; less strong tea with milk	Regular coffee, strong tea; colas, alcohol
Fats (use in moderation)	Margarine; butter, cream; vegetable oils; mild salad dressings, mayonnaise, oil and vinegar with herbs	Highly seasoned dressings
Sauces, gravies	Mildly flavored, less strong meat bases	Strongly seasoned, especially with pepper, hot peppers, and sauces
Miscellaneous	Salt in moderation (iodized); flavorings; herbs, spices; mustard, catsup, vinegar in moderation, as tolerated	Strongly flavored condiments; popcorn; nuts, coconut as tolerated

such as fruits, vegetables, and whole grains. During alternate periods of diarrhea or excessive flatulence, the fiber content may need to be decreased. Supportive therapy will help reduce stress factors.

Constipation

Americans spend a quarter of a billion dollars for laxatives each year for their so-called problem of "regularity." However, "regularity" of elimination is highly individual, and it is not necessary for good health to have a bowel movement daily. Usually this common short-term problem results from various sources of nervous tension and worry or changes in social setting such as vacations and altered routines. Also, it may be caused by prolonged use of laxatives or cathartics, low-fiber diets, or lack of exercise, which can cause decreased intestinal muscle tone. Improved exercise, dietary, and bowel habits are usually sufficient to remedy the situation. The diet should include increased fiber and naturally laxative fruits, as well as inceased fluid. If chronic constipation persists, agents that increase stool bulk may be necessary. These include bran, cellulose, and hemicellulose materials. Any laxative habit on a regular basis should be avoided.

Diarrhea

Functional diarrhea usually results from general dietary excesses with fermentation of sugars involved or excess fiber stimulation of intestinal muscle function. It may result in some cases from intolerance to specific nutrient factors. For example, *lactose intolerance* is a rather widespread condition in which lactose cannot be digested because of lactase deficiency (see p. 435). Diarrhea in infants is a more serious problem, especially if it is prolonged and associated with infection. The infant's relatively high water content and large area of intestinal mucosa in proportion to body surface area cause rapid fluid and electrolyte loss.

Organic Diseases

Organic diseases of the intestine may be classified in three general groups: (1) anatomic changes such as in diverticulosis, (2) malabsorption syndromes, as in celiac disease (sprue), and (3) inflammatory bowel disease with infectious mucosal changes, as in ulcerative colitis or in Crohn's disease (regional enteritis).

Diverticulosis

Diverticula (L. *diverticulare,* to turn aside) are small pouchlike protrusions from the intestinal lumen, usually the colon, and produce a condition called *diverticulosis.* More often it occurs in older people and develops at points of weakened musculature in the bowel wall. It is periodically symptomatic and requires nutritional therapy.

Clinical symptoms The condition is usually without symptoms unless the diverticula becomes inflamed, a state called *diverticulitis.* Fecal residue causes increased irritation. Increased hypermotility and intraluminal pressures from **luminal segmentation** cause pain. This pain and tenderness is usually localized in the lower left side of the abdomen and is accompanied by nausea, vomiting, and distension, intestinal spasm, and fever. If the process continues, intestinal obstruction or perforation may necessitate surgery.

Nutritional therapy Current studies and clinical practice have demonstrated better management of diverticular disease with a high-residue diet than with former practices using restricted amounts of residue (see p. 48). The type of fiber used apparently also plays a part. Some studies have indicated that fibers of a coarse type have a more significant effect on stool weight, increased intestinal transit, and reduced intraluminal pressure in the colon than do the fine types of bran. Thus, used as dietary

Luminal segmentation Formation of divisions, or segments, along the alimentary canal. In diverticulitis, this may occur at the site of diverticuli and increase the motility of the gastrointestinal tract, promoting diarrhea.

fiber, the texture of bran may be important in relationship to its clinical effectiveness. The relationship of dietary fiber and diverticular disease is further reinforced by studies of populations, such as in Japan since the current "Westernizing" of its culture.

Malabsorption Syndrome–Celiac Disease (Sprue)

Malabsorption syndrome occurs when there is poor absorption caused by damage to mucosal villi.

Celiac disease
Malabsorption syndrome brought on by eating gluten-rich foods (wheat, rye, barley, and oats). Characterized by steatorrhea, distention, flatulence, weight loss, and malnutrition because of poor absorption associated with damage to the mucosal villi. May be a hereditary condition.

Sprue Alternate term for adult celiac disease, a malabsorption syndrome.

Gluten-sensitive enteropathy A disorder characterized by the inability to absorb *gluten,* a protein found in wheat, barley, oats, and rye. Commonly found in *celiac disease* and *sprue.*

Cause Adult **celiac disease (sprue)** is similar in nature to the related childhood syndrome. Most adult patients give a history of having had episodes of celiac disease as a child. In this condition of **gluten-sensitive enteropathy** (or celiac disease), the offending agent in the gluten protein is the *gliadin* fraction, which is toxic to sensitive individuals. As little as 3 g/day of this fraction can produce diarrhea and steatorrhea in celiac patients who are in remission. When these peptides of gliadin, derived from digestion of wheat protein, enter the mucosal epithelial cell, they cannot be further broken down. Increased amounts of these peptides in the cells then interfere with normal cell metabolism. The damaged mucosa becomes permeable to other wheat and milk proteins. In turn these substances may be antigenic, participating in antigen-antibody reactions. In some cases of celiac disease, this process may diffusely involve the entire intestinal mucosa, with more severe effect on the upper small bowel. As a result, the absorption area is greatly impaired for all nutrients, especially fat. Malabsorption of sugar, protein, vitamins, and minerals may also be present.

Clinical symptoms The characteristic diarrhea consists of multiple foamy, malodorous, bulky, and greasy stools. Poor absorption of fat is evident in the large amounts appearing in the stools as fatty acids and soaps (fatty acids saponified with calcium salts). Poor absorption of iron produces a microcytic-hypochromic anemia. In some persons a lack of folic acid produces a macrocytic anemia. Poor absorption of vitamin K may lead to hemorrhagic tendencies. Poor calcium absorption may produce a disturbed calcium/phosphorus ratio with resulting tetany (see p. 146). The condition varies widely in severity of symptoms and nature of treatment.

Nutritional therapy Since the discovery that gluten is the important factor in the cause of celiac disease, a low-gluten, gliadin-free diet has been widely used with marked remission of symptoms. Gluten is a protein found mainly in wheat, with additional amounts of rye and oats. The gliadin fraction is the offending agent in sensitive individuals. General guidelines for restricting food sources of these offending materials is given on p. 428.

Inflammatory Bowel Disease

U.S. incidence rates of Crohn's disease are 4 to 6/100,000 adults/year, with prevalence rates of 40 to 100/100,000. Incidence is highest among teenagers, with a secondary peak at ages 55 to 60.

The term *inflammatory bowel disease* is used to apply to both *ulcerative colitis* and *Crohn's disease.* Their related condition, *short-bowel syndrome,* results from repeated surgical removal of sections of the intestine as the disease progresses. The incidence of these diseases, especially Crohn's disease, has increased worldwide. The two diseases have similar clinical and pathologic features. They are particularly prevalent in industrialized areas of the

Gluten-Free Diet for Adult Celiac Disease (Sprue)

Characteristics

■ All forms of wheat, rye, oat, buckwheat, and barley are omitted, except gluten-free wheat starch.
■ All other foods are permitted freely, unless specified otherwise by the physician.
■ The diet should be high in protein, calories, vitamins, and minerals.

Foods	Allowed	Not Allowed
Milk (2 glasses or more)	As desired	
Cheese	Any, as desired	
Eggs (1 or 2 daily)	As desired	
Meat, fish, fowl (1 or 2 servings)	Any plain meat	Breaded, creamed, or with thickened gravy; no bread dressings
Soups	All clear and vegetable soups; cream soups thickened with cream, cornstarch, or potato flour only	No wheat flour-thickened soup; no canned soup except clear broth
Vegetables (2 servings of green or yellow daily, at least)	As desired, except creamed	No cream sauce or breading
Fruits (at least 2 or 3 daily, including 1 citrus)	As desired	
Bread	Only that made from rice, corn, or soybean flour, or gluten-free wheat starch	All bread, rolls, crackers, cake, and cookies made from wheat and rye, Ry-Krisp, muffins, biscuits, waffles, pancake flour, and other prepared mixes, rusks, Zwiebach, pretzels; any product containing oatmeal, barley, or buckwheat; no breaded food or food crumbs
Cereals	Cornflakes, cornmeal, hominy, rice, Rice Krispies, Puffed Rice, precooked rice cereals	No wheat or rye cereals, wheat germ, barley, buckwheat, kasha
Pastas		No macaroni, spaghetti, noodles, dumplings
Desserts	Jell-O, fruit Jell-O, ice or sherbet, homemade ice cream, custard, junket, rice pudding, cornstarch pudding (home-made)	Cakes, cookies, pastry; commercial ice cream and ice cream cones; prepared mixes, puddings; homemade puddings thickened with wheat flour

CAUTION: **Read labels on all packaged and prepared foods.**

world, suggesting that pathogenic agents in the environment play a significant role.

Causes Both ulcerative colitis and Crohn's disease have severe, often devastating nutritional consequences, but they can be distinguished by two main differences: (1) *anatomic distribution* of the inflammatory process, and (2) the nature of *tissue changes* involved.[4] First, Crohn's disease can occur in any part of the intestinal tract. But ulcerative colitis is confined to the colon and rectum. Second, in Crohn's disease, the inflammatory tissue changes become chronic and can involve any part of the intestinal wall and may penetrate the entire wall. Often this extensive tissue involvement leads to partial or complete obstruction and to *fistula* formation. The tissue changes in ulcerative colitis, on the other hand, are usually acute, lasting for brief periods, and are limited to the mucosal and submucosal tissue layers of the intestine.

Clinical symptoms A chronic bloody diarrhea is the most common clinical symptom, occurring at night as well as during the day (see Issues and Answers, pp. 450-451). Ulceration of the mucous membrane of the intestine leads to various associated nutritional problems such as anorexia, nutritional edema, anemia, avitaminosis, protein losses, negative nitrogen balance, dehydration, and electrolyte disturbances. Clinicians have observed evidence of specific deficiencies of zinc and vitamin E, with improvement occurring when supplements of the particular nutrient involved are taken. There is general weight loss, often general malnutrition, fever, skin lesions, and arthritic joint involvement.

Medical management Restoring positive nutrition is a basic requirement for tissue healing and health. Drug therapy includes antibacterial and antinflammatory medication, adrenal **corticosteroids**—mercaptopurine or azathioprine in continuing Crohn's disease—together with general supportive care.[5]

Nutritional therapy Two goals are paramount in nutritional therapy: (1) supporting the tissue-healing process and (2) avoiding nutritional deficiency states. In serious conditions, management includes elemental diets. These elemental formulas are composed of absorbable isotonic preparations of amino acids, glucose, fat, minerals, and vitamins. In patients who tolerate these supplements, there is diminished gastrointestinal protein loss and improved nutrition, accompanied by clinical remission. In cases where the small bowel has been shortened or the disease process is extensive, as in Crohn's disease, **parenteral** intravenous hyperalimentation (total parenteral nutrition, TPN) is most effective, particularly in childhood to prevent severe growth retardation. Nutritional repletion improves symptoms: diminished gastrointestinal secretion and motility, decreased disease activity, relief of partial intestinal obstruction, occasional closure of enteric fistulas, and renewed immunocompetence. Supplements help avoid deficiencies in agents such as zinc, copper, chromium, selenium, and other nutrients.

General continuing dietary management Emphasis of treatment should be on restoring optimal nutrient intake, removing deficits, preventing local trauma to inflamed areas, and controlling less easily absorbed material such as fats. To help secure additional kilocalories, medium-chained triglycerides (MCT), as in the commercial preparations Portagen or MCT oil, may be used instead of regular fats. The focus of the diet centers on protein and energy, minerals and vitamins, and texture.

High protein In inflammatory bowel disease, there are large losses of protein from the intestinal mucosal tissue by exudations and bleeding, as well as losses associated with impaired intestinal absorption. Healing can occur only if adequate protein is provided. Through elemental formulas or protein supplements with food as tolerated, the diet must supply adequate protein—about 100 g/day—for needed tissue synthesis and healing. Tasteful ways of including protein foods of high biologic value (eggs, meat, cheese) can be devised to tempt poor appetites. Milk causes diffi-

Corticosteroid A steroid (hormonal substance) secreted by the adrenal cortex that influences the metabolism of nutrients, electrolytes, and water. Clinically, corticosteroids are given to reduce (among other things) inflammation, as in inflammatory bowel disease such as Crohn's disease or ulcerative colitis.

Parenteral Not through the alimentary canal. Given by injection through a subcutaneous, intramuscular, intravenous, or other route.

culty with many patients, so it is usually omitted at first, then gradually added in cooked forms.

High energy About 2500 to 3000 kcal/day are needed to restore nutritional deficits from daily losses in the stools and consequent weight loss. Also the negative nitrogen balance can be overcome only if sufficient kilocalories are present to spare protein for tissue-building.

Increased minerals and vitamins When anemia is present, iron supplements can be used (see p. 161). Sometimes oral iron preparations are poorly tolerated, and blood transfusions may be used during critical periods. Extra vitamins needed for healing and metabolism of the increased kilocalories and protein should be added. These are the B vitamins—thiamin, riboflavin and niacin—and ascorbic acid. Trace minerals such as zinc, which participate in tissue synthesis, are needed along with vitamin E, which contributes to tissue integrity. Supplements of these vitamins and

Low-Residue Diet

Foods	Allowed	Not Allowed
Beverages	Only 2 glasses of milk, if allowed, boiled or evaporated; fruit juices, coffee, tea, carbonated beverages	Alcohol
Eggs	Prepared in any manner, except fried	Fried eggs
Cheese	Cottage, cream, milk American, Tillamook (use in small amounts)	Highly flavored cheeses
Meat or poultry	Roasted, baked, or broiled tender beef, bacon, ham, lamb, liver, veal, fish, chicken, or turkey	Tough meats, pork; no fried or highly spiced meats
Soup	Bouillon, broth, strained cream soups from the foods allowed	Any others
Fats	Butter, margarine, oils, 30 ml (1 oz.) cream daily	None
Vegetables	Canned or cooked strained vegetables, such as asparagus, beets, carrots, peas, pumpkin, squash, spinach, young string beans, tomato juice	Raw or whole cooked vegetables
Fruits	Strained fruit juices, cooked or canned apples, apricots, Royal Anne cherries, peaches, pears; dried fruit puree; ripe banana and avocado; all without skins or seeds	All other raw fruits, other cooked fruits
Bread and crackers	Refined bread, toast, rolls, crackers	Pancakes, waffles, whole-grain bread or rolls
Cereals	Cooked cereal such as Cream of Wheat, Maltomeal, strained oatmeal, cornmeal, cornflakes, puffed rice, Rice Krispies, puffed wheat	Whole-grain cereals; other prepared cereals
Potatoes or substitute	Potatoes, white rice, macaroni, noodles, sphagetti	Fried potato, potato chips, brown rice
Desserts	Gelatin desserts, tapioca, angel food or sponge cake, plain custards, water ice or ice cream without fruit or nuts, rennet or simple puddings	Rich pastries, pies, anything with nuts or dried fruits
Sweets	Sugar, jelly, honey, syrups, gumdrops, hard candy, plain creams, milk chocolate	Other candy; jam, marmalade
Miscellaneous	Cream sauce, plain gravy, salt	Nuts, olives, popcorn, rich gravies, pepper, spices, vinegar

minerals are routine. Potassium therapy may be indicated if undue losses from diarrhea and tissue destruction occur causing hypokalemia.

Low residue To avoid irritation of the mucosal lining until healing is well established, the diet should be fairly low in residue. In acute stages it may be almost residue free through the use of elemental formulas or residue-free foods. A low-residue diet (see box on p. 430) may be used initially, with additional protein and kilocalorie additions given in interval feedings. As soon as tolerated, a regular diet with high-protein feedings is indicated. Only heavy roughage need be avoided. The primary concern is supplying the necessary nutrition in as appetizing a manner as possible.

Perhaps no other condition better illustrates the need for a close working relationship among the team of physician, clinical dietitian, nurse, and patient than does inflammatory bowel disease. The person's appetite is poor, but adequate nutritional intake is imperative. In creative ways, individually explored and implemented, the fundamental therapeutic needs must be met. This can be done through vigorous nutritional care using a range of feeding modes, combined with constant supportive warmth and encouragement.

Food Allergies, Sensitivities, and Intolerances

Immunocompetence The ability to produce antibodies in response to an antigen.

A number of conditions may cause certain food allergies or intolerances. These may be conditions of **immunocompetence** or of specific genetic origin. The resulting difficulty in handling certain foods may lie at the point of digestion in the intestine or at the metabolic level in the cell.

Food Allergies

The word "allergy" comes from the Greek words, *allos* (other) and *ergon* (work). Thus the name implies an unusual or inappropriate response to a stimulus. An allergic condition results from a disorder of the immune system. It is immunity gone wrong.[6]

Food Allergy

Food allergy Specific term for immunologic sensitivity reactions.

Food sensitivity General term for adverse nutrient reactions.

The term **food allergy** should be used only for hypersensitivity that is caused by normal immunologic reaction to specific constituents of food or their digestive products. The term **food sensitivity** is a general nonspecific term more correctly used for nonallergic food sensitivities, though it is sometimes used synonomously with food allergies. Food allergy is distinct from other food intolerances or sensitivities, which are caused by nonimmunologic mechanisms, such as lack of digestive enzymes or cell enzymes. In general there are three basic approaches to the diagnosis and treatment of adverse reactions to foods: (1) clinical assessment, (2) dietary manipulation, and (3) laboratory tests. Appropriate dietary counseling is essential.

Common Food Allergens

A wide variety of environmental, emotional, and physical factors influence reaction, and a suitable regimen is sometimes difficult to find. Since sensitivity to protein substances is a common basis for food allergy, the early foods of infants and children are frequent offenders. Children tend to become less allergic as they grow older.

Milk Cow's milk has long been a common cause of allergic disease in infants. In sensitive children it causes gastrointestinal difficulties such as vomiting, diarrhea, and colic, or respiratory and skin problems. The problem is generally identified by clinical symptoms, family history, and a trial on a milk-free diet, using a substitute formula such as a soybean preparation. Freedom from symptoms on a milk-free diet iss usually followed by a retrial on milk to determine if it causes the symptoms to reappear. Only then is the diagnosis of milk allergy established. Often symptoms appear and disappear spontaneously, regardless of dietary changes. But they tend to be more often caused by food if gastrointestinal problems are present.

Eggs, wheat, and other foods The albumin in egg white is a potential allergen, so it is usually added to the infant's diet following earlier use of egg yolk. Wheat is also a fairly common food allergen among allergic children. The specific biochemical sensitivity to gluten, a protein found in wheat, in the child with gluten-induced celiac disease (see p. 427) may be considered an example, although the biochemical defects in the mucosal cell in celiac disease represent a different sensitivity mechanism.

In an allergic child's diet solid foods are usually added slowly to the original formula, with common offenders excluded in early feedings. The following is a general list of foods that have been frequent offenders and may be avoided initially:

eggs	**bacon**
fish	**citrus fruits**
wheat	**nuts**
strawberries	**peanut butter**
tomatoes	**chocolate**
pork	**pineapple**
milk or milk products	

In some cases a series of diagnostic food elimination diets are used to identify offending foods. A core of less-often offending foods is used initially, with gradual addition of other single foods one at a time to test the response. If a given food causes return of the allergy, the food is then identified as an offending allergen and is eliminated from use. It may be retested later to determine if it is still an allergen. Guidance in the substitution of special food products and in the use of special recipes can be provided. In some cases, additives such as food dyes and colors used in food processing cause allergic responses.

Family Education

A knowledge and understanding of the allergic state and the many factors that influence it is essential. If specific foods have been definitely identified as offenders, careful guiidance to eliminate these from the diet is needed. The common use of the offending food in daily meal patterns and its occurrence in a number of commercial products and other hidden sources should be discussed. Label reading and recipe adaptation are important. As an allergic child grows older, reaction to the given food may wane, and it can be gradually added in the diet.

Genetic Disease

Certain food intolerances may also stem from underlying genetic disease.

Nature of Genetic Disease

The gene pattern of the original chromosomes we receive at conception from our parents determines our inheritied physical traits or genetic disease pattern. Genes in each cell control not only common hereditary characteristics but also the metabolic functions of the cell. They regulate the synthesis of some 1000 or more *specific* cell enzymes that control metabolism within the cell. Each of these enzymes is a *specific* protein synthesized by a *specific* DNA pattern in a *specific* gene. When a specific gene is abnormal (mutant), the enzyme whose systhesis it controls cannot be made. In turn the metabolic reaction controlled by that specific enzyme cannot take place. A specific genetic disease then manifests symptoms connected with those reaction products. As primary examples, we will look briefly at two such genetic diseases: (1) *phenylketonuria*, which affects amino acid metabolism, and (2) *galactosemia*, which affects carbohydrate metabolism. Both are detected by newborn screening procedures, mandatory now by law.

Phenylketonuria (PKU)

Phenylketonuria results from a missing cell enzyme, *phenylalanine hydroxylase,* which oxidizes *phenylalanine,* an essential amino acid, to tryosine, another amino acid. Phenylalanine therefore accumulates in the blood, and its alternate metabolites, the phenyl acids, are excreted in the urine. One of these acids *phenylpyruvic acid,* is a phenylketone; hence the term *phenylketonuria (PKU).* The condition may exist as classical PKU or as one of the several *hyperphenylalanemia variants (HPV).* More recent work over the past decade has shown that phenylalanine hydroxylase is not a single enzyme but a mixture of four factors, one or more of which may be active. Untreated PKU can produce devastating effects, but present dietary management can avoid these results.

Clinical symptoms In past years, before current newborn screening and treatment practices, the most profound effect observed in persons with *untreated* phenylketonuria was mental retardation. The IQ of affected persons was usually below 50 and frequently less than 20. Central nervous system damage caused irritability, hyperactivity, convulsive seizures, and bizarre behavior.

Dietary management PKU can now be well controlled by dietary means. After screening at birth, a special low-phenylalanine diet effectively controls the serum phenylalanine levels so they are maintained at appropriate amounts to prevent clinical symptoms, especially central nervous system damage.[7] Since phenylalanine is an essential amino acid necessary for growth, it cannot be totally removed from the diet. Blood levels of phenylalanine are constantly monitored, and the metabolic team nutritionist calculates the diet to allow a limited amount of phenylalanine tolerated by the individual child. Based on extensive studies, guidelines for dietary management of PKU are currently being used effectively. This management is built on two basic components, (1) a substitute for milk, the infant's first food, and (2) guidelines for adding solid foods.

Milk-substitute formula Milk has a relative high phenylalanine content, so a special formula is necessary. In the United States the formula is usually made from Lofenalac, a special casein hydrolysate product balanced with fats, carbohydrates, vitamins, and minerals. A small, designated measure of milk, usually evaporated milk, is added to the Lofenalac formula to adjust the phenylalanine content. Other products, Milupa PKU 1 and 2, European formulas now marketed in the United States, are component-type formulas. These are phenylalanine-free mixtures of amino acids, useful to allow a greater variety of foods to make up the limited phenylalanine allowance in the diet. Also, in most cases, although it requires more effort and hence commitment, the mother who wishes to breast-feed her baby can do so with careful team guidance and support.

Expanded low-phenylalanine diet As the infant grows, at about 6 months of age solid foods are added to the diet, calculated according to their phenylalanine content. These food additions are selected from a list of phenylalanine food-exchange groups or equivalents.[8] The individual child's diet is prescribed by the clinical nutritionist and physician according to the child's blood phenylalanine test as well as age and weight. The nutritionist then calculates the nutrient and energy levels and outlines the food plan in terms of numbers of food choices, or exchanges, allowed daily from each food group. Then a general meal pattern of feedings is determined to guide the mother in food choices for the child. There may be some relaxing of the diet during school years, but most authorities emphasize the need for continued control. This is especially needed for girls as they approach childbearing years. Guidelines have been developed for management of maternal PKU during pregnancy.[9]

Family counseling Initial education and support of the parents is essential, since dietary management of PKU is the only known effective method of treatment. Dietary control during the first year of life is directly related to three factors: (1) the parents' understanding of the diet, (2) the appropriateness of the dietary prescription for the needs of the individual infant, and (3) the frequency of infection. A number of teaching guides and materials have been developed and are available to help in family counseling and education.[10] Parents must understand and accept the absolute necessity of following the diet carefully. This requires patience, understanding, and continued reinforcement. Frequent home visits by the nutritionist and nurse may be a source of guidance and support as the child grows older. Other family members and any subsequent siblings should also be tested for PKU. The PKU team, together with wise parents, provides initial and continuing care so that the PKU child will grow and develop normally (Figure 19-2). Such a child, diagnosed at birth by widespread screening programs, can have a healthy and happy adulthood ahead, instead of the profound disease consequences experienced in the past.

Galactosemia

This genetic disease, also caused by a missing cell enzyme, affects carbohydrate metabolism. The missing enzyme controls the conversion of *galactose* to glucose. Milk, the infant's first food, contains a large amount of the precursor *lactose* (milk sugar), (see p. 44). After galactose is initially

Figure 19-2
PKU. This child is a delightful, perfectly developed 2-year-old. Screened and diagnosed at birth, she has eaten a carefully controlled low-phenylalanine diet and is growing normally.

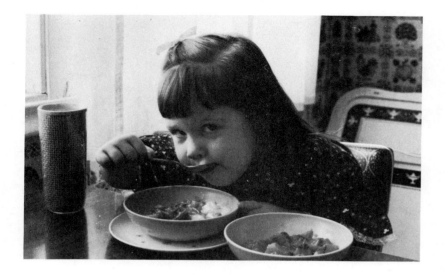

Hepatomegaly Enlargement of the liver.

Ascites Accumulation of fluid in the abdominal cavity.

combined with phosphate to begin the metabolic conversion to glucose, it cannot proceed further in the galactosemic infant. Galactose rapidly accumulates in the blood and in various body tissues.

Clinical symptoms In the past the excess tissue accumulations of galactose caused rapid damage to the untreated infant. The child failed to thrive, and clinical symptoms were apparent soon after birth. Continued liver damage brought jaundice, **hepatomegaly** with cirrhosis, enlargement of the spleen, and **ascites.** Without treatment, death usually resulted from liver failure. If the infant survived, continuing tissue damage and hypoglycemia in the optic lens and the brain caused cataracts and mental retardation. Now, however, with newborn screening programs, these infants are detected immediately and provided with special dietary management. With this vital nutritional therapy, they continue to grow and develop normally.

Dietary management The main indirect source of dietary galactose is milk. Therefore, *all* forms of milk and lactose must be removed from the diet. In this instance a *galactose-free diet* is used. Any needed amount of galactose for certain body structures can be synthesized by the body. A soy-base milk-substitute formula, such as Isomil or Prosobee, is used. Breast-feeding, of course, cannot be used. Later, as solid foods are added to the infant's diet at about 6 months of age, careful attention must be given to avoiding lactose from other food sources. Parents are carefully instructed to check labels on all commercial products to detect any lactose or lactose-containing substances.

Lactose Intolerance

A deficiency of any one of the disaccharidases in the intestine—lactase, sucrase, or maltase—may produce a wide range of gastrointestinal problems and abdominal pain because the specific sugar involved cannot be digested (see p. 462). Of these, lactose intolerance is the most common. It

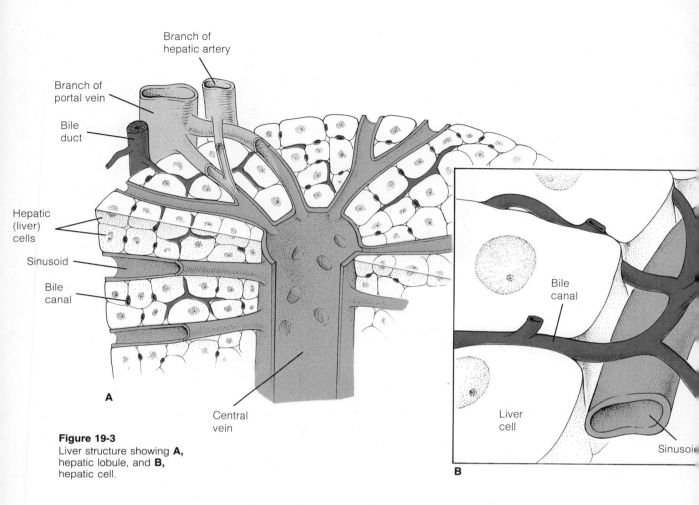

Branch of
hepatic artery

Branch of
portal vein

Bile
duct

Hepatic
(liver)
cells

Sinusoid

Bile
canal

A

Central
vein

Bile
canal

Liver
cell

Sinusoi

B

Figure 19-3
Liver structure showing **A,**
hepatic lobule, and **B,**
hepatic cell.

Hypermotility Excessive
perstalsis activity along the
alimentary canal.

is frequently seen in adults and may also occur in children. The accumulated concentration of undigested lactose in the intestine creates osmotic pressure and draws from the gut, thus stimulating **hypermotility** and resulting in abdominal cramping and diarrhea. Milk treated with lactase enzyme, lactose-hydrolyzed milk, can be tolerated by these persons without the difficulty encountered with regular milk. A diet similar to that used for galactosemia is required, although the underlying cause of the difficulty is quite different. Milk and all products containing lactose are carefully avoided, unless treated with lactase enzyme. Soy milk products are used for children.

Problems of the Accessory Organs

Three major accessory organs lie adjacent to the gastrointestinal tract and produce important digestive agents that enter the intestine and aid in the handling of food substances. Specific enzymes are produced for each of the major nutrients, and bile is added to assist the enzyme digestion of fats. These three organs are the liver (Figure 19-3), gallbladder, and pancreas. Diseases of these organs can easily affect gastrointestinal function and cause problems of interference with the normal handling of specific types of food.

Diseases of the Liver
Hepatitis

Acute hepatitis, usually a self-limiting inflammatory condition, is caused by viruses, alcohol, drugs, or toxins. In infectious hepatitis the viral agent is transmitted by the oral-fecal route, a common one in many epidemic diseases. The usual entry is through contaminated food or water. In other cases the virus may be transmitted in infected blood used for transfusions or by contaminated instruments, such as syringes or needles.

Necrosis Cell death.

Clinical symptoms The viral agents of hepatitis produce diffuse injury to liver cells, especially the parenchymal cells. In milder cases the liver injury is largely reversible, but with increasing severity more extensive necrosis occurs. In some cases massive necrosis may lead to liver failure and death. A cardinal symptom of hepatitis is *anorexia,* contributing to the risk of malnutrition. Varying clinical symptoms appear depending on the degree of liver injury. *Jaundice,* a major symptom, may be obvious or not, depending on the severity of the disease (see box, pp. 438-439). There is evidence that malnutrition and impaired immunocompetence contribute to the development of spontaneous infections and continuing liver disease. General symptoms—in addition to the main sign of anorexia—include malaise, weakness, nausea and vomiting, diarrhea, headache, fever, enlarged and tender liver, and enlarged spleen. When jaundice develops it usually occurs for an initial period of 5 to 10 days, deepens for 1 to 2 weeks, then levels off and decreases. After this crisis point there is sufficient recovery of injured cells and convalescence of 3 weeks to 3 months follows. Optimal care during this time is essential to avoid relapse.

Treatment Bedrest is essential. Physical exercise increases both the severity and duration of the disease. A daily intake of 3000 to 3500 ml of fluid guards against dehydration and gives a general sense of well-being and improved appetite. Optimal nutrition is the major therapy and provides foundation for recovery of the injured liver cells and overall return of strength.

Nutritional therapy The principles of diet therapy relate to the liver's function in metabolizing each nutrient:

High protein Protein is essential for liver cell regeneration. It also provides lipotropic agents such as methionine and choline (see p. 92) for the conversion of fats to lipoproteins and removal from the liver, thus preventing fatty infiltration. The diet should supply from 75 to 100 g of high-quality protein daily.

High carbohydrate Sufficient available glucose must be provided to restore protective glycogen reserves and to meet the energy demands of the disease process. Also, an adequate amount of glucose ensures the use of protein for vital tissue regeneration, the so-called protein-sparing action of carbohydrate. The diet should supply from 300 to 400 g of carbohydrate daily.

Moderate fat An adequate amount of fat in the diet makes the food more palatable and therefore encourages the anorexic patient to eat. A moderate amount of easily used fat, such as whole milk, cream, butter, margar-

Clinical Application

Jaundice: When to Expect It, What to Do About It

As jaundice is not usually a life-threatening condition, it is easy for health workers to take it lightly. After all, the yellow-to-orange skin color that arises in this disorder is harmless, so it would seem. But it reflects an accumulation of excessive bile pigments in the blood that results from a rise in *bilirubin,* a product of heme that is released when red blood cells are destroyed. The underlying condition causing the hemolysis is the major issue of medical treatment.

In a broader psychological sense, however, the condition can be devastating. The embarrassment of an altererd body image, with accompanying depression and withdrawal, can affect appetite and willingness to comply with therapy recommended for the underlying illness. To promote a healthy recovery, health workers must treat jaundice as seriously as these effects dictate. Several actions are helpful:

Explain the Reason for Jaundice
Jaundice can be discussed in three phases—prehepatic, hepatic, and posthepatic:

- **Prehepatic jaundice.** Most often this phase is caused by a massive breakdown in red blood cells. It is seen most often in Rh factor sensitization, hemolytic anemias, sickle cell anemia, massive lung infarctions, transfusion reactions, and septicemia. The result is an excessive amount of bilirubin in a form that cannot be excreted— i.e., fat-soluble. The body's bilirubin transport system, based on albumin, then deposits the excess in the patient's skin.
- **Hepatic jaundice.** In this case, the liver cannot convert fat-soluble bilirubin into the water-soluble form required for its removal from the blood. This condition is seen in hepatitis, cirrhosis, metastatic cancer, and prolonged drug use, especially of drugs broken down by the liver.
- **Posthepatic jaundice.** This phase occurs when the flow of bile into the duodenum is blocked. Since bile carries water-soluble excretable bilirubin, this blockage can cause it to back up, resulting in a backlog of bilirubin in the blood. Blockage often occurs with inflammation, scar tissue, stones, or tumors in the liver, bile, or pancreatic systems.

Identify Nutrition-Related Problems
Jaundice is often associated with anorexia, indigestion, nausea, and vomiting.

Help Resolve Nutrition-Related Problems
To overcome indigestion or anorexia, recommend small meals providing some of the patient's favorite foods. To overcome nausea or vomiting, simple foods may be necessary. Foods rich in fat and caffeine should also be avoided.

Clinical Application—cont'd

Encourage the Patient to Discuss Personal Feelings and Concerns

Such information is essential to develop a treatment plan designed to meet each patient's unique needs. Counseling helps the patient feel psychologically stronger and ready to help the health care process.

Discuss Pertinent Patient Needs With Family and/or Friends

Often "significant others" avoid the patient with discolored skin out of embarrassment or a lack of understanding. A discussion of the patient's need for support may help other persons accept the patient socially and support efforts to resolve underlying health problems.

Make Referrals to Outside Agencies, as Needed

If jaundice is caused by alcohol or drug abuse, the patient and family may require special counseling. Referral to community programs after hospital discharge may help provide continuing support.

References

Gannon, R.B., and Pickett, K.: Jaundice, Am. J. Nursing **83**:404, 1983.

---

ine, vegetable oil, and cooking fat, is beneficial. The diet should incorporate about 100 to 150 g of such fat daily.

High energy From 2500 to 3000 kcal are needed daily to furnish energy demands of the tissue regeneration process, to compensate for losses resulting from fever and general debilitation, and to renew strength and recuperative powers.

Meals and feedings The problem of supplying a diet adequate to meet the increased nutritive demands for a patient whose illness makes food almost repellent calls for creativity and supportive encouragement. The food may need to be in liquid form at first, using concentrated commercial or blended formulas (Table 19-2) for frequent feedings. As the patient can better tolerate solid food, appetizing and attractive food is needed. Since nutritional therapy is the key to recovery, a major nutrition and nursing responsibility requires devising ways to encourage an optimal food intake. The clinical dietitian and the nurse should work together closely to achieve this goal.

Cirrhosis

The French physician Laennec first named the disease, from the Greek word *kirrhos,* meaning "orange," because the cirrhotic liver has a firm, fibrous mass and orange-colored nodules projecting from its surface. The nutritional or alcoholic form of cirrhosis bears his name, *Laennec's cirrhosis.*

Liver disease may advance to the chronic state of cirrhosis (Figure 19-4). Some forms of cirrhosis result from biliary obstruction or liver necrosis from undetermined causes. In some cases it results from previous viral hepatitis. The most common problem, however, is fatty cirrhosis associated with malnutrition and alcoholism. This relentless malnutrition, together with impaired immunocompetence, accounts for the frequent occurrence of infectious relapses. An increasingly poor intake, as the alcoholic person continues to drink excessively, leads to multiple nutri-

Table 19-2
Principles of Dietary
Management for Children with
Cystic Fibrosis

Principle	Reason
High calorie	Energy demands of growth and compensation for fecal losses; large appetite usually ensures acceptance of increased amounts of food
High protein	Usually tolerated in large amounts; excess above normal growth needs required to compensate for losses
Moderate carbohydrate	Starch less well tolerated, simple sugars easily assimilated
Low to moderate fat, as tolerated	Fat poorly absorbed, but tolerance varies widely
Generous salt	Food generously salted to replace sweat loss; salt supplements in hot weather
Vitamins	Double doses of multivitamins in water-soluble form (vitamin E supplements sometimes used as low blood levels of the vitamin have been observed); vitamin K supplements with prolonged antibiotic therapy
Pancreatic enzymes	Large amounts given by mouth with each meal (may be mixed with cereal or applesauce for infants) to compensate for pancreatic deficiency—powdered pancreas extract containing steapsin, trypsin, and amylopsin (Pancreatin, or other pancreatic extracts such as Cotazyme or Viokase).

tional deficiencies. However, alcoholism can cause cirrhosis and death not only because it promotes malnutrition but also because alcohol and its metabolic products disturb liver metabolism and damage liver cells directly. Damage to the liver cells occurs as fatty infiltration causes cellular destruction and fibrotic tissue changes.

High-Protein, High-
Carbohydrate, Moderate-Fat
Daily Diet

1 L (1 qt) of milk

1 to 2 eggs

224 g (8 oz) lean meat, fish, poultry

4 servings vegetables:
   2 servings potato or substitute
   1 serving green leafy or yellow vegetable
   1 to 2 servings of other vegetables, including 1 raw

3 to 4 servings fruit (include juices often)
   1 to 2 citrus fruits (or other good source of ascorbic acid)
   2 servings other fruit

6 to 8 servings bread and cereal (whole grain or enriched)
   1 serving cereal
   5 to 6 slices bread, crackers

2 to 4 tbsp butter or fortified margarine

Additional jam, jelly, honey, and other carbohydrate foods as patient desires and is able to eat them

Sweetened fruit juices increase both carbohydrate and fluid

Figure 19-4
Comparison of normal liver and liver with cirrhotic tissue changes. **A,** Anterior view of organ, **B,** cross section, **C,** tissue structure.

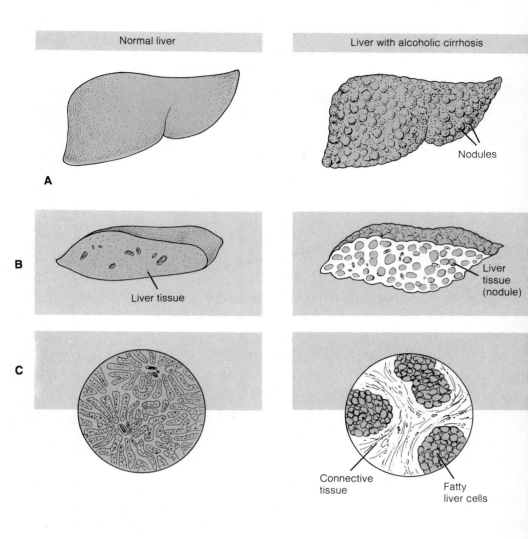

Normal liver

Liver with alcoholic cirrhosis

Nodules

A

B

Liver tissue

Liver tissue (nodule)

C

Connective tissue

Fatty liver cells

Macrocytic anemia An anemia characterized by red cells that are larger and paler than normal.

Clinical symptoms Early signs of cirrhosis include gastrointestinal disturbances such as nausea, vomiting, loss of appetite, distention, and epigastric pain. In time jaundice may appear. There is increasing weakness, edema, ascites, and anemia from gastrointestinal bleeding, iron deficiency, or hemorrhage. A specific **macrocytic anemia** from folic acid deficiency is also frequently observed. Steatorrhea is a common symptom. Essentially, the major symptoms are caused by a basic protein deficiency and its multiple metabolic problems: (1) plasma protein levels fall leading to failure of the capillary fluid shift mechanism, causing ascites (see p. 172), (2) lipotropic agents are not supplied for fat conversion to lipoproteins and damaging fat accumulates in the liver tissue, (3) blood clotting mechanisms are impaired since factors such as prothrombin and **fibrinogen** are not adequately produced, and (4) general tissue catabolism and negative nitrogen balance continue the overall degenerative process.

Fibrinogen A fraction of human plasma given via transfusion to increase coagulation of the blood.

As the disease progresses, the increasing fibrous scar tissue impairs blood circulation through the liver, and portal hypertension follows. Con-

Varices Enlarged veins.

tributing further to the problem is the continuing ascites. The impaired portal circulation with increasing venous pressure may lead to *esophageal* **varices,** with danger of rupture and fatal massive hemorrhage.

Treatment When alcoholism is the underlying problem, treatment is difficult. Each patient requires individual supportive care and approach (see Issues and Answers, pp. 450-451). Therapy is usually aimed at correcting fluid and electrolyte problems and providing nutritional support to encouraging hepatic repair as much as possible.

Nutritional therapy Nutritional therapy for cirrhosis should include the following:

Protein according to tolerance In the absence of impending hepatic coma, about 80 to 100 g protein/day is needed to correct severe undernutrition, regenerate functional liver tissue, and replenish plasma proteins. However, if signs of hepatic coma appear, protein should be adjusted to individual tolerance.

Low sodium Sodium is usually restricted to 500 to 1000 mg/day to help reduce fluid retention (see p. 465).

Texture If esophageal varices develop, it may be necessary to give soft foods that are smooth in texture to prevent the danger of rupture.

Optimal general nutrition The remaining overall diet principles outlined for hepatitis are continued for cirrhosis for the same reasons. Kilocalories, carbohydrates, and vitamins, especially B-complex vitamins plus folic acid, are supplied according to individual need and deficiency. Moderate fat is used. Alcohol is strictly forbidden.

Hepatic Encephalopathy

As cirrhotic changes continue in the liver and portal blood circulation diminishes, collateral circulation develops, bypassing the liver. The normal liver has a major function of removing ammonia from the blood by converting it to urea for excretion. In the diseased liver these normal reactions cannot take place. Therefore ammonia-laden blood, carrying the products of protein metabolism, approaches the liver but cannot follow the usual portal pathways and is detoured around the liver through the collateral circulation. Then it reenters the systemic blood flow and produces ammonia intoxication and coma. The resulting hepatic **encephalopathy** brings changes in consciousness, behavior, and neurologic status.

Encephalopathy Any degenerative disease of the brain.

Clinical symptoms Typical response involves disorders of conciousness and alterations in motor function. There is apathy, confusion, inappropriate behavior, and drowsiness, progressing to coma. The speech may be slurred or monotonous. A coarse, flapping tremor is observed in the outstretched hands. The breath may have a fecal odor.

Treatment The fundamental objective of treatment is removal of the sources of excess ammonia. A more recent drug has largely replaced neomycin as the primary medical treatment for reducing blood ammonia. This is *lactulose,* a nonabsorbable synthetic disaccharide. It acts by trapping nitrogen in the stools, thus decreasing ammonia production. It is usually effective in most patients and improves the encephalopathy in 1 to 2 days. In addition, recent therapy for hepatic disease has also included the use of *branched-chain amino acids*. These three essential amino acids, leucine, isoleucine, and valine (see p. 90), are not catabolized by the liver but are taken up by other tissues. Thus they can be metabolized without dependance on healthy liver tissue, as is the case with other amino acids. Mixtures of these amino acids have therefore been successfully used to maintain adequate nitrogen balance and reduce the encephalopathy.

Nutritional therapy Nutritional therapy for hepatic encephalopathy should include:

Low protein Protein intake is reduced as individually necessary to restrict the dietary sources of nitrogen in amino acids. The amount of restriction will vary with the circumstances. The unconscious patient will receive no protein, but the usual amounts given range from 15 to 50 g daily, depending on whether symptoms are severe or mild. A simple method for

Low-Protein Diets—15 g, 30 g, 40 g, and 50 g Protein

General description

- The following diets are used when dietary protein is to be restricted.
- The patterns limit foods containing a large percentage of protein, such as milk, eggs, cheese, meat, fish, fowl, and legumes.
- Meat extractives, soups, broth, bouillon, gravies, and gelatin desserts should also be avoided.

Basic Meal Patterns (contain approximately 15 g of protein)

Breakfast	Lunch	Dinner
½ cup fruit or fruit juice	1 small potato	1 small potato
½ cup cereal	½ cup vegetable	½ cup vegetable
1 slice toast	salad (vegetable or fruit)	salad (vegetable or fruit)
Butter	1 slice bread	1 slice bread
Jelly	Butter	Butter
Sugar	1 serving fruit	1 serving fruit
2 tbsp cream	Sugar	Sugar
Coffee	Coffee or tea	Coffee or tea

For 30 g Protein

Add: 1 cup milk
28 g (1 oz) meat, 1 egg, or equivalent

For 40 g Protein

Add: 1 cup milk
70 g (2½ oz) meat, or 1 egg and 42 g (1½ oz) meat

For 50 g Protein

Add: 1 cup milk
112 g (4 oz) meat, or 2 eggs and 56 g (2 oz) meat

Examples of Meat Portions

28 g (1 oz) meat = 1 thin slice roast, 4 × 5 cm (1½ × 2 in)
1 rounded tbsp cottage cheese
1 slice American cheese

70 g (2½ oz) meat = Ground beef patty (5 from 448 g [1 lb])
1 slice roast

112 g (4 oz) meat = 2 lamb chops
1 average steak

controlling dietary protein uses a base meal pattern containing approximately 15 g of protein, adding small items of protein foods according to the level of total protein desired, is given in the box on p. 443.

Kilocalories and vitamins The amounts of kilocalories and vitamins are prescribed according to need. An intake of 1500 to 2000 kcal/day is sufficient to prevent tissue breakdown, which would be a source of more amino acids and available nitrogen. Carbohydrates and fats sufficient for energy needs are essential. Vitamin K is usually given parenterally, along with other vitamins that may be deficient. Close attention is also given to possible mineral deficiencies.

Fluid intake Fluid intake/output is carefully controlled.

Diseases of the Gallbladder
Functions of the Gallbladder

The liver produces daily about 600 to 800 ml of bile, which the gallbladder normally concentrates fivefold to tenfold and stores in its small 40- to 70-ml capacity.

The main function of the gallbladder is to concentrate and store bile. Its powers of such concentration are great. Through the *cholecystokinin (CCK) mechanism* (see p. 65), the presence of fat in the duodenum stimulates contraction of the gallbladder with the release of bile into the common duct and then into the small intestine.

Cholecystitis and Cholelithiasis

Inflammation of the gallbladder, *cholecystitis,* usually results from a low-grade chronic infection. Normally cholesterol in bile, which is insoluble in water, is kept in solution by the other bile ingredients. However, when the absorbing mucosal tissue of the gallbladder is inflamed or infected, changes occur in the tissue. The absorptive powers of the gallbladder may be altered, affecting the solubility of the bile ingredients. Excess water may be absorbed, or excess bile acids may be absorbed. Under these abnormal absorptive conditions, cholesterol may precipitate, forming gallstones composed of almost pure cholesterol. This condition is called *cholelithiasis.* High dietary fat intake over a long period of time predisposes a person to gallstone formation because of the constant stimulus to produce more cholesterol as a necessary bile ingredient to metabolize the fat.

Clinical symptoms When inflammation, stones, or both are present in the gallbladder, contraction from the cholecystokinin mechanism causes pain. Sometimes the pain is severe. There is fullness and distention after eating and particular difficulty with fatty foods.

Treatment Surgical removal of the gallbladder, *cholecystectomy,* is usually indicated. However, the surgeon may wish to postpone surgery until the inflammation has subsided. If the patient is obese, as many persons with gallbladder disease are, some weight loss before surgery is advisable. Thus the supportive therapy is largely dietary. Recently a new drug, chenodiol, has been used successfully to dissolve small gallstones and may prove to be an effective alternative to surgery in some cases.

Nutritional therapy Nutritional therapy for diseases of the gallbladder should include:

Fat Because dietary fat is the principal cause of contraction of the diseased organ and subsequent pain, it is usually reduced. Kilocalories for

Low-Fat Diet

General description

- This diet contains foods that are low in fat.
- Foods are prepared without the addition of fat.
- Fatty meats, gravies, oils, cream, lard, and desserts containing eggs, butter, cream, nuts, and avocados are avoided.
- Foods should be used in amounts specified and only as tolerated.
- The sample pattern contains approximately 85 g protein, 50 g fat, 220 g carbohydrate, and 1670 kilocalories.

	Allowed	Not allowed
Beverages	Skim milk, coffee, tea, carbonated beverages, fruit juices	Whole milk, cream, evaporated and condensed milk
Bread and cereals	All kinds	Rich rolls or breads, waffles, pancakes
Desserts	Jell-O, sherbet, water ices, fruit whips made without cream, angel food cake, rice and tapioca puddings made with skim milk	Pastries, pies, rich cakes and cookies, ice cream
Fruits	All fruits, as tolerated	Avocado
Eggs	3 allowed per week, cooked any way except fried	Fried eggs
Fats	3 tsp butter or margarine daily	Salad and cooking oils, mayonnaise
Meats	Lean meat such as beef, veal, lamb, liver, lean fish and fowl, baked, broiled, or roasted without added fat.	Fried meats, bacon, ham, pork, goose, duck, fatty fish, fish canned in oil, cold cuts
Cheese	Dry or fat-free cottage cheese	All other cheese
Potato or substitute	Potatoes, rice, macaroni, noodles, sphaghetti, all prepared without added fat	Fried potatoes, potato chips
Soups	Bouillon or broth, without fat; soups made with skimmed milk	Cream soups
Sweets	Jam, jelly, sugar, sugar candies without nuts or chocolate	Chocolate, nuts, peanut butter
Vegetables	All kinds as tolerated	The following should be omitted if they cause distress: broccoli, cauliflower, corn, cucumber, green pepper, radishes, turnips, onions, dried peas, and beans
Miscellaneous	Salt in moderation	Pepper, spices; highly spiced food, olives, pickles, cream sauces, gravies

Suggested Menu Pattern

Breakfast	**Lunch and Dinner**
Fruit	Meat, broiled or baked
Cereal	Potato
Toast, jelly	Vegetable
1 tsp butter or margarine	Salad with fat-free dressing
	Bread, jelly
Egg 3 times per week	1 tsp butter or margarine
Skim milk, 1 cup	Fruit or dessert, as allowed
Coffee, sugar	Skim milk, 1 cup coffee, sugar

Fat-Free Diet

General Description

The following additional restrictions are made to the low-fat diet to make it relatively fat free.
1. Meat, eggs, and butter or margarine are omitted.
2. A substitute for meat at the noon and evening meal is 84 g (3 oz) of fat-free cottage cheese.

energy needs should come principally from carbohydrate foods, especially during acute phases. Although for cholecystitis, some hospitals may not serve patients a special diet labeled "low fat," nonetheless attention is needed to moderate the fat intake and curtail foods causing pain or discomfort. Certainly a limit of fat to 25% to 30% of the total kilocalories is prudent. A diet plan for a low-fat regimen is given on p. 445.

Kilocalories If weight loss is indicated, kilocalories will be reduced according to need. Principles of weight-reduction food plans are given in Chapter 15. Usually such a restricted diet will have a low-fat ratio and meet the needs of the patient for fat restriction.

Cholesterol and "gas formers" Two additional modifications usually found in traditional diets for gallbladder disease concern restriction of foods containing cholesterol and foods labeled "gas formers." Neither modification has a valid rationale. The body synthesizes daily several times more cholesterol than is present in an average diet. Thus restriction of cholesterol in food has no appreciable effect on reducing gallstone formation. Total dietary fat reduction is more to the point. Also, blanket restriction of so-called gas formers is unwarranted, since food tolerances are highly individual (see p. 423).

Diseases of the Pancreas
Pancreatitis

Acute inflammation of the pancreas, *pancreatitis,* is caused by the digestion of the organ tissues by the very enzymes it produces, principally trypsin. Normally enzymes remain in an inactive form until the pancreatic juice reaches the lumen of the duodenum (see p. 28). However, gallbladder disease may cause a gallstone to enter the common bile duct and obstruct the flow of pancreatic juice or cause a reflux or bile from the common duct into the pancreatic duct. This mixing of digestive materials activates the powerful pancreatic enzymes within the gland. In such activated form, they begin their damaging effects on the pancreatic tissue itself, causing acute pain. Sometimes infectious pancreatitis may occur as a complication of mumps or a bacterial disease. Also, the excessive use of alcohol may be another factor in the disease. Mild or moderate pancreatitis may subside completely; but it has a tendency to recur.

Treatment Care consists of measures recommended for acute disease involving shock. These measures include intravenous feeding at first, replacement therapy of fluid and electrolytes, blood transfusions, antibiotics and pain medications, and gastric suction.

Nutritional therapy In initial stages oral feedings are withheld because entry of food into the intestines stimulates pancreatic secretions. As healing progresses and oral feedings are resumed, a light diet is used to avoid excessive stimulation of pancreatic secretions. Alcohol and excess use of coffee should also be avoided to decrease pancreatic stimulation.

Cystic Fibrosis of the Pancreas

Cystic fibrosis is a generalized hereditary disease of children that involves the exocrine glands, particularly the pancreas, and thus affects many tissues and organs. In past years its prognosis was poor. Few children with an early onset survived past 10 years of age. However, with better knowledge of the disease, improved diagnostic tests, clinical treatment, and antibiotic therapy, prognosis has improved.

Clinical symptoms Cystic fibrosis usually produces characteristic clinical symptoms: (1) pancreatic deficiency with greatly diminished digestion of food caused by the absence of pancreatic enzymes, (2) malfunction or mucus-producing glands with accumulation of thick viscid secretions and subsequent respiratory difficulties and chronic pulmonary disease, (3) abnormal secretions of the sweat glands, containing high electrolyte levels, and (4) possible cirrhosis of the liver arising from biliary obstruction and increased by malnutrition or infection.

Treatment Treatment is based on three factors: (1) control of respiratory infections, (2) relief from the effects of an extremely viscid bronchial secretion, and (3) the maintenance of sound nutrition. The digestive deficiency and malabsorptive character of cystic fibrosis is evident in the nature of the child's stools. They are similar to those in celiac disease (typically bulky, mushy, greasy, foul, and foamy), but they also contain more undigested food. Only about half, 50% to 60%, of the child's food is broken down and absorbed. Thus the child with cystic fibrosis has a much more voracious appetite.

Nutritional therapy The basic objective is to compensate for the loss of nutrient material resulting from insufficiency of pancreatic enzymes. Protein hydrolysates, split fats (emulsified simple fats), and simple sugars are used more easily. There is a wide variation, however, in tolerance for fat, and the amount of fat intake is usually prescribed according to the character of the stools. Large increases of protein seem to be well tolerated and are needed for the replacement of losses and for growth. Diet guides for cystic fibrosis are similar to those outlined for celiac disease (see p. 428), with food forms varying according to the age of the child. The diet differs, however, in that gluten sources need not be restricted, and there is greater emphasis on quantity of food. The important principles of dietary management for children with cystic fibrosis are summarized in Table 19–3.

To Sum Up

The nutritional management of gastrointestinal disease is based on careful consideration of four major factors: (1) *secretory functions,* providing the chemical agents and environment necessary for digestion, (2) *neuromuscular functions,* required for motility and mechanical digestion, (3) *absorptive function,* transporting nutrients into the circulatory system, and (4) *psychological factors,* reflected by changes in gastrointestinal function.

Esophageal problems vary widely from simple dysphagia to serious disease or obstruction. Nutritional therapy varies according to degree of dysfunction.

Peptic ulcer, a common gastrointestinal problem, is an erosion of the mucosal lining of the duodenum and less commonly the stomach. It results in such nutritional problems as low plasma protein levels, anemia, and weight loss. Medical management consists of drug therapy, rest, and individual nutritional therapy.

Intestinal diseases include anatomic changes such as diverticulosis and malabsorption problems, such as are found in celiac disease, ulcerative colitis or Crohn's disease. Nutritional therapy involves modification of the diet's protein and energy content, food texture, increased vitamins and minerals, and fluid and electrolyte replacement, with continuous adjustment of the diet according to need.

Common liver disorders include hepatitis, usually caused by viral infection, and cirrhosis, an inflammatory condition resulting from tissue damage by such toxins as excessive alcohol. Uncontrolled cirrhosis leads to a another major liver disorder, hepatic encephalopathy. Nutrient and energy levels required vary with each condition.

Diseases of the gallbladder include cholecystitis, inflammation that interferes with the absorption of water or bile acids, and cholelithiasis, or gallstone formation. Treatment involves a generally reduced fat diet and removal of the gallbladder surgically.

Questions for Review

1. What is the basic principle of diet planning for patients with esophageal problems? Outline a general nutritional care plan for a patient with reflux esophagitis caused by a hiatal hernia.

2. In current practice what are the basic principles of diet planning for patients with peptic ulcer disease? How do these principles differ from traditional therapy?

3. Outline a course of nutritional management for a person with peptic ulcer disease, based on the liberal individual approach. How would you plan nutrition education for continuing self-care and avoidance of recurrence?

4. Describe the causes, clinical signs, and treatment of each of the following diseases: diverticulosis, celiac disease, and inflammatory bowel disease.

5. What is the rationale for treatment in the spectrum of liver disease—hepatitis, cirrhosis, and hepatic encephalopathy?

6. Develop a 1-day food plan for a 45-year-old male, 183 cm (6 ft, 1 in) tall, weighing 90 kg (200 lb), with infectious hepatitis; another plan for a similar patient with cirrhosis of the liver; and another for a patient with hepatic encephalopathy. What principles of diet therapy apply for each?

7. What are the principles of nutritional therapy for gallbladder disease? Write a 1-day meal plan for a 30-year-old woman, 165 cm (5 ft, 6 in) tall, weighing 81 kg (180 lb), who has an inflamed gallbladder with stones and is awaiting a cholecystectomy.

References

1. National Institutes of Health: The prevalence of dental caries in United States children, The National Dental Caries Prevalence Survey 1979-80, U.S. Dept. of Health and Human Services Pub. No., 82-2245, NIH, Washington, D.C., 1981, Government Printing Office.
2. Leveille, G.A., and Coccodrilli, G.D.: Cariogenicity of foods: current concepts, Food Technol. **36:**93, 1982.
3. Rydning, A., and others: Prophylatic effect of dietary fibre in duodenal ulcer disease, Lancet **2:**736, 1982.
4. Farthing, M.J.G.: Gastrointestinal dysfunction in inflammatory bowel disease, Clin. Nutr., Suppl., **2**(4):5, 1983.
5. Kirsner, J.B., and Shorter, R.G.: Recent developments in nonspecific inflammatory bowel disease, I., N. Engl. J. Med. **306:**775, 1982.
6. Buisseret, P.D., Allergy, Sci. Am. **247**(2):86, 1982.
7. Schneider, A.J.,: Newborn phenylalanine/tyrosine metabolism: Implications for screening for phenylketonuria, Am. J. Dis. Child **137:**427, 1983.
8. Schuett, V.E., Low protein food list, Madison, Wisconsin, 1981, University of Wisconsin.
9. Acosta, P.B., and others: Nutrition in pregnancy of women with hyperphenylalaninemia, J. Am. Diet. Assoc. **80**(5):443, 1982.
10. Williams, S.R.: Nutrition and diet therapy, ed. 5, St. Louis, 1985, The C.V. Mosby Co., p. 542, A89.

Further readings

Buisseret, P.D.: Allergy, Sci. Am. **247**(2):86, 1982.

For those interested in expanded background on the relation of allergy to the body's immune system. Numerous applications to food allegies. Excellent illustrations to clarify basic concepts.

Kosel, K., and others: Total pancreatectomy and islet cell autotransplantation, Am. J. Nurs. **82:**568, 1982.

Excellent review by a skilled team of nurses of an accessory organ to the gastrointestinal tract and the problems related to pancreatitis, its surgical treatment, and follow-up care.

Makhlouf, G.M.: Function of the gallbladder, Nutr. Today **17:**10, 1982.

Modern view of the gallbladder, with many excellent graphics to depict its structure and functions.

Paige, D.M., ed.: Diarrhea, Clin. Nutr. Suppl., **3**(1):2–33, 1984.

Entire issue is devoted to the topic of diarrhea. Its four articles provide excellent current background on nutrition-diet diarrhea issues: food sensitivity and intolerance, food-borne infections and poisonings, oral hydration and feeding, and the importance of breast feeding. Many helpful tables and graphs.

Phillips, S.F., and Stephen, A.M.: The structure and function of the large intestine, Nutri. Today **16**(6):4, 1981.

Excellent graphics and readable text clarifying structures, functions, and diseases of the large intestine. Good view of actions of dietary fiber.

Synder, J.D., From pedialyte to popsicles: a look at oral rehydration therapy used in the United States and Canada, Am. J. Clin. Nutr. **35**(1):157, 1982.

Good brief reference with tables for comparative values of many commonly used oral rehydration fluids used in pediatric practices.

Issues and Answers

Nutritional Aspects of Diarrhea

Gastrointestinal diseases often present barriers to efficient nutrient absorption. So nutritional deficiencies are automatically planned for. But these conditions also lead frequently to diarrhea, which only compounds the problem of nutrient loss. All types of diarrhea result in loss of fluids and electrolytes, with replacement therapy an initial primary concern. However, different types of diarrhea also present other problems that require different modes of treatment related to the disease the diarrhea accompanies. We will examine first three common types of diarrhea: watery, fatty, and small volume.

Types of Diarrhea

Watery diarrhea occurs when the amount of water and electrolytes moving into the intestinal mucosa exceeds the amount absorbed into the bloodstream. This movement of water and electrolytes may be secretive or osmotic. *Secretive* movement of water and electrolytes into the mucosa may be active or passive: (1) *Active movement* occurs with excessive gastric hydrochloric acid secretion or enterotoxic infections (e.g., **cholera**) and (2) *passive movement* occurs with a rise in hydrostatic pressure that accompanies such infectious diseases as salmonellosis or tuberculosis, nonbacterial infections, fungal infections, renal failure, irradiation **enteritis,** and inflammatory bowel disease. Other conditions that are associated with watery diarrhea include hyperthyroidism and thyroid carcinoma and hypermotility of the gastrointestinal tract. *Osmotic* movement of water and electrolytes into the mucosa occurs when nutrients are not absorbed because intolerable levels of nonabsorbable particles are present in the intestinal **chyme.** Such particles include: (1) *lactose* in lactase-deficient individuals, (2) *gluten* in persons with gluten-sensitive enteropathy, (3) large amounts of *magnesium* frequently used in antacid therapy for individuals with peptic ulcers, or (4) *iron.* It also occurs in people with a reduced gastrointestinal transit time caused by the removal of part of the intestine.

Cholera An acute infectious disease characterized by severe diarrhea, acidosis, vomiting, muscle cramps, and prostration. Associated with drinking contaminated water.

Enteritis Inflammation of the intestine.

Chyme A semifluid, creamy, hemogeneous material that forms when gastric secretions digest food.

    Fatty diarrhea, or *steatorrhea*, occurs with maldigestion or malabsorption. *Maldigestion* involves a lack of enzymatic activity required to completely digest food, e.g., reduced pancreatic exocrine activity (release of intestinal enzymes from the pancreas) caused by pancreatic insufficiency. *Malabsorption* means that digested materials do not make it across the intestinal mucosa to enter the bloodstream. This failure occurs in conditions in which the intestinal villi are destroyed (e.g., radiation therapy, celiac disease).

    Small volume diarrhea occurs mainly when the rectosigmoid area of the colon is irritated, e.g., in inflammatory bowel disease (Crohn's disease or ulcerative colitis). It also occurs when inflammatory conditions affect areas adjacent to the colon, as in pelvic inflammatory disease, diverticulitis, appendicitis, or hemorrhagic ovarian cysts.

Issues and Answers—cont'd

Syncope A brief loss of consciousness associated with, among other things, reduced levels of extracellular fluid, as occurs during uncontrolled diarrhea.

Hypokalemia Low potassium levels in the blood

"Dumping" syndrome A number of physical problems (nausea, vomiting, sweating, palpitations, syncope, diarrhea, etc.) that occur when stomach contents are emptied at an abnormally fast rate. Occurs when part of the stomach or intestinal tract is removed.

Specific Nutritional Therapy

If uncontrolled, each of these types of diarrhea bring similar metabolic results: **syncope, hypokalemia,** *acid-base imbalances,* and *hypovolemia* with resulting *renal failure.* They may also be accompanied by low levels of fat-soluble vitamins, B_{12} or folic acid, or eventually lead to protein-energy malnutrition. But in addition to these general conditions, each type also manifests specific problems associated with the specific disorders they accompany, requiring differing treatment in each case.

Watery diarrhea often accompanies inflammatory bowel conditions, such as Crohn's disease, for which diet therapy involves: (1) increased protein and kilocalories, (2) low residue fats, and lactose, (3) avoidance of foods that stimulate peristalsis. Thus, *secretive diarrhea* is reduced by eliminating foods that may stimulate gastric acid secretion, and all types of watery diarrhea can be avoided by reducing the motility of the gastrointestinal tract. In other conditions in which *osmotic diarrhea* occurs, e.g., **dumping syndrome,** this problem is avoided by giving fluids *between* meals to avoid any extreme difference in osmotic pressures on either side of the intestinal wall. Small frequent meals also help prevent this problem as well as any painful distention.

Fatty diarrhea frequently accompanies conditions associated with maldigestion, such as chronic pancreatitis. The dietary management of this disease involves: (1) frequent meals, high in protein and carbohydrate, low in fat; (2) consumption of medium-chain triglycerides (MCT), which are more easily absorbed under adverse conditions; and (3) avoiding gastric stimulants (especially caffeine and alcohol). Fatty diarrhea also accompanies conditions of malabsorption, such as gluten-sensitive enteropathy. In addition, this type of diarrhea also requires the removal of items that will damage the mucosal villi, items such as lactose and gluten and products containing them. Sometimes it requires restricting fat. In both cases, the primary need is to monitor fats that would otherwise appear in the feces. As the therapy progresses, the fat content of the meal can be increased, as tolerated, to normal levels to improve palatability.

Small volume diarrhea may accompany diverticulosis of the colon. A high-residue diet is recommended to increase fecal bulk, thereby preventing diarrhea. To prevent flatulence and distention, however, the fiber (such as wheat bran, fruits, vegetables) should be added to the diet gradually.

All types of diarrhea can result in malnutrition because of loss of electrolytes and fluids. But it is also important to identify the *type* of diarrhea occurring with each patient. Only then can an effective nutritional management strategy be designed to (1) replace fluid-electrolyte losses and (2) eliminate or prevent other possible nutrition-related problems specific for each case.

References
Chernoff, R., and Dean, J.A.: Medical and nutritional aspects of intractable diarrhea, J. Am. Diet. Assoc. **76:**161, 1980.

Chapter 20
Coronary Heart Disease and Hypertension

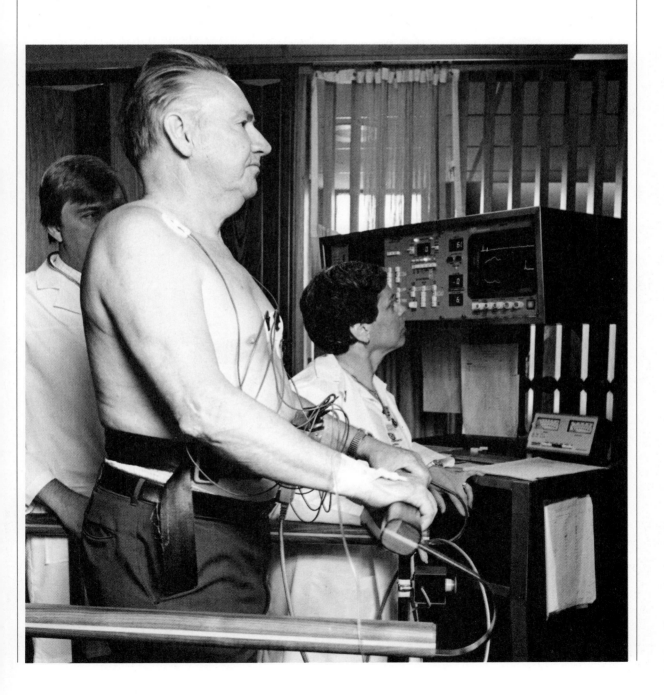

Preview

For the past 50 years diseases of the heart and blood vessels have been the major cause of death in the United States and in most other Western societies. The magnitude of this health care problem is enormous. Every day an estimated 3400 Americans, more than two each minute, suffer a heart attack. Every day approximately 1600 persons suffer cerebrovascular accidents (strokes). Every day more than 100,000 children and 1.7 million adults continue to suffer from various forms of rheumatic and congestive heart disease.

Despite a decline in general cardiovascular mortality during the past decade, the leading cause of death in the United States remains coronary heart disease. As more and more is learned about this disease process, it is now clear that not one but many factors, including hypertension, are involved and increase a person's risk of developing heart disease.

Chapter Objectives

After study of this chapter, the student should be able to:

1. Identify the factors related to heart disease and account for their effect on the underlying disease process involved.

2. Describe the relationship of hypertension to heart disease.

3. Describe possible nutrition factors in heart disease.

4. Relate current knowledge of heart disease to a reasonable plan for nutritional care in its prevention and treatment.

Coronary Heart Disease

Arteriosclerosis Group of cardiovascular diseases characterized by a thickening of the arterial walls and a loss of elasticity.

Atheroma Tumor-type growths on inside lining of blood vessels, composed of lipid-material (largely cholesterol) and cellular debris.

Plaque A patch or flat area forming on a tissue.

Intima Innermost layer of a blood vessel.

Atherosclerosis A form of heart disease in which blood vessels are blocked by atheroma (plaque) deposits on the inner lining.

Embolus A circulating blood clot, which may come to lodge in a blood vessel, causing an *embolism.*

Ischemia Deficiency of blood to a body part because of constriction or actual obstruction of a blood vessel.

Infarct The death of tissue caused by a loss of blood flow to that area, usually caused by a thrombus (clot) clogging the artery feeding the area.

Myocardial infarction (MI) Death of heart tissue caused by blockage preventing the flow of blood to or through its coronary arteries.

Coronary Referring to the arteries that carry nutrients and oxygen to the heart muscle.

Thrombosis Development of a blood clot (thrombus) that lodges in a blood vessel and cuts off the blood supply at that point.

The Problem of Atherosclerosis
The Disease Process

Atherosclerosis, the major **arteriosclerosis** disease and underlying pathologic process in coronary heart disease, remains an unsolved problem in modern medicine. The characteristic lesions involved, **atheromas,** are raised fibrous **plaques** (Figure 20-1). They appear on the interior surface, the **intima**, of the blood vessel as discrete lumps, elevated above the unaffected surrounding area. The plaque usually contains fatty material, such as lipoproteins, the carriers of cholesterol in the blood, which are found both inside and outside of the cells. Crystals of cholesterol can be seen with the unaided eye in the softened cheesy debris of advanced lesions. It is this fatty debris that suggested the original name **atherosclerosis**, from the Greek *athera* (gruel) and *sclerosis* (hardening). This fatty degeneration and thickening narrows the vessel lumen and may allow a blood clot to develop, or an **embolus**, from its irritating presence. Eventually the clot may cut off blood flow in the involved artery. If the artery is a critical one, such as a major coronary vessel, a heart attack occurs. The tissue area serviced by the involved artery is deprived of its vital oxygen and nutrient supply, (**ischemia**) and the cells die. The localized area of dying or dead tissue is called an **infarct**. Since the artery involved is one supplying the cardiac muscle, or *myocardium,* the result is called an acute **myocardial infarction**. The two major **coronary** arteries, with their many branches, are so named because they lie across the brow of the heart muscle and resemble a crown.

Three major theories have developed concerning the cause of fatty plaques:[1]

Injury and blood clot This view holds that injury to the blood vessel wall occurs first from some mechanical damage or physical condition, leading to rupture of small capillary blood vessels and formation of a blood clot or **thrombosis**. This physical injury may result from elevated blood pressure, chemical damage from cigarette smoking and resultant carbon monoxide in the blood, or from some mechanical trauma.

Genetic factors This view holds that genetic and environmental factors cause mutation of a single smooth muscle cell from near the side of the plaque, and the cells of the plaque are its offspring. The plaque is comparable, then, to a benign tumor of the artery wall. The same kinds of agents or conditions may be involved that transform cells and initiate cancers in a similar process.

Lipid disorder This view holds that serum lipids, especially serum cholesterol, are the chief cause of the plaque formation and thus of coronary heart disease. Since the fatty plaques involved in the underlying disease process consist mainly of lipid material, especially cholesterol crystals, much investigation has focused upon lipid metabolism. In this chapter we will look at this theory and review the basis for current nutritional therapy being used for persons with heart disease.

Relation to Lipid Metabolism

In the frustrating search for the cause of atherosclerosis, a number of nutrient factors have been investigated and have been found to have vary-

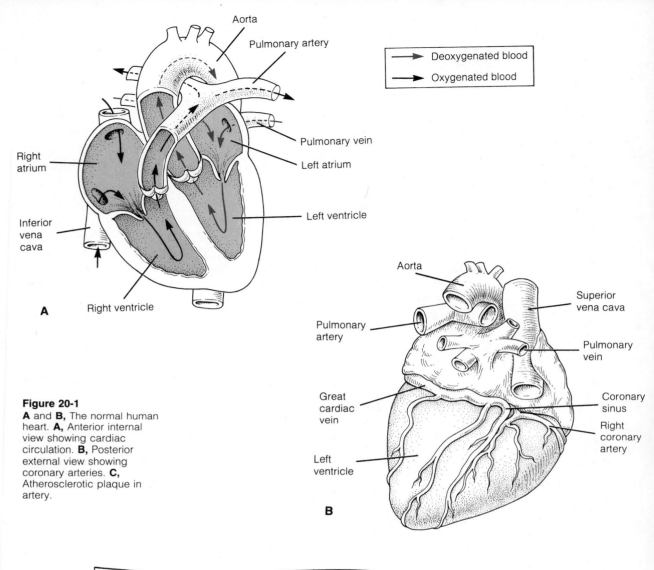

Deoxygenated blood

Oxygenated blood

A, Aorta, Pulmonary artery, Right atrium, Inferior vena cava, Pulmonary vein, Left atrium, Left ventricle, Right ventricle

B, Aorta, Pulmonary artery, Great cardiac vein, Left ventricle, Superior vena cava, Pulmonary vein, Coronary sinus, Right coronary artery

Figure 20-1
A and **B,** The normal human heart. **A,** Anterior internal view showing cardiac circulation. **B,** Posterior external view showing coronary arteries. **C,** Atherosclerotic plaque in artery.

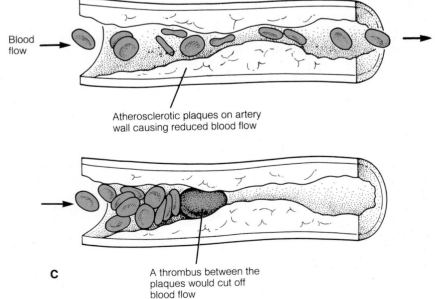

Blood flow

Atherosclerotic plaques on artery wall causing reduced blood flow

A thrombus between the plaques would cut off blood flow

C

ing associations with the disease process. Remember, however, that to demonstrate *association* is not to prove *cause*. Nevertheless, three lipid substances are involved in the disease process:

Dietary fat (triglycerides) A number of large-scale studies have shown a definite association between amount and types of dietary fat and elevated blood lipid levels.[2] This association has been repeatedly demonstrated.

Polyunsaturated A carbon chain containing more than one double bond.

Cholesterol Dietary substitution of foods high in **polyunsaturated** fatty acids for foods high in saturated fatty acids has produced a lowering of blood cholesterol. However, the significance of these lowered blood cholesterol levels in terms of the disease process is unclear.[3]

Lipoprotein Complex of lipids and protein carriers.

Lipoproteins Increased concentrations of certain **lipoproteins** in plasma have been associated in a number of studies with an increased risk of atherosclerotic heart and peripheral vascular disease. Lipoproteins are the major transport forms of lipids in the blood. An increase in one or more of these lipoproteins creates the condition **hyperlipoproteinemia**. A more general term referring to elevated blood lipids is *hyperlipidemia*.

Hyperlipoproteinemia Elevation of lipoproteins in the blood.

At this point, we do know several things about atherosclerosis: (1) it is a multiple-risk factor disease process (Table 20-1), (2) elevated serum cholesterol *is* one of the major risk factors for the disease process, and (3) dietary fat *can* affect serum cholesterol.

Table 20-1
Multiple Risk Factors in Cardiovascular Disease

Personal Characteristics (no control)	Learned Behaviors (intervene and change)	Background Conditions (screen-treat)
Sex	Stress/coping	Hypertension
Age	Smoking cigarettes	Diabetes mellitus
Family history	Sedentary life	Hyperlipidemia (especially
	Obesity	hypercholesterolemia)
	Food habits	
	Excess fat	
	Excess sugar	
	Excess salt	

Classes of Lipoproteins

The lipoproteins in the blood are produced mainly in two places: (1) *intestinal wall* after initial ingestion, digestion, and absorption of dietary fat from a meal and (2) *liver,* from endogenous fat sources. These endogenous lipoproteins carry fat and cholesterol to the tissues for use in energy production and for interchange with other products of cell metabolism. The lipoproteins are classified according to their fat content and thus their density.

Chylomicron Lowest density lipoprotein; contains the highest amount of fat, mainly triglycerides.

Lipoprotein lipase An enzyme that helps remove triglycerides from chylomicrons.

Chylomicrons Highest lipid content, lowest density, composed mostly of dietary triglycerides (TG), with a small amount of carrier protein. They accumulate in portal blood following a meal and are efficiently cleared from the blood by the specific enzyme, **lipoprotein lipase**.

Table 20-2
Characteristics of the Classes of Lipoproteins

Characteristic	Chylomicrons	Very Low Density (VLDL)	Intermediate Density (IDL)	Low Density (LDL)	High Density (HDL)
Composition					
Triglycerides (TG)	80%-95%; diet, exogenous	60%-80%; endogenous	40%; endogenous	10%-13%; endogenous	5%-10%; endogenous
Cholesterol	2%-7%	10%-15%	30%	45%-50%	20%
Phospholipid	3%-6%	15%-20%	20%	15%-22%	25%-30%
Protein	1%-2%	5%-10%	10%	20%-25%	45%-50%
Function	Transport dietary TG to plasma and tissues, cells	Transport endogenous TG to cells	Continue transport of endogenous TG to cells	Transport cholesterol to peripheral cells	Transport free cholesterol from membranes to liver for catabolism
Place of synthesis	Intestinal wall	Liver	Liver	Liver	Liver
Size, density					
Description	Largest, lightest	Next largest, lightest	Intermediate size, lighter	Smaller, heavier	Smallest, most dense, heaviest
Density	0.095	0.095-1.006	1.00-1.03	1.0191.063	1.063-1.210
Size in nanometers (nm)	75-100	30-80	25-40	10-20	7.5-10
Electrophoretic equivalent	Origin (nonmigrating)	Prebeta	Broad beta	Beta	Alpha

Very low–density lipoprotein (VLDL) A lipoprotein whose name is derived from its position in electrophoresis, a method used in analyzing lipoprotein fractions in the blood.

Intermediate-density lipoprotein (IDL) Lipoprotein that is approximately 30% cholesterol; it carries triglycerides to body cells.

Low-density lipoprotein (LDL) A lipoprotein that carries at least 66% of the total amount of cholesterol in plasma.

Familial hypercholesterolemia Presence of defective low-density lipoprotein (LDL) receptors, resulting in an increase in LDL-cholesterol.

Very low–density lipoproteins (VLDL) Still carry a large lipid (TG) content but include about 10% to 15% cholesterol. These lipoproteins are formed in the liver from endogenous fat sources.

Intermediate-density lipoproteins (IDL) Continue the delivery of endogenous triglycerides to cells and carries about 30% cholesterol.

Low-density lipoproteins (LDL) Carry in addition to other lipids about two thirds or more of the total plasma cholesterol. They are formed in the serum from catabolism of VLDL.

High-density lipoproteins (HDL) Carry less total lipid and more carrier protein. They are formed in the liver from endogenous fat sources. Since HDL carries cholesterol from the tissues to the liver for catabolism and excretion, higher serum levels are considered protective against cardiovascular disease. The "normal" (statistic) range for HDL-cholesterol is 30 to 80 mg/dl. Thus a value below 30 mg/dl implies significant risk, and a value of 75 or above contributes definite protection and decreased risk.

The characteristics of these classes of lipoproteins are summarized in Table 20-2. Note the comparative functions of LDL and HDL. Since LDL carries cholesterol to the peripheral cells, it contributes the "cholesterol of concern" in **familial hypercholesterolemia** (type II) and is a more valid measure of risk status than is the total cholesterol value.

Classification of Lipid Disorders

Lipid disorders have been classified traditionally in a descriptive typing system, but more currently they have been given a functional classification:

Traditional descriptive typing system An initial *descriptive* typing system for lipid disorders was proposed by Fredrickson and others:[4]

Type I	chylomicrons elevated, rare
Type IIa	LDL elevated, common
Type IIb	LDL and VLDL elevated, common
Type III	IDL elevated, uncommon
Type IV	VLDL elevated, common
Type V	LDL and chylomicrons elevated, uncommon

This descriptive classification is limited, however, and has not been accepted by all clinicians.[5]

Current functional classification Current research and practice has begun to concentrate on the protein fractions of the lipoprotein molecules and a more comprehensive *functional* classification has developed.[6,7] In comparison with the former descriptive typing system, it reveals two additional important factors: (1) increased recognition of the *genetic factors* involved and (2) increased focus on the role of *apoproteins* in the process of lipoprotein formation, transport, and destruction. The term **apoprotein** refers to the protein portion of a combined protein (from the Gr. **apo**, from). It is this apoprotein component that helps to form the special spheric droplets of lipid material for transportation in the blood stream (see p. 457). When lipoproteins are synthesized in the intestinal wall, the liver, and the serum, the protein component is made up of varying kinds of apoprotein parts. These apoproteins and their corresponding *apolipoproteins* have been identified. The class designations in current common use are apoprotein A, B, C, and E. In turn, each class consists of several different proteins, for example, A-I, -II, -III, and -IV and C-I, -II, -III. Table 20-3 lists these various classes of apoproteins associated with specific classes of lipoproteins. This current functional approach classes lipid disorders in four major groups based on the underlying functional problem: (1) defects in apolipoprotein synthesis, (2) enzyme deficiencies, (3) LDL-receptor deficiency, and (4) other inherited hyperlipidemias. The summary of these lipid disorders in Table 20-4 provides a review of the basic related conditions and nutritional therapies.

Apoprotein Protein part of a compound, such as a lipoprotein.

Apo- Prefix implying separation or being derivative from.

Table 20-3
Apoproteins in the Structure of Human Plasma Lipoproteins

Apoprotein	Related Lipoprotein	Functions
A-I	HDL, chylomicrons, intestinal VLDL	Activates the plasma enzyme lecithin-cholesterol acyltransferase (LCAT)
A-II	HDL	Transports HDL
A-III	Subfraction of HDL	Catalyzes transfer of cholesterol esters among lipoproteins
B	LDL, VLDL, IDL, chylomicrons, chylomicron remnants	Unclear
C-I	VLDL, HDL, chylomicrons	Activates LCAT
C-II	VLDL, HDL, chylomicrons	Activates lipoprotein lipase
C-III	VLDL, HDL, chylomicrons	Several different forms and functions, depending on structure
E (rich in arginine)	VLDL, HDL, chylomicrons, chylomicron remnants	Excess amount present in beta-VLDL of persons with type III hyperlipoproteinemia

Table 20-4
Functional Classification of Lipid Disorders

Type of Defect	Lipid Disorder	Abnormal Lipid Pattern	Clinical Characteristics	Nutritional Therapy	Corresponding Type in Former Descriptive Classification (Frederickson)
Defective synthesis of apolipoproteins	Apolipoprotein A deficiency	Decreased HDL Increased tissue cholesterol Decreased serum cholesterol Increased serum triglyceride (TG)	Rare Genetic Tangier disease	Low cholesterol Low fat	
	Apolipoprotein B deficiency	High mucosal tissue fat No lipoprotein synthesis possible	Rare Genetic Serious prognosis for child Malabsorption Steatorrhea	Very low fat	
	Apolipoprotein E deficiency	Increased chylomicron remnants Decreased serum LDL Increased cholesterol Increased TG	Relatively uncommon Genetic Xanthomas Premature atherosclerosis	Low cholesterol (<300 mg) Low saturated fat Increased substitution of polyunsaturated fat Weight reduction	Type III
Enzyme deficiency	Lipoprotein lipase deficiency	Increased chylomicrons	Rare Genetic Early childhood Abdominal pain (pancreatitis) Lipemia, retinalis Xanthomas Hepatosplenomegaly	Very low fat (20 g) High carbohydrate Medium-chain triglycerides (MCT)	Type I
	Lecithin-cholesterol acyltransferase (LCAT) deficiency	Overall abnormal lipid pattern: all lipoproteins have low amounts of cholesterol esters and high concentrations of free cholesterol and lecithin Accumulation of large LDL particles rich in unesterified cholesterol	Rare Genetic Abnormal cornea Anemia Kidney damage	Low cholesterol Low fat	
LDL-receptor deficiency	Familial hypercholesterolemia	Increased LDL Increased total cholesterol Increased VLDL	Common Genetic Increased atherosclerosis All ages Xanthomas	Low cholesterol (<300 mg) Low saturated fat Substitution of polyunsaturated fat	Type II

Table 20-4, cont'd
Functional Classification of Lipid Disorders

Type of Defect	Lipid Disorder	Abnormal Lipid Pattern	Clinical Characteristics	Nutritional Therapy	Corresponding Type in Former Descriptive Classification (Frederickson)
Other inherited hyperlipidemias	Familial hypertriglyceridemia	Increased VLDL Increased TG Increased cholesterol Sometimes increased blood sugar	Common Genetic Glucose intolerance Possible type II (noninsulin-dependent) diabetes mellitus Obesity Accelerated atherosclerosis	Weight reduction Low, simple carbohydrates Low saturated fat Low cholesterol	Type IV
	Familial multiple hyperlipoproteinemia	Increased VLDL Increased LDL	Fairly common Genetic Adult Xanthomas; vascular disease	Low cholesterol (<300 mg) Low saturated fat Substitution of polyunsaturated fat Weight reduction	Type IIb
	Familial type V hyperlipoproteinemia	Increased chylomicrons Increased VLDL Increased cholesterol Increased TG	Rare Glucose intolerance Obesity Abdominal pain (pancreatitis) Hepatosplenomegaly	Weight reduction Controlled carbohydrate and fat High protein	Type V

Nutritional Therapy—Fat-Controlled Diets

Two factors are of concern in a fat-controlled diet: (1) the total amount of fat in the diet and (2) the kind of fat used. These two principles are applied here in the generally used approach of the "prudent" food pattern, as originally proposed by the American Heart Association (Table 20-5).

Amount of Fat

Almost half the kilocalories of the average American's diet is contributed by fat. It is recommended currently that this amount be moderated to about 30% of the total kilocalories or lower.

Kind of Fat

About two thirds of the total fat in the American diet is of animal origin and therefore mainly saturated fat. The remaining one-third has come from vegetable sources and is mainly unsaturated fat. However, this ratio has gradually been changing over the past few years with the use of less animal and more plant fat.

The Prudent Diet

This changed ratio of dietary fat is the general goal of the prudent diet as indicated in Table 20-5. The fat-controlled diet reduces animal fat and

Table 20-5
The Prudent Diet as
Compared with the Usual
American Diet

	Prudent Diet	Usual American Diet
Total kilocalories	Sufficient to maintain ideal body weight	Often excessive for need
Cholesterol	300 mg	600-800 mg
Total fats (% of kilocalories)	30%-35%	40%-45%
Saturated	10% or less	15%-20%
Monounsaturated	15%	15%-20%
Polyunsaturated	10%	5%-6%
P/S ratio (polyunsaturated/saturated fat in the diet)	1-1.5 = 1	0.3 = 1
Carbohydrate (% of kilocalories)	50%-55%	40%-45%
Starch (complex CHO)	30%-35%	20%-25%
Simple sugars	10%	15%-20%
Proteins (% of total kilocalories)	12%-20%	12%-15%
Sodium	130 mEq	200-250 mEq

Polyunsaturated/saturated (P:S) ratio Ratio of polyunsaturated to saturated fat (fatty acids) in a diet.

uses plant fat instead. A simplified fat-controlled diet with emphasis on polyunsaturated fatty acids (PUFA) is the guideline, as illustrated here by the **polyunsaturated/saturated (P:S) ratio** for fats. When obesity is present, kilocalories are lowered.

The Problem of Acute Cardiovascular Disease

Objective—Cardiac Rest

In the initial acute phase of cardiovascular disease, a myocardial infarction or heart attack usually requires additional dietary modifications. The basic clinical objective is *cardiac rest.*

Nutritional Therapy

All care, including nutritional therapy, is directed toward ensuring that this requirement for cardiac rest is followed, so that the damaged heart may be restored to normal functioning. The diet therefore should be modified in *energy value* and *texture,* as well as being modified continually in fat and sodium.

Kilocalories A brief period of undernutrition during the first few days after the heart attack reduces the workload of the damaged heart. The metabolic demands for digestion, absorption, and metabolism of food require a generous cardiac output volume. Thus, to decrease the level of metabolic activity to one that the weakened heart can accommodate, small feedings are spread over the day. The patient can progress to more food as healing occurs. During the initial recovery stages, the diet may be limited to about 1200 to 1500 kcal to continue cardiac rest from metabolic workloads. Afterward, if the patient is obese, this kilocalorie level will continue to help the patient begin very gradually to lose excess weight.

Texture Early feedings should generally include foods soft in texture or easily digested to avoid excess effort in eating. Smaller meals served more frequently may give needed nutrition without undue strain or pressure. Temperature extremes in foods, both solids and liquids, should be avoided.

Fat The general "prudent" diet (Table 20-5) will control amount and kind of fat for most patient needs. If the patient has a diagnosed lipid disorder, additional specific modifications of lipid components such as cholesterol may be added according to individual needs. Previously prohibited foods such as eggs and shellfish may be used (see Issues and Answers, pp. 475-476).

Sodium General attention to a reduced sodium content in the foods selected is also emphasized. This will help control any tendency to fluid accumulation in the body tissues. Added tissue fluid requires more work from the heart to maintain an increased blood volume circulation.

The Problem of Chronic Heart Disease
Congestive Heart Failure

In chronic coronary heart disease a condition of *congestive heart failure* may develop over time. The progressively weakened heart muscle, the myocardium, is unable to maintain an adequate cardiac output to sustain normal blood circulation. The resulting fluid imbalances cause *edema*, especially **pulmonary edema**, to develop. This condition brings added problems in breathing and places more stress on the laboring heart.

Pulmonary edema Fluid accumulation in the lungs.

Cardiac Edema: Sodium and Water Metabolism

The fluid imbalances bringing on edema are caused by three events:

Imbalance in capillary fluid shift mechanism As the heart fails to pump out the returning blood fast enough, the venous return is retarded, and a disproportionate amount of blood accumulates in the vascular system that is concerned with the right side of the heart. As a result venous pressure rises, overcoming the balance of filtration pressures necessary to maintain the normal capillary fluid shift mechanism (see p. 172). This mechanism is the basic means of maintaining the normal flow of fluids throughout the body. Body fluids must travel from the blood vessels into the tissues to service the cells and then back into circulation in the vessels. As a result of the failure of the mechanism to operate properly in congestive heart failure, the fluid that normally would flow between the tissue spaces and the blood vessels is held in the tissue spaces, rather than being returned to circulation. This accumulation of fluid in the tissues is called *edema*.

Renin Enzyme secreted by the juxtaglomerular cells of the kidney.

Angiotensin Powerful vasopressor hormone and stimulator of the hormone aldosterone from the adrenal cortex.

Aldosterone Hormone secreted by the adrenal cortex to regulate sodium, potassium, and water balance.

Hormonal influences Two basic hormonal mechanisms that normally control water balance in the body actually contribute to the cardiac edema in congestive heart failure. These are the aldosterone and ADH mechanisms.

Aldosterone mechanism This mechanism, described more completely as the **renin-angiotensin-aldosterone** *mechanism* is a life-saving sodium- and, hence, water-conserving mechanism. However, in this instance it only compounds the edema problem. As the heart fails to propel the blood circulation forward, the deficient cardiac output effectively reduces the blood flow through the kidney nephrons. Increased renal blood pressure triggers the renin-angiotensin mechanism, which in turn causes the adrenals to produce aldosterone. Aldosterone is the hormone that causes the kidney tubules to reabsorb more sodium and, following it, water. As a result, still more water is held in the tissues.

ADH mechanism This water-conserving hormonal mechanism also adds to the edema. The cardiac stress and the reduced renal flow cause the release of the **antidiuretic hormone (ADH)**, also known as **vasopressin**, from the pituitary gland. This hormone stimulates still more water reabsorption in the nephrons of the kidney.

Increased free-cell potassium As the reduced blood circulation depresses cell metabolism, cell protein is broken down and releases its bound potassium in the cell. As a result, the amount of free potassium is increased inside the cell, which increases osmotic pressure. Sodium ions in the fluid surrounding the cell then also increase in number to balance the increase within the cell and hence prevent cell dehydration. The larger amount of sodium in time eventually causes still more water retention.

Nutritional Therapy—Sodium-Restricted Diet

Because of the role of sodium in water balance, the diet used to treat cardiac edema restricts the sodium intake. Four levels of dietary sodium restriction have been outlined by the American Heart Association. Three of these are in common use; one is too severely restricted to be realistic or useful. Compare these levels with sodium in the general diet.

Sodium in the General Diet

The taste for salt is an acquired one. Some persons salt food heavily and habituate their taste to high salt levels. Others acquire a taste for less salt and use smaller amounts. Common daily adult intakes of sodium range widely, according to habit, from about 3 to 4 g to as high as 10 to 12 g with heavy use.

Levels of Sodium-Restricted Diets

The main source of dietary sodium is common table salt—sodium chloride. Many other lesser-used sodium compounds, such as baking powder and baking soda, and especially the large amount of sodium compounds in processed foods, contribute additional amounts. Thus the label "salt free" does not mean "sodium free," nor does "low salt" mean "low sodium." The remaining dietary source of sodium is the naturally occurring sodium in certain foods as one of its minerals. The four levels of sodium-restricted diets increasingly delete food items or ways of food preparation that involve sodium:

Mild sodium restriction (2 to 3 g) Salt may be used *lightly* in cooking, assuming use of fresh foods, but *no added salt* is allowed. In some hospitals, this diet level is often called "no added salt" (NAS) and ordered as such. But this is a less helpful generalized label since an increasing amount of salt is already in frozen convenience foods as processed and purchased for hospital menus and each such item must be evaluated individually. Obviously salty foods in which salt has been used as a preservative or a flavoring agent are omitted. These foods would include such items as pickles, olives, bacon, ham, and potato chips. A general deletion list for mild sodium restriction is shown in the box opposite.

Antidiuretic hormone (ADH) Hormone produced by the pituitary to reduce urine formation.

Vasopressin Hormone secreted by the hypothalamus to stimulate muscular contraction, raise blood pressure, and concentrate urine.

Table salt—sodium chloride (NaC1)—is about 40% (actually 39.34%) sodium (Na).

Restrictions for a Mild Low-Sodium Diet (2 to 3 g sodium)

Do not use

- Salt at the table (use salt lightly in cooking)
- Salt-preserved foods such as salted or smoked meat (bacon and bacon fat, bologna, dried or chipped beef, corned beef, frankfurters, ham, kosher meats, luncheon meats, salt pork, sausage, smoked tongue); salted or smoked fish (anchovies, caviar, salted and dried cod, herring, sardines), sauerkraut, olives
- Highly salted foods such as crackers, pretzels, potato chips, corn chips, salted nuts, salted popcorn
- Spices and condiments such as bouillon cubes,* catsup,* chili sauce,* celery salt, garlic sauce, onion salt, monosodium glutamate, meat sauces, meat tenderizers,* pickles, prepared mustard, relishes, Worcestershire sauce, soy sauce
- Cheese,* peanut butter*

*Dietetic low-sodium kinds may be used.

Moderate sodium restriction (1000 mg) There is no salt used in cooking, no added salt, and no salty foods. Beginning with this level some control of natural sodium foods is instituted. Vegetables that are higher in sodium are limited in use, salt-free canned vegetables are substituted for regular canned ones, salt-free baked products are used, and meat and milk are used in only moderate portions. A general deletion list for moderate sodium restriction is shown the box below.

Restrictions for a Moderate Low-Sodium Diet (1000 mg sodium)

Do not use

- Salt in cooking or at the table
- Salt-preserved foods such as salted or smoked meat (bacon and bacon fat, bologna, dried or chipped beef, brains, corned beef, frankfurters, ham, kosher meats, luncheon meats, salt pork, sausage, smoked tongue, kidneys), salted or smoked fish (anchovies, caviar, salted and dried cod, herring, sardines, frozen fish fillets, canned salmon,* tuna*), sauerkraut, olives
- Highly salted foods such as crackers, pretzels, potato chips, corn chips, salted nuts, salted popcorn
- Spices and condiments such as bouillon cubes,* catsup,* chili sauce,* celery salt, garlic salt, onion salt, monosodium glutamate, meat sauces, meat tenderizers,* pickles, prepared mustard, relishes, Worcestershire sauce, soy sauce
- Cheese,* peanut butter*
- Buttermilk (unsalted buttermilk may be used) instead of skim milk
- Canned vegetables* or canned vegetable juices*
- Frozen peas, frozen limas, frozen mixed vegetables, or any frozen vegetables to which salt has been added
- More than one serving of any of these vegetables in one day—artichokes, beet greens, beets, carrots, celery, dandelion greens, kale, mustard greens, spinach, Swiss chard, turnips (white)
- Regular bread, rolls,* crackers*
- Dry cereals,* except puffed rice, puffed wheat, and shredded wheat
- Quick-cooking Cream of Wheat
- Shellfish (clams, crab, lobster, shrimp); oysters may be used
- Salted butter, salted margarine, commercial French dressings,* mayonnaise,* or other salad dressings*
- Regular baking powder,* baking soda or anything containing them; self-rising flour
- Prepared mixes (pudding,* gelatin,* cake, biscuit)
- Commercial candies

*Dietetic low-sodium kinds may be used.

Restrictions for a Strict Low-Sodium Diet (500 mg sodium)

Do not use

- Salt in cooking or at the table
- Salt-preserved foods such as salted or smoked meat (bacon and bacon fat, bologna, dried or chipped beef, brains, corned beef, frankfurters, ham, kosher meats, luncheon meats, salt pork, sausage, smoked tongue, kidneys), salted or smoked fish (anchovies, caviar, salted and dried cod, herring, sardines, frozen fish fillets, canned salmon,* tuna*), sauerkraut, olives
- Highly salted foods such as crackers, pretzels, potato chips, corn chips, salted nuts, salted popcorn
- Spices and condiments such as bouillon cubes,* catsup,* chili sauce,* celery salt, garlic salt, onion salt, monosodium glutamate (MSG, Accent, and so on), meat sauces, meat tenderizers,* pickles, prepared mustard, relishes, Worcestershire sauce, soy sauce
- Cheese,* peanut butter*
- Buttermilk (unsalted buttermilk may be used) instead of skim milk
- More than 2 cups skim milk a day, including that used on cereal
- Any commercial foods made of milk (ice cream, ice milk, milk shakes)
- Canned vegetables* or canned vegetable juices*
- Frozen peas, frozen limas, frozen mixed vegetables, or any frozen vegetables to which salt has been added
- Artichokes, beet greens, beets, carrots, celery, dandelion greens, kale, mustard greens, spinach, Swiss chard, turnips (white)
- Regular bread,* rolls,* crackers*
- Dry cereals,* except puffed rice, puffed wheat, and shredded wheat
- Quick-cooking Cream of Wheat
- Shellfish (clams, crab, lobster, shrimp); oysters may be used
- Salted butter, salted margarine, commercial French dressings,* mayonnaise,* or other salad dressings*
- Regular baking powder,* baking soda or anything containing them; self-rising flour
- Prepared mixes (pudding,* gelatin,* cake, biscuit)
- Commercial candies

*Dietetic low-sodium kinds may be used.

Sodium restricted diets: Conversion of mg to mEq
Equivalent weight (Eq) of an element equals its atomic weight or gram-molecular weight (mol wt) divided by its valence. (Consult the periodic table of elements in any chemistry book for atomic weights and valences.) Thus for sodium (Na) and potassium (K):

$$1 \text{ Eq Na} = \frac{23 \text{ g (mol wt of Na)}}{1 \text{ (valence of Na)}} = 23 \text{ g}$$

or

$$1 \text{ mEq Na} = 23 \text{ mg}$$

$$1 \text{ Eq K} = \frac{39 \text{ g (mol wt of K)}}{1 \text{ (valence of K)}} = 39 \text{ g}$$

or

$$1 \text{ mEq K} = 39 \text{ mg}$$

Essential Hypertension

Essential hypertension High blood pressure of unknown cause.

Strict sodium restriction (500 mg) In addition to the deletions thus far, meat, milk, and eggs are used in smaller portions. Milk is limited to two cups total in any form, meat to 5 or 6 ounces total daily, and eggs to no more than one. Vegetables with higher sodium content are deleted. A general deletion list for strict sodium restriction is shown in the box above.

Severe sodium restriction (250 mg) This level is too restrictive to be nutritionally adequate, realistic, or helpful and is rarely used, if at all. No regular milk is used; low-sodium milk is substituted. Meat is limited to 2 to 4 ounces a day, and eggs are limited to about 3 a week.

The Problem of Hypertension

Incidence

High blood pressure presents a problem in the lives of some 60 million Americans. At least 95% of these persons have **essential hypertension,** meaning that its cause is unknown. It has become the fourth largest public health problem in America. It carries no overt signs and has potentially serious implications if not treated and controlled. Both treatment and control can be accomplished. However, despite a wealth of research in past years, there are few clues to its cause and our lack of information leaves us more confused than enlightened.

Public Awareness

In the past few years, two major events have stimulated increased research interest and public concern about hypertension. First, the National Heart, Lung, and Blood Institute of the National Institutes of Health conducted an educational campaign through the National High Blood Pressure Education Program to inform Americans about the serious problem of hypertension. But this effort reached only a limited number of persons and many others remain uninformed and untreated. Nonetheless, it was a significant stimulus to needed work. Second, clinical trials of the Hypertension Detection and Follow-up Program clearly demonstrated high blood pressure can effectively be treated, even in its milder forms.[8] In this study the intensive treatment plan generally lowered mortality by 17% when compared to a "regular care" approach. In a mild hypertensive group, with diastolic pressure 90 to 104 mm Hg, the mortality reduction rate was 20%.

Nondrug Approaches

A significant result of these studies has been a renewed focus on nonpharmacologic approaches to the control of hypertension, and the U.S. National Heart, Lung, and Blood Institute has increased its emphasis on nondrug therapies.[9] The report urged that these therapies, such as diet, exercise, and behavior modification, be "pursued aggressively" in treating not only mild hypertension but also as an important adjunct in more severe cases. The goal of all therapies is to reduce as much as possible the quantity of drugs required. Thus nutritional therapy has a fundamental role in the care of persons with hypertension.

Blood Pressure Controls
Arterial Pressure

Systolic Referring to the heart's period of contraction.

Diastolic Referring to the heart's period of dilation; the "relaxation" phase of the heartbeat.

As commonly measured, blood pressure is an indication of the arterial pressure in the vessels of the upper arm. This measure is obtained by an instrument for determining the force of the pulse, a *sphygmomanometer*. The upper figure recorded is the **systolic** pressure from the contraction of the heart muscle. The lower figure recorded is the **diastolic** pressure, produced during the relaxation phase of the cardiac cycle. Thus the upper limit of a normal adult blood pressure would be recorded 150/89. Several factors contribute to maintaining the fluid dynamics of normal blood pressure: (1) increased pressure on the forward blood flow, (2) increased resistance from the containing blood vessels, and (3) increased viscosity of the blood itself, making movement through the vessels more difficult. Of these factors, increased blood viscosity is a rare event. Thus in discussing high blood pressure in general terms, we are dealing with the first two factors, the pumping pressure of the heart muscle propelling the blood forward and the resistance to its forward flow presented by the blood vessel walls.

Muscle Tone of Blood Vessel Walls

In hypertension the body's finely tuned mechanisms to maintain fluid dynamics are not operating effectively. Normally, these systems include several agents that act to variously dilate and constrict the blood vessels to meet whatever need is present at a given time. In a hypertensive person, however, the dilation or constriction of blood vessels does not occur in its normal manner. If not effectively treated, uncontrolled elevated blood pressure results. The body systems that operate to help maintain normal blood pressure include: (1) neuroendocrine functions of the sympathetic nervous system, (2) hormonal systems such as the renin-angiotensin-aldosterone effect, and (3) enzyme systems which control materials that act to dilate or contrict smooth muscle as needed.[10]

Step-Care Treatment Approach

Based on the national studies indicated and widespread community screening programs, current medical treatment centers on an improved "step-care" method of identifying types of blood pressure levels and matching standard treatment programs to these diagnosed types. Increased emphasis is given to nondrug therapies and to limited use of drugs. The identification of patients with hypertension according to degree of severity has improved the basic approach to care. These steps of care are termed mild, moderate, or severe:

Mild hypertension Diastolic pressure is 90 to 104 mm Hg in this mild form. Initial consideration is given to other risk factors such as weight or stress. Individual treatment is initiated using nondrug approaches and centers on nutritional therapies of weight loss, sodium restriction, and behavioral techniques.

Moderate hypertension Diastolic pressure is 105 to 119 mm Hg with moderate hypertension. Prompt evaluation and treatment is indicated. A combination of drugs may be used: (1) a diuretic agent to decrease the blood volume and (2) a blocking agent to decrease muscle constriction of blood vessel walls. The basic nutritional therapy already outlined serves as support, with the goal of reducing the quantity of medication required.

Severe hypertension Diastolic pressure is 120 to 130 mm Hg and above. Immediate evaluation and vigorous drug therapy is demanded. Diuretic and beta-blocker agents are continued and a third drug may be added, a peripheral vasodilator to assist in reducing arterial resistance to blood flow. In all cases the implications for diet therapy revolve around potassium replacement and the use of diuretics and nutritional support for weight management and sodium modification. In addition to supportive nutritional therapy, additional nondrug therapies include physical exercise and stress reduction activities, such as biofeedback and meditation.

Principles of Nutritional Therapy

There is no question that nutritional therapy plays a large role in the treatment of hypertension, although some controversy centers on the restriction of sodium.[11] In general, however, the focus of current nutritional therapy is on weight management, sodium control, general nutrient balance, and an individualized food plan.

Weight Management

Body weight reflects the individual's energy balance. The energy input in food is balanced with the energy output in physical activity, with a desirable lean weight maintenance reflecting this balance. In practice weight management is not quite this simple. But because the overweight state has been closely associated with hypertension risk factors, a careful and wisely planned individualized program of weight reduction is a cornerstone of therapy (see Chapter 15).

Sodium Control

At present the prevailing concensus is that some measure of sodium control is indicated for persons with hypertension.[12] Recent studies have shown that sodium restriction accompanied by weight reduction can effectively control mild or moderate arterial pressures.[9] Generally two of the sodium restriction levels recommended by the AHA are used for hypertensive patients: the mild 2 g and the moderate 1 g levels (see p. 465).

General Nutrient Balance

Other nutrient factors are involved in planning the diet for hypertensive patients. These include other minerals and the ratio of the energy nutrients.

Other minerals In addition to sodium control, adequate intakes of two other minerals have been discussed in relation to elevated blood pressure. These are *potassium* and *calcium*. As sodium's balancing electrolyte partner, potassium is also involved in the hypertensive process in patients at risk. The renin-angiotensin-aldosterone mechanism (see p. 172) affects both sodium and potassium balance. It operates to reabsorb sodium in a direct ion exchange with potassium and thus tends to produce a low-potassium state. This factor, together with a low-potassium intake, contributes to the development of hypertension in susceptible individuals. Recent studies, though controversial, have suggested that inadequate calcium intake in susceptible individuals also promotes hypertension, because of a defect in the sodium-calcium exchange system through which calcium enters the cell when sodium leaves it.[13,14]

Ratio of energy nutrients The ratio of protein, carbohydrate, and fat in the overall diet for the person with hypertension is an important consideration. Since all three of these nutrients contribute kilocalories, they are important in the overall goal of weight management. The relative ratio suggested by the U.S. Dietary Goals provides a reasonable basis for distributing the total kilocalories in the diet among these three nutrients: 1. *Carbohydrates* should have the largest allowance, 50% to 55% of the total kilocalories, with a large portion of complex carbohydrate. 2. *Protein* should make up about 15% to 20%, with monitoring of excess protein intake, which usually carries animal fat with it. 3. *Fat* should be modified to take up only 25% to 30% of the total kilocalories, with emphasis on unsaturated fat. Some extreme diets may actually provide too little fat—10% or less.

Food Plan

A realistic and effective individual food plan must provide clients with assistance and guidance in food preparation and selection of food products.

Food preparation Reliance on potassium-based salt substitutes or products containing them is unwise, nor is the result particularly palatable.

Clinical Application

**The Spice of Life:
Breaking Up the
Salt Monopoly**

If you counsel with persons on sodium-restricted diets, you probably spend a lot of time answering the question, "Is there life without salt?" To which the standard reply is something like, "Of course there is. You'll just have to get used to the natural flavor of foods." This answer usually falls flat.

We learn to like the taste of salt. It is a taste that "accumulates" over the years. That's why it's unreasonable, for example, to expect a middle-aged man who has just discovered he has hypertension to suddenly give up the seasoning habits of a lifetime. It's overly optimistic to expect anyone raised on hot dogs, potato chips, and TV dinners to fall in love with the flavor of fresh broccoli overnight. There is hope, however. Subjects in one study developed a lower tolerance for salty foods after following a low sodium diet for 5 months. So if you can convince clients to reduce their salt intake for a significant period of time, you might get them to fall out of love with the taste of salt.

There is still the problem of getting clients to use less salt to begin with. Answer: introduce them to the world of salt-free seasonings. Some persons are already familiar with a variety of alternative seasonings and only need some recipes that show how to use them creatively. Others think that gourmet cooking means just using pepper instead of salt. These individuals need a little extra help in selecting and using salt-free seasonings successfully. Here are some suggestions for guidelines:

- Stop adding salt at the table. It's pure habit. Get rid of the shaker—throw it away, hide it, or get it out of sight—anything to remove the reminder.
- If foods taste too fresh without added salt, sprinkle them with fresh lemon juice—not salt.
- When cooking, cut the amount of salt in the recipe in half and avoid other sodium-rich seasonings.
- If you're already a good cook, or even if you're not, refer to guides for hints on spicing up old favorites without salt.
- If you're not the world's greatest chef, enroll in a basic cooking class at a local adult education center or community college and use these guidelines when preparing meals at home. You may also want to check the Foods section of your local newspaper for listings of special low-sodium cooking classes offered by local health organizations.
- Relax for a moment while dinner is simmering on the stove and enjoy the wonderful new aromas filling your kitchen. Sodium reduction can introduce you to a flavorful new adventure with food.

References
Bertino, M., Beauchamp, G.K., and Engleman, K., Long-term reduction in dietary sodium alters the taste of salt, Am. J. Clin. Nutr. **36**:1134, 1982.
Wylie-Rossett, J., Spices to the rescue, Prof. Nutr. **14**:4, 1982.

Numerous guides for good preparation of primary foods with alternative seasonings to salt are available, as summarized in the salt-free food guides in the Appendix. A variety of condiments (avoiding high-sodium ones) and such flavor aides as herbs, spices, lemon, wine, onion, and garlic can help train the taste for less salt (see box, p. 470). A reduced use of higher-sodium soft drinks and mineral waters (see Appendixes, E and F), as well as other processed foods, will eliminate still more salt.

Food products Close attention to food product labeling is important in a person's effort to control sodium. Current labeling regulations, although not perfect, do provide additional information for the consumer who wishes to control sodium and other food additives. The food industry has responded to current consumer and FDA concerns about the sodium content of food products and is providing needed information.

Special needs Individual adaptation of nutritional therapy principles is fundamental to all nutrition counseling. In particular special attention should be given to those types of ethnic diets, such as the Chinese, that are traditionally high in sodium.[15] Guidelines have been prepared to assist in counseling with such clients.[12]

Education and Prevention

Effective education for preventing hypertension-related health problems such as coronary heart disease must start early, focus on high-risk groups, and use a variety of resources.

Start Early

Prevention of hypertension begins in childhood, especially with children of high-risk families. With close attention to meeting general growth needs, some preventive measures related to weight control and avoidance of high-sodium food habits should be included. Prevention in childhood, when food habits are developing, is easier than trying to change adult habits that have become entrenched. In these developmental years families can build sound health habits with a general focus on good nutrition, including attention to food behaviors related to fat, sugar, and salt and promotion of a physically active life. Also, for adults with heart disease, learning should be an integral part of therapy. For example, for the adult hospitalized with myocardial infarction learning should not begin with so-called discharge instructions. Such a process fails to build sound knowledge for personal decision-making or to provide stress-reducing support. Rather the learning process should begin early in convalescence to give the patient and family a clear knowledge of positive needs. It should focus on positive behavior changes, to reinforce sound self-care within the limits of individual capacity and avoid the negative anxiety of a "cardiac cripple."

Focus on High-Risk Groups

Real contributions can be made by support learning in families with strong histories of familial lipid disorders (see p. 460). Hypertension has been closely associated with certain high-risk groups—including Black Americans, persons with a family history of hypertension, and those who are obese. Education concerning the risks of hypertension and coronary heart disease should be directed particularly to persons in these groups.

Use a Variety of Resources

Many excellent resources for individual and family patient education are provided by the American Heart Association (AHA) through their national and regional offices. Practical discussions need to center on such aspects as food buying and preparation to make the diets palatable and enjoyable. Explore your own community to discover agencies, programs, and materials that provide broad resources on hypertension and heart disease. In addition to the AHA, a number of resource persons and programs may be found in most communities to assist persons with hypertension in planning a program of care. These include various weight management programs, registered dietitians in private practice or in health care centers who provide nutritional counseling, and a number of special cookbooks and cooking classes creatively designed to develop kilocalorie- and sodium-controlled cuisines. Low-sodium cooking guides and informational materials may also be obtained in public bookstores and libraries. Community screening programs sponsored by industry provide educational guidance for employees. Local health care centers teach hypertension clients and their families self-blood–pressure monitoring skills so they may assume more control in managing their own health.

To Sum Up

Coronary heart disease remains the leading cause of death in the United States. *Atherosclerosis,* its underlying pathology, involves the formation of plaque, a fatty substance that builds up along the interior surfaces of blood vessels, interfering with blood flow and damaging blood vessels. If this buildup becomes severe, it cuts off supplies of oxygen and nutrients to tissue cells, which in turn begin to die. When this occurs in a coronary artery, the result is a *myocardial infarction,* or heart attack.

The risk for atherosclerosis increases with the amount and type of blood lipids (lipoproteins) available. There is increasing evidence that the *apoprotein* portion of lipoproteins may be as important a factor as the lipid components in the disease process. Elevated *serum cholesterol* is also considered to be a risk factor in atherosclerotic development.

Dietary recommendations for acute *cardiovascular disease* (heart attack) include caloric restriction, soft-texture foods, and small, frequent meals to reduce the demands of digestion, absorption, and metabolism of foods and to achieve ideal body weight. Also fat, saturated fat, cholesterol, and sodium should be restricted. Persons with chronic *coronary heart disease* and *hypertension* benefit from weight control, exercise, and sodium restriction to overcome cardiac edema and help control elevated blood pressure.

Current dietary recommendations to help prevent coronary heart disease involve reducing weight, limiting fats to 25% to 30% of all kilocalories, increasing the ratio of polyunsaturated fats, limiting sodium intake to 2 to 3 g per day, and increasing exercise.

Questions for Review

1. Which types of hyperlipoproteinemia occur most often? Identify the lipids that are elevated in each case, as well as predisposing factors. Describe the types of diet recommended for each.
2. Identify four dietary recommendations that should be made for the patient with a heart attack. Describe how each recommendation helps recovery.
3. Discuss the four levels of sodium restriction, describing general food choices and preparation methods.
4. What dietary changes could the average American make to reduce saturated fats and to substitute polyunsaturated fats?
5. What does the term *essential hypertension* mean? Why would weight management and sodium restriction contribute to its control? What other nutrient factors may be involved in hypertension?

References

1. Crooke, M.B.: Diet lipids and coronary heart disease—proof or prudence, J. NZ Dietet. Assoc. **36**(1):8, 1982.
2. Gordon, D.J., and others: Dietary determinants of plasma cholesterol change in the recruitment phase of the Lipid Research Clinics Coronary Primary Prevention Trail, Arteriosclerosis **2**(6):537, 1982.
3. Vessby, B., Lithell, H., and Boberg, J.: Will serum lipid lowering treatment reduce the incidence of coronary heart disease? Artery **9**(5):372, 1981.
4. Frederickson, D.S., and others: Dietary management of hyperlipoproteinemia, DHEW Pub. No. (NIH) 76-110, Washington, D.C., 1975.
5. Grouse, L.D.: A medical misdemeanor: I harbored evil thoughts about the Frederickson fat classification, JAMA **244**:2090, 1980.
6. Maciejko, J.J., and others: Apolipoprotein A-1 as a marker of angiographically assessed coronary-artery disease, N. Engl. J. Med. **309**(7):385, 1983.
7. Kolata, G.: Cholesterol-heart disease link illuminated, Science **221**(4616):1164, 1983.
8. Friedwald, W.T.: Current nutrition issues in hypertension, J. Am. Dietet. Assoc. **80**(1):17, 1982.
9. Dunstand, H.: NHLB-HTN New NIH report, Arch. Int. Med. **144**:1045, 1984.
10. Frohlich, E.D.: Physiological observations in essential hypertension, J. Am. Dietet. Assoc. **80**(1):18, 1982.
11. Wilber, J.A.: The role of diet in the treatment of high blood pressure, J. Am. Dietet. Assoc. **80**(1):25, 1982.
12. Stamler, J., and others: Prevention and control of hypertension by nutritional-hygienic means, J. Am. Dietet. Assoc. **243**(18):1819, 1980.
13. McCarron, D.A.: Low serum concentration of ionized calcium in patients with hypertension, N. Engl. J. Med. **307**:226, 1982.
14. McCarron, D.A., Morris, C.D., and Cole, C.: Dietary calcium in human hypertension, Science **217**:267, 1982.
15. Chew, T.: Sodium values of Chinese condiments and their use in sodium-restricted diets, J. Am. Dietet. Assoc. **82**(4):397, 1983.

Further readings

Friedwald, W.T., ed.: Current nutrition issues in hypertension, J. Am. Diet. Assoc. **80**(1):17, 1982.

Entire issue presents "state of the science" from hypertension's physiology to sodium in food processing. Good background reading with many charts, tables, references.

Kris-Etherton, P.M., and others: Teaching principles and cost of sodium-restricted diets. J. Am. Dietet. Assoc., **80**(1):55, 1982.

Report of class project—planning, teaching, and evaluating a community class on salt-free diets. Tables include alternative seasonings, sample menus, and costs.

Morisky, D.E., and others: Five-year blood pressure control and mortality following health education for hypertensive patients, Am. J. Pub. Health **73**(2):153, 1983.

This study demonstrates the effectiveness of a continuing patient education program, based on needs assessment, in a high-risk population of urban poor hypertensive patients.

Shank, F.R., and others: Perspective of Food and Drug Administration on dietary sodium, J. Am. Dietet. Assoc. **80**(1):29, 1982.

FDA scientists review the various initiatives of this federal agency to monitor the sodium content of the national food supply: information includes both sodium and potassium intakes of Americans and regulatory actions of FDA related to sodium and potassium content of our food supply.

Wilber, J.A.: The role of diet in the treatment of high blood pressure, J. Am. Diet. Assoc. **80**(1):25, 1982.

Good review of medical treatment of hypertension and common types of diuretics used. Emphasizes role of nutrition professionals and other health team members in all successful programs of control.

Issues and Answers

Recent Risk-Factor Findings

Recent research findings regarding "old" and "new" risk factors for coronary heart disease may affect the advice you give clients about details regarding foods. Some formerly "forbidden" items have been given a reprieve and others need even stricter control.

Relax About These Items

Eggs Eggs are no longer considered a major risk factor in heart disease. Many individuals with heart disease have given up eggs to keep their cholesterol levels low. Even healthy individuals stay away from this food to avoid "heart trouble." Eggs gained the reputation of being enemies of good health because of their high cholesterol content—approximately 250 mg/yolk. Studies have shown that eating large amounts of eggs can raise cholesterol levels under controlled conditions. However, in free-living conditions, the intake is much more moderate (about 3/week) and doesn't affect cholesterol levels.

The fear of eggs has been based partially on misinformation, or worse, "semi-information" about heart disease that focuses on dietary cholesterol as the main culprit. The truth is that cholesterol alone is not a risk factor for many people. It is a high-risk factor for persons who have the genes for the risk, which is only about 15% to 25% of the American public. Moreover, food intake alone is not the only risk factor in heart disease. So, give eggs a break. No single food should ever be so maligned for causing a health problem—short of allergies, metabolic intolerances, or poisoning. Instead of eliminating eggs, discuss *all* of the sources of cholesterol in each individual's diet. Help each client develop a personal meal plan low in cholesterol as well as saturated fats, to reduce the risk of developing atherosclerotic plaques.

Shellfish It is also now "safe" to include shrimp, crab, and other edible crustaceans to a low cholesterol diet. These foods were assigned high cholesterol levels in the 1940s when the analysis techniques were still very crude. More efficient methods now indicate that the cholesterol level of the oyster, for example, has "dropped" from about 200 mg/3½ oz to 50 mg. With these new findings, plus a knowledge that shellfish are rich in polyunsaturated fats, you can now reassure shrimp-loving clients that their favorite seafood is no longer taboo.

Milk Have your milk-loving clients stated that they would rather give up their favorite beverage than switch to skim? Some of them may not have to. A 1982 report on the effects of whole, low-fat (2% butterfat) milk, skim fluid milk, and fermented milks in the forms of yogurt, buttermilk, and sweet acidophilus milk indicated that none of these milk products affected serum lipids in 68 healthy persons. Only yogurt resulted in a small rise in triglyceride levels. The study did show, however, that skim milk had the greatest cholesterol-lowering effect. With this in mind, you will want to advise high-risk clients

Continued.

Issues and Answers—cont'd

with heart disease to make the switch to skim. Clients with normal blood lipid levels who are concerned mainly with prevention could be told that moderate use of whole milk probably won't increase their chances of developing disease.

Tighten Control of These Items

Coffee Heavy coffee-drinking *does* have an effect on blood cholesterol levels. It also disrupts normal heart rhythms. Serious effects have been seen even in healthy persons after drinking nine or more cups of coffee or tea a day. These same affects were seen in patients with a history of abnormal heart rhythms after only two cups. The basic recommendation is that persons with coronary heart disease should avoid caffeine. Clients concerned with prevention should be advised to reduce their intake as much as possible.

Alcohol Several studies have indicated that a moderate alcohol intake raises HDL-cholesterol levels, which in turn reduces the risk of developing atherosclerotic plaque. However, in animal studies, it was found that taking large amounts of alcohol over an 18-month period interrupts heart rhythms. You may advise clients who want to drink to do so in moderation. Few problems have been found in research subjects drinking less than 6 oz/day of a light beverage alcohol such as beer or wine.

Cigarettes Cigarette smokers have lower HDL-cholesterol levels than nonsmokers, even when their body weight is lower. Strongly urge individuals at risk to quite smoking. Some clients will benefit from a referral to a local Heart Association or other health agency to join an education or behavior modification group.

References

Dawber, T.R., and others: Eggs, serum cholesterol, and coronary heart disease, Am. J. Clin. Nutr. **36**(4):617, 1982.

Dobmeyer, D.L., and others: The arrhythmogenic effects of caffeine in human beings, N. Engl. J. Med. **308**(38):814, 1983.

Gordon, T., and others: Alcohol and high-density lipoprotein cholesterol, Circulation **64**(suppl. III):63, 1981.

Hjermann, I., and others: Effect of diet and smoking intervention on the incidence of coronary heart disease: Lancet **2**(8259):1303, 1981.

Marano, H.E.: Cholesterol: shellfish off the hook, Am. Health **2**(2):28, 1983.

Rodgers, J.: Cholesterol: eggs-onerated? Am. Health **2**(4):28, 1983.

Thompson, L.U., and others: The effect of fermented and unfermented milks on serum cholesterol, Am. J. Clin. Nutr. **36**:1106, 1982.

Chapter 21
Renal Disease

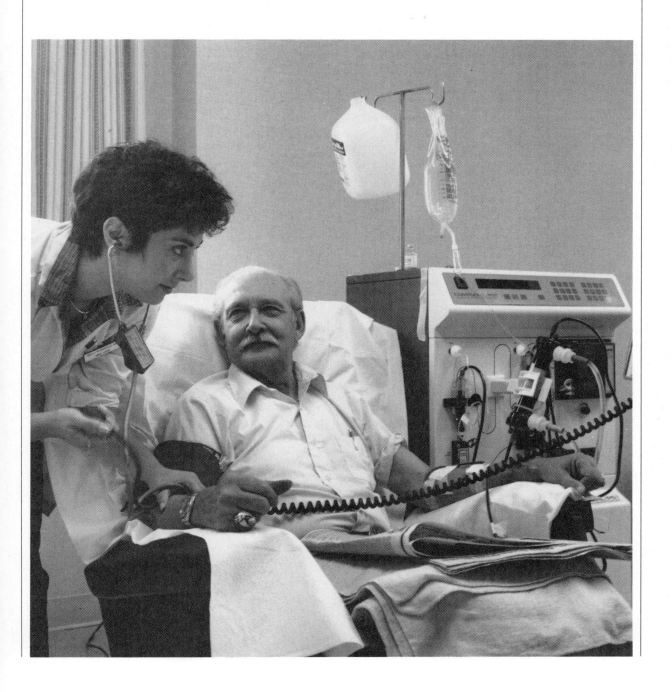

Preview

Kidney diseases affect the lives of more than 8 million Americans and kill 60,000 a year. Another 3 million or more have related infections, many of which go undetected. In all, these kidney problems are a leading cause of lost work time and pay. They are the fourth leading health problem in America.

The recent advent of renal dialysis technology and kidney transplant techniques have prolonged the lives of the 50,000 persons in the United States today who develop kidney failure each year. This survival is not without human and monetary cost. A scarcity of organ donors and rejection problems continue to plague successful transplant surgery. Also, time-consuming dialysis, although life extending, exacts an emotional and physical toll on persons with irreversible chronic renal failure. The treatment costs American taxpayers some $1.4 billion each year via Medicare. Thus although kidney disease may not be considered as much a killer as heart disease or cancer, it is still a serious national and personal health problem.

Chapter Objectives

After study of this chapter, the student should be able to:

1. Identify dietary factors that contribute to basic tissue changes in long-standing renal disease and describe the nature of these changes.

2. Compare nutritional care of patients with glomerulonephritis and nephrosis in terms of disease process, renal function, and diet modifications.

3. Describe the effects of changes in renal function that accompany chronic renal failure and plan nutritional therapy for a patient on hemodialysis.

4. Relate types of renal calculi to nutritional therapy indicated in each case.

Physiology of the Kidney

Nephron The functional unit of the kidney, located in the cortex; site of the proximal tubule, descending and ascending portions of the Loop of Henle, and the distal and collecting tubules.

Glomerulus A convoluted cluster of blood vessels in the cortex of the kidney at the head of the nephron; site of cell-free filtrate formation.

Bowman's capsule A cupped membrane surrounding the glomerulus; site of cell-free filtrate formation.

Basic Renal Functions
Basic Functional Unit—the Nephron

Knowledge of the normal functions of the kidney forms an essential background for understanding therapy in renal disorders based on the organ's impaired functioning in disease. The basic functional unit of the kidney is the **nephron.** Major advances today in treating kidney disease are based on providing maximal support for these vital nephron functions[1] (Figure 21-1). We are provided at birth with far more of these filtering-reabsorbing nephron units than we need, about 2 million of them. But we begin to lose them gradually after age 30.[2] The nephron is an exquisite example of a highly complex, minute tissue unit. It is adapted in fine detail to its vital function—maintaining an internal fluid environment compatible with life. These vital units of the kidney are the master chemists of our bodies. We have the kind of body fluids and tissues that we have not merely because of what the mouth takes in but because of what the kidneys keep. Only because they work in the way they do has it become possible for us to have specific tissues of a specific nature to do specific tasks.

Specific Integrated Nephron Functions

Each kidney contains some 1 million nephrons. As the body fluid flows through these finely structured units, the nephrons perform four significant functions to support life:

1. Filtration of most constituents from the entering blood except red cells and proteins.
2. Reabsorption of needed substances as the filtrate continues along the winding tubules.
3. Secretion of additional ions to maintain acid-base balance.
4. Excretion of unneeded materials in a concentrated urine.

Nephron Structures

Specific nephron structures perform unique metabolic tasks to maintain body balance. These key structures include the **glomerulus** and the tubules.

Glomerulus

At the head of each nephron, blood enters in a single capillary and then branches into a group of collateral capillaries. This tuft of collateral capillaries is held closely together in a cup-shaped membrane. This cup-shaped capsule is named **Bowman's capsule,** for the young English physician, Sir William Bowman, who in 1843 first clearly established the basis of plasma filtration and consequent urine secretion based on this intimate relationship of blood-filled glomeruli and enveloping membrane. The filtrate formed here is cell free and virtually protein free. Otherwise it carries the same constituents as does the entering blood.

Tubules

Continuous with the base of Bowman's capsule, the nephron tubule winds in a series of convolutions towards its terminal in the renal pelvis. Specific reabsorption functions are performed by the four sections of the tubule:

Figure 21-1
The nephron—functional unit
of the kidney.

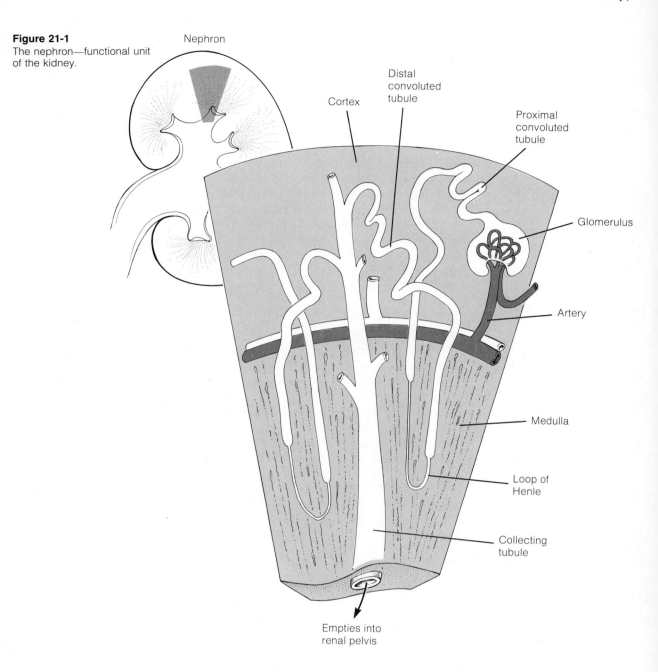

Empties into
renal pelvis

Proximal tubule In the first section nearest the glomerulus, major nutrient reabsorption occurs. Essentially 100% of the glucose and amino acids and 80% to 85% of the water, sodium, potassium, chloride, and most other substances are reabsorbed. Only 15% to 30% of the filtrate remains to enter the next section.

Loop of Henle This is the midsection of the renal tubule. Here the tubule narrows, and its thin loop dips into the central renal **medulla.** Through a balanced system of water and sodium exchange in the limbs of the loop,

Medulla Innermost portion of the kidney; site of the Loop of Henle.

important fluid density is created surrounding the loop. This area of increased density is important to concentrate the urine by osmotic pressure as it later passes through this same area of the kidney in the collecting tubule.

Distal tubule   The latter portion of the tubule functions primarily in providing acid-base balance through secretion of ionized hydrogen. It also conserves sodium by reabsorbing it under the influence of aldosterone (see p. 172).

Collecting tubule   In the final section of the tubule, water is absorbed under the influence of the hormone ADH and the osmotic pressure of the more dense surrounding fluid. The resulting volume of urine now concentrated and excreted is only 0.5% to 1% of the original filtered water and its solutes.

Nephron Disease Problems

General Causes of Renal Disease

A number of disease conditions may interfere with the normal functioning of the nephrons, the vital functional units of the kidney.

Inflammatory and Degenerative Disease

Inflammation of the small blood vessels and membranes in the nephrons may be short term, as in acute glomerulonephritis. In other cases it may diffusely involve entire nephrons or nephron segments, disrupting normal function. Nephrotic lesions develop, leading to progressive chronic renal failure. Nutritional disturbances in the metabolism of protein, electrolytes, and water follow.

Infection and Obstruction

Bacterial infection of the urinary tract may range from occasional mild, uncomfortable bladder infection to more involved chronic recurrent disease and obstruction from kidney stones. This obstruction anywhere in the urinary tract blocks drainage causing further infection and tissue damage.

Damage from Other Diseases

Circulatory disorders such as prolonged hypertension, often associated with the renin-angiotensin-aldosterone mechanism (see p. 172), can cause degeneration of the small renal arteries and curtail efficient function. A vicious cycle ensues. The demand on the kidney in turn causes more hypertension and still more damage. Other diseases, such as diabetes and gout, may also damage kidney function. Abnormalities present from birth may lead to poor function, infection, or obstruction.

Damage from Other Agents

Environmental agents such as insecticides, solvents, and similar materials are poisons that can damage the kidneys. Some drugs may also harm renal tissue.

   In the treatment of renal disease, nutritional therapy is based on impaired renal function and resulting clinical symptoms. In this chapter we will focus primarily on the more serious degenerative processes of glomerulonephritis, nephrosis, and renal failure. Then we will briefly review the more common problems that occur in the urinary tract—obstructive kidney stones and urinary tract infection.

Glomerulonephritis
Disease Process

Glomerulonephritis is an inflammatory process affecting the glomeruli, the small blood vessels in the head of the nephron. It is most common in its acute form in children 3 to 10 years of age, although 5% or more of the initial attacks occur in adults past age 50. The most common cause is a previous streptoccocal infection. It has a more or less sudden onset, a brief course in its acute form, and is usually completely cleared in a year or two. In other cases it progresses to a chronic form, involving an increased amount of renal tissue and eventually requiring dialysis and other support treatments. Recent immunologic studies and electron microscopy have demonstrated the underlying process as an immune-complex disease. **Antigen-antibody** complexes form lumpy deposits between the epithelial cells of the nephron capsule and the basement membrane of the glomeruli. Lesions develop leaving scar tissue and obstructing the circulation through the glomerulus. Fatty degeneration and necrosis of the conjoined tubules follow, and ultimate destruction of the nephron results. The net result if the disease becomes progressive is a reduction in the number of functioning nephrons available.

Clinical Symptoms

Classic symptoms include gross **hematuria** and proteinuria. There may be varying degrees of edema (see p. 172), with shortness of breath resulting from sodium and water retention and circulatory congestion. Also, there may be moderate *tachycardia* and mild or marked elevation of blood pressure. The patient is generally anorexic, which contributes to feeding problems. If the disease progresses to renal insufficiency, there is **oliguria** or **anuria,** which signals development of acute renal failure.

Nutritional Therapy

The plan for nutritional care depends on the course of the disease:

General care in uncomplicated disease The general treatment is symptomatic and designed to provide optimal nutritional support. In short-term acute cases in children, pediatricians and nutritionists favor overall optimal nutrition with adequate protein, unless symptoms of oliguria or anuria develop. These complications usually last no more than 2 or 3 days and are managed by conservative treatment. Salt is usually not restricted unless complications of edema, hypertension, or oliguria become dangerous. Thus in most patients with acute uncomplicated disease, especially in children with poststreptococcal glomerulonephritis, diet modifications are not crucial. The main treatment centers on bed rest and antibiotic drug therapy. The fluid intake will be adjusted to output as a rule, including losses in vomiting or diarrhea.

Specific therapy in progressive disease If the disease process advances, however, more specific nutritional therapy measures are indicated. The

---

Glomerulonephritis Inflammation of the capillary glomeruli in the kidney. May result after a streptococcus infection.

Antigen Any substance that stimulates the production of an antibody specifically designed to interact with it. Examples of antigens include toxins, bacteria, foreign proteins, etc.

Antibody An animal protein made up of a specific sequence of amino acids that is designed to interact with a specific *antigen* during an allergic response or to prevent infection, etc.

Hematuria Presence of blood in the urine.

Oliguria Reduced amount of urine in comparison with fluid intake.

Anuria Complete lack of urine secretion by the kidneys. Also known as *anuresis.*

nutrient factors most involved are protein, carbohydrate, sodium, potassium, and water:

Protein If the **blood urea nitrogen (BUN)** is elevated and oliguria is present, dietary protein must be restricted. Usually the diet contains 0.5 protein/kg of ideal body weight. Some patients may use 1 g/kg as long as renal function is adequate to maintain a normal BUN level.

Carbohydrate To provide sufficient energy from kilocalories, carbohydrates should be given liberally. This will also reduce the catabolism of tissue protein and prevent starvation ketosis.

Sodium The restriction of sodium varies with the degree of oliguria. If renal function is impaired, the sodium will be restricted to 500 to 1000 mg/day. As recovery occurs, sodium intake can be increased.

Potassium With severe oliguria, renal clearance of potassium is impaired. Potassium intoxication may occur, requiring dialysis. Thus potassium intake is monitored carefully according to disease progression.

Water Fluids are restricted according to the ability of the kidney to excrete urine. If restriction is not indicated, fluids can be consumed as desired.

Nephrotic Syndrome
Disease Process

The nephrotic syndrome, or **nephrosis,** is characterized by a group of symptoms resulting from kidney tissue damage and impaired nephron function. The most evident symptoms are massive **edema** and **proteinuria.** This condition may be caused by progressive glomerulonephritis. It may also be associated with other diseases, such as diabetes or connective tissue disorders—**collagen disease.** In some cases, it may result from drug reactions, exposure to heavy metals, or even from reaction to toxic venom following a bee sting. The primary degenerative lesion is in the capillary basement membrane of the glomerulus, permitting excape of large amounts of protein into the filtrate. The tubular changes that occur are because of the high protein concentration in the filtrate, with some protein uptake from the tubule lumen. Both filtration and reabsorption functions are disrupted.

Clinical Symptoms

The cardinal symptom of massive edema is apparent. **Ascites** (see p. 172) is common. The abdomen becomes increasingly distended as fluid collects in the serous cavities. Often **striae** (stretch marks) appear on the stretched skin of the extremities. The massive edema is largely caused by the gross loss of protein, principally albumin, in the urine, some 4 to 10 g/day. This means that the plasma protein is greatly reduced. The albumin fraction is largely responsible for maintaining the capillary fluid shift mechanism. Thus fluid balance between tissue fluid and circulating fluid is decreased to less than 4 g/dl. Also, the serum lipid levels are elevated, with cholesterol over 300 mg/dl. Free fat, oval fat bodies, or fatty droplets are found in the urine. Protein losses are also indicated by the presence of urinary globulins and specialized binding proteins for thyroid and iron, producing

Blood urea nitrogen (BUN) Blood test used to identify any disorder in kidney function.

Nephrosis Inflammation of the nephron.

Edema The presence of abnormally large amounts of fluid in the intercellular tissue spaces.

Proteinuria Presence of abnormally high levels of serum protein in the urine.

Collagen disease Connective tissue diseases such as rheumatoid arthritis, scleroderma, lupus erythematosus, and others.

Ascites Outflow and accumulation of fluid in the abdominal cavity. Also known as *abdominal* or *peritoneal dropsy.*

Striae Streaks or lines on stretched skin caused by weakening of the elastic tissue by constant tension.

Pedal edema Edema in the feet.

signs of hypothyroidism and anemia. As serum protein loss continues, tissue proteins are broken down and general malnutrition ensues. Fatty tissue changes in the liver and general sodium retention further contribute to the edema. Severe ascites and **pedal edema** mask the gross tissue-wasting.

Nutritional Therapy

Nutritional therapy is directed toward control of the major symptoms, edema and malnutrition, resulting from the massive protein losses.

Protein Replacement of the prolonged nitrogen deficit is a fundamental and immediate need. As indicated, the plasma albumin level may have been reduced to 20% or less of its normal value. This is a major factor in the development of nephrotic ascites and edema. Daily protein needs vary according to need, from 1 g/kg/day to larger amounts in extreme cases.

Kilocalories Sufficient kilocalories must always be provided to ensure protein use for tissue synthesis. High daily intakes of 50 to 60 kcal/kg are essential. Since appetite is usually poor, much encouragement and support are needed. The food must be as appetizing as possible and in a form most easily tolerated.

Sodium Sodium levels in the diet must be sufficiently reduced to combat the massive edema. Usually a 500-mg sodium diet (see p. 166) is sufficient to help initiate **diuresis.**

Diuresis Increased urination.

The dietary management is similar to that given for hepatitis (see p. 432), with additional need for sodium restriction. There is no need for potassium restriction. Iron and vitamin supplements may be helpful.

Chronic Renal Failure
Disease Process

There are two types of renal failure—chronic and acute—which are characterized by a number of symptoms.

Acute renal failure Total shutdown of renal function, requiring emergency treatment.

Acute renal failure Renal failure may occur as an acute phase with sudden shutdown of renal function following some metabolic insult or traumatic injury to normal kidneys. The situation is often life threatening and is a medical emergency in which the nutritionist and nurse play important supportive roles. **Acute renal failure** may be caused by various events: (1) severe injury such as extensive burns or crushing injuries that cause widespread tissue destruction, (2) infectious diseases such as peritonitis, or (3) toxic agents in the environment such as carbon tetrachloride, poisonous mushrooms, or in sensitive individuals certain drugs such as penicillin. The major sign of such an acute renal failure is *oliguria*. This diminished urine output is brought on by the underlying tissue problems that characterize acute renal failure.[3] There is usually blockage of the tubules caused by cellular debris from tissue trauma or urinary failure with backup retention of filtrate materials.

Chronic renal failure The course of renal failure may become chronic with progressive degenerative changes in renal tissue and marked depression of all renal functions.[4] At this stage, few functioning nephrons remain and these gradually deteriorate (see box, opposite). Chronic renal in-

Clinical Application

The Aging Western Kidney

Cortex An outer layer. The renal cortex contains the glomeruli and tubules.

Renal disease typically follows a progressive downhill course. Why should this be? The work of Brenner's group at Harvard indicates that the stage may well have been set in our distant evolutionary past as an adaptation of the kidney to meet the nitrogenous excretion needs of our hunter/scavenger meat-eating ancestors.

Because these ancient ancestors of ours were carnivores, their protein intake was transient and intermittent. They could only eat after a successful hunting expedition. Thus, at these times of surfeit, a large number of "extra" nephrons had to be available to meet their needs for the prompt excretion of waste products, largely urea, and the conservation of fluid and electrolytes until the next meal became available. They achieved this metabolic task mainly by *hyperfiltration* through increased use of their large number of "extra" superficial glomeruli, largely in the outer part (**cortex**) of the kidney, which normally maintains a "resting state." It was only in the past 5000 to 10,000 years, when population groups developed agriculture and herding, that a more continuous food intake pattern became possible. Now, in many Western countries, our adult diet averages approximately 3000 kcal and more than 100 g of protein—largely meat—*daily*.

Thus, the answers to our initial questions—Why do we have far more nephrons than we seem to need? Why do we begin losing some of these nephrons through a "normal aging" process of glomerular sclerosis after age 30? Why is renal disease so inexorably progressive?—lie in a fundamental mismatch between the evolutionary design of our kidneys and the functional burden we place on them by our modern eating habits. Our sustained protein excesses, along with other solutes, impose demands for sustained increases in renal blood flow and glomeruli filtration rates. This requires that our "extra" reserve glomeruli of the outer renal cortex be in more or less continuous use and predisposes even healthy persons to observed progressive glomerular sclerosis over time with deterioration of normal kidney function. In healthy persons, this deterioration poses no problem because we have so many extra nephrons. But when renal disease occurs, the burden is compounded. The disease accelerates the deterioration process and makes coping no longer possible. The downhill course inevitably ensues. The aging and vulnerable Western kidney, then, seems to be related inevitably to our lifetime of large protein meals.

References
Brenner, B.M., Meyer, T.W., and Hostetter, T.H.: Dietary protein intake and the progressive nature of kidney disease, N. Engl. J. Med. **307**(11):652, 1982.

sufficiency may result from a variety of diseases that involve the nephrons: primary glomerular disease, metabolic diseases with renal involvement such as diabetes, type I, exposure to toxic substances, infections, renal vascular disease, renal tubular disease, chronic phylonephritis, or congenital abnormality of both the kidneys. Depending on the nature of the predisposing renal disease, there is extensive scarring of renal tissue. This distorts the kidney structure and brings vascular changes from the prolonged hypertension involved.

Clinical Symptoms

The symptom complex of advanced renal insufficiency is commonly called **uremia**. Symptoms result from the progressive loss of nephrons and the consequent decreased renal blood flow and glomerular filtration. As the nephrons are lost one by one, the remaining nephrons gradually lose their ability to maintain body water balance, concentration of solutes in body fluids (osmolality), and electrolyte and acid-base balance. This continuing loss of nephrons brings many metabolic insults.

Uremia Presence in the blood of large amounts of byproducts of protein metabolism. Caused by impaired nephron function leading to the inability to excrete urea and other products. A toxic condition characterized by headache, nausea, vomiting, diminished vision, convulsions, or coma.

Water balance The increased load of solutes causes an osmotic diuresis. Increasingly the kidney cannot excrete a normal concentrated urine. Dehydration follows and may become critical. On the other hand, water intoxication may occur if there is excess fluid intake.

Electrolyte balance A number of imbalances among electrolytes result from the decreasing nephron function:

Sodium With osmotic diuresis, sodium loss contributes to a decreasing extracellular fluid volume (see p. 168). As the plasma volume decreases, renal filtration declines further, worsening the renal failure. In this state the kidney cannot respond appropriately to maintain sodium balance. Any sudden increase in sodium intake cannot be excreted readily and causes still more edema.

Potassium The balance of potassium is usually not impaired as readily until the oliguria becomes severe or acidosis increases.

Phosphate, sulfate, and organic acids With reduced nephron function there is reduced filtration and excretion of these materials produced by the metabolism of food. Thus these anions become concentrated in body fluids, with subsequent displacement of bicarbonate (see p. 168), causing metabolic acidosis.

Calcium and phosphate Metabolism of these electrolytes is greatly disturbed as a consequence of renal tissue loss. Two metabolic functions of the kidney—activation of vitamin D and the action of the parathyroid hormone in controlling the serum calcium-phosphorus levels (see p. 144)—cannot proceed at normal levels. The impaired vitamin D activation results in a bone disease called **osteodystrophy**. This disturbance causes bone pain, various bone deformities, awkward gait, and in children impaired growth. Also, there may be calcification of soft tissues, which further hinders renal function.

Osteodystrophy A disease often accompanying renal failure in which calcium is lost from the bones; poor bone formation. *Renal osteodystrophy* is a result of chronic kidney disease which may begin in childhood and can result in *renal dwarfism*.

Nitrogen retention Increasing loss of nephron function brings elevated amounts of nitrogenous metabolites such as urea and creatinine. The urea load results from dietary protein metabolism, whereas creatinine load results from increasing catabolism of muscle mass.

Anemia The normal kidney participates in the production of red blood cells, through action of a specific enzyme. The damaged kidney cannot accomplish this task, and there is depressed red blood cell production. The red cells that are produced survive a shorter time but have a usual size and hemoglobin content.

Hypertension When blood flow to renal tissue is increasingly impaired, the resulting *ischemia* (see p. 455) brings increasing hypertension through the nephrons' close relationship to the renin-angiotensin mechanism (see p. 172). In turn hypertension causes cardiovascular damage and further deterioration of the kidney.

Azotemia The elevated blood urea nitrogen (BUN), serum creatinine, and serum uric acid levels are reflected in the characteristic laboratory finding of **azotemia**.

General signs and symptoms The increasing loss of renal function brings progressive weakness, shortness of breath, general lethargy, and fatigue. There is thirst, anorexia, weight loss, and gastrointestinal irritability with diarrhea or vomiting. Increasing capillary fragility brings skin, nose, oral, and gastrointestinal bleeding. Nervous system involvement brings muscular twitching, burning sensations in the extremities, or uremic convulsions. Cheyne-Stokes respiration (irregular, cyclic type of breathing) indicates acidosis. There is ulceration of the mouth, a persistent bad or metallic taste, and fetid breath. Malnutrition lowers resistance to infection. Osteodystrophy continues with aching and pain in bone and joints.

Nutritional Therapy

Treatment must be individual, adjusted according to progression of the illness, type of treatment being used, and the patient's response. In general, however, basic therapy objectives are to:
- Reduce and minimize protein breakdown
- Avoid dehydration or hydration
- Correct acidosis carefully
- Correct electrolyte depletions and avoid excesses
- Control fluid and electrolyte losses from vomiting and diarrhea
- Maintain optimal nutritional status
- Maintain appetite, general morale, and sense of well-being
- Control complications such as hypertension, bone pain, and central nervous system abnormalities
- Retard progression of renal failure, postponing the ultimate necessity of dialysis

These general measures of treatment involve nutritional care as a major role. The nutritionist becomes an indispensible member of the renal care team. Principles of therapeutic nutrition for chronic renal failure involve variable nutrient adjustments according to individual need:

Protein The crucial problem is to provide sufficient protein to prevent protein breakdown, yet avoid an excess that would elevate urea levels. General limitations of protein are 0.5 g/kg/day, to help reduce azotemia.

Azotemia Term meaning nitrogen, referring to an excess of urea and other nitrogenous substances in the blood.

Creatinine End-product of the breakdown of body tissue. Found in muscles and blood; excreted in urine. High levels indicate abnormally high catabolism of body proteins, and possibly inadequate intake of carbohydrate and fat, which have a protein-sparing effect.

Some clinicians recommend adjustments of protein according to **creatinine** clearance. There is no need to restrict protein intake until the creatinine clearance falls below 40 ml/minute. Thereafter the dietary protein must be regulated according to the declining renal function (Table 21-1). If there is liberal caloric intake, patients may be maintained in nitrogen balance for prolonged periods on as little as 35 to 40 g protein/day.[5] If the blood urea level is very high, however, protein intake needs to be reduced to 20 g. Only essential amino acids are supplied by milk and egg protein and the patient is not burdened with nonessential amino acids that make demands on the body for disposal of their nitrogenous waste products and do little to counteract the tissue-protein breakdown. In any case protein will be closely controlled according to individual need ranging in quantity from 20 to 70 g and having a high biologic value to supply essential amino acids.

Table 21-1
Protein and Nitrogen Needs in Chronic Renal Failure

Creatinine Clearance (ml/min)	Nitrogen* (g/day)	Protein (g/day)
40 and above	Unrestricted	Unrestricted
10-40	9.6	60
5-20	6.4	40†
2-10	2.5-3.0 (+1.3-2.6)	20 (+ EAA/analogues)†
8 and below	Transplantation Dialysis	
5 and below	Dialysis	

*Total protein/6.25.
†EAA, Essential amino acids/alpha-keto-, alpha-hydroxy-analogues of EAA.

Amino acid supplements Currently promising approaches to protein replacement are being developed using mixtures of essential amino acids or if amino acid precursors. Other supplements have a relatively high proportion of nitrogen-free analogues of essential amino acids, especially *branched-chained amino acids* (see p. 90).[6]

Kilocalories Adequate kilocalories are mandatory. Carbohydrate and fat must supply sufficient nonprotein kilocalories to spare dietary protein for tissue-protein synthesis and to supply energy. About 300 to 400 g of carbohydrate is the average daily need. Sufficient fat, 75 to 90 g, is added to give the patient 2000 to 2500 total kcal daily.

Water Total fluid intake is guarded to avoid water intoxication from overloading or dehydration from too little water. With predialysis patients, the fluid intake should be sufficient to maintain an adequate urine volume.

Sodium The need for sodium intake varies. Both severe restriction and excess are to be avoided. The dietary need is closely related to the patient's handling of water. If hypertension and edema are present, the sodium intake needs to be restricted. Usually, the sodium intake will vary between 500 to 2000 mg (see p. 464).

Potassium The patient's potassium levels may be depressed or elevated. Adjustment of intake is made accordingly to maintain normal levels. If significant losses occur with severe vomiting or diarrhea, *careful* supplementation with potassium may be needed. In general the damaged kidney cannot clear potassium adequately. Thus the daily dietary intake is kept at about 1500 mg.

Hyperparathyroidism Greater-than-normal levels of activity by the parathyroid glands, which regulate calcium and phosphorus. High calcium levels increases the chances of developing calcium-containing urinary calculi.

Phosphate and calcium Abnormal serum levels of these electrolytes results from the secondary **hyperparathyroidism** caused by the damaged kidney function. Phosphate intake should therefore be restricted to slow down or prevent this developing imbalance, which leads to the complicating bone disease, osteodystrophy. Moderate dietary restriction of both protein and phosphorus is an effective means of delaying progression of functional renal deterioration.[7] Further control of phosphate levels is ensured by use of aluminum hydroxide gel to bind phosphate in the intestinal tract and thus prevent its absorption. A calcium supplement such as calcium lactate tablets relieves the hypocalcemia and its resultant tetany effects (see p. 146). In some cases calcium carbonate is used because it also buffers the accompanying metabolic acidosis.

Vitamins In more restricted protein diets, supplementary vitamins are usually advisable since a diet supplying 40 g or less of protein does not contribute the full daily spectrum of all the vitamins. A multivitamin tablet or capsule is usually added to the diet of renal patients on protein restriction. To help correct the bone disease present, an activated form of vitamin D_3—1,25-dihydroxycholecalciferol—may be used with caution.[8]

Maintenance Kidney Dialysis

Dialysis Separatingsubstances in solution by taking advantage of the different rates at which they pass through a semipermeable membrane.

Since the advent of the artificial kidney machine, patients with progressive chronic renal failure have been treated both at **dialysis** centers and at home. These treatments, however, are expensive. Currently much of the cost is now paid under a provision of Medicare. Some 18,000 patients receive this needed artificial kidney care.

Hemodialysis Removal of toxic substances from the blood by passing it through a machine that contains a semipermeable membrane and a liquid into which the substances will be diffused.

The diet of a patient on **hemodialysis** is a very important aspect of maintaining biochemical control. Several basic objectives govern each individually tailored diet: (1) maintaining protein and kilocalorie balance, (2) preventing dehydration or fluid overload, (3) maintaining normal potassium and sodium blood levels, and (4) maintaining acceptable serum phosphorus and calcium levels. Control of infection is an underlying goal. Nutritional therapy in most cases can be planned with more liberal nutrient allowances.

Protein For most adult dialysis patients, a standard protein allowance of 1 g/kg lean body weight provides for nutritional needs, maintains positive nitrogen balance, does not produce excessive nitrogenous waste, and replaces the amino acids lost during each dialysis treatment. At least 75% of this daily protein allowance should consist of protein of high biologic value, such as eggs, meat, fish, and poultry but little if any milk. Milk is restricted because it adds more fluid and has a high content of potassium, sodium, and phosphate.

Kilocalories Carbohydrates and fats (depending on blood lipid levels) are supplied in generous amounts to provide the needed energy for daily activities and to prevent tissue protein breakdown. The usual prescription is for 40 kcal/kg lean body weight. In selecting carbohydrate foods, a majority of the kilocalories should be supplied by simple carbohydrates, with control of complex carbohydrates. The complex carbohydrates contribute protein of lower biologic quality and should not take up large amounts of the protein allowance.

Water balance Fluid is usually limited to 400 or 500 ml/day plus an amount equal to urinary output, if any. The total intake must account for additional fluids in the foods consumed and in water derived from the catabolism or oxidation of foods, as well as fecal fluid losses. Even with this restriction there may be a mild fluid retention between dialysis treatments, with a daily weight gain in that period of about 0.45 kg (1 lb).

Sodium To control body fluid retention and hypertension, sodium should be limited to 1000 to 2000 mg daily. This restriction helps to prevent pulmonary edema or congestive heart failure from fluid overload.

Potassium Potassium restriction is imperative to prevent hyperkalemia, which can become a problem. Potassium accumulation can easily cause cardiac arrhythmias or cardiac arrest. Therefore, a daily dietary restriction of 1500 to 2000 mg is usually followed.

Vitamins During the dialysis treatments, water-soluble vitamins from the blood are lost in the dialysate filtered out of the circulating blood. A daily supplement of all the water-soluble vitamins is therefore usually given. However, the fat-soluble vitamins, especially vitamins A and D, may build up. Thus multivitamin preparations used usually exclude these vitamins.

Ambulatory Dialysis

An alternate form of treatment some patients can use is Continuous Ambulatory Peritoneal Dialysis (CAPD). This is a home dialysis process that introduces dialysate directly into the peritoneal cavity, where it can be exchanged for fluids that contain the metabolic waste products. This is done by attaching a disposable bag containing the dialysate to a catheter permanently inserted into the peritoneal cavity, waiting 20 to 30 minutes for the solution exchange, then lowering the bag to allow the force of gravity to cause the waste-containing fluid to drain into it. When the bag is empty, it can be folded around the waist or tucked into a pocket, allowing the user mobility. They are not only free to move, but with good self-care they are also free from some of the extensive dietary restrictions placed on hemodialysis patients.

As a guide for patient counseling, you may find it helpful to use a dietary regimen followed by nutritionists at a number of clinics:

- Increase protein intake to provide 1.2 to 1.5 g/kg body weight
- Limit phosphorus intake to 1200 mg/day by restricting phosphorus-rich foods, such as nuts and legumes, to 1 serving/wk and dairy products, including eggs, to a half-cup portion or 1 egg or its equivalent each day
- Increase potassium intake by eating a wide variety of fruits and vegetables each day

- Encourage liberal fluid intake to prevent dehydration
- Avoid sweets and fats to control triglyceride and HDL levels
- Maintain lean body weight by incorporating the kilocalories provided by the dialysate into the total meal plan

Another important factor to keep in mind is that hemodialysis patients often lose their appetite. Thus the most basic aspect of your efforts to help CAPD clients adjust to this new system is to encourage them to eat.[9]

Kidney Transplant

The transplantation of kidneys from one person to another has been limited because of rejection of the foreign organ by the recipient in many cases, except when the donor and the recipient are identical twins. Now, however, a new drug, *cyclosporine,* is providing more success with organ transplants. This drug not only helps to suppress the recipient's immune system cells that attack the transplanted kidney as foreign but also helps to fight off infections.[10] Nutritional support for the surgical procedure would be an important adjunct to therapy (see p. 509). Such successful transplantation has given new life to many patients with chronic renal failure. The quality of this extended life becomes a significant aspect of patient and family counseling (see Issues and Answers, pp. 504-505).

Urinary Tract Problems

Renal Calculi

Disease Process

The basic cause of renal calculi is unknown, but many factors contribute directly or indirectly to their formation. These factors relate to the nature of the urine itself or to the conditions of the urinary tract environment. According to the concentration of urinary constituents, the major stones formed are calcium stones, struvite stones, uric acid stones, and cystine stones (Figure 21-2).

Calcium stones By far the majority of kidney stones—about 96%—are composed of calcium compounds, usually calcium oxalate or calcium oxalate mixed with calcium phosphate.[11] In persons who form stones, which is a familial tendency, the urine produced is supersaturated with these crystalloid elements, and there is a lack of normal urine substances that prevent the crystals from forming stones. Excessive urinary calcium may result from the following:

1. **Excess calcium intake** that may come from prolonged use of large amounts of milk and alkali therapy for peptic ulcer or the use of hard water.
2. **Excess vitamin D** that may cause increased calcium absorption from the intestine as well as increased calcium withdrawal from bone.
3. **Prolonged immobilization,** as in body casting or immobilization in extended illness or diability, that may lead to withdrawal of bone calcium and increased urine concentration.
4. **Hyperparathyroidism** that causes excess calcium excretion. About two thirds of the persons with this endocrine disorder have renal stones, but this disorder accounts for only about 5% of total calcium stones.
5. **Renal tubular acidosis** that causes excess excretion of calcium because of defective ammonia formation.

Figure 21-2
Renal calculi: stones in
kidney, pelvis, and ureter.

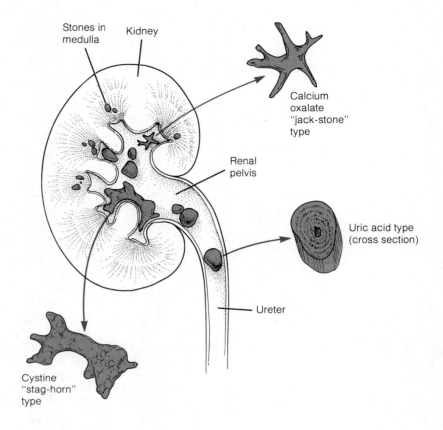

Stones in
medulla

Kidney

Calcium
oxalate
"jack-stone"
type

Renal
pelvis

Uric acid type
(cross section)

Ureter

Cystine
"stag-horn"
type

6. **Idiopathic calciuria** that may cause some persons, even those on a low-calcium diet, for unknown reasons to excrete as much as 500 mg of calcium daily.

7. **Oxalate** compounded with calcium that, because of some error in handling oxalates, accounts for about half of the calcium stones. Oxalates occur naturally in only a few food sources (see opposite).

8. **Animal protein** that has been linked to increased excretions of calcium, oxalate, and urate. A vegetarian-type diet has been recommended by some investigators as a wise choice for stone-forming patients.[12]

Struvite stones Urinary
stones made up of ammonia
magnesium phosphate, a
very hard crystal.

Struvite stones Next to calcium stones in frequency are **struvite stones,** composed of a single compound—magnesium ammonium phosphate ($MgNH_4PO_4$). These are often called infection stones because they are associated with urinary tract infections. The offending organism is *Proteus mirabilis.* This is a urea-splitting bacterium that contains urease, an enzyme that hydrolyzes urea to ammonia. Thus the urinary pH becomes alkaline. In the ammonia-rich environment struvite precipitates and forms large, staghorn calculi. Surgical removal is usually indicated.

Uric acid stones Excess uric acid excretion may be caused by an impairment in the intermediary metabolism of purine, such as occurs in gout. It may also result from rapid tissue breakdown in wasting disease.

Food Sources of Oxalates

Fruits	Vegetables	Nuts	Beverages	Other
Berries, all	Baked beans	Almonds	Chocolate	Grits
Currants	Beans, green and wax	Cashews	Cocoa	Tofu, soy products
Concord grapes	Beets	Peanuts	Draft beer	Wheat germ
Figs	Beet greens	Peanut butter	Tea	
Fruit cocktail	Celery			
Plums	Chard, Swiss			
Rhubarb	Chives			
Tangerines	Collards			
	Eggplant			
	Endive			
	Kale			
	Leeks			
	Mustard greens			
	Okra			
	Peppers, green			
	Rutabagas			
	Spinach			
	Squash, summer			
	Sweet potatoes			
	Tomatoes			
	Tomato soup			
	Vegetable soup			

Cystinuria A hereditary condition in which large amounts of cystine and other amino acids (lysine, ornithine and arginine) are secreted in the urine. May result in the formation of urinary cystine calculi.

Cystine stones A hereditary metabolic defect in renal tubular reabsorption of the amino acid cystine causes this substance to accumulate in the urine. This condition is called **cystinuria.** Since this disorder is of genetic origin, these patients are characterized by early onset age and a positive family history. This is one of the most common metabolic disorders associated with renal stones in children.

Urinary Tract Conditions

Two major factors cause urinary tract conditions leading to the formation of renal stones: (1) *physical changes in the urine* and (2) *an organic stone matrix.* Susceptible persons form stones when physical changes in the urine predispose to such formation. Such physical changes occur because of (1) *urine concentration* that results from a lower water intake or excess water loss, as in prolonged sweating, fever, vomiting, or diarrhea and (2) *urinary pH changes,* from the normal mean of 5.85 to 6.00, that may be influenced by diet or altered by the ingestion of acid or alkali medications. The second factor in renal stone formation is the organic matrix. This necessary core around which crystals may precipitate is a mucoprotein-carbohydrate complex. Possible sources of these organic materials include: (1) bacteria masses from recurrent urinary tract infections, (2) renal epithelial tissue of the urinary tract that has sloughed off, possibly because of vitamin A deficiency, and (3) calcified plaques (Randall's plaques) formed beneath the renal epithelium in hypercalcinuria. Irritation and ulceration of overlying tissue cause the plaques to slough off into collecting tubules.

Clinical Symptoms

Severe pain and numerous urinary symptoms may result with renal stone formation, along with general weakness and sometimes fever. Laboratory examination of urine and chemical analysis of any stone passed help determine treatment.

Treatment

Treatment should include a number of considerations:

Fluid intake A large fluid intake produces a more dilute urine and is a foundation of therapy. The dilute urine helps to prevent concentration of stone constituents.

Urinary pH An attempt to control solubility is made by changing the urinary pH to an increased acidity or alkalinity, depending on the chemical composition of the stone formed. An exception is calcium oxalate stones, since the solubility of calcium oxalate in urine is not pH dependent. Conversely, however, calcium phosphate is soluble in an acid urine.

Stone composition Possible dietary constituents of the stone can be controlled to reduce the amount of substance available for precipitation.

Binding agents Materials that bind the stone elements and prevent their absorption in the intestine can help to cause fecal excretion. For example, sodium phytate is used to bind calcium, and aluminum gels are used to bind phosphate. Glycine and calcium have a similar effect on oxalates.

Nutritional Therapy

The plan of nutritional care is directly related to the stone chemistry:

Calcium stones A low-calcium diet of about 400 mg daily is usually given (see opposite). This amount is half of an average adult intake of 800 mg. This lower level is achieved mainly by removal of milk and dairy products. Other calcium food sources affected are leafy vegetables and whole grains. If the stone is calcium phosphate, phosphorus foods would also be reduced (see p. 496). This can also be accomplished mainly by removal of milk and dairy products. Sometimes a test diet of 200 mg calcium may be used to rule out hyperparathyroidism as a causative factor (see p. 497).

Since calcium stones have an alkaline chemistry, an acid ash diet may also be used to create a urinary environment less conducive to precipitation of the basic stone elements. Food groups are based on the pH of the metabolic ash produced (see p. 497). An acid ash diet would increase the amount of meat, grains, eggs, and cheese (see p. 498). It would limit the amount of vegetables, milk, and fruits. An alkaline ash diet would recommend opposite use of these foods.

The use of cranberry juice has been promoted as assisting in acidification of the urine. Some studies have found significant decreases in mean urinary pH with the use of cranberry juice. However, the concentrations and volumes of juice used in such studies are not practical for clinical use.[13] The commercially prepared cranberry juices on the consumer market are too dilute to be effective, since they contain only about 26% cranberry juice. Thus a very large volume would be required to achieve any

	Foods allowed	Foods not allowed
Low-Calcium Diet (approximately 400 mg calcium)		
Beverage	Carbonated beverage, coffee, tea	Chocolate-flavored drinks, milk, milk drinks
Bread	White and light rye bread or crackers	
Cereals	Refined cereals	Oatmeal, whole-grain cereals
Desserts	Cake, cookies, gelatin desserts, pastries, pudding, sherbets, all made without chocolate, milk, or nuts; if egg yolk is used, it must be from one egg allowance.	
Fat	Butter, cream (2 tbsp daily) French dressing, margarine, salad oil, shortening	Cream (except in amount allowed), mayonnaise
Fruits	Canned, cooked, or fresh fruits or juice except rhubarb	Dried fruit, rhubarb
Meat, eggs	224 g (8 oz) daily of any meat, fowl, or fish except clams, oysters, or shrimp; not more than one egg daily including those used in cooking	Clams, oysters, shrimp, cheese
Potato or substitute	Potato, hominy, macaroni, noodles, refined rice, spaghetti	Whole-grain rice
Soup	Broth, vegetable soup made from vegetables allowed	Bean or pea soup, cream or milk soup
Sweets	Honey, jam, jelly, sugar	
Vegetables	Any canned, cooked, or fresh vegetables or juice except those listed	Dried beans, broccoli, green cabbage, celery, chard, collards, endive, greens, lettuce, lentils, okra, parsley, parsnips, dried peas, rutabagas
Miscellaneous	Herbs, pickles, popcorn, relishes, salt, spices, vinegar	Chocolate, cocoa, milk gravy, nuts, olives, white sauce

*Depending on calcium content of local water supply. In instances of high calcium content, distilled water may be indicated.

Hyperoxaluria Excretion of high levels of oxalate in the urine. Oxalates, found in several vegetables (e.g., spinach, tomatoes, rhubarb) combine with calcium to form urinary stones.

consistent effectiveness as a urinary acidification agent. Instead, to achieve a sustained acidification of urinary pH, most physicians rely on drugs.

Calcium oxalate stones resulting from **hyperoxaluria** would be treated by dietary avoidance of foods high in oxalates (see p. 493). Persons with calcium oxalate stones should avoid taking vitamin C supplements because about one half of the ingested vitamin is converted to oxalic acid. However, this is not always the case, and more studies of patients with renal calculi are needed before precise conclusions can be reached.

Uric acid stones About 4% of the total incidence of renal calculi are uric acid stones. Since uric acid is a metabolic product of *purines,* dietary control of this precursor is indicated (see pp. 498-499). Purines are found in

Low-Phosphorus Diet (approximately 1 g phosphorus and 40 g protein)		Foods Allowed	Foods Not Allowed
	Milk	Not more than 1 cup daily; whole, skim, or buttermilk or 3 tbsp powdered, including the amount used in cooking	
	Beverages	Fruit juices, tea, coffee, carbonated drinks, Postum	Milk and milk drinks except as allowed
	Bread	White only; enriched commercial, French, hard rolls, soda crackers, rush	Rye and whole-grain breads, cornbread, biscuits, muffins, waffles
	Cereals	Refined cereals, such as Cream of Wheat, Cream of Rice, rice, cornmeal, dry cereals, cornflakes, spaghetti, noodles	All whole-grain cereals
	Desserts	Berry or fruit pies, cookies, cakes in average amounts; Jell-O, gelatin, angel food cake, sherbet, meringues made with egg whites, puddings if made with one egg or milk allowance	Desserts with milk and eggs, unless made with the daily allowance
	Eggs	Not more than one egg daily, including those used in cooking; extra egg whites may be used	
	Fats	Butter, margarine, oils, shortening	
	Fruits	Fresh, frozen, canned, as desired	Dried fruits such as raisins, prunes, dates, figs, apricots
	Meat	One large serving or two small servings daily of beef, lamb, veal, pork, rabbit, chicken, or turkey	Fish, shellfish (crab, oyster, shrimp, lobster, and so on), dried and cured meats (bacon, ham, chipped beef, and so on), liver, kidney, sweetbreads, brains
	Cheese	None	Avoid all cheese and cheese spreads
	Vegetables	Potatoes as desired; at least two servings per day of any of the following: asparagus, carrots, beets, green beans, squash, lettuce, rutabagas, tomatoes, celery, peas, onions, cucumber, corn; no more than 1 serving daily of either cabbage, spinach, broccoli, cauliflower, brussels sprouts, or artichokes	Dried vegetables such as peas, mushrooms, lima beans
	Miscellaneous	Sugar, jams, jellies, syrups, salt, spices, seasonings; condiments in moderation	Chocolate, nuts, nut products such as peanut butter, cream sauces

Sample Menu Pattern

Breakfast	Lunch	Dinner
Fruit juice	Meat 56 g (2 oz)	Meat 56 g
Refined cereal	Potato	Potato
Egg	Vegetable	Vegetable
White toast	Salad	Salad
Butter	Bread, white	Bread, white
½ cup milk	Butter	Butter
Coffee or tea	½ cup milk	Dessert
	Dessert	Coffee or tea
	Coffee or tea	

Low-Calcium Test Diet (200 mg calcium)

	Grams	Milligrams Calcium
Breakfast		
Orange juice, fresh	100	19.00
Bread (toast), white	25	19.57
Butter	15	3.00
Rice Krispies	15	3.70
Cream, 20% butterfat	35	33.95
Sugar	7	0.00
Jam	20	2.00
Distilled water, coffee, or tea*		0.00
TOTAL		81.22
Lunch		
Beef steak, cooked	100	10.00
Potato	100	11.00
Tomatoes	100	11.00
Bread	25	19.57
Butter	15	3.00
Honey	20	1.00
Applesauce	20	1.00
Distilled water, coffee, or tea		0.00
TOTAL		56.57
Dinner		
Lamb chop, cooked	90	10.00
Potato	100	11.00
Frozen green peas	80	10.32
Bread	25	19.57
Butter	15	3.00
Jam	20	2.00
Peach sauce	100	5.00
Distilled water, coffee, or tea		0.00
TOTAL		60.89
TOTAL MILLIGRAMS CALCIUM		198.68

*Use distilled water only for cooking and for beverages.

active tissue such as glandular meat, other lean meat, meat extractives, and in lesser amounts in plant sources such as whole grains and legumes. An effort to produce an alkaline ash to increase the urinary pH would be indicated.

Cystine stones About 1% of the total stones produced are cystine, caused by a relatively rare genetic disease. Cystine is a nonessential amino acid

Acid and Alkaline Ash Food Groups

Acid ash	Alkaline ash	Neutral
Meat	Milk	Sugars
Whole grains	Vegetables	Fats
Eggs	Fruits (except cranberries, prunes, plums)	Beverages (coffee, tea)
Cheese		
Cranberries		
Prunes		
Plums		

Acid Ash Diet

The purpose of this diet is to furnish a well-balanced diet in which the total acid ash is greater than the total alkaline ash each day. It lists (1) unrestricted foods, (2) restricted foods, (3) foods not allowed, and (4) sample of a day's diet.

Unrestricted Foods: Eat as much as desired of the following foods.

- Bread: any, preferably whole grain; crackers, rolls
- Cereals: any, preferably whole grain
- Desserts: angel food or sunshine cake; cookies made without baking powder or soda; cornstarch pudding, cranberry desserts, custards, gelatin desserts, ice cream, sherbet, plum or prune desserts; rice or tapioca pudding
- Fats: any, as in butter, margarine, salad dressings, Crisco, Spry, lard, salad oils, olive oil
- Fruits: cranberries, plums, prunes
- Meat, eggs, cheese; any meat, fish, or fowl, two servings daily; at least one egg daily
- Potato substitutes: corn, hominy, lentils, macaroni, noodles, rice, spaghetti, vermicelli
- Soup: broth as desired; other soups from foods allowed
- Sweets: cranberry or plum jelly; sugar, plain sugar candy
- Miscellaneous: cream sauce, gravy, peanut butter, peanuts, popcorn, salt, spices, vinegar, walnuts

Restricted Foods: Do not eat any more than the amount allowed each day.

- Milk: 2 cups daily (may be used in other ways than as beverage)
- Cream: 1/3 cup or less daily
- Fruits: one serving of fruit daily (in addition to prunes, plums, cranberries); certain fruits listed under "Sample menu" are not allowed at any time
- Vegetables including potato: two servings daily; certain vegetables listed under "Foods not allowed" are not allowed at any time

Foods Not Allowed

- Carbonated beverages, such as ginger ale, cola, root beer
- Cakes or cookies made with baking powder or soda
- Fruits: dried apricots, bananas, dates, figs, raisins, rhubarb
- Vegetables: dried beans, beet greens, dandelion greens, carrots, chard, lima beans
- Sweets: chocolate or other candies than those under "Unrestricted foods"; syrups
- Miscellaneous: other nuts, olives, pickles

Sample Menu

Breakfast	Lunch	Dinner
Grapefruit	Creamed chicken	Broth
Wheatena	Steamed rice	Roast beef, gravy
Scrambled eggs	Green beans	Buttered noodles
Toast, butter, plum jam	Stewed prunes	Sliced tomato
Coffee, cream, sugar	Bread, butter	Mayonnaise
	Milk	Vanilla ice cream
		Bread, butter

Low-Purine Diet (approximately 125 mg purine)

General Directions

- During acute stages use only list 1.
- After acute stage subsides and for chronic conditions, use the following schedule:
Two days a week, not consecutive, use list 1 entirely.
The remaining days add foods from list 2 and 3, as indicated.
Avoid list 4 entirely.
- Keep diet moderately low in fat.

Low Purine Diet—cont'd

Typical Meal Pattern

Breakfast	Lunch	Dinner
Fruit	Egg or cheese dish	Egg or cheese dish
Refined cereal and/or egg	Vegetables, as allowed (cooked or salad)	Cream of vegetable soup, if desired
White toast	Potato or substitute	Starch (potato or substitute)
Butter, 1 tsp	White bread	Colored vegetable, as allowed
Sugar	Butter, 1 tsp	White bread, butter, 1 tsp, if desired
Coffee	Fruit or simple dessert	Salad, as allowed
Milk, if desired	Milk	Fruit or simple dessert
		Milk

Food List 1

May be Used as Desired; Foods that Contain an Insignificant Amount of Purine Bodies

Beverages
  Carbonated
  Chocolate
  Cocoa
  Coffee
  Fruit juices
  Postum
  Tea
Butter*
Bread: White and crackers, cornbread
Cereals and cereal products
  Corn
  Rice
  Tapioca
  Refined wheat
  Macaroni
  Noodles

Cheese of all kinds*
Eggs
Fats of all kinds* (moderation)
Fruits of all kinds
Gelatin, Jell-O
Milk: buttermilk, evaporated, malted, sweet
Nuts of all kinds,* peanut butter
Pies* (except mincemeat)
Sugar and sweets
Vegetables
  Artichokes
  Beets
  Beet greens
  Broccoli
  Brussels sprouts
  Cabbage
  Carrots

Celery
Corn
Cucumber
Eggplant
Endive
Kohlrabi
Lettuce
Okra
Parsnips
Potato, white and sweet
Pumpkin
Rutabagas
Sauerkraut
String beans
Summer squash
Swiss chard
Tomato
Turnips

Food List 2

One Item Four Times a Week; Foods that Contain a Moderate Amount (up to 75 mg) of Purine Bodies in 100 g Serving

Asparagus	Finnan haddie	Mushrooms	Salmon
Bluefish	Ham	Mutton	Shad
Bouillon	Herring	Navy beans	Spinach
Cauliflower	Kidney beans	Oatmeal	Tripe
Chicken	Lima beans	Oysters	Tuna fish
Crab	Lobster	Peas	Whitefish

Food List 3

One Item Once a Week; Foods that Contain a Large Amount (75-150 mg) of Purine Bodies in 100 g Serving

Bacon	Duck	Perch	Sheep
Beef	Goose	Pheasant	Shellfish
Calf tongue	Halibut	Pigeon	Squab
Carp	Lentils	Pike	Trout
Chicken soup	Liver sausage	Pork	Turkey
Codfish	Meat soups	Quail	Veal
	Partridge	Rabbit	Venison

Foods List 4

Avoid Entirely; Foods that Contain Very Large Amounts (150-1000 mg) of Purine Bodies in 100 g Serving

Sweetbreads	825 mg	Kidneys (beef)	200
Anchovies	363 mg	Brains	195 mg
Sardines (in oil)	295 mg	Meat extracts	160-400 mg
Liver (calf, beef)	233 mg	Gravies	Variable

*High in fat.

Low-Methionine Diet

	Foods Allowed	Foods Not Allowed
Soup	Any soup made without meat stock or addition of milk	Rich meat soups, broths, canned soups made with meat broth
Meat or meat substitute	Peanut butter sandwich, spaghetti, or macaroni dish made without addition of meat, cheese, or milk; one serving per day; chicken, lamb, veal, beef, pork, crab, or bacon (3)	Fish and those not listed above
Beverages	Soy milk, tea, coffee	Milk in any form
Vegetables	Asparagus, artichoke, beans, beets, carrots, chicory, cucumber, eggplant, escarole, lettuce, onions, parsnips, potatoes, pumpkin, rhubarb, tomatoes, turnips	Those not listed as allowed
Fruits	Apples, apricots, bananas, berries, cherries, fruit cocktail, grapefruit, grapes, lemon juice, nectarines, oranges, peaches, pears, pineapple, plums, tangerines, watermelon, cantaloupe	Those not listed as allowed
Salads	Raw or cooked vegetable or fruit salad	
Cereals	Macaroni, spaghetti, noodles	
Bread	Whole wheat, rye, white	
Nuts	Peanuts	
Desserts	Fresh or cooked fruit, ices, fruit pies	
Eggs		In any form
Cheese		All varieties
Concentrated sweets	Sugar, jams, jellies, syrup, honey, hard candy	
Concentrated fats	Butter, margarine, cream	
Miscellaneous	Pepper, mustard, vinegar, garlic, oil, herbs, spices	

produced from the essential amino acid *methionine*. Thus a diet low in methionine is used (see above and opposite). This diet is used with high fluid and alkali therapy.

The nutritional therapy principles in renal stone disease are outlined in Table 21-2.

Urinary Tract Infection
Disease Process

The term *urinary tract infection (UTI)* refers to a wide variety of clinical infections in which a number of microorganisms are present in any portion of the urinary tract. A most common form is **cystitis**, an inflammation of the bladder prevalent in young women. The condition is called recurrent UTI if three or more bouts are experienced in a year. The majority of cases are caused by aerobic members of the fecal flora, especially *Escherichia coli*. The presence of these organisms in the urine is termed **bacteriuria**. Urine produced by the normal kidney is sterile and remains so as it travels to the bladder. In UTI, however, the normal urethra has microbial flora, so that any voided urine in normal persons contains many

Cystitis Inflammation of the bladder. Can be caused by allergy, bacteria, gonorrhea, and other conditions. Often characterized by frequent voiding and burning. Untreated, it may lead to stone formation.

Bacteriuria Presence of bacteria in the urine.

Low-Methionine Diet—cont'd

Meal Pattern

Breakfast	Lunch	Dinner
1 cup fruit juice	1 serving soup	56 g (2 oz) meat
½ cup fruit	1 serving sandwich	1 med starch
1 slice toast	1 cup fruit	½ cup vegetable
1½ pats butter	240 ml (8 oz) soy milk*	1 serving salad
2 tsp jelly	3 tsp sugar	1 tbsp dressing
1 tbsp sugar	1 tbsp cream	1 slice bread
Beverage	Beverage	1 serving dessert
1 tbsp cream		1 tbsp sugar
		1 tbsp cream
		1½ pats butter
		Beverage

Sample Menu

Breakfast	Lunch	Dinner
Orange juice	Vegetable soup, vegetarian	Chicken, roast
Applesauce	Peanut butter sandwich	Baked potato
Whole-wheat	Canned peaches	Artichoke
toast	Soy milk*	Sliced tomatoes
Butter	Sugar	French dressing
Jelly	Cream	Whole-wheat bread
Sugar	Coffee or tea	Fruit ice
Coffee		Sugar
Cream		Cream
		Butter
		Coffee or tea

Adapted from Smith, D.R., Kolb, F.O., and Harper, H.A.: The management of cystinuria and cystine-stone disease. J. Urol. **81**:61, 1959.

*Optional: use in children to include protein intake. Omit if urine calcium is elevated in adults.

bacteria. Bacteriuria is present when the quantity of organisms is more than 100,000 bacterium/ml urine. The female anatomy is more conducive to entry of these bacteria into the urinary tract. Recurrent cystitis occurs mostly in young and otherwise healthy women who have infections that usually correspond with sexual activity and who are diaphragm users. In most cases simply having the diaphragm refitted to a smaller size or changing to another birth control method will solve the problem.

Clinical Symptoms

Cystitis is characterized by frequent voiding and burning on urination. Untreated, it may lead to stone formation.

Table 21-2
Summary of Diet Principles in Renal Stone Disease

Stone Chemistry	Nutrient Modification	Diet Ash
Calcium	Low calcium (400 mg)	Acid ash
Phosphate	Low phosphorus (1000-1200 mg)	
Oxalate	Low oxalate	
Struvite ($MgNH_4PO_4$)	Low phosphorus (1000-1200 mg) (associated with urinary infections)	Acid ash
Uric acid	Low purine	Alkaline ash
Cystine	Low methionine	Alkaline ash

Treatment

Currently antibiotic treatment has been cut back a great deal. Studies show that a single dose of antibiotic is just as effective as the usual 7- to 10-day course treatment in 90% of all women who have uncomplicated cystitis.[14] General nutritional measures include acidifying the urine by taking vitamin C, since cranberry juice is not effective, and drinking a large amount of fluids to produce a dilute urine. Control of UTI is an important measure, since it is a risk factor in stone formation.

To Sum Up

Through its unique functional units, the nephrons, the kidneys act as a filtration system, reabsorbing substances the body needs, secreting addtional ions to maintain a proper pH balance in the blood, and excreting unnecessary materials in a concentrated urine. Renal function can be impaired by a variety of conditions. These include inflammatory and degenerative diseases, infection and obstruction, chronic diseases (hypertension, diabetes mellitus, gout), environmental agents (insecticides, solvents, toxic substances) and some medications, and trauma. Some clinical conditions affecting structure and function include glomerulonephritis, nephrotic syndrome, acute and chronic renal failure, renal calculi, and urinary tract infections. In many cases, except nephrotic syndrome, dietary protein may need to be reduced as part of the nutritional care plan. Water, electrolytes, and kilocalorie intake should also be closely monitored to match individual needs.

Chronic kidney disease at its end stage is treated by *dialysis* and *kidney transplant*. Dialysis patients must be monitored closely for protein, water, and electrolyte balance. Nutritional support of transplant patients is needed primarily as support for the surgical procedure; a normal diet is often well tolerated after surgery and convalescence.

Renal diseases have predisposing factors. For example, untreated urinary tract infections may lead to renal calculi, and progressive glomerulonephritis may lead to nephrotic syndrome. The Western diet is suspect as a predisposing factor in the development of chronic renal failure. Excess protein intake may overtax human nephrons, which were not originally designed to handle a steady diet of protein-rich foods.

Questions for Review

1. For each of the following conditions, outline the nutritional components of therapy, explaining the impact of each on kidney function: glomerulonephritis, nephrotic syndrome, and chronic renal failure.
2. Identify four clinical conditions that can impair renal function. Give an example of each, describing its effect on various structures in the kidney.
3. List the nutritional factors that must be monitored in individuals undergoing renal dialysis.
4. Outline the medical and nutritional therapy used for patients with various types of renal calculi. Describe each type of stone and explain the rationale for each aspect of therapy.
5. For what condition is a urinary tract infection a predisposing factor? What general nutritional principles are recommended in the treatment of such infections?

References

1. Treichel, J.A.: Advances in treating kidney disease, Science News **123**(10):150, 1983.

2. Brenner, B.M., Meyer, T.W., and Hostetter, T.H.: Dietary protein intake and the progressive nature of kidney disease, N. Engl. J. Med. **307**(11):652, 1982.

3. Hermreck, A.S.: The pathophysiology of acute renal failure, Am. J. Surg. **144**(6):605, 1982.

4. Report: Diet and the progression of chronic renal failure, Lancet **2**(8311):1314, 1982.

5. Burton, B.T., and Hirschman, G.H.: Current concepts of nutritional therapy in chronic renal failure: an update, J. Am. Dietet. Assoc. **82**(4):359, 1983.

6. Mitch, W., Abras, E., and Walser, M.: Long-term effects of a new ketoacid–amino acid supplement in patients with chronic renal failure, Kidney Int. **22**(1):48, 1982.

7. Machio, G., and others: Effect of dietary protein and phosphorus restriction on the progression of early renal failure, Kidney Int. **22**(4):371, 1982.

8. Hodsman, M.B., and others: Preliminary trials with 24,25-dihydroxyvitamin D_3 in dialysis osteomalacia, Am. J. Med. **74**(3):407, 1983.

9. Bodnar, D.M.: Rationale for nutritional requirements for patients on continuous ambulatory peritoneal dialysis J.Am. Diet. Assoc. **80**(3):247, 1982.

19. Treichel, J.A.: Advances in treating kidney disease, Science News, **123**(10):150, 1983.

11. Metheny, N.: Renal stones and urinary pH, Am. J. Nurs. **82**:1372, 1982.

12. Brockis, J.G., Levitt, A.J., and Cruthers, S.M.: The effects of vegetable and animal protein diets on calcium, urate, and oxalate excretion, Brit. J. Urol. **54**:590, 1982.

13. Report: Cranberries and urinary infections, Nutrit. and the MD **VIII**(8):4, 1982.

14. Report: Cystitis: less drastic solutions, Health Facts **8**(51):2, 1983.

Further Readings

Batterman, C., Atcherson, E., and Roy, C.: Restrictions and recreation for patients with renal failure, J.Am. Dietet. Assoc. **83**(3):333, 1983.

Interesting "mini-vacation trip" experience of renal care practitioners (a dietitian and two social workers) with a group of dialysis patients. Illustrates how food planning was used as a teaching tool and a means of building a stronger cooperative working relationship to improve diet habits.

Burton, B.T., and Hirschman, M.D.: Current concepts of nutritional therapy in chronic renal failure: an update, J. Am. Diet. Assoc. **82**(4):359, 1983.

Nutritional therapy in chronic renal failure is in a constant state of flux. This article provides comprehensive background for current practices. Good charts.

Metheny, N.: Renal stones and urinary pH, Am. J. Nurs. **82**:1372, 1982.

Excellent reference for further understanding of distinguishing features and treatment of different types of kidney stones. Preventive nursing measures. Comprehensive chart with pictures.

Issues and Answers

Renal Disease: Technology vs. the Quality of Life

Imagine spending up to 18 hours a week hooked up to a machine to which you literally owed your life. Imagine having a 40% chance of never being able to work outside the home again, leading a life of poverty and restricted mobility—all because of that machine. This is probably hard for most of us to imagine. Yet, for approximately 55,000 Americans on maintenance dialysis, this is the reality of their everday lives. And all of us on the medical-nutrition-nursing renal care team must also deal with this reality daily in our work with these persons and their families. Especially is this sensitivity needed in nutrition couseling and teaching. Food is tied up with so many personal values that when it must be drastically changed—or when choice is gone altogether—it's as if a part of self has been diminished.

Researchers, physicians, and other renal team members, as well as patients, are becoming increasingly concerned with the *quality* of life rather than merely the *length* of life available to the person on dialysis. The only alternative currently available is kidney transplantation. On the surface, this method could be considered preferable to hemodialysis or even peritoneal dialysis because it frees the individual from any mechanical device. However, researchers are beginning to investigate the quality of life a kidney transplant provides to determine whether either method is preferable to the other.

The first issue of greatest concern is, of course, the effect of the treatment method on lifespan. Mortality rates for individuals on dialysis (8% to 15%) are in the same range as those for people receiving their first kidney transplant from a parent or a sibling (10% to 15%). However, rates among young dialysis patients with no extrarenal disease can drop as low as 2%, in contrast with rates that can soar to 30% among individuals recieving kidneys from cadavers. Still, some people feel that the benefits of increased mobility outweigh the drawbacks of a possible reduction in lifespan.

In one study, life quality measures (sleep habits, food habits, energy level, sexual activity, changes in income and/or employment, satisfaction with marriage, etc.) were examined among individuals on dialysis compared with successful transplant operations and unsuccessful operations. As expected, subjects who had had sucessful operations reported a near-normal quality of life—they were less tired, less inconvenienced by frequent medical treatments, and had better incomes and/or more full-time employment following renal failure than other renal patients.

Also as expected, individuals whose transplant operations were not successful indicated that the quality of their lives was the lowest of all subjects. For example, none of these subjects reported full-time employment since renal failure. They were mainly recipients of kidneys from cadavers. Thus, this process is assumed to be the least desirable of all possible alternatives.

Issues and Answers—cont'd

A surprising result of this study was that dialysis patients who never received a transplant felt that the quality of their lives was also near normal. Researchers admit that the reason for this probably includes denial or accommodation. However, they also acknowledge that human response to life experiences is an extremely complex issue, one that is difficult to assess with current "immature" research methods available for evaluating the quality of life in general.

The health care team responsible for the individual with renal failure may have its own set of parameters for determining the quality of life each mode of treatment may provide. The results of this study suggest that patients' own evaluation of their lives may involve factors much more complex than those to which the professional has been exposed. The study serves as a reminder that professionals must be open to the concerns and viewpoints of the individual faced with such major choices in treatment and relate their care planning in all areas to these personal concerns.

References
Johnson, P.J., McCauley, C.R., and Copley, J.B.: The quality of life of hemodialysis and transplant patients, Kidney Int. **22**(3):286, 1982.

Chapter 22
Nutritional Care of Surgery Patients

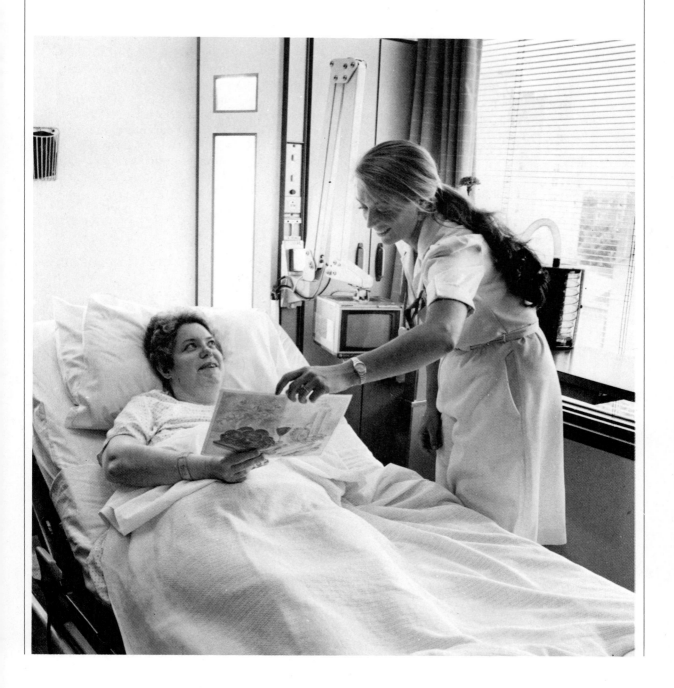

Preview

A high incidence of malnutrition among hospitalized patients has been increasingly observed over the past few years. A large number of these malnourished persons are surgical patients. In numerous surveys in both American and European hospitals nearly 50% of the surgical patients have had clinical evidence of protein-energy malnutrition. Effective nutritional support can reverse this malnutrition, markedly improve prognosis, and speed recovery. A spectrum of feeding modes, both enteral and parenteral, have helped to provide these remarkable means.

Surgery itself places physiologic and psychologic stress on patients. This state of stress brings added nutritional demands. Deficiencies can accrue easily and may lead to serious clinical problems. Careful attention to preoperative preparation of the patient facing surgery, together with vigorous postoperative nutritional support, can reduce complications and provide resources for better healing and more rapid recovery.

Chapter Objectives

After study of this chapter, the student should be able to:

1. Describe the relation of malnutrition to the outcome of surgical treatment and identify means of avoiding this complicating condition.
2. Relate nutritional therapy to tissue healing.
3. Identify special nutritional problems of gastrointestinal surgery and outline an appropriate plan of care in each case.
4. Describe parenteral modes of feeding to meet unusual nutritional needs.

Nutritional Needs of General Surgery Patients

Preoperative Nutritional Care
Nutrient Stores

Nutritional resources fortify the patient for the demands of surgery. When time permits, nutritional preparation should correct any nutrient deficiencies. It should also provide reserves for the surgery itself and for the immediate postoperative period until regular feedings can be resumed.

Protein The most common nutritional deficiency in surgical patients is that of protein. Tissue and plasma reserves are imperative to prepare the patient for blood losses during surgery and for tissue breakdown in the immediate postoperative period.

Energy Sufficient kilocalories must be provided to build up any deficit. Carbohydrate is needed for glycogen stores and to spare protein for tissue synthesis.

Persons with bleeding tendencies may be given added vitamin C before surgery.

Vitamins and minerals Normal tissue stores of vitamins are needed for the added metabolism of carbohydrates and protein. Any deficiency state such as anemia should be corrected. Electrolytes and fluids should be in balance and correction made of any dehydration, acidosis, or alkalosis.

Immediate Preoperative Period

In the usual preparation for surgery, nothing is given by mouth for at least 8 hours before surgery. This ensures that the stomach has no retained food at the time of the operation. In case of emergency surgery, if the patient has recently eaten a meal, gastric suction is used. Food in the stomach may be vomited or aspirated during surgery or recovery from anesthesia. Also, any food present may increase the possibility of postoperative gastric retention and dilation. It may also interfere with the procedure itself, especially in abdominal surgery. Before gastrointestinal surgery, a low-residue (see p. 430) or residue-free diet may be followed for several days to clear the operative site of any residue. Low-residue, chemically defined formulas, or **elemental formulas**, can provide a complete diet in liquid form. Such formulas, if palatable enough, can be taken orally in sufficient amounts to maintain nutritional resources. Otherwise they may be fed by tube.

Elemental formula Formula whose components cannot be broken down into simpler parts.

Postoperative Nutritional Care

Healthy body tissues undergo continuous turnover, with small physiologic losses being constantly replenished by nutrients in the food eaten. In disease, however, especially surgical disease, losses are greatly increased. At the same time replacement from food is diminished or even absent for a brief or extended period. Nutritional support, therefore, becomes all the more significant as a means of aiding recovery.

Protein

Exudate Material that escapes from blood vessels and is deposited in tissues, or tissue surfaces; characterized by a high content of protein, cells, or other cellular solid matter.

Adequate protein intake in the postoperative recovery period is of primary therapeutic concern to replace losses and supply increased demands. In addition to protein losses from tissue breakdown, added loss of plasma proteins can occur through hemorrhage, wound bleeding, and **exudates**. Increased metabolic losses of protein can also result from extensive tissue

A negative nitrogen balance of as much as 20 g/day may occur after surgery. This represents an actual loss of tissue protein of over 1 lb/day.

destruction and inflammation or from infection and trauma. If any degree of prior malnutrition or chronic infection existed, the patient's protein deficit may actually become severe and cause serious complications. There are a number of reasons for this increased protein demand:

Tissue synthesis in wound healing Tissue protein can be synthesized only by essential amino acids brought to the tissue by the circulating blood (see p. 90). The necessary essential amino acids must come either from the diet protein or by intravenous feeding. Tissue protein deficiencies are best met by oral feeding. As early as possible an intake of 100 to 150 g daily should be attempted to restore lost protein tissues and synthesize new tissue at the wound site. Although tissue protein is broken down more rapidly during stress, fortunately it is also built up more rapidly, provided sufficient amino acids are present to supply the anabolic demand. If oral feedings are possible, although appetite is poor, palatable concentrated liquid drinks or commercial formulas are useful (see p. 513).

Avoidance of shock A reduction in blood volume (hypovolemia), from a loss of plasma proteins and a decrease in circulating red blood cell volume contribute to the potential danger of shock (see p. 172). When protein deficiencies exist, this danger is increased.

Control of edema When the serum protein is low, edema develops as a result of the loss of colloidal osmotic pressure required to maintain the normal shift of fluid between the capillaries and the surrounding interstitial tissues (see p. 172). This general edema may affect heart and lung action. Local edema at the surgical site also delays closure of the wound and hinders normal healing processes.

Callus Unorganized meshwork of newly grown, woven bone developed on pattern of original fibrin clot (formed after fracture) and which is normally replaced by hard adult bone.

Bone healing In orthopedic surgery, extensive bone healing is involved. Protein is essential for proper **callus** formation and calcification. A sound protein matrix is mandatory for the anchoring of mineral matter.

Resistance to infection Amino acids are necessary constituents of the proteins involved in body defense mechanisms. These defense agents include antibodies, special blood cells, hormones, and enzymes. Tissue integrity itself is a first line of defense against infections.

Lipid transport Protein is necessary for the transport of lipids in the body (see p. 457). They provide essential materials to form lipoproteins, the transport form of fat. Proteins thus protect the liver, a main site of fat metabolism, from danger caused by fatty infiltration.

Multiple clinical problems may easily develop following surgery when protein deficiencies exist. There may be poor wound healing, or **dehiscence**, delayed healing of fractures, anemia, failure of gastrointestinal stomas to function, depressed lung and heart function, reduced resistance to infection, extensive weight loss, liver damage, and increased mortality risks.

Dehiscence Splitting open, separation of the layers of a surgical wound.

Water

Water balance is a vital concern after surgery. Adequate fluid therapy is necessary to prevent dehydration. Large water losses may occur from vomiting, hemorrhage, exudates, diuresis, or fever. When drainage is involved, as is common in many surgeries, there is still more fluid loss. Intravenous therapy will supply initial needs, but oral intake should begin as soon as possible and be maintained in sufficient quantity, according to individual needs, to avoid both extremes of dehydration and water intoxication. Daily weight of the patient provides a guideline for meeting fluid requirements.

Energy

As is always the case when increased protein is demanded for tissue rebuilding, sufficient nonprotein energy kilocalories must be supplied to protect the protein. Adequate amounts of *carbohydrate* are essential to ensure the use of protein for necessary tissue protein synthesis and to supply the energy required for increased metabolic demands. As protein is increased, the total kilocalories must be increased as well, since sufficient caloric intake is essential and often critical to the successful outcome of surgical procedures. About 2800 kcal/day must be provided before protein can be used for tissue repair and not be diverted to help provide energy. In acute stress, as in extensive surgery or burns, when protein needs may be as high as 200 g/day, 4000 to 6000 kcal may be required. In addition to its protein-sparing action, carbohydrate also helps to avoid liver damage from depletion of glycogen reserves. *Fat* must be adequate to maintain body tissue fat reserves but it must not be excessive.

Vitamins

All of the vitamins play important roles in the healing process. Vitamin C is imperative for wound healing. It is necessary for the formation of cementing material in the ground substance of connective tissue, in capillary walls, and in the building up of new tissue. Extensive tissue regeneration such as occurs in burns or radical surgeries may require an additional vitamin C supplementation. As kilocalorie and protein intake are increased, the B vitamins must also be increased. They provide essential coenzyme factors for protein and energy metabolism. Vitamin K is essential to the blood-clotting mechanism.

Minerals

Replacing mineral deficiencies and ensuring continued adequacy is essential. In tissue breakdown, potassium and phosphorus are lost. Electrolyte losses, especially sodium and chloride, accompany fluid losses. Iron-deficiency anemia may develop from blood loss or malabsorption.

General Dietary Management

Enteral Feeding (Oral)

The majority of general surgical patients can and should progress to oral feeding as soon as possible to provide adequate nutrition. Remember that routine postoperative intravenous fluids are intended to supply hydration needs and electrolytes, not to sustain nutritional needs. Ordinary postsurgical intravenous therapy cannot supply full nutrient needs or compete with oral feedings. A rapid return to regular eating should be encouraged and maintained.

Parenteral Feeding

In cases of major tissue trauma or damage or when a patient is unable to obtain sufficient nutrients orally, parenteral feeding may be necessary. It provides crucial nutritional support from solutions containing higher percentage glucose, amino acids, electrolytes, minerals, and vitamins, with lipid emulsions fed separately about twice a week through a Y-tube connection, for needed kilocalories (see p. 511). Such solutions may be fed for brief periods by peripheral vein feeding or for longer periods of more severe nutritional needs by central vein feeding—*total parenteral nutrition (TPN)* (see p. 521).

Routine Postoperative Diets

Oral intake of solid foods should be encouraged and supported as soon as possible after surgery to hasten recovery.

As rapidly as possible, as soon as intestinal peristalsis returns, water and *clear liquids* such as tea, coffee, broth, and juice may be given to help supply important fluids and some sodium and chloride. These initial liquids also help stimulate normal gastrointestinal function and early return to a full diet. Progression fo *full liquids* should soon follow. Milk and milk products—including puddings, cream soups, high-protein beverages, and ice cream—supply much vital protein and carbohydrate. Each patient will progress to solid food in *soft to regular diets* according to individual tolerance.

Special Nutritional Needs for Gastrointestinal Surgery Patients

Head and Neck Surgery

Surgery involving the mouth, throat, or neck will require modification in the manner of feeding. The patient usually cannot chew or swallow normally.

Enteral Feeding (Oral)

Concentrated feedings in liquid form will need to be planned. These feedings may consist of special enteral formulas of protein hydrolysates or amino acids with added carbohydrate, fat, vitamin, and minerals. As tolerated, milk-based beverages, soups, fruit juices with lactose, and eggnogs can supply frequent reinforced oral nourishment. A milkshake-type blended formula, supplemented with skim milk powder or other protein concentrate, can supply 20 g of protein and 400 kcal (see p. 419).

Enteral Feeding (Tube)

Patients who are comatose or severely debilitated or who have undergone radical neck or facial surgery may require tube feeding. New developments in small-bore feeding tubes have made this method of feeding easier.[1] In cases of long-term need, rapid development of sophisticated delivery systems and standardized formulas has made continued home enteral nutrition possible for many patients.[2] A wide variety of feeding tubes for enteral nutrition are available. Usually a nasogastric tube is used (see p. 551). In cases of esophageal obstruction, surgical insertion of a special tube may be made through the abdominal wall. In other cases a special Moss tube may be placed during surgery for short-term postsurgical feeding to allow early intake of an elemental formula and avoid postoperative **paralytic or adynamic ileus**.[3] The tube may be removed 2 days after surgery and can be followed by oral elemental formula and a full low-residue

Paralytic or adynamic ileus Obstruction of the intestines, resulting from inhibition of bowel motility.

Commercial formulas provide the advantages of convenience, formulation to meet special needs, and sanitation. They have disadvantages of cost (especially with long-term use) and osmolality problems with concentration of materials in solution.

Intact nutrient A nutrient in its natural undigested form, such as protein.

Elemental nutrient A single nutrient component as rendered normally by digestion, such as an amino acid.

Blended food formulas provide the advantages of lower cost, calculation to meet personal tolerances, usually less problems with osmolality, and the psychological advantage of being "real food." They have the disadvantage of problems with sanitation in mixing and storing.

Vagotomy Interruption of the impulses carried by the vagus nerve(s), resulting in prevention of increased flow or acidity of gastric secretions.

diet soon thereafter. In general the tube feeding formula will be prescribed according to the patient's need and tolerance. Small amounts of formula are used at first and gradually increased. Usually 2 L of formula are sufficient for a 24-hour period. The feeding should not exceed 240 to 360 ml (8 to 12 oz) in each 3- to 4-hour interval. Two general types of formula may be used:

Commercial formulas A number of commercial formulas of different types are available for selection and use according to individual need.[5,6] These products may be made from **intact nutrient** sources for use with an intact bowel able to digest and absorb them. Others may use predigested or **elemental nutrients,** which are readily absorbed with only minimal residue. Still others may be formulas designed for special problems, or single-nutrient modules of protein, carbohydrate, and fat, which may be mixed together to meet the patient's specific needs.

Blended food mixtures Sometimes blended food mixtures are preferred by some persons, especially older patients at home who feel comforted by "regular food."[6] Any food that will liquify in a high-speed blender can be used, or strained baby food may be added to simplify the mixing process. Ingredients may include a milk base, with added egg, strained meat, vegetable, fruit, fruit juices, nonfat dry milk, cream, vitamins, or minerals as needed. Some patients may wish to use blended food mixtures because of the cost factor involved in long-term use of enteral formula products. Close nutritional monitoring of such blended formulas is necessary, however. Sometimes when they are diluted to go through the tube, the nutrient density may not compare with that of a commercial formula. Although long-term tube feeding may well meet physiologic needs for the patient, it also carries psychologic burdens. Support for the quality of life must also be a part of patient care planning.

Stomach Surgery
Nutrition Problems

A number of nutrition problems may develop following gastric surgery, depending on the type of surgical procedure employed (Figure 22-1) and the patient's response. A partial gastrectomy may create little postoperative difficulty. A total gastrectomy is another matter, however, since there is complete excision of the stomach and the remaining portion of the esophagus is joined to the jejunum—*anastomosis.* This resectioning may produce serious nutritional deficits and requires careful diet planning. When a **vagotomy** is also performed, there is increased gastric fullness and distention. The stomach becomes atonic and empties poorly, so that food fermentation follows, producing flatus and diarrhea. After gastric surgery about 50% of the patients fail to regain weight to optimal levels. The nutritional care of patients who have had gastric surgery primarily falls into two phases: the immediate postoperative period and a later "dumping syndrome" period.

Immediate Postoperative Period

Generally, after surgery, frequent small oral feedings are resumed according to the patient's tolerance. A typical pattern of simple dietary progres-

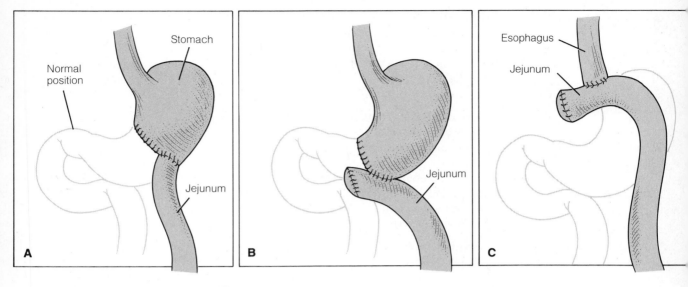

Figure 22-1
Gastric surgery. **A,** Partial gastrectomy, Bilroth I. **B,** Partial gastrectomy, Bilroth II. **C,** Total gastrectomy.

sion may cover about a 2-week period. The basic principles of such general diet therapy for the postgastrectomy period involve (1) keeping the *size* of meals small and frequent and (2) keeping the food simple, easily digested, mild, and low in bulk. Increasingly, however, surgeons are using recently developed techniques and equipment such as a needle-catheter jejunostomy procedure to provide earlier nutritional support with an elemental formula.[7]

Later "Dumping Syndrome"

This complication is sometimes encountered after initial recovery from a gastrectomy when the patient begins to eat food in greater volume and variety. Increasing discomfort may be experienced after meals. About 10 to 15 minutes after eating, the patient has a cramping, full feeling, rapid pulse, weakness, cold sweating, and dizziness. Frequently the patient becomes nauseated and vomits. Such a distressing reaction to food intake increases anxiety. Less and less food is eaten, bringing continuing weight loss and increased malnutrition. This postgastrectomy complex of symptoms may be termed more precisely the *jejunal hyperosmolic syndrome*. It is more likely to occur in the patient who has had total gastrectomy. These symptoms of shock result when a meal containing a large portion of readily soluble carbohydrates rapidly enters the jejunum, which has been attached to the small remaining portion of the stomach during surgery. This rapidly entering food mass is a concentrated hyperosmolar solution in relation to the surrounding circulating blood. To achieve osmotic balance, therefore, water is drawn from the blood into the intestine, causing a rapid shrinking of the vascular fluid compartment. As a result the blood pressure drops and signs of cardiac insufficiency appear—rapid pulse, sweating, weakness, and tremors. A second series of events may follow

Diet for Postoperative Gastric Dumping Syndrome

General Description

- Five or six small meals daily.
- Relative high fat content to retard passage of food and help maintain weight.
- High protein content (meat, egg, cheese) to rebuild tissue and maintain weight.
- Relatively low carbohydrate content to prevent rapid passage of quickly utilized foods.
- No milk; no sugar, sweets, or desserts; no alcohol or sweet carbonated beverages.
- Liquids between meals only; avoid fluids for at least 1 hour before and after meals.
- Relatively low-roughage foods; raw foods as tolerated.

Meal Pattern

Breakfast
   2 scrambled eggs with 1 to 2 tbsp butter or margarine
   ½ to 1 slice bread or small serving cereal with butter or margarine
   2 crisp bacon strips
   1 serving solid fruit*

Midmorning sandwich of:
   1 slice bread
   Butter or margarine
   56 g (2 oz) lean meat

Lunch
   112 g (4 oz) lean meat with 1 or 2 tbsp butter or margarine
   ½ to 1 slice bread with butter or margarine
   ½ banana or other solid fruit*

Midafternoon
   Same snack as midmorning

Dinner
   112 g lean meat with 1 or 2 tbsp butter or margarine
   Green or colored vegetable† with butter or margarine
   ½ to 1 slice bread with butter or margarine (or small serving starchy vegetable substitute)
   1 serving solid fruit*

Bedtime
   56 g meat or 2 eggs or 56 g cheese or cottage cheese
   1 slice bread or 5 crackers
   Butter or margarine

*Fruit choice: applesauce, baked apple, canned fruit (drained), banana, orange or grapefruit sections.
†Vegetable choice: asparagus, spinach, green beans, squash, beets, carrots, green peas.

Postprandial Occurring after dinner, or after a meal.

about 2 hours later. The concentrated solution of carbohydrate is rapidly digested and absorbed, causing a consequent **postprandial** rise in the blood glucose. The glucose load in the blood then stimulates an overproduction of insulin, which in turn leads to an eventual drop in the blood sugar below normal fasting levels. Symptoms of mild hypoglycemia result. Dramatic relief of these distressing symptoms and gradual regaining of lost weight follows careful control of the diet. Characteristics of this diet are given in the box above.

Gallbladder Surgery
Nutrition Problems

Cholecystitis Inflammation of the gallbladder.

Cholelithiasis Formation of gallstones.

For patients suffering from acute **cholecystitis** and **cholelithiasis** (Figure 22-2), the treatment is usually surgical removal of the gallbladder—*cholecysectomy*. Following surgery, control of fat in the diet aids wound healing

Figure 22-2
Gallbladder with stones
(cholelithiasis).

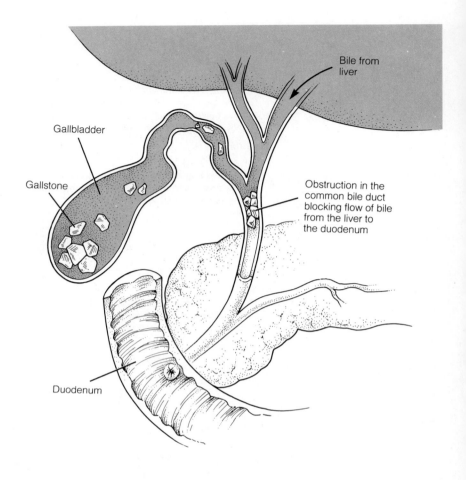

Gallbladder

Gallstone

Bile from
liver

Obstruction in the
common bile duct
blocking flow of bile
from the liver to
the duodenum

Duodenum

**Cholicystokinin
mechanism** Hormone
secreted by mucosa of upper
intestine, which stimulates
contraction of the
gallbladder.

and comfort. The presence of fat in the duodenum continues to stimulate the **cholecystokinin mechanism** (see p. 444), which causes contraction and pain in the surgical area. There is also a period of readjustment needed to the more aqueous supply of liver bile available to assist fat digestion and absorption.

Dietary Management

Depending on individual tolerance and response, a relatively low-fat diet may need to be followed for a brief time with moderate fat use thereafter. The low-fat regimen outlined for gallbladder disease (see p. 455) may serve as a guide.

Ileostomy and Colostomy

In cases of intestinal lesion or obstruction or when chronic inflammatory bowel disease (see p. 427) involves the entire colon, the treatment of choice is usually resection of the intestine to remove the diseased portion. An *ileostomy*, usually permanent but sometimes temporary, may also be established. In this procedure the end of the remaining small intestine, the ileum, is attached to an opening in the abdominal wall and a stoma is

Figure 22-3
A, Ileostomy. **B,** Colostomy.

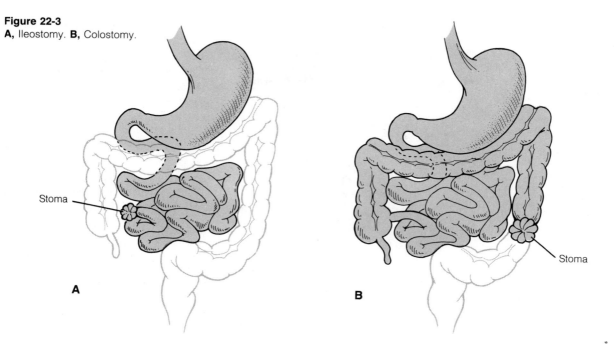

formed to provide for discharge of the intestinal contents (Figure 22-3). In a *colostomy,* which can be temporary or permanent, the colon is resected, and a stoma is made with the proximal sigmoid or descending colon.

Nutrition Problems

An ileostomy and a colostomy produce different problems in nutrition management. With an ileostomy, problems with fluid-electrolyte imbalance from loss of unabsorbed intestinal contents is common, requiring replacement therapy. The intestinal contents at the point of the ileus are unformed, irritating, and even errosive to the skin. There is free, almost continuous, drainage, and the stoma should not be irrigated. Establishment of controlled functioning is difficult. Many patients, however, do develop a reasonable degree of regularity in regard to meals, but some sort of appliance is necessary to hold the discharge. With a colostomy, management is easier. Normal contents of the intestine at this point in the colon are solid or semisolid, since more water and electrolytes have been absorbed by the proximal colon. The consistency of the discharge is less irritating and creates fewer control problems. Often a sigmoid colostomy can be adequately controlled by simple dietary measures and periodic irrigation, so that in many cases no protective appliance is needed. Coping with any ostomy is difficult at best, however, and patients need much support and practical help in learning about self-care.[8]

Dietary Management

A low-residue diet (see p. 430) is usually used in the immediate postoperative period. As soon as possible the diet should be advanced to a regular pattern of food to provide (1) optimal nutrition and physical rehabilitation and (2) an additional means of psychologic support. Diet counseling with the patient and family helps to establish the most successful pattern of meals and avoidance of foods that may cause individual discomfort. In general, persons with ostomies should eat regular diets of foods that agree with them, sufficient in quantity and nutrient value to maintain proper weight and energy. The low-residue diet may be used occasionally when diarrhea occurs.

Rectal Surgery
Nutrition Problems

For a brief period following rectal surgery—*hemorrhoidectomy*—there is pain on elimination. Thus bowel movement should be delayed until initial healing is begun.

Dietary Management

A clear fluid or nonresidue diet is indicated for initial use. The basic foods used are almost completely digested and absorbed in the small intestine, leaving minimal residue for elimination by the colon. In some cases a non-residue commercial formula may be used during the initial postoperative period.

Special Nutritional Needs for Patients with Burns

Nutritional Support Base
Treatment and Prognosis

The burned patient, especially one with extensive burns, presents a tremendous nutritional challenge. Nutritional care is often the determining factor in survival and healing. The plan of care and its outcome depend on several factors: (1) *age*—elderly persons and very young children are more vulnerable, (2) *health condition*—the presence of any preexisting condition, such as diabetes, heart or renal disease, or any other associated injuries, complicates care, and (3) *burn severity*—the location and severity of the burn wounds and the time elapsed before treatment are significant.

Degree and Extent of Burns

The depth of the burn wound affects its healing process:; (1) *first degree* burns—**erythema**—involve cell necrosis above the basal layer of the epidermis, (2) *second degree* burns involve erythema and blistering, and necrosis within the dermis, and (3) *third degree* burns result in a full-thickness skin loss, including the fat layer. Second- and third-degree burns covering 15% to 20% or more of the total body surface, or even 10% in children and elderly persons, usually cause extensive fluid loss and require intravenous fluid therapy. Burns of severe depth covering more than 50% of the body surface area are often fatal, especially in infants and older persons. Patients with major burn injuries are usually transferred for care to a specialized burn care facility.

Erythema Redness of the skin produced by congestion of the capillaries, resulting from a variety of causes, one of which can be radiant heat, i.e., burns.

Stages of Nutritional Care

The nutritional care of the patient with massive burns is adjusted to individual needs and responses. At all times attention to amino acid needs is vital,[9] in addition to critical fluid-electrolyte balance and energy (kilocalorie) support.[10] Generally three periods of care can be identified.

Immediate Shock Period

Massive flooding edema occurs at the burn site during the first hours after a burn to about the second day. Loss of enveloping skin surface and exposure of tissue fluids lead to immediate loss of water and electrolytes—mainly sodium—and large protein depletion. In an effort to balance this loss, water shifts from surrounding tissue spaces in the body, only adding to the continuous loss at the burn site. As a result the water circulating in the blood is withdrawn, thus decreasing the blood volume (**hypovolemia**) and pressure. Blood concentration and diminished urine output occur as a result. Cell dehydration follows as cell water is drawn out to balance the tissue fluid losses. Cell potassium is also withdrawn, and circulating serum potassium levels rise. Immediate intravenous fluid therapy replaces water and electrolytes by use of a salt solution such as **lactated Ringer's solution**. With such immediate care, shock can be prevented. Renal failure is a rare occurrence when resuscitation is started early. During the first part of this initial shock period—the first 12 to 14 hours following the injury—**colloid** solutions such as albumin or plasma are not effective since most of such solutions are lost in fluids at the burn site. Usually vascular endothelial permeability returns to normal after the first day, however, and colloid solutions can then be used to help restore plasma volume. During this initial period, no attempt is made to meet nutritional requirements in protein and kilocalories because (1) glucose-free, balanced electrolyte solutions are needed since infusion of glucose at this time may result in hyperglycemia and (2) an *adynamic ileus* develops after the injury and precludes any use of the gastrointestinal tract at this time.

Recovery Period

After about 48 to 72 hours, tissue fluids and electrolytes are gradually reabsorbed into the general circulation, balance is established, and the pattern of massive tissue loss is reversed. At this point a sudden **diuresis** occurs, indicating successful therapy. The patient returns to preinjury weight by about the end of the first week. A careful check of fluid intake and output is essential, with constant checks for signs of dehydration or over hydration.

Secondary Feeding Period

Toward the end of the first postburn week, adequate bowel function returns, and a vigorous feeding period must begin. At this point, despite the patient's depression and anorexia, life may well depend on rigorous nutritional therapy. Several factors necessitate this increased intake:

1. Tissue destruction The massive burn injury has brought large losses of protein and electrolytes that must be replaced.

2. Tissue catabolism Tissue protein breakdown has followed the injury, with consequent loss of lean body mass and nitrogen.

3. Increased metabolism Increased metabolic demands arise from additional needs. **Sepsis** or fever make extra kilocalories necessary for energy needs. Extra carbohydrate and B vitamins are needed for energy as the body resources mobilize to meet basal metabolic requirements. Tissue regeneration requires extra protein and key vitamins such as ascorbic acid. The success of follow-up *skin grafting* requires optimal tissue health.

Hypovolemia An abnormally low volume of circulating blood plasma.

Lactated Ringer's solution Sterile solution of calcium chloride, potassium chloride, sodium chloride and sodium lactate in water given to replenish fluid and electrolytes.

Colloid Glutinous, gluelike; a dispersion of matter throughout a medium.

Diuresis Increased urine excretion.

Sepsis Presence in the blood or other tissues of pathogenic microorganisms or their toxins—the condition associated with such presence.

Nutritional Therapy

Successful nutritional therapy during this critical feeding period is based on vigorous energy and protein therapy.

High energy From 3500 to 5000 kcal, with a high percentage of carbohydrate, is necessary to spare protein essential for tissue regeneration and to supply the greatly increased metabolic demands for energy.

High protein Depending on the extent of the burn injury, individual needs will vary from 150 g to as high as 400 g. Children will require 2 to 4 times the normal RDAs of protein for age. In general, most adults require an increased amount of protein—2 to 3 g/kg of body weight—to achieve nitrogen balance.

High vitamins From 1 to 2 g of vitamin C may be needed for tissue regeneration. Increased thiamin, riboflavin, and niacin are necessary to metabolize the extra carbohydrate and protein.

Dietary Management

To meet these crucial nutrient demands, either enteral or parenteral modes of feeding may be used.

Enteral feeding To achieve the necessary intake of increased nutrient density indicated, a careful intake record must be maintained. Oral feedings are desirable if at all tolerated by the patient. Concentrated oral liquids must be given using protein hydrolysates or amino acids to ensure adequate intake. Commercial formulas are usually used to supply large amounts of nourishment. Solid foods according to individual food preferences are added by about the second week. Tube feeding may be required by some patients in the beginning to ensure adequate intake. In this case low-bulk defined formula solutions may be given through small-bore feeding tubes. In either case, continuous support and encouragement are necessary. Food should be made as attractive and appetizing as possible, supplying items particularly liked and respecting disliked foods.

Parenteral feeding For some patients, oral intake and tube feedings may be inadequate to meet the accelerated demands or may be impossible because of associated injuries or complications. In these cases parenteral feeding is needed to provide essential nutritional support.

Follow-up Reconstruction

Continuous vigorous nutrition is essential to maintain tissue integrity for successful skin grafting or plastic reconstructive surgery. The patient will need not only physical rebuilding of body resources but also much personal support to rebuild the human spirit and will, since there may be disfigurement and disability. Health team members can do much to help instill the courage and confidence the patient must have to face the future again. Whatever the future demands, however, optimal physical stamina gained through persistent, supportive care—medical, nutritional, and nursing—will help the patient rebuild the personal resources needed to cope.

Total Parenteral Nutrition—Care of the Malnourished or Hypermetabolic Patient

TPN Development and Use
TPN Development

In nutritional therapy, the term *parenteral* means any feeding method other than by the normal gastrointestinal route. In current usage it refers to special feeding using central and peripheral veins to achieve necessary nutritional support when the gastrointestinal tract cannot be used. Since the development of this basic surgical technique over the past decade, it has provided a major advance in critical patient care. The complete sustaining of increased nutritional requirements through intravenous feeding has been termed *total parenteral nutrition (TPN)*. Also *peripheral vein parenteral nutrition (PPN)* can be used in many cases as a viable alternative.[11] It may be used in conjunction with enteral feeding, such as oral intake or tube feeding, as is frequently the case in transition feeding.[12] A clinical nutritionist with special advanced training designs and calculates these special feedings according to individual needs. Presently the clinical nutrition specialist and the physician have available a wide spectrum of formulas and delivery systems from which to plan individual nutritional therapy according to the clinical problems presented.

Indications for TPN Use

Three basic factors govern decisions concerning the use of TPN. Since there are risks involved, careful assessment of each of these factors is necessary.

Availability of gastrointestinal tract If major abdominal injury renders the gut totally unavailable for use, an alternative means of sustaining nutrition is an obvious necessity. In other cases the gut may be unavailable because of obstruction, **fistulas**, or malignant disease. Or the patient may be unable to eat because of coma, severe anorexia, or mental disturbance.

Fistula Abnormal passage, usually between two internal organs, or leading from an internal organ to the surface of the body.

Degree of malnutrition If a patient is malnourished, any medical treatment attempted will have less chance of success. Studies indicate that there is far more general malnutrition among hospitalized patients than was previously assumed. Also, it is clear that disease states impose an even greater threat to positive nutritional status. Thus the assessment of nutritional status becomes an important part of overall care, especially for hospitalized patients (see p. 356). For the more severely malnourished patient, more serious consideration of TPN is indicated.

Degree of hypermetabolism or catabolism If a patient is suffering from major trauma or severe sepsis or from malignant disease, the rate of catabolism takes a devastating toll on the body resources. This toll may be measured by nitrogen balance studies, with a loss ranging up to 15 g of nitrogen over 24 hours. Catabolic periods follow surgery, with more extensive surgery bringing the greatest losses of body resources. Malignant disease and its radiation treatment and chemotherapy (see p. 545) or any critical illness place additional demands on the body's metabolism.

Basic rules for use of TPN Using the three basic factors mentioned previously, most clinicians have formed general rules to guide the choice of TPN as a preferred means of therapy. Combinations of these factors in-

Table 22-1
Patient Situations Imposing
Need for TPN

Patient with Limited or Impossible Use of Gut	Metabolic Rate, Degree of Catabolism (nitrogen loss per 24 hr)	Degree of Malnutrition*
Situation 1	Normal (0-8) g)	Severe
Situation 2	Moderate (8-15) g)	Moderate
Situation 3	Severe (15 g)	Normal

*In terms of percent of normal standards of nutritional assessment.

dicating need for TPN are given in Table 22-1. Two basic rules form the basis for choice of TPN:

The "rule of five" If a patient has been unable to eat for 5 days and is highly likely to be unable to eat for at least another week, TPN should be considered *then* rather than waiting until malnutrition exists.

Weight loss rule Any patient who has lost 7% of the usual body weight over 2 months or who has been deprived of oral nutrition for 5 to 7 days or longer is a candidate for TPN.

Patient Candidate for TPN

Based on these considerations, candidates for vigorous nutritional therapy through TPN can be identified. These candidates include (1) *severely malnourished patients who are being prepared for surgery,* such as those with cancer of the esophagus or stomach, (2) *patients with postoperative complications,* such as those with fistulas or short bowel syndrome, (3) *patients with inflammatory bowel disease,* such as those with acute Crohn's disease, radiation enteritis, or ulcerative colitis, and (4) *patients with malabsorption or inadequate oral intake,* such as those with chronic malnutrition, major trauma as in burns, malignant neoplasms, or acute and chronic relapsing pancreatitis.

Nutrition Assessment
General Assessment

Initial individual nutrition assessment provides the necessary basis for (1) identifying patients requiring special therapy, (2) calculating their nutritional requirements, and (3) determining the specific nutrient formula to meet these requirements. This is the task of the clinical nutritionist on the TPN team. This initial assessment is done by standard methods: anthropometric measures, biochemical laboratory data, clinical observations, and dietary evaluations, together with a detailed history. These general methods are described in Chapter 16 and can be reviewed there.

Specific TPN Procedures

According to individual patient needs and clinical situations, specific guidelines for TPN nutritional assessment include the following procedures:

Degree of weight loss Use measures of current body weight and height. Interpret these measures in terms of desirable lean body weight for

Table 22-2
Indications of Severe Protein-Calorie Malnutrition According to Percentage of Recent Weight Loss

% Body Weight Loss	Time Period
2%	1 week
5%	1 month
7.5%	3 months
10%	6 months

height, usual body weight, and amount of recent weight change. Compare patient's amount of recent weight change with the values indicating malnutrition given in Table 22-2.

Body fat stores and skeletal muscle mass Using caliper measures of triceps skinfold (TSF) and standard reference tables for TSF data, estimate the patient's body fat stores. Using the midarm circumference (MAC) measure, calculate the midarm muscle circumference (MAMC) and compare with standard reference tables: MAMC (cm) = (MAC (cm) − [0.314 × TSF mm]).

Lean body mass Using amount of creatinine output in a 24-hour urine collection, determine the creatinine-height index using standard tables.

Degree of catabolism Using amount of urea nitrogen output in a 24-hour urine collection and the nitrogen value of the diet during the same 24-hour period, calculate the overall nitrogen balance for that period: N balance = N intake (protein intake/6.25) − N loss (urinary urea N + 4).

Immune function Use total lymphocyte count or percentage of lymphocytes in total white blood cell count to determine general function of patient's immune system. Skin testing for sensitivity to common recall antigens can also give immune function data.

Plasma protein compartment Use the serum albumin level as a measure of the body's visceral protein mass. Also, using laboratory data for total iron-binding capacity (TIBC), calculate the value for transferrin, the body's iron transport compound: transferrin (mg/dl) = (TIBC [μg/dl] × 0.8) −43. A reference for determination of protein-kilocalorie malnutrition using these plasma values is given in Table 22-3. Monitoring of these nutritional assessment data continues throughout therapy.

Table 22-3
Determination of Protein-Calorie Malnutrition by Plasma Values

Laboratory Data	Normal Values	Degree of Malnutrition Moderate	Severe
Serum albumin (g/dl)	3.5	2.1-3.0	<2.1
Serum transferrin (mg/dl)	180-260	100-150	<100
Total lymphocyte count Per mm³ % of WBC	1500-4000 20%-53%	800-1200	<800

Nutrition Requirements: TPN Prescription

Energy Requirements

In health about 35 kcal/kg body weight are required for maintenance, whereas in catabolic illness it is about 50 to 60 kcal/kg.

$$\text{Nitrogen} = \frac{\text{Total protein}}{6.25}$$

The kilocalorie needs of the critically ill patient will range from 2000 to as much as 5000 or 6000 kcal/day in major trauma or sepsis. The great difference is seen in comparing health and illness needs. This large energy input is necessary to meet the increased basal metabolic demands and the large energy cost of catabolism, fever, malnutrition, and any physical activity.

Protein Requirements

Protein is needed to maintain nitrogen balance and provide essential amino acids. In addition, an adequate ratio of nitrogen to nonnitrogen kilocalories is necessary to protect the nitrogen sources for use in tissue protein synthesis. For meeting the metabolic stress of illness, the ratio should be 150 to 200 kcal/g of nitrogen. In terms of protein intake the patient needs a minimum of 1.2 to 1.5 g protein/kg body weight. Compare this increased requirement with the usual maintenance adult requirements in health: 0.8-1.0 g protein/kg.

Electrolyte Requirements

Individual monitoring data are used to determine electrolyte balances and needs. An example of the electrolyte composition of a basic TPN formula is given in Table 22-4.

Table 22-4
Example of Basic TPN Formula Components

Components	Amounts
Basic solution	
Crystalline amino acids	2.75%
Dextrose	25%
Additives	
Electrolytes	
Na	50 mEq/L
Cl	50 mEq/L
K	40 mEq/l
HPO_4	25 mEq/L
Ca	5 mEq/L
Mg	8 mEq/L
Vitamins	
Multiple (MVI)	1.7 mlconc./L
Vitamin C (day)	500 mg
Trace elements solution (day)	
Zn	3 mg
Cu	1.6 mg
Cr	2 μg
Se	120 μg
Mn	2 μg
I	120 μg
Fe	1.5 μg
Other additives (as needed)	
Regular insulin	0-25 units/L
Heparin	1000 units/L

Vitamin and Mineral Requirements

Added vitamin and mineral needs are created by hypermetabolic effects and depleted states. An evaluation of the extent of these needs is based on invididual assessment data. Particular attention is paid to trace elements. These needs are reflected in Table 22-4.

Preparation of TPN Solutions

With the development of the TPN technique, products for use in TPN nutrient solutions have also been developing. They are used by the TPN team in formulating nutritional needs for each patient, based on the nutritional requirements for protein, energy, electrolytes, vitamins, and minerals.

Protein-Nitrogen Source

Remember that 6.25 g protein, amino acids, equals 1 g nitrogen. Currently the nitrogen source of choice is crystalline amino acids, both essential and nonessential. A number of commercial products are available in a variety of compositions and dilutions. After the individual patient prescription is determined by the TPN team physician and clinical dietitian, the pharmacist on the team mixes accurate solutions for each patient as indicated. However, all team members should know about these solutions and keep up with the various commercial product changes. For example, the usual amino acid need is supplied by a 3.5% or 4.25% dilution. This dilution is achieved by use of 1 L of a standard 7.0% or 8.5% amino acid solution mixed with 1 L of dextrose solution.

Nonprotein Energy Source—Kilocalories

Nonprotein kilocalories to protect protein for tissue synthesis demands are supplied by glucose and fat solutions.

Glucose (dextrose) Dextrose solutions range from the 5% solution, used traditionally in peripheral intravenous support of fluid and electrolytes postsurgically, to the hypertonic 70% available for TPN formulations. The usual solution used for TPN is 50% dextrose. When this solution is mixed with amino acid solution, it renders a 25% dextrose solution in the formula. Dextrose solutions given intravenously do not deliver the classic 4 kcal/g. In the *anhydrous* form, these solutions are 91% calorigenic, providing 3.75 kcal/g. Thus a final solution of 25% dextrose would provide 850 kcal. For example, a liter of 25% glucose per 2.7% amino acid (Travasol) would provide 4.63 g nitrogen and a kilcalorie/nitrogen ratio of 183:1. This ratio will vary with different solutions. In common TPN dextrose solutions using the *monohydrate* form, the energy value of the dextrose is a little less: 3.4 kcal/g.

Fat Emulsions of fat provide a concentrated source of nonprotein kilocalories and ensure a necessary supply of the main essential fatty acid, linoleic acid (see p. 61). Two products are currently available: Intralipid and Liposyn. Both come in 10% (1.1 kcal/ml) and 20% (2.0 kcal/ml) concentrations. They are fat emulsions derived from soy oil (Intralipid) and safflower oil (Liposyn). Both contain neutral triglycerides of predominantly unsaturated fatty acids. They are usually used as a supplement to the main TPN solution, provided separately according to need, usually one to two bottles a week for adults. They are administered separately through a Y-connector tube. They are never mixed with the main dextrose–amino acid solution because the fat emulsion would break down.

Electrolytes

The formulation of electrolytes is based on the usual requirements for normal electrolyte balance with adjustments according to individual patient monitoring. A general ratio of electrolytes is shown in Table 22-4.

Vitamins

Multivitamin formulas are available for use in TPN solutions, as are individual vitamins for formulating the solution according to patient needs. Multiple formulas such as MVI (multiple vitamin injection) supply water-soluble B-complex vitamins and vitamin C as well as water-soluble forms of vitamins A, D, and E. Since vitamins B_{12}, folate, and K may alter their form when added to the rest of the vitamin formula, they are added separately and not on a daily basis, as indicated in Table 22-4.

Minerals

Precipitate To cause a substance in solution to settle down in solid particles.

Caution is needed in adding minerals to the TPN solution. Incompatabilities of certain electrolytes and other components may result in the formation of an insoluble **precipitate**, depending on factors such as ion concentration and solution pH. More attention has been given recently to the need for added trace minerals,[13] as well as the need for close monitoring of calcium balance.[14]

Figure 22-4
Catheter placement for total parenteral nutrition (TPN) made by feeding via subclavian vein to superior vena cava.

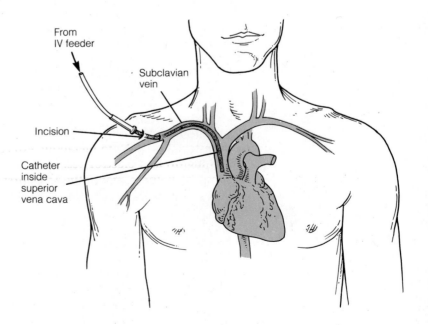

From
IV feeder

Subclavian
vein

Incision

Catheter
inside
superior
vena cava

Mixing the Formula

The pharmacist on the TPN team mixes the components of the specific solution for patient's prescription according to a rigid protocol. A laminar flow hood provides an aseptic environment in which the solutions, open medication vials, and other materials can be handled safely. To ensure stability, the individual solution formulas are ordered and mixed on a daily basis.

Administration of TPN
TPN Team

The insertion of the central vein TPN line is a surgical procedure done by the physician (Figure 22-4). It is usually performed at the bedside following strict aseptic procedures. The nurse on the TPN team has special training in care of the patient on TPN and is responsible for administering the formula (see box below) and maintaining the rigid protocols developed to avoid infection or other complications. The clinical nutrition specialist on the TPN team is responsible for nutrition assessment, interpretation of data, and calculating formula needs in close collaboration with the physician. The pharmacist is responsible for mixing the formulas according to individual prescription worked out by the physician and the clinical nutritionist. In the hands of a well-trained TPN team, risks have been minimized and complications can be controlled by team effort.

Home TPN for Long-Term Use

Experience from home use of other long-term medical care equipment, such as that for renal dialysis, has led to the concept of self-infusion of

---

Clinical Application

Administration of TPN Formula

Careful administration of TPN formulas is essential. Specific protocols will vary somewhat. Usually, however, they include the following points:

- **Start slowly** Give time to adapt to the increased glucose concentration and osmolality of the solution.
- **Schedule carefully** During the first 24 hours, 1 to 2 L is given by continuous drip, the slow rate regulated usually by an infusion pump.
- **Monitor closely** Note metabolic effects of glucose (not to exceed 200 mg/dl) and electrolytes.
- **Increase volume gradually** After first day, increase by 1 L/day to reach desired daily volume.
- **Make changes cautiously** Watch the effect of all changes and proceed slowly.
- **Maintain a constant rate** Keep the correct hourly infusion rate, with no "catch up" or "slow down" effort to meet original volume order.
- **Discontinue slowly** Take patient off of TPN feeding gradually, reducing rate and daily volume about 1 L/day.

parenteral nutrients at home. (See Issues and Answers, pp. 530-531). Home TPN can greatly reduce the cost of such treatment. In the hands of selected, well-trained patients and families it allows mobility and travel. It offers special promise in long-term management of such conditions as severe abdominal injury or chronic severe inflammatory bowel disease. Special equipment, solutions, and guidelines for training selected patients and families have been developed and are successfully being used in a number of cases.[15]

To Sum Up

The nutritional demands of surgery begin before the patient reaches the operating table. Preoperatively the task is to correct any existing deficiencies and build nutrient reserves to meet surgical demands. Postoperatively it is to replace losses and support recovery. The additional task of encouraging eating is often required during this period.

Pre- and postsurgical feedings are given in a variety of ways. The oral route is always preferred, but damage to the intestinal tract or a poor appetite may require other enteral or parenteral feedings. Diets are modified according to the surgical procedure performed. For the depleted surgical patient, nutritional support relies heavily on biomedical technology to facilitate enteral or parenteral feedings administered by specially trained TPN team members.

Questions for Review

1. Describe the general impact of imbalances of the following nutritional factors during the pre-, immediate post-, and postoperative periods; protein, kilocalories, vitamins and minerals, and fluids.
2. Describe the major surgical effects for which nutritional therapy must be planned following these procedures: mouth, throat, or neck surgery; gastric resection; cholecystectomy; and rectal surgery.
3. Write a 1-day meal plan for a person experiencing the postgastrectomy "dumping syndrome." What general dietary guidelines are used?
4. Describe the difference in care between ileostomy and a colostomy. What are the dietary implications of each?
5. Outline the nutritional care of a burn patient from treatment for immediate shock through recovery and tissue reconstruction.
6. What is TPN? For whom is it usually recommended? Why?

References

1. Rodgers, L., Moss, J., and Wright, R.: New developments in enteral feeding techniques, Nutr. Support Serv. **2**(10):17, 1982.
2. Jensen, T.: Home enteral nutrition, Dietet. Currents **9**(4):1, 1982.
3. Moss, G.: Maintenance of gastrointestinal function after bowel surgery and immediate enteral full nutrition, II. Clinical experience with objective demonstration of intestinal absorption and motility, J. Parent. Enter. Nutr. **5**:215, 1981.
4. Shils, M., Bloch, A., and Chernoff, R.: Liquid formulas for oral and tube feeding, New York, 1979, Memorial Sloan-Kettering Cancer Center.
5. Chernoff, R.: Nutritional support: formulas and delivery of enteral feeding, J. Am. Dietet. Assoc. **79**(4):426, 1981.
6. Ross, G.: Geriatric enteral hyperalimentation, Part I, Nutr. Support Serv. **1**(6):29, 1981.
7. Page, C.P.: Needle-catheter jejunostomy, Clin. Consultations **1**(3):5, 1981.
8. Knebel, F.: Diet for smooth digestion, Am. Health **2**(4):72, 1983.
9. Cynober, L., and others: Plasma and urinary amino acid pattern in severe burn patients—evolution throughout the healing period, Am. J. Clin. Nutr., **36**(3):416, September, 1982.
10. Desai, M.H., and Teres, D.: New high caloric density supplement for enteral nutrition in burned patients, Nutr. Support Serv. **2**:20, 1982.
11. Kelly, S.E.: Peripheral vein TPN: a viable alternative to the central venous approach, Clin. Consultations **1**(2):1, 1981.
12. Wade, J.E.: Transitional enteral feeding, Clin. Consultations **1**(2):10, 1981.
13. Solomons, N.: Zinc nutriture in total parenteral nutrition, Clin. Nutr. **2**(3):8, 1983.
14. Allen, L.H.: Calcium nutriture in total parenteral nutrition, Clin. Nutr. **2**(3):18, 1983.
15. Chrysomilides, S.A., and Kaminski, M.V.: Home enteral and parenteral nutritional support: a comparison, Am. J. Clin. Nutr. **34**:2271, 1981.

Further Readings

Fleeman, C.M., and Wright, R.A.: Concepts of home parenteral nutrition, Nutr. Support Serv. **1**(6):16, 1981.

Outlines a patient selection and training program for home TPN—describes equipment, detailed procedures, and benefits.

Grant, J.P.: Administration of parenteral nutrition solutions in Handbook of total parenteral nutrition, Philadelphia, 1980, W.B. Saunders Co.

General reference manual for use in the assessment, prescription, administering, monitoring of parenteral nutrition solutions.

Kirkpatrick, J.R., and Nelson, R.: Preoperative nutritional support: indications and strategies, Nutr. Support Serv. **1**(6):28, 1981.

Provides basis for attention to patient's nutritional status *before* surgery and ways of building up nutritional resources.

Knebel, F.: Diet for smooth digestion, Am. Health **2**(4):72, 1983.

A heart-warming account by a man with a colostomy who learns how to cope. He describes in highly personal fashion how life without a rectum teaches you to manage your food with fiber and supplements.

Munster, A.M.: The early management of thermal burns, Surgery **87**:29, 1980.

Describes immediate post-burn state and importance of early resuscitation and management of nutritional, physical, and metabolic needs.

Special issue: Nutrition for surgical patients, Surg. Clin. N. Am., 1981.

The articles in this special issue relate nutrition in surgery to metabolism, trauma, infection, enteral and parenteral nutrition, nutrition assessment. Excellent reference for clinical practice and basis for therapies to meet nutritional needs.

Issues and Answers

**The Challenge of
Long-Term TPN
Therapy**

The purpose of any non-oral feeding method is to restore the patient, if possible, to the oral feeding state. How long this will take varies according to the original nutritional and health status of the patient, as well as the extent of the illness. Persons with inflammatory bowel syndrome (see Chapter 19) may require 2 to 3 months to reap the clinical benefits of "bowel rest" afforded by TPN; at least one individual with "no-bowel" syndrome has done very well on TPN for more than a decade! While this makes TPN's potential for long-term use seem tremendous, it is not without its drawbacks.

First of all, the intestinal effects of TPN suggest potential hazards with long-term use. The lack of food in the alimentary canal results in: (1) reduced secretion of hormones and enzymes into the gastrointestinal tract, (2) cholestasis because of an increased viscosity of bile that is *not* secreted into the gastrointestinal tract, (3) mucosal atrophy and hypoplasia caused by possibly reduced levels of cholecystokinin, and (4) less insulin secreted in response to the same amount of glucose obtained orally. These difficulties do not interfere with the ability to digest foods for 2 to 3 months.

But what if the patient graduates to oral or tube feedings after that? Will there be difficulties with: (1) undigested foods, (2) a higher risk for gallstones, (3) impaired nutrient absorption across an atrophied mucosa, or (4) a risk of hyperglycemia? These questions indicate the need for *very* careful monitoring and *gradual* refeeding for such patients.

Other problems regarding long-term TPN *have* been verified and measured. These problems have more to do with the nature of the formula solution rather than with the bowel. Their potential for causing malnutrition warrants careful control and prevention methods on the part of the health care professional. The TPN process uses solutions of glucose and amino acids, as well as vitamin and mineral supplements, with additional fat emulsion used as needed. During the use of these solutions, blood levels of key nutrients must be carefully monitored:

Glucose Solutions

Glucose levels must be carefully monitored, since excessive amounts may result in: (1) *hyperglycemia,* (2) *respiratory distress,* especially in critically ill patients—excessive glucose intake raises the respiratory quotient (RQ = $CO_2:O_2$) by increasing CO_2 production, or (3) *lipogenesis,* which may or may not be desirable in individual patients. The best defense against such problems is to use solutions that provide half of the total nonprotein energy from fats and half from glucose.

Amino Acid Solutions

Several deficiencies have been associated with amino acid use:

- **Carnitine** Carnitine is an amino acid that helps incorporate fatty acids into the cell for energy use. One patient on TPN for a year developed muscle weakness, high bilirubin levels, and hypoglycemia. Plasma carnitine levels were found to be low.

Issues and Answers—cont'd

Symptoms subsided after he was given 400 mg l-carnitine for 7 days. To avoid further problems, he was maintained on a dose of 60 mg/day.

- **Aluminum** Amino acids were originally provided by solutions of hydrolysates. Casein hydrolysate solutions also contained large amounts of aluminum, apparently in the water added to prepare the hydrolysate. In the body, aluminum is believed to contribute to a painful bone disease characterized by osteomalacia. Fortunately, most hydrolysate solutions are no longer manufactured by major pharmaceutical companies.
- **Calcium** Amino acid solutions provide extra sulfur (e.g., methionine and cysteine), which binds with calcium and promotes its excretion. As a result, premature infants on TPN may develop osteomalacia, a painful bone disease associated with calcium deficiency.

Vitamin and Mineral Supplements

These additional supplements may create a problem because of difficulty in being released from solution or variability in requirements among patients:

- **Iron** The supplement frequently used in TPN solutions, iron dextran, does not release iron as easily as desired. Ferrous citrate is recommended by at least one study, which found that 74% to 81% of its iron was readily available for binding with ferritin in the blood.
- **Biotin** One patient, who developed **delirium tremens**, dermatitis, severe depression, anorexia, nausea, and vomiting, was relieved of his symptoms after one week of biotin supplementation at 300 μg/day.

Delirium tremens Mental disturbance marked by delirium with trembling and great excitement.

Thus, for maximum promotion of the nutritional status of patients requiring long-term TPN, health care professionals should (1) carefully monitor a *gradual* refeeding program to avoid problems created by reduced gastrointestinal secretions and mucosal atrophy, (2) provide sufficient fats (as half of the nonprotein kcals) to prevent respiratory distress in very ill patients and spare protein for tissue repair and development, (3) be aware of deficiency symptoms and potential effects of "undesirable" additives (sulfur, ammonia, etc.) found in amino acid solutions and be prepared to adjust the solution accordingly, (4) adjust vitamin and mineral levels to suit individual needs, and (5) select solutions from which nutrients are readily available.

References

Cole, D., and Zlotkin, S.: Increased sulfate as an etiological factor in the hypercalciuria associated with total parenteral nutrition, Am. J. Clin. Nutr. **37**:108, 1983.

Hallberg, D., and others: Parenteral nutrition: goals and achievements, Part II, Nutr. Support Serv. **2**(8):35, 1982.

Klein, G.L., and others: Aluminum loading during total parenteral nutrition, Am. J. Clin. Nutr. **35**(6):1425, 1982.

Levenson, J.L.: Biotin-responsive depression hyperalimentation, J. Parent. Enter. Nutr. **7**:181, 1983.

Sayers, M.H., and others: Supplementation of total parenteral nutrition solutions with ferrous citrate, J. Parent. Enter. Nutr. **7**:117, 1983.

Worthly, L., Fishlock, R., and Snoswell, A.: Carnitine deficiency with hyperbilirubinemia, generalized skeletal muscle weakness, and reactive hypoglycemia in a patient on long-term total parenteral nutrition: treatment with intravenous l-carnitine, J. Parent. Enter. Nutr. **7**:176, 1983.

Chapter 23
Nutrition and Cancer

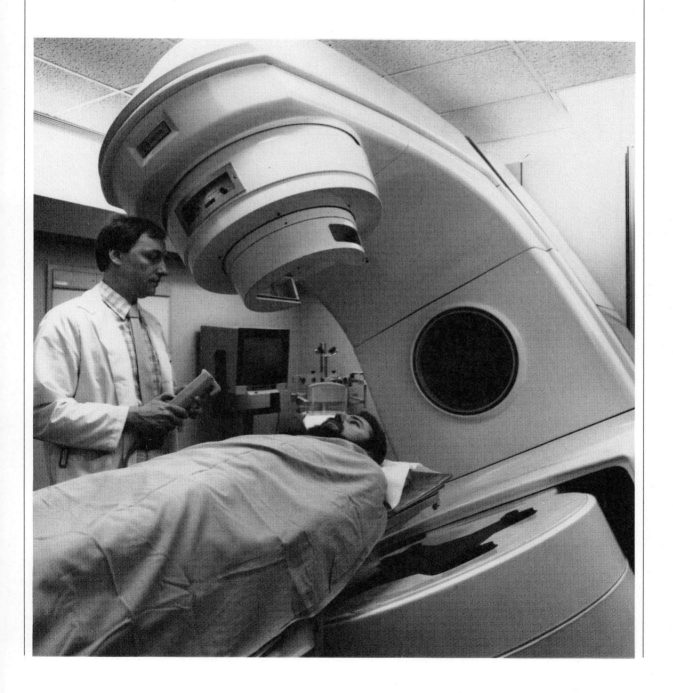

Preview

The American Cancer Society estimates that approximately 440,000 Americans die of cancer each year, with about 114,000, or 25%, dying of lung cancer. In its multiple forms cancer has become one of our major public health problems. It is second only to heart disease and accounts for about 20% of the total deaths in the United States each year. In current study and practice, although published results are conflicting, important nutritional relationships seem to exist in two basic areas: (1) *prevention,* related to the environment and to the body's defense system; and (2) *therapy,* related to nutritional support for medical treatment and rehabilitation. To understand these nutritional relationships, we must clarify them in terms of cancer's nature as a growth process, cancer's physiologic basis in the structure and function of cells, and the body's defense systems, both in immunity and the healing process.

Chapter Objectives

After study of this chapter, the student should be able to:

1. Relate nutrition to development of a cancer cell and to the body's defense system.

2. Identify nutritional effects of the various medical therapies for cancer and describe ways of handling related eating problems.

3. List ways cancer affects nutritional requirements and outline dietary management to meet these needs.

Process of Cancer Development

Cancer Cellular tumor whose natural course is fatal; unlike benign tumor cells, cancer growths are invasive and spread easily.

Neoplasm Any new or abnormal growth; uncontrolled or progressive growth. Also called a tumor.

Difficulties in the study of cancer have arisen from its varying nature and its multiple forms. The term **cancer** is used to designate a malignant tumor or **neoplasm** (new growth). There are many different forms of cancer, however, varying worldwide and changing with population migrations. There are multiple causes and conflicting research results because of the large number of variables involved. Thus it is clear that we are dealing with a wide range of malignant tumors collectively known as cancer. We would be more correct, then, to use the plural term "cancers" in discussing this great variety of neoplasms. To better understand cancer development, therefore, we should view it as a growth process that has its physiologic basis in the structure and function of cells. Since nutrition is fundamental to all tissue growth, we need to look briefly at the cancer cell to understand the relationship of nutritional factors to cancer. This "misguided cell" and its tumor tissue represent normal cell growth that has "gone wild."

The Cancer Cell

The marvel of human life is that the process of cell growth and reproduction goes on almost flawlessly over and over again, guided by the cell's genes. In adult humans some 3 to 4 million cells complete the normal life-sustaining process of cell division every second, largely without mistake, guided by the genetic code.[1] The specific genetic material in the cell nucleus is arranged as chromosomes and genes, which hold the controlling agent, *deoxyribonucleic acid (DNA)*. Specific sites along the chromosomes are called genes. Each gene carries specific genetic information that controls synthesis of specific proteins and transmits genetic heritance. A single chromosome thread is made up of hundreds of genes arranged end to end, and each gene of DNA is made up of some 600 to several thousand smaller subunits called nucleotides. The nucleic acids, DNA and its companion, *ribonucleic acid (RNA)*, compose the controlling system by which both the cell and the organism sustain life. The structure of DNA is that of a very large polynucleotide made up of many individual mononucleotides, each one of which has three parts: a sugar (deoxyribose), a phosphate, and a specific nitrogenous base—adenine, cytosine, guanine, or thymine. It is the pairing of these nitrogenous bases, as indicated in Figure 23-1, that incorporates the "genetic code" and enables the DNA to transmit messages to guide specific protein structure. The DNA appears as a twisted ladder or spiral staircase in structure and is thus called a "helix" (spiral).

Gene Control

Cells arise only from preexisting cells by division and carry the cell's genetic pattern. Normally the various cell structures and functions operate in an orderly manner under gene control, directing the cell's specific processes of protein synthesis. Gene action, however, can be switched on and off, depending on the position of a cell in the body, the stage of body development, and the external environment. Specific regulator genes control such function by producing a repressor substance as needed to regulate operator genes and structural genes. This orderly regulation of induction and repression in cell activity, however, can be lost with mutation

Figure 23-1
Diagram of a portion of DNA structure. Note the components. The sugar deoxyribose and phosphate form the parallel bars of the ladderlike structure (a double helix); the connecting nitrogenous bases (the pyrimidines, thymine and cytosine, and the purines, adenine and guanine) form the rungs (*A,* adenine; *T,* thymine; *C,* cytosine; *G,* guanine; *S,* sugar—deoxyribose; *P,* phosphate). The dotted lines represent the hydrogen bonding between the nitrogenous bases.

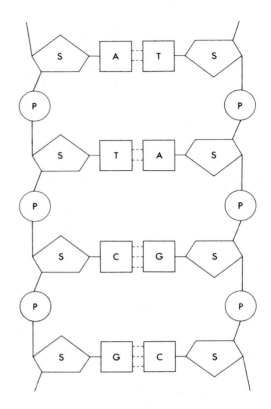

of these regulatory genes. Control is also lost when a specific gene for some reason moves from its position to another location on the chromosome. A cell may become malignant when one of these potentially cancer-causing genes is translocated and reinserted into a highly active part of the DNA.[2]

Cancer Cell Derivation

The cancer cell is derived, then, from a normal cell that has lost control over cell reproduction and is thereby transformed from a normal cell into a cancer cell (Figure 23-2).

Cancer Tumor Types

Based on the differentiation of cells and their specific nature, cancer tumors may be classified according to two factors: (1) the type of *originating tissue,* with tumors arising from connective tissues called **sarcomas** and those from epithelial tissue called **carcinomas**, and (2) *degree of cell tissue change,* with tumor stages defined in relation to rate of growth, degree of autonomy, and invasiveness.

Relation to Aging Process

Since the incidence of cancer increases with age, a relationship exists between cancer cell development and the aging process in cells, tissues, and organ systems.

Sarcoma Tumor, usually malignant, arising from connective tissue.

Carcinoma Tumor, usually malignant, arising from epithelial tissue.

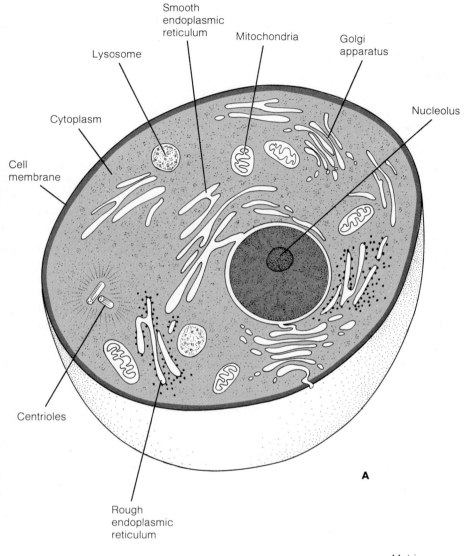

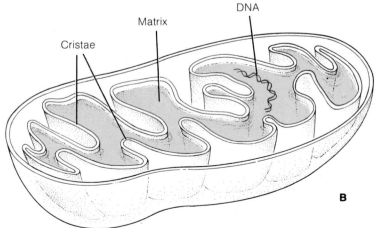

Figure 23-2
A, Diagram of major cell structures, showing organelles associated with cell nutrition and metabolism. **B**, Structure of a mitochondrion, the "powerhouse" of the cell.

Causes of Cancer Cell Development

The underlying cause of cancer, as indicated previously, is the fundamental loss of control over normal cell reproduction. A number of contributory causes to this loss have been suggested by various investigations and can be seen as interrelated in their actions:

Mutations Mutations are caused by loss of one or more of the regulatory genes in the cell nucleus. Such a mutant gene may be inherited, although some environmental agent may contribute to its expression.

Chemical carcinogens A number of chemical carcinogens (hydrocarbons) can interfere with the structure or function of regulatory genes. Exposure to such agents may be by individual choice, such as in cigarette smoking, or by exposure to general environmental substances. Possible cancer-causing actions of such substances may be mutation, effect on regulation of gene function, or activation of a dormant virus.

Radiation In some instances radiation may be sufficient to cause chromosome breakage and incorrect rejoining. Radiation damage may come from x rays, radioactive materials, atomic exhausts or wastes, or from sunlight. The overexposure to sunlight is related to skin cancer, rapidly on the rise in the United States and Europe, afflicting younger and younger persons. The common forms on the head and neck are usually basal cell carcinoma and are easily cured by surgical removal. However, a far more lethal form, *malignant melanoma,* strikes more than 15,000 Americans a year, killing some 45% of them.[3]

Oncogenic viruses Oncogenic, or tumor-inducing, viruses that interfere with the function of regulatory genes have been identified in animals and are the focus of much current research. Although oncogenes were first found in viruses, their evolutionary history indicates that they are also present and functioning in normal vertebrate cells as well. It is their abnormal expression that can lead to cancerous growth. A virus is little more than a packet of genetic information encased in a protein coat. It contains a small chromosome, DNA or RNA, with a relatively small number of genes, usually fewer than five and never more than several hundred. In contrast, cells of complex organisms have thousands of genes. Disease viruses act as parasites, taking over the cell machinery to replicate themselves.

Epidemiologic Factors

Studies of cancer distribution and occurrence in relation to such factors as race, diet, region, sex, age, heredity, and occupation show variable and conflicting results. The specific role of diet in cancer etiology is still unclear (see Issues and Answers, pp. 556-558). However, the incidence of cancer does vary a great deal from country to country and that of specific cancer types varies from 6- to 300-fold.[4] Although our cancer incidence rates have not changed markedly over the past few decades, cancer is *endemic* in our population. The U.S. incidence rates for cancer are appreciably greater than those for many other countries.[5] Racial incidence of cancer seems to change as population groups migrate and acquire the different cancer characteristics of the new population. Although it has been difficult to pinpoint specific dietary factors in the cause of cancer, worldwide epidemiologic studies do show significant correlation of mortality from breast cancer with the consumption of dietary fats in countries around the world.[6] Currently a large study involving 7000 postmenopausal women, with a subgroup having stage II breast cancer, is underway in the United States to help determine the nature of the relationship of dietary fat to breast cancer.[7]

Stress Factors

The idea that emotions may play a part in malignancy is not new, Galen, a second century Greek physician, wrote of such relationships, as have many different kinds of "healers" since that time. However, these relationships are difficult to measure. Even with great technologic and scientific advances, Western medicine holds fast to the scientific method and its basic tenet that a thing must be measurable under controlled conditions to be said to exist. Nonetheless, increasing observations are being made of relationships between cancer and less measurable factors. Clinicians and researchers have reported that psychic trauma, especially the loss of a central relationship, does seem to carry with it a strong cancer correlation. The cause of a possible relationship between psychic trauma and cancer may lie in two physiologic areas: (1) damage to the thymus gland and the immune system and (2) hormonal effects mediated through the hypothalymus, pituitary, and adrenal cortex. This cascade of physiologic events may provide the neurologic currency that converts anxiety to malignancy. Such a stressful state may also make a person more vulnerable to other factors present, influencing the integrity of the immune system, food behaviors, and the nutritional status.

The Body's Defense System

The human body's defense system is remarkably efficient and complex. Several components of special type cells protect not only against external invaders such as bacteria and viruses but also against internal "aliens" such as malignant tumor cells.

Components of the Immune System

Cellular immunity Specific, acquired immunity in which the role of the T-lymphocytes predominates.

Humoral immunity Acquired immunity in which the role of antibodies (produced by B-lymphocytes and plasma cells) predominates.

Two major populations of cells provide the immune system's primary line of defense for detecting and destroying malignant cells that may arise daily in the body. These cells mediate specific **cellular immunity** and **humoral immunity,** as well as providing supportive backup biologic systems. These two populations of lymphoid cells, or *lymphocytes* (a type of white blood cell), develop early in life from a common stem cell in fetal liver and bone marrow (Figure 23–3). They then differentiate and populate the peripheral lymphoid organs during the latter stages of gestation. One type are called *T cells*, traced from thymus-derived cells, and the other *B cells*, traced from bursa-derived cells. Both T and B lymphocytes are derived from precursor cells in the bone marrow.

T cells After precursor cells migrate to the thymus, the T cell population is differentiated in this small gland (which lies posterior to the sternum and anterior to the great vessels partly covering the trachea). The majority of the circulating small lymphocytes in blood, lymph, and certain areas of

Figure 23-3
Development of the T and B cells, lymphocyte components of the body's immune system.

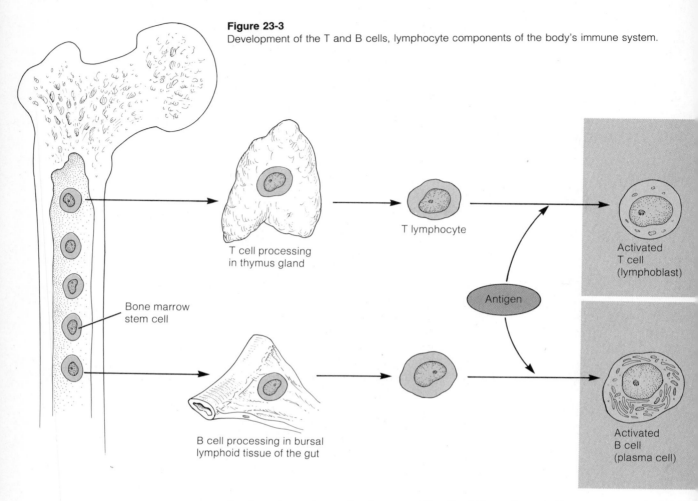

T cell processing
in thymus gland

T lymphocyte

Bone marrow
stem cell

Antigen

Activated
T cell
(lymphoblast)

B cell processing in bursal
lymphoid tissue of the gut

Activated
B cell
(plasma cell)

The thymus is a small organ, weighing about 14 g (½ oz) at birth. It reaches its largest size of 37 g (1⅓ oz) at puberty, and reduces in older age to 7 g (¼ oz).

the lymph nodes and spleen are T cells. When these cells meet an antigen (alien substance), they proliferate and initiate specific cellular immune responses: (1) they activate the *phagocytes,* special cells that have intracellular killing and degrading mechanisms for destroying invaders, and (2) they initiate an inflammatory response through chemical mediators released by the antigen-stimulated T cells. Scientists have now discovered that some T lymphocytes can do even more, not only proliferating in response to an antigen but also attacking it. These special T cells are called "helper cell-independent cytotoxic T lymphocytes," abbreviated more graphically to the name *HIT cells.*[8]

B cells The B cell population matures first in the marrow and then, following migration, in the solid peripheral lymphoid tissues of the body—the lymph nodes, spleen, and gut. These cells are responsible for synthesis and secretion of specialized protein known as *antibodies.* When the B cells contact an antigen, they increase and initiate specific humoral immune responses: (1) they produce specific antibodies in the blood, and (2) they produce a particular antibody secretion in the bowel and upper respiratory mucosa. This combination of antigen and antibody then attracts phagocytes and initiates the inflammatory response for healing. Recently teams of researchers and clinicians have been able to develop specially tailored proteins, called *monoclonal antibodies,* and then use them to diagnose and treat a number of diseases, including cancer.[9] As their name implies, these special antibodies are produced by identical descendents, or clones, of a single cell through specific techniques involving injection and development in laboratory mice. These controlled products are specific antibodies for specific targets.

Relation to Nutrition

Nutritional support is necessary to maintain the integrity of this efficient human immune system. Severely malnourished populations have displayed changes in the structure and function of the immune system because of atrophy of basic tissues involved: liver, bowel wall, bone marrow, spleen, and lymphoid tissue. The role of nutrition in maintaining normal immunity and in combating sustained attacks in malignancy is fundamental.

The Healing Process

Tissue integrity, essential for the healing process, is maintained through protein synthesis. Such strength of tissue is a front line of the body's defense system. This process of healing through protein synthesis for tissue integrity demands optimal nutritional intake. Specific nutrients—protein and key vitamins and minerals, as well as nonprotein energy sources—must constantly be supplied. Wise and early use of vigorous nutritional support for cancer patients has been shown to provide recovery of normal nutritional status, including **immunocompetence,** thereby improving their response to therapy and prognosis.[10]

Immunocompetence The ability or capacity to develop an immune response, such as antibody production or cell-mediated immunity, following exposure to antigen.

Nutritional Support for Cancer Therapy

Current cancer therapy takes three major forms: *surgery, radiation,* and *chemotherapy.* Nutritional support for any form of cancer therapy enhances its potential success.

Surgery
Operable Tumors

Early diagnosis of operable tumors has led to successful surgical treatment of a large number of cancer patients. As with any surgery, but particularly with cancer patients because their general condition may be weakened, optimal nutritional status preoperatively and maximal nutritional support postoperatively are fundamental to the healing process.

Nutrition Relationships

Nutrition has both general and specific relationships: (1) support of the general healing process and overall body metabolism and (2) specific modifications of nutrient factors, texture, or feeding method according to the surgical site and organ function involved. Prevention of problems through early detection and surgical treatment has significantly increased cancer cure rates. Surgical treatment may also be used with other forms of therapy for removal of single metastases or for prevention and alleviation of symptoms.

Radiation
Treatment Role

Following the discovery of **radiation** in the 19th century, scientists soon found that it could damage body tissue. Continued study of its use and control revealed that normal tissue could largely withstand an amount of radiation that would damage or destroy cancer tissue. The subsequent role of radiation in cancer treatment has developed around controlled use with two types of tumor: (1) those responsive to therapy within a dose level tolerable to health of normal tissue and (2) those that can be targeted without damage to overlying vital organ tissue.

Forms

Radiation used in cancer therapy is produced from three main sources: (1) *x rays*, the oldest form of cancer treatment, or electromagnetic waves similar to heat and light rays, with varying penetration according to the speed at which the electrons strike the target, (2) *radioactive isotopes*, such as cobalt 60, and (3) *atomic particles*, derived from radioactive materials.

Effects

Radiotherapy may be used alone or in conjunction with other therapies both for curative and **palliative care** for some 50% of all cancer patients at some time during the course of their disease. Radiation effects will influence nutritional status and therapy a great deal, depending on site and intensity of treatment: (1) *head and neck* radiation will affect the oral mucosa and salivary secretions, as well as the esophagus, influencing taste sensations and sensitivity to food temperature and texture, while (2) radiation of *abdomen*, may produce denuded bowel mucosa, loss of villi and absorbing surface area, vascular changes from intimal thickening, thrombosis, ulcer formation, or inflammation. Obstruction, fistual formation, or strictures may further contribute to general malabsorption, compounded by curtailment of food intake resulting from anorexia and nausea.

Chemotherapy

Although chemotherapy has been recognized as a valid cancer therapy over the past few decades, the most effective agents currently in use have largely been developed only within the past few years.

Principles of Action

Intensive research in the past few years has resulted in the development of a large number of effective *antineoplastic drugs*. Their therapeutic use is based on two general principles related to rate and mode of action:

Rate of action The so-called cell or log (logarithm)-kill hypothesis of the action of chemotherapeutic agents on tumors indicates that a single dose can only be as much as 99.9% effective in killing the tumor cells. Thus if as large a tumor as is compatible with life can be treated with a drug tolerable at a toxicity level that is 99.9% effective, the tumor is gradually reduced with successive doses that cause "fractional killing" with each dose. This process finally brings the tumor within the capability of the body's own immune system to take over and make the final kill and cure. The smaller the tumor, either because of early detection or initial treat-

Radiation Electromagnetic phenomenon that has properties combining both wave and particle functions. Spans the entire spectrum from low-frequency radio waves, through white light, to high-frequency gamma rays.

Palliative care Care that gives relief but no cure.

ment by surgery or radiation, the greater the possible effectiveness of the chemotherapeutic agents. Also, two other principles of dosage rate for greater effectiveness are important: (1) aggressive use of maximal tolerable dosages in repeated series and (2) use of several drugs together for a *synergistic* effect.

Mode of action Chemotherapeutic agents are effective because they disrupt the normal processes in the cell responsible for cell growth and reproduction. Some agents interfere with DNA synthesis. Others disrupt DNA structure and RNA replication. Others prevent cell division by mitosis, or cause hormonal imbalances, or make unavailable the specific amino acids necessary for protein synthesis. It is this diversity in mode of action that provides a basis for grouping these drugs into certain classes of chemotherapeutic agents: (1) alkaloids, (2) alkylating agents, (3) antibiotics, (4) antimetabolites, (5) enzymes, and (6) hormones. They are usually used in combined therapy or as adjuvant therapy in conjunction with surgery or radiation.

Toxic effects Chemotherapeutic agents have the same effects on rapidly reproducing normal cells as they do on rapidly reproducing cancer cells. Interference with normal function is most apparent in normal cells of the bone marrow, the gastrointestinal tract, and the hair follicles, accounting for a number of the toxic side effects and problems in nutritional management:

1. **Bone marrow effects,** including interference with production of red cells (anemia), white cells (infections), and platelets (bleeding).
2. **Gastrointestinal effects,** including nausea and vomiting, **stomatitis,** anorexia, ulcers, and diarrhea.
3. **Hair follicle effects,** including alopecia (baldness) and general hair loss.

Stomatitis Inflammation of the oral mucosa.

Nutritional Therapy

In general, in caring for the patient with cancer, nutritional therapy is directed toward two types of problems: (1) those related to the disease process itself and (2) those related to the medical treatment of the disease. Thus the objective of a strong nutrition program in cancer therapy is twofold: (1) to meet the hypermetabolic demands of the disease and thus prevent extensive catabolic effects on the body and (2) to alleviate symptoms of the disease or side effects of the treatment by adapting both food forms and the feeding process according to individual responses and needs.

Problems Related to the Disease Process

General feeding problems pose a great challenge to the nutritionist who is planning care and to the nurse who is providing supportive assistance. These problems relate to the overall systemic effects of the neoplastic disease process itself and to the specific individual responses to the type of cancer involved.

General Systemic Reactions

Anorexia Lack or loss of appetite.

The disease process causes three basic systemic effects: (1) **anorexia,** (2) a hypermetabolic state, and (3) a negative nitrogen balance. These effects are often accompanied by a continuing weight loss. The extent of these effects may vary widely with individual patients, from mild, scarcely discernable responses to the extreme forms of debilitating **cachexia** (see p. 549) seen in advanced disease. This extreme weight loss and weakness is caused by abnormalities in glucose metabolism. The cancer patient's body in this state cannot produce glucose efficiently from carbohydrates and instead feeds off its own tissue protein and converts it to glucose instead.[11] A new drug, hydrazine sulfate, is now being used and appears to correct this metabolic error, allowing patients to conserve more energy.[12] The anorexia is frequently accompanied by depression or discomfort during normal eating. This further contributes to a limited nutrient intake at the very time the disease process causes an increased metabolic rate and nutrient demand. Often this imbalance of decreased intake and increased demand creates a negative nitrogen balance, an indication of body-tissue wasting. Sometimes a true tissue loss of protein is masked by outward nitrogen equilibrium as the growing tumor retains nitrogen at the expense of the host, further compounding the problem.

Cachexia Profound and marked state of bodily disfunction; general ill health and malnutrition.

Specific Responses Related to Type of Cancer

Interrelated functional and metabolic problems stem from specific types of cancer and their effects on the body. All of these factors contribute to nutritional depletion. In addition to the primary nutritional deficiencies induced by the disease process itself, secondary difficulties in ingestion and use of nutrients relate to specific tumors that cause obstructions or lesions in the gastrointestinal tract or adjacent tissue. Thus these conditions curtail intake or absorption of adequate nutrients.

Problems Related to Cancer Treatment

Each of the medical treatments for cancer entails physiologic stress, toxic tissue effects, or changes in normal body function. Thus the benefit achieved is not without attendant problems. Nutritional support seeks to alleviate these problems.

Surgery

Beyond the regular nutritional needs surrounding any surgical procedure and its healing process, gastrointestinal surgery poses special problems for normal eating and digestion and absorption of food nutrients. In head and neck surgery, or resections in the oropharyngeal area, sometimes necessitated by cancer, food intake is greatly affected. A creative variety of food forms and semiliquid textures as well as modes of feeding must be devised.[13] Often the mechanical problems of eating make long-term tube feeding necessary. Gastrectomy may cause numerous postgastrectomy "dumping" problems requiring frequent, small, low-carbohydrate feedings. *Vagotomy* contributes to gastric stasis. Various intestinal resections or tumor excisions may cause steatorrhea because of general malabsorption, fistulas, or **stenosis.** Pancreatectomy causes loss of the digestive enzymes, induced insulin-dependent diabetes mellitus, and general weight loss.

Stenosis Narrowing or contraction of a duct or opening.

Radiation

Radiation to the oropharyngeal area often produces a loss of taste sensation, with increasing anorexia and nausea. Other means of tempting ap-

Endarteritis Inflammation of
the inner lining of an artery.

petite through food appearance and aroma, as well as texture, must be developed. Abdominal radiation may cause intestinal damage, with tissue edema and congestion, decreased peristalsis, or **endarteritis** in small blood vessels. In the intestinal wall there may be fibrosis, stenosis, necrosis, or ulceration. General malabsorption or fistulas may develop, as well as hemorrhage, obstruction, and diarrhea, all contributing to nutritional problems. The liver is somewhat more resistant to damage from radiation in adults, but children are more vulnerable.

Chemotherapy

The major nutritional problems during chemotherapy relate to (1) the gastrointestinal symtoms caused by the effect of the toxic drugs on the rapidly developing mucosal cells, (2) the anemia associated with bone marrow effects, and (3) the general systemic toxicity effect on appetite. Stomatitis, nausea, diarrhea, and malabsorption contribute to many food intolerances. Antiemetic drugs such as prochlorperazine (Compazine) may be used (Table 23-1). Such drugs act on the vomiting center in the brain to prevent the nausea response. Prolonged vomiting seriously affects fluid and electrolyte balance. Certain chemotherapeutic drugs also have special effects. For example, monoaminoxidase (MAO) inhibitors may be used for pretreatment relief of mental or emotional depression or for palliative therapy. These antidepressant drugs cause well-known pressor effects when used with tyramine-rich foods. Thus these foods should be avoided when using such drugs (see p. 547).

Principles of Nutritional Therapy for Cancer

Two important principles of vigorous nutritional therapy in cancer care emerge: (1) personal nutrition assessment for each patient and (2) optimum nutritional therapy to maintain sound nutritional status and thus support medical treatment.

Nutrition Assessment

It is far more difficult to replenish a nutritionally depleted patient than to maintain a good nutritional status from the outset of the disease process. Therefore a primary goal in nutritional therapy is to prevent a depleted state. Both initial assessment for baseline data and regular monitoring thereafter during treatment are necessary. A detailed personal history is essential to determine individual needs, desires, and tolerance. Review all of these procedures in Chapter 16.

Nutritional Therapy and Plan of Care

The nutritionist, in consultation with the physician, develops an individual plan of nutritional care based on interpretation of the nutrition assessment data. This nutritional therapy outline is then incorporated into the nursing care plan as the nutritionist works with the nursing staff to carry it out. Primary care provided by the experienced clinical nutritionist on a regular basis is a necessary part of the oncology team practice. This vigorous care often makes the difference in the success rate of medical therapy. Thus the clinical nutritionist can assess individual patient needs, determine nutritional requirements, plan and manage nutritional care,

Table 23-1
Medications Used to Control Nausea and Vomiting in Patients Receiving Chemotherapy*

Antiemetic Drug/Action	Cancer Chemotherapeutic Drug Couteracted	Dosage Used	Side Effects	Comments
Phenothiazines Action: blocks CTZ stimulation by dopamine	Moderate emetic-potential drugs			
Examples Compazine (prochlorperazine) Torecan (thiethylperazine) Phenergan (promethazine)		5–10 mg, orally or parenterally before chemotherapy; every 4–6 hr after, for 24–48 hr	Sedation Orthostatic hypertension	Less effective when given on an "as needed" basis
Droperidol (inapsine) Action: sedative and antiemetic	Cisplatin	0.5 mg intravenously 1 hr before chemotherapy; every 4 hr after	Somnolence	Some patients given up to 1.5 mg intravenously developed a tolerance for the drug
Corticosteroids Dexamethasone (Hexadrol, Decadron)	Cyclophosphamide Doxorubicin	10 mg intramuscularly before chemotherapy	Perianal stinging if given too rapidly	Moderate to high relief in 70% of the patients
Methylprednisolone (SoluMedrol)	Nitrogen mustard Mitomycin Methyl-CCNU	250 mg intravenously every 6 hr for 4 doses beginning 2 hr	Swelling Facial rash Weakness, lethargy	Effects of methylprednisolone considered disappointing
Tetrahydrocannabinol (THC, marijuana)	Variety of agents studied Methotrexate 5-FU Methyl-CCNU Cyclophosphamide Doxorubicin Nitrosoureas Mechlorethamine Cisplatin	10 mg/m²	Somnolence Visual hallucinations	Patients (usually older) not used to THC refused to continue it because of CNS effects Response associated with extent of THC-induced "high" Most effective with flurouracil, cyclophosphamide, methotrexate, doxorubicin "High" blocked by giving a phenothiazine
Metoclopramide (Reglan) Widely used in Europe; not approved currently for use in United States	Cisplatin	Single 20 mg dose, given orally halfway through a 6 hr infusion of cisplatin (100 mg/m²); higher doses might be possible intravenously (1–3 mg/kg/dose)	Sedation	Works well for patients who do not respond to other antiemetic drugs

*Data modified from studies reported by Huber, S.L., and Ballentine, R.: Nutr. Support Serv. **2**(10):30, 1982.

Tyramine-Restricted Diet

General directions

- Designed for patients on monoamine oxidase (MAO) inhibitors, drugs that have been reported to cause hypertensive crises when used with tyramine-rich foods. These include foods in which aging, protein breakdown, and putrefaction are used to increase flavor. Studies indicate that as little as 5 to 6 mg tyramine can produce a response, and 25 mg is a danger dose.
- Food sources of other pressor amines such as histamine, dihydroxyphenylalanine, and hydroxytyramine are also avoided.
- Avoid all foods listed. Limited amounts of foods with a lower tyramine amount such as yeast bread may be included in a specific diet.
- Avoid over-the-counter drugs such as decongestants, cold remedies, and antihistamines.

Foods to avoid		Additional foods to avoid
(Representative tyramine values in µg/g or ml)		Other aged cheeses
	1416	Blue
	516	Boursault
Cheeses	466	Brick
N.Y. state cheddar	225	Cheddars (other)
Gruyére	180	Gouda
Stilton	86	Mozzarella
Emmentaler	50	Parmesan
Brie		Provolone
Camembert		Romano
Processed American	25.4	Roquefort
Wines	3.6	Yeast and products made with yeast
Chianti	0.6	Homemade bread
Sherry	0.4	Yeast extracts such as soup cubes, canned
Riesling	4.4	meats, and marmite
Sauterne	2.3	Italian broad beans with pod (fava beans)
Beer, ale—varies with brand	1.8	Meat
Highest		Aged game
Average		Liver
Least		Canned meats with yeast extracts
		Fish (salted dried)
		Herring, cod, capelin
		Pickled herring
		Other
		Cream, especially sour
		Yogurt
		Soy sauce, vanilla, chocolate
		Salad dressings

monitor progress and responses to therapy, and make adjustments in care according to status and tolerances.

Nutritional Needs

Although individual needs will vary, of course, guidelines for nutritional therapy must meet increased nutrient needs.

Energy Great energy demands are placed on the cancer patient. These demands result from the hypermetabolic state of the disease process and the tissue-healing requirements. Of this total dietary kilocaloric value, there must be sufficient carbohydrate to spare protein for vital tissue synthesis. For an adult patient with good nutritional status, about 2000 kcal/

day will provide for maintenance needs. A more malnourished patient may require 3000 to 4000 kcal, depending on the degree of malnutrition and body trauma.

Protein Tissue protein synthesis, a necessary component of healing and rehabilitation, requires essential amino acids and nitrogen. Efficient protein use, which depends on an optimum protein/kilocalorie ratio, promotes tissue building, prevents tissue wastage (catabolism), and helps make up tissue deficits. An adult patient with good nutritional status will need about 80 to 100 g/day of protein to meet maintenance needs and assure anabolism. A malnourished patient will need more, 100 to 200 g to replenish tissue and restore positive nitrogen balance.

Vitamins and minerals Key vitamins and minerals control protein and energy metabolism through their roles in cell enzyme systems. They also play a necessary part in structural development and tissue integrity. Hence an optimum intake of vitamins and minerals, at least to the recommended dietary allowances (RDA) levels but frequently to the higher-potency therapeutic levels, is indicated. Depending on individual nutritional status, supplements to dietary sources may be needed.

Fluids Adequate fluid intake is important for two reasons: (1) to replace gastrointestinal losses or losses caused by infection and fever and (2) to help the kidneys dispose of the metabolic breakdown products from destroyed cancer cells as well as from the toxic drugs used in treatment. For example, some toxic drugs such as cyclophosphamide (Cytoxan), require as much as 2 to 3 L of forced fluids daily to prevent hemorrhagic cystitis.

Nutritional Management

The specific feeding method used depends on the individual patient's condition. However, the classic dictum of nutritional management should prevail: *"If the gut works, use it."* The spectrum of management approaches include four feeding methods—two enteral forms and two parenteral forms.

Enteral Feeding: Oral Diet and Nutrient Supplementation

An oral diet with supplementation is the most desired form of feeding, of course, whenever it is possible. A carefully designed personal plan of care based on nutrition assessment data and including adjustments in texture, temperature, food choices, and tolerances can often meet needs. Personal food tolerances will vary according to the current treatment and nature of the disease. A number of adjustments in food texture, temperature, amount, timing, taste, appearance, and form can be made to help alleviate symptoms stemming from common problems in successive parts of the gastrointestinal tract.[13] Eating problems may be caused by loss of appetite, difficulties in the mouth or with swallowing, or various gastrointestinal problems.

Loss of appetite Anorexia is a major problem and curtails food intake when it is needed most. It is a general systemic effect of the cancer disease process itself. Loss of appetite is further induced by the cancer treatment and progressively enhanced by personal anxiety, depression, and stress of the illness. Such a vicious cycle, if not countered by much effort, can lead to more malnutrition and the well-recognized starvation or "cancer cachexia," a syndrome of emaciation, debilitation, and malnutrition.[11, 12] A vigorous program of eating, *not dependent on appetite for stimulus*, must be planned with patient and family. The overall goal is to provide food with as much *nutrient density* as possible so that "every bite will count."

Mouth problems Various problems contributing to eating difficulties may stem from sore mouth, stomatitis, or taste changes. *Sore mouth* often results from chemotherapy or radiation to the head and neck area. It is increased by any state of malnutrition or from infections such as **candidiasis** (thrush), with numerous ulcerations of the oral and throat mucosa. Frequent small meals and snacks, soft in texture, bland in nature, and cool to cold in temperature, are often better tolerated. Chemotherapy or head and neck radiation may also cause alterations in the tongue's taste buds, causing taste distortion ("taste blindness") and inability to distinguish the basic tastes of salt, sweet, sour, or bitter, with consequent food aversions. Since the aversion is often toward basic protein foods, a high-protein liquid supplement may be needed.[14] *Dental problems* may also contribute to mouth difficulties and should be corrected. *Salivary secretions* are also affected by cancer therapy, so foods with a high liquid content should be used. Solid foods may be swallowed more easily with use of sauces, gravies, broth, yogurt, or salad dressings. A food processor or blender can render foods in semisolid or liquid forms and make them easier to swallow. If the swallowing problem is especially severe because of tumor growth or therapy, guides for a special swallowing training program, including progressive food textures, exercises, and positions, can be followed.[15]

Gastrointestinal problems Eating difficulties may include nausea and vomiting (see box, p. 550), general indigestion, bloating, or specific surgery responses such as the postgastrectomy "dumping" syndrome. Nausea is often enhanced by foods that are hot, sweet, fatty, or spicy, so these can be avoided according to individual tolerance. Frequent small feedings of cold foods, soft to liquid in texture may be more appealing. These can be eaten slowly with rests in between. Antinausea drugs may be prescribed to help with food tolerance (Table 23-1). Other food problems may include general diarrhea, constipation, flatulence, or specific lactose intolerance or surgery responses, such as occur with intestinal resections and various ostomies.[16] The effect of chemotherapy or radiation treatment on the mucosal cells secreting lactase contributes to lactose intolerance. In such cases a nutrient supplement formula with a nonmilk protein base may be used.

A number of commercial nutrient supplement products are available. A comparative review of these products will provide the basis for developing a formulary in the hospital setting for a limited number of such products. A food processor can be used at home to produce creative solid and liquid food combinations from regular foods for interval liquid supplementation.

Enteral Feeding: Tube

When the patient is unable to eat but the gastrointestinal tract can still be used, tube feedings may be needed to provide the necessary nutritional

Candidiasis Superficial fungus infection (genus: *Candida*) of moist parts of the body (infection of oral mucuous membranes is called *thrush*).

Clinical Application

Controlling Nausea and Vomiting in Patients Receiving Chemotherapy

Chemotherapy creates an almost "catch-22" situation in terms of the nutritional management of patients with cancer. On the one hand, it works best in the patient who is well-nourished. On the other hand, it often triggers nausea and vomiting to such a degree that the patient cannot consume enough food to be well-nourished. The resulting course of malnutrition may be further aggravated by alterations in taste acuity. To help prevent this problem of malnutrition, there are several things you may do:

- **Obtain a detailed history of emesis** Include data about onset, duration, and severity. Estimate the severity by degree of weight loss, electrolyte depletion, and retching. Also record factors aggravating or relieving emesis.
- **Limit food intake** Do this selectively and carefully to avoid taste aversions to foods previously enjoyed by the patient.
- **Evaluate emetic effect of antiemetic drugs** Note drugs used in patient's medical chemotherapy, anticipating possible emetic effects, as well as effectiveness of any anti-emetic drugs being used to control the nausea (Table 23-1). Relate personal food plan and support counseling with patient and family about these effects.
- **Identify potential psychogenic causes** These are suspected when emesis occurs before the drug is administered, or just as it is administered. Anticipatory nausea and vomiting has also been associated with the office or clinic visit itself, a person (e.g., the physician or nurse), or an event associated with treatment. This is most often seen in patients on chemotherapy for more than 6 months.
- **Identify other illnesses** Congestive heart failure, influenza, bowel obstruction may also be responsible for nausea and vomiting.
- **Identify other drugs, treatments** Use of other emetic drugs (e.g., antibiotics, digitalis, narcotics) or radiation therapy may aggravate nausea and vomiting during chemotherapy.

The nausea itself occurs when an area in the medulla of the brain—the vomiting center (VC)—is stimulated directly or indirectly by messages sent from the gastrointestinal tract or the cerebral cortex. The chemoreceptor trigger zone (CTZ), located near the VC, can also transmit stimuli induced by chemotherapy drugs. These three stimulatory routes suggest that the control of nausea and vomiting lies in a careful evaluation of three factors: (1) ingested food items, (2) psychological influences, and (3) the emetic effects of any and all drugs, treatments, or illnesses occurring simultaneously.

References
Huber, S.L., and Ballentine, R.: Therapeutic trends in the management of chemotherapy-induced nausea and vomiting, Nutr. Support Serv. **2**(10):30, 1982.

Figure 23-4
Types of tube feeding. **A**, Common nasogastric feeding tube; **B**, gastrostomy-jejunal enteral feeding tube.

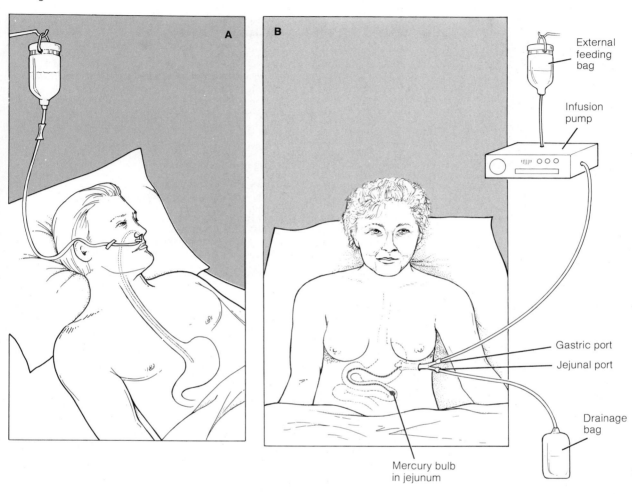

support (Figure 23-4). A number of individual problems, however, surround the use of tube feedings. Many patients have negative attitudes toward nasogastric tubes (Table 23-2). Such an unnatural feeding method carries with it emotional problems for the patient. However, there is better acceptance with the newer small-caliber feeding tubes.[17] Some highly motivated patients have even learned to pass their tubes themselves. Patients can be fed in some instances by pump-monitored slow drip during the night and be freed from the tube during the day. The development of sophisticated enteral formulas and delivery systems has also made home enteral nutrition both feasible and practical.[18] The concentration of the formula, its *osmolality,* is an important consideration in the effort to avoid imbalances in the gastrointestinal fluid and electrolyte circulation. Many commercial formulas are available, but they must be selected with care. Blended food formulas are rarely used by hospitals because there are too

Table 23-2
Problem-Solving Tips for
Patients Receiving Enteral
Nutrition

Problem	Suggested Solutions
Thirst, oral dryness	Lubricate lips Chew sugarless gum Brush teeth Rinse mouth frequently CAUTION: use lemon drops sparingly because of cariogenic effects
Tube discomfort	Gargle with a mixture of warm water and mouth wash Gently blow nose Clean tube regularly with water or water-soluble lubricant If persistent, pull tube out gently, clean it, and reinsert Request smaller tube
Tension, fullness	Relax, breathe deeply after each feeding
Loud stomach noises	Take feedings in private
Limited mobility	Change positions in bed or chair Walk around the house or hospital corridor

Gustatory distress
  General dissatisfaction
  with feeding
	Warm or chill feedings
	CAUTION: Feedings that are too cold may cause diarrhea
	Serve favorite foods that have been liquified

Persistent hunger	Chew a favorite food, then spit it out Chew gum Suck lemon drops (sparingly)
Inability to drink	Rinse mouth frequently with water and other liquids

many uncontrolled factors. For example, hospital use of raw egg for patient fare is banned by most state health regulations and powdered egg white is a substitute item. But for home use, some patients prefer a blended formula composed of regular food items. Sometimes this is better tolerated, provides psychologic support, and is less costly than long-term use of commercial formula products. But it must be carefully prepared and controlled.

Parenteral Feeding

When the gastrointestinal system cannot be used and nutritional support is vital, two additional modes of parenteral feeding may be needed. First, *peripheral vein feeding* can be used for brief periods to administer solutions of dextrose, amino acids, vitamins, and minerals, with intermittent fat emulsions. Second, to meet greater nutritional support requirements, a larger central vein may be used for feeding a more concentrated formula of these ingredients. This *total parenteral nutrition (TPN)* process requires a surgical technique and careful assessment and administration. (These procedures are reviewed in Chapter 22.) The use of TPN with cancer patients has been questioned by some practitioners. In many cases, however, it has been a significant means of turning cancer patients' metabolic status from catabolism to anabolism, often avoiding the serious development of cancer cachexia.

To Sum Up

Cancer is a term applied to abnormal, malignant growth in various body tissue sites. The cancerous cell is derived from a normal cell that loses control over reproduction. Cancer cell development occurs via mutation, carcinogens, radiation, and oncogenic viruses. It is also influenced by many epidemiologic factors such as diet, alcohol consumption, and smoking, as well as physical and psychologic stress factors. Cell development is mediated by the body's immune system, primarily its T cells, a type of white cell found in blood, lymph, and certain parts of the lymph nodes and spleen, and B cells, which manufacture and secrete antibodies.

Cancer therapy consists primarily of surgery, radiation, and chemotherapy. Supportive nutritional therapy for the cancer patient should be highly individualized and depends on the response of each body system to the disease and to the treatment itself. It is based on a thorough nutritional assessment and provided by a number of routes (oral, tube feeding, peripheral vein, TPN). The oral route is preferred if at all possible. In some cases nutrient and kilocaloric supplements are required. These requirements must be designed for specific physical and psychologic needs of individual patients.

Questions for Review

1. What is cancer? Identify and describe several major causes of cancer cell formation.
2. How does your body attempt to defend itself against cancer? What nutritional factors may diminish this ability?
3. List and describe the rationale and mode of action of the types of therapies used to treat cancer.
4. Differentiate those factors challenging cancer recovery that are associated with the disease process vs. the type of therapy used.
5. Outline the general procedure for the nutritional management of a cancer patient.

References

1. Kahn, C.: DNA's mysterious master, Health **13**(10):40, 1981.
2. Miller, J.: Cancer genes and chromosome changes, Science News **122**(21):326, 1983.
3. Wallis, C.: Bring back the parasol, Time, May 30, 1983, p. 46.
4. Doll, R., and Peto, R.: The causes of cancer: quantitative estimates of avoidable risks of cancer in the United States today, J. Natl. Cancer Inst. **66**:1191, 1981.
5. Brown, R.R.: The role of diet in cancer causation, Food Technol. **37**:49, 1983.
6. Carroll, K.K.: Neutral fats and cancer, Cancer Res. **41**:3695, 1981.
7. Report: Study will look at diet as a cancer treatment, Health Facts, **8**(51):2, 1983.
8. Miller, J.: Double duty cells in human immune system, Science News, **123**(20):308, 1983.
9. Langone, J.: Monoclonals: the super antibodies, Discover **4**(6):68, 1983.
10. Kaminski, M.V., and others: Nutritional status, immunity and survival in neoplastic disease, Nutr. Support Serv. **2**(4):7, 1982.
11. Wollard, J.: Nutritional management of the cancer patient, Food Technol. **37**:69, 1983.
12. Seligmann, J., and Witherspoon, D.: A new, old cancer drug, Newsweek, June 6, 1983, p. 95.
13. Bloch, A.: Practical hints for feeding the cancer patient, Nutr. Today **16**(6):23, 1981.
14. Chernoff, R.: Nutritional support: formulas and delivery of enteral feeding, J. Am. Diet. Assoc. **79**(4):426, 1981.
15. Rosenbaum, E.H.: and others: Nutrition for the cancer patient, Palo Alto, CA, 1980, Bull Publishing Co.
16. Mullen, B.D.: The ostomy book: living comfortably with colostomies, ileostomies, and urostomies, Palo Alto, CA, 1980, Bull Publishing Co.
17. Rodgers, L., and Wright, R.A.: New developments in enteral feeding techniques, Nutr. Support Serv. **2**(10):17, 1982.
18. Jensen, T.G.: Home enteral nutrition, Dietet. Currents, **8**(4):1, 1982.

Further Readings

Darbinian, J.A., and Coulston, A.M.: Parenteral nutrition in cancer therapy: a useful adjunct? J. Am. Diet. Assoc. **82**(5):493, 1983.
  and
Hushen, S.C.: Questioning TPN as the answer, Am. J. Nurs. **82**:852, 1982.
  and
Copeland, E.M.: Intravenous hyperalimentation and chemotherapy: an update, J. Parent. Enter. Nutr. **6**(3):236, 1982.

These sources point up some of the controversy surrounding use of TPN with cancer patients. In the first two, experienced clinical nutritionists and a nurse clinican raise questions with case histories about the usefulness of TPN for cancer patients, especially in end-stage disease. Conversely, a leading physician in the field provides a positive update and identifies those patients who can benefit from this therapy.

Decker, J., and Goldstein, J.C.: Risk factors in head and neck cancer, N. Engl. J. Med. **306**(19):1151, 1982.
  and
Larsen, G.L.: Rehabilitation for the patient with head and neck cancer, Am. J. Nurs. **82**:119, 1982.
  and

Fleming, S.M., Weaver, A.W., and Brown, J.M.: The patient with cancer affecting the head and neck: problems in nutrition, J. Am. Diet. Assoc. **70**:391, 1977.

Cancer of the head and neck presents special communication and feeding problems. In this trio of articles, specialists in these areas—speech pathologists, physicians, and nutritionists—review prevention through control of environmental risk factors and problems in personal and nutritional rehabilitation.

Eating hints: recipes and tips for better nutrition during cancer treatment, Office of Cancer Communications, National Cancer Institute, Bethesda, M.D., 20205.

This free little book provides a well-organized resource for cancer patients and families. It is full of practical ways to help the patient eat well and enjoy it, despite problems caused by treatment.

Shils, M.E.: How to nourish the cancer patient, Nutr. Today **16**(3):4, 1981.
and
Bloch, A.S.: Practical hints for feeding the cancer patient, Nutr. Today, **16**(6):23, 1981.

This series of two articles give a comprehensive review of nutritional support for cancer patients. Excellent illustrations, also available on slides as a teaching aid.

Issues and Answers

**Dietary Guidelines
for Cancer
Prevention**

The American public is always searching for a means of preventing devastating diseases before they start. At the turn of the century, it sought relief from killer infections that now have become virtually nonexistent. Today, the battle is being waged against disease, cancer, and stroke. The medical community has responded, establishing dietary and other lifestyle guidelines to reduce the risk of hypertension and coronary heart disease, both of which may lead to a stroke. The lay community has been anxiously awaiting guidelines for cancer prevention as well.

Recently, such public guidelines were reported. A National Research Council (NRC) panel of nutrition scientists—clinicians, researchers, and educators—issued these guidelines, based on current knowledge and expert opinion. In the report from NRC, the recommended dietary allowances (RDA) took the form of a set of six "interim" dietary guidelines intended to reduce the risk of developing a variety of cancers:

- Reduce fat intake to 30% of total kcal in the diet.
- Include fruit (especially, citrus), vegetables (especially, carotene-rich), and whole grains in the diet daily.
- Avoid foods preserved by pickling or smoking.
- Avoid food contamination with carcinogens of any source (intentional additives, unintended contaminants, or naturally-occurring compounds).
- Continue efforts to identify mutagens in foods, test their carcinogenic properties and, if it can be done without reducing the nutritive value of the food, remove them or limit their content in that food.
- Avoid excessive alcohol intake.

If these diet and cancer guidelines sound familiar, it is because most of them are. They have already been included in the U.S. Dietary Goals issued earlier by the USDA. These U.S. Dietary Goals were developed primarily to reduce the risk of heart disease, diabetes mellitus, hypertension, and other related chronic disease. The two new statements added are common sense warnings: (1) avoid carcinogen-contaminated foods and (2) identify, test, and limit the use of carcinogenic mutagens. Here, however, they are directed at regulatory agencies and the food industry rather than the public.

However, this NRC report and its recommended "interim guidelines" have been criticized by some persons in the scientific community. Also, some ask, since these guidelines have been presented before, and today are considered "common sense" nutrition, why they were offered by such a prestigious body as the National Research Council?

Some critics charge that the NRC's Committee on Diet, Nutrition and Cancer felt "pressured" into providing information that would

Issues and Answers—cont'd

meet the public's demand for preventive measures against chronic disease. These critics do not take issue with the guidelines *per se*. However, they feel that the suggestion is made that the guidelines *will*, without complete certainty, prevent cancer, when in most cases this is not entirely known. But the Executive Summary of the NRC Committee's findings states clearly that evidence regarding the effect of many of their recommendations is inconclusive:

Fats are strongly associated with cancer of the breast, prostate, and bowel, in per capita as well as case-control studies; an increase of 10% to 40% of total kcal as fat increases tumor incidence. Yet no one yet knows *how* fats induce tumor formation.

Citrus fruits are recommended for vitamin C, which is associated with a lower risk of stomach and esophageal cancers. Vitamin C *has* inhibited the *in vivo* and *in vitro* formation of carcinogenic N-nitroso compounds in laboratory tests. But it has not been shown to have any effect on *preformed* tumors.

Carotene-rich vegetables are recommended for vitamin A which, in epidemiological studies, shows an inverse relationship with cancer of the lung, bladder, and larynx. Unfortunately, no one yet knows whether this effect is due to vitamin A itself, the carotenoids (vitamin A precursors) or other factors in food, or the retinoids (synthetic analogues of vitamin A that lack its toxic effects, but also inhibit neoplasms). Despite its "anti-cancer" effect, large vitamin A supplements cannot be recommended because the vitamin (1) is highly toxic in large amounts and (2) may not be effective if carotene (found only in food) is the primary preventive agent.

Whole grains are recommended for the "anti-cancer" properties of the fiber they contain. Specific components (bran and cellulose) of fiber have been associated with inhibiting cancer formation or growth, especially in the colon. However, the Committee indicates that the evidence thus far associating total fiber intake to cancer prevention is not entirely conclusive.

Pickled and smoked foods are associated with cancer of the stomach and esophagus in China, Japan, Iceland, and elsewhere. Processing produces high levels of compounds or mutagens (polycycline aromatic hydrocarbons and N-nitroso compounds) that can change the genetic material in cells in bacteria and animals. They are suspected of being carcinogenic in humans.

Contamination with carcinogens occurs when a large amount of an additive is purposefully used, environmental additives (pesticides, industrial chemicals) enter the food supply, or naturally-occurring toxins develop from molds (aflatoxin) or from bacterial action (nitrosamine formation). Control over such contamination is primarily up to the food industry and the government's enforcement of the Delaney Clause (p. 203), which prohibits addition of any

Continued.

Issues and Answers—cont'd

substance having carcinogenic properties. This recommendation is beyond the control of the general public, other than by political action (boycotts against offending food companies, lobbying Congress).

Mutagens are substances that change part of the genetic material in cells and are always suspect for being carcinogenic. Some mutagens occur naturally in foods and others occur during the cooking process, especially in high-heat processes such as charcoal broiling. The Committee itself believes that no one can determine how these mutagens actually contribute to the incidence of cancer.

Alcohol is recommended in limited quantities, based on limited evidence associating heavy beer-drinking with colorectal cancer and alcohol-induced cirrhosis with liver cancer. In combination with cigarette smoking, alcohol has certainly contributed to the risk of cancer of the mouth, larynx, esophagus, and respiratory tract. However, the key question to alcohol limitation remains: How much is *too* much?

Critics further contend that the NRC Committee was somewhat "selective" in its formation of guidelines. For instance, even though an inverse relationship was found between stomach cancer and milk consumption, no recommendation was made to increase milk intake.

The irony of this situation is the fact that no critic can take issue with any of the recommendations made, based on the general principle of health promotion. Whether or not the advice is harmful—and this certainly is *not* the case here—critics feel that the Council is really "telling the public what it wants to know" without yet having firm enough evidence, which may mislead some persons seeking dietary "cures" and preventions. Nonetheless, they are all reasonable statements, given the extent of our knowledge and experience.

References
National Research Council, Executive summary: Diet, nutrition and cancer, Nutr. Today, **17**(4):20, July/Aug, 1982
Harper, A.E., A matter of opinion: Firm recommendations, infirm basis, Nutr. Today, **17**(4):16, July/Aug, 1982.

Chapter 24

Computers in Nutrition Practice

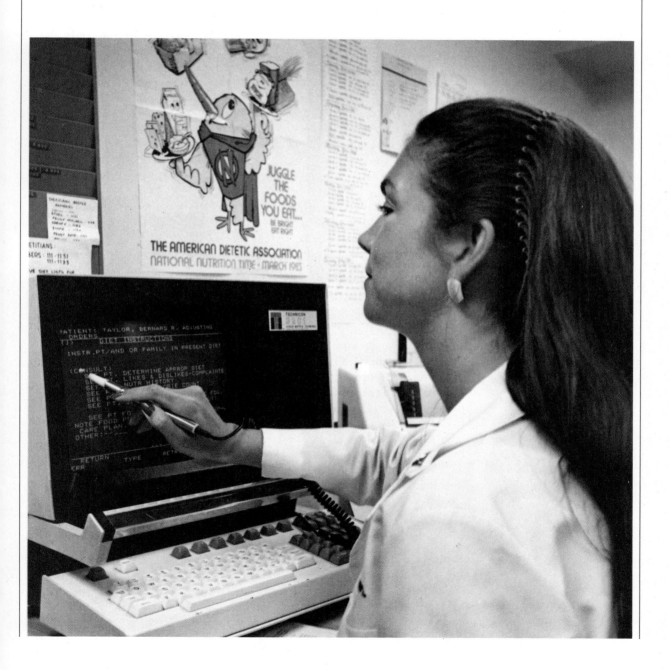

Preview

Our society appears to be moving rapidly from an economy based largely on products of an earlier industrial era into a time of increasing focus on human services. Computer literacy is becoming increasingly essential to us all, not only in our personal lives, but also in our professional practices. All the while, however, as we see our society becoming more and more dependent on the computer for survival, we must prevent the human being—ourselves and our clients/patients—from becoming prisoner, at social and psychologic cost, to its technology. Instead, we must use the computer as we would a fine tool, constantly refining and developing our own systems to meet our own special needs. In health care in general and in nutritional care in particular, our management information systems require both the development of the components to meet our needs and our ability to use them with skill and wisdom.

In this chapter we introduce some current applications of computer systems in nutrition practice. Whet your own appetite to delve further because the computer is here to stay. The heart of its technology—tiny miracle chips smaller than postage stamps—now touch almost all aspects of our lives.

Chapter Objectives

After study of this chapter, the student should be able to:

1. Identify both advantages and possible problems of computer system use in health care practice.

2. Describe specific computer applications in nutritional practice and education, research and writing, and management of services.

3. Identify database resources available for nutrition services and how they are accessed and used.

What Computers Can and Cannot Do

Mainframe computer
Largest type of computer system; used by large institutions, research centers, universities, and corporations.

Minicomputers Larger than a microcomputer but smaller than a standard mainframe computer though based on the same system as the mainframe; main unit ranges in size from that of a desk to a refrigerator.

Microcomputers Smallest computers, developed around 1975; microcomputers today have as much or more computing ability as earlier mainframe computers.

Hardcopy Printed sheets of paper one can hold in the hand as opposed to information displayed only on a monitor screen.

MODEM Contraction of the terms *"modulator-demodulator"*; device that converts and reconverts data and signals transmitted over telephone lines allowing computers to "speak" with each other.

The advent of the microprocessor chip has made a tremendous difference in computer size and cost. As a result, multiple applications of computer technology have developed in many fields. The former limited access available only in large costly **mainframe computers** has expanded to newer **minicomputers** and to rapid generations of small affordable **microcomputers** designed for many professional, business, and personal uses. Over the past two decades, applications of this computer capability have been developed in the fields of health care and nutrition. This impact is only beginning to be felt. But of one thing we can be sure—this impact will continue to grow and assume multiple applications. This rapid growth will require increased knowledge and skill on the part of all practitioners. Thus in this final chapter we will look briefly at (1) some of the many ways computers can help us with our work, (2) the human factor that only we can supply, and (3) some applications of these computer capabilities in nutrition practice management.

General Information Management

Whether it be number-crunching or word wizardry, the computer can perform innumerable functions in handling units of information.

Data Input

The computer can store large amounts of data, depending on its capacity. These data are then in the computer's "memory" for use according to need. These pieces of information may be in the form of numbers or words, as well as directions for use of these units.

Data Output

Whether called up to be viewed on a screen or printed out as **hardcopy,** the computer output is made up of pieces of data that it gives back to the user. Initial stored data may be retrieved for use as is or analyzed by the computer according to a directing program with the results returned to the user.

Data Analysis

The computer can perform a number of functions on data it has received from the user. It can sort, file, tabulate, calculate, edit, rewrite, reformat, compare, contrast, project, cost, and plan according to "what if" scenarios provided.

Data Communications

Anyone with a personal microcomputer can send messages via "electronic mail" to another person with a microcomputer by use of a **MODEM** (telephone hookup) and dialing one of several nationwide "electronic mailbox" networks, such as Telenet. Also, a local network of personal computers at various work stations may be set up in almost any environment. Data and equipment can thus be shared with gains in productivity and economy. Connections may also be made between microcomputers and a large mainframe computer within an organization, thus unlocking the larger power of the mainframe computer for wider use.

Basic Computer System Development

Hardware Mechanical equipment comprising a computer system and necessary for its operation.

Software Computer programs; so named because they have no electronic circuits or other "hard" ware.

Types of Systems

The development of either a large or a small computer system depends largely on an initial analysis of what the objectives for its use by a particular practitioner or organization may be.[1] Comprehensive *minicomputer* systems are used in large medical centers to coordinate all aspects of patient care. Persons who will be using the system should be involved in its planning. The wide range of application of computers in nutrition makes it important for the nutritionist and the nurse to become involved with the information systems team in purchasing equipment and making sure it suits specific needs and in training staff for its proper use. Although it may not be necessary to become a computer expert, basic knowledge can go a long way in getting the most for your money in **hardware** and **software.** For example, one important fact to know is that software programs are computer hardware–specific and won't work on just any system. This consumer problem reflects the highly competitive nature of the computer market.

Types of Tasks

First, basic questions must be asked in considering components for a computer system: What do you want the system to do? What management needs will it serve? What are your work activities and cost objectives? What specific tasks must the system be able to do? By and large, the types of tasks required in providing nutritional services may include the following:

Business management Whether the activity is food service or patient care, business management principles must underlie its operation. These include fiscal responsibility such as accounting, forecasting, budgets, and cost control. Also scheduling working activities, including both material and human resources, is a necessary activity.

Primary client/patient care Business management principles are also involved in daily patient care. Activities involved include handling cost-effectiveness studies, program planning, and evaluation.

Education Computer-assisted instruction finds use in both patient education and professional/staff education, as well as employee training.

Research Research concerning clinical problems and the most cost-effective methods of providing services are necessary working activities.

Writing Word-processing capabilities of the computer provide support for a variety of writing tasks, including records and reports, communications, articles, or educational materials or books.

User-friendly Easy to use; self-explanatory; systems that are more tolerant of human error or carelessness.

Multiple-purpose Computer term used to designate those microcomputers that have multiple applications or task capacities, as compared with single special-purpose instruments.

In designing a computer system to accomplish such tasks, the second phase of study requires consideration of hardware and software components best suited to serve these identified needs. The terms **user-friendly** and **multiple-purpose** are current buzzwords applied to desirable computer systems, especially microsystems. In essence, for the greatest efficiency and cost-effectiveness, the system operation should be neither difficult to learn nor increase anxiety of the user, and it should serve a variety of identified purposes.

The "machinery"

Since the computer is a machine that handles data, its major parts are concerned with getting data into the machine (terminal), processing the data (memory), storing data (disks), and making a hardcopy of the results (printer). The key to success is finding the parts best suited to your overall needs. Here are some principles that apply to selection of a computer system:

Terminal The **terminal** is the simplest part. It provides a viewing screen and a keyboard for punching in information. Terminals can get fancy and have detachable keyboards, reversible (white-on-black) letters, or upper and lower case letters to make the screen easy to read. These options have no effect on your ability to enter information into the computer itself.

Memory This is the amount of information that can be processed by computers. It is measured in three ways: (1) **bit** (binary digit)—a unit of information that results from the computer making a choice between two alternatives (for example, *yes* or *no,* (2) **byte**—approximately 8 bits, and (3) *character*—a letter, number, or other symbol appearing on the keyboard. It is important to remember that every bit, byte, and character is not available to you. Some of them are taken up by the computer's **operating system,** information "built in" by the manufacturer so that the computer will know what to do with the information fed into it. Thus a 36 **K (kilobyte)** memory will only have 24 K available to you if 12 K is used up just in telling the computer how to work.

Disk A disk may be either the **floppy disk** (diskette), which is a round, flat, plastic "pancake" on which information is stored, or a *hard disk,* also called a Winchester disk, which has a much greater capacity. In purchasing a **disk drive**—the compartment into which the disk is placed so that information can be recorded on it—you should consider whether speed is really important, how long you intend to keep the information, and whether disks will be mailed or relocated frequently. You will also need to consider the volume of data you intend to store on each disk and the file size. A **file** is an index or number of key words or symbols used to find information that is needed quickly or on a regular basis (for example, to update data). It may consist of such items as client names, chart numbers, formulas, or medical conditions. The file often increases your volume needs if an extensive data base, for example, th USDA nutrient databank, is used in the program. One last word about disks: *back-ups are essential.* An extra copy of important information must always be made and stored in a safe place. This practice preserves your files from accidental or intentional destruction. Files should be copied and stored away from the computer room. This is easiest to do if your computer can copy data from one disk to another quickly and accurately.

Printer Before selecting a **printer,** think about how much information must be printed and how often. Slower speed printers, gauged by characters per second (cps), may cost only half as much as faster printers, gauged by lines per minute (1pm). Thus, unless you must produce reports rapidly and often, you may save money with a slower printer.

Terminal Computer system component, usually including a keyboard and display screen, through which one can send or receive information.

Bit (Binary digit) Smallest unit of computer information; several bits make up a letter, number, or word. Eight bits = one byte.

Byte Group of adjacent bits forming a specific part of a binary word. One byte = eight bits.

Operating system Program that provides specific commands for operating a computer; helps the computer to operate more easily.

(K) kilobyte 1024 bytes, or characters, of memory storage. Thus, 4 K = 4,096 bytes of memory and 64 K = 65,536 bytes of memory.

Floppy disk (diskette) Thin, flexible, circular mylar disks coated for magnetic recording of information. Comes in either 8 in or 5¼ in diameters.

Disk drive Electromechanical device that houses and spins the information carrying disks (floppy or hard), transferring the data from the disk to the working memory of the computer.

File A body of related information recorded on a computer disk.

Printer Major component of a computer system; prints output from the computer. Two main types are dot-matrix and letter quality impact (daisy wheel) printers.

Obviously, cost is not the only bottom line when it comes to selecting a computer. Volume, frequency of use, efficiency, and many other factors must be considered. However, one must be practical. Equipment becomes obsolete very quickly at the rate of development occurring in computer technology today. Before investing in any "can't-to-withouts" right away, ask yourself a few questions: What will my data processing needs be 5 years from now? Can the equipment I'm about to buy be expanded to include any new needs? Will I really benefit by having **printouts** quickly? Your responses will indicate whether you even need to buy the equipment now. Carefully evaluate its ability to meet your needs for accuracy and speed for the next 3 to 5 years. You may decide that leasing equipment for immediate needs is your wisest way to go until you test results and determine your overall eventual requirements.

Printout Hardcopy computer output printed on paper.

The Human Factor

Computers can help us in many ways with our work. However, there is one thing that computers cannot do. They cannot supply the human factor. This far-reaching new information technology itself is viewed by many as being neutral, with its meaning lying in user applications. But in another very real sense this technology is *not* neutral. It changes and influences our view of our work and our experience with it. It shapes the very nature of our work. It changes the way we approach our tasks and provides opportunities to develop new approaches to our work organization. But the transition to a computer system form of management and work situation is not an easy one.

General User Anxiety

First-time users of computer equipment often experience *techostress,* an anxiety based on concerns about the effect of computers on their lives. These new procedures require new learning. There are altered tasks and different roles. But the pay-offs are enormous. We can reassure ourselves of the human values involved by remembering this apt phrase concerning the use of computers: "Without me you're nothing."[2] Nonetheless, there are possible social and psychologic costs of a proliferation of electronic helpers, and importance of computer literacy is growing.

Professional Resistance

There has been resistance on the part of some practitioners toward the application of computer technology in clinical practice. But analysis of the clinical encounter indicates that little occurs that is not related in some way to obtaining information, processing it, or applying it to patient problems. The question of application of the powerful information-management tool provided by the computer is not one primarily of technical feasibility but of practitioner acceptance.[3] Critics worry that the human touch will be lost when computers are used. But perhaps the opposite is true. When computers do the tedious and laborious time-consuming tasks of information management, the clinician is freed to focus undivided interest and attention on the patient as a *person.*

Confidentiality

A real concern in any practice, of course, is confidentiality of patient information. Thus automated medical records systems are of particular concern. Though not totally immune to abuses, computers provide safeguards by use of electronic locks, passwords, and other protective measures. These measures provide better security than do our traditional, sometimes chaotic, methods of handling medical records that provide very little protection against unauthorized use.

Patient/Client Response

Some patients have reacted negatively to the use of computers in aspects of patient care such as history-taking or counseling. In general, however, patients and clients do respond positively to the increased individual attention from practitioners who are freed of other diverting laborious tasks.

Computer Applications in Nutrition Practice

The earliest and most extensive applications of computer-managed services in nutrition and dietetics have been in the area of food service systems. However, many other areas of application in clinical nutrition practice, community nutrition, nutrition education and research are currently being developed (see Issues and Answers, pp. 576-577). Some examples of applications in these practice areas are described here.

Clinical Nutrition: The Hospital Setting
Computer System Development

Network Interconnected group of computers, terminals, or telephones.

Microprocessor Small, integrated circuit chip holding all the circuits or the "brains" of a computer.

By and large, most of the computer **networks** used by hospital dietetic and nursing departments in large medical centers have been designed around the large hospital-wide minicomputer system (see p. 562). The rapid advance in **microprocessor** technology, however, has made it possible for smaller health care facilties and individual practitioners to develop computer capabilities. These smaller systems offer flexibility and programming, multiple uses, and lower cost, together with constant uninterrupted access.[4,5] Some leaders in the computer industry believe that the large minicomputer, which has long been a cornerstone of business and professional operations of many kinds, will find some of its operations taken over by newer generations of microcomputers. The advances in local area networking and high-capacity media storage alone allow the microcomputer to provide most of the services needed at far less cost and with much more flexibility. Bigger and more expensive isn't always better.

Clinical Nutrition: Patient Care

The first basic area of computer application in nutrition practice is in clinical care in the hospital setting. The work of a clinical nutritionist/dietitian in patient care, closely integrated with that of the nurse and other members of the health care team, presents many opportunities for computer applications. The practitioner-patient encounter demands obtaining a wealth of detailed information, which well-designed computer systems can help manage. The clinician is constantly involved in the basic aspects of patient care: assessment, analysis, intervention, implementation, and evaluation. The patient care team uses computer management systems in constantly coordinating communications. This is essential in planning all aspects of patient care, including nutritional assessment and support services, nutritional analysis, and nutritional therapy.

Communications in Patient Care

In large hospital settings the primary health care team uses sophisticated computer systems in all phases of patient care. The computer's coordinating control program is usually a broad automated hospital information system (AHIS) such as the IBM Patient Care System.[6,7] Such systems have applications in various aspects of patient care: (1) storage and retrieval of clinical and statistical data, (2) a base of educational materials that may be consulted in patient care problems, (3) guidance for patient care planning, (4) patient care audits to ensure quality standards, and (5) clinical research. A computerized dietary order entry system instantly communicates orders/messages from the patient care units to the floor diet offices. Nursing personnel record information into the patient database from their own terminal located on each patient care unit. The corresponding messages are printed immediately in the appropriate floor diet office. Message changes are made on any CRT terminal by using a **light pen** and preformatted display screens. Daily reports are generated automatically via a high-speed printer in the hospital information systems department. In addition to the dietary order entry **module,** additional application modules in the system support patient care: clinic scheduling/patient registration, census, financial management, clinical laboratory recording, electrocardiogram evaluation, medical record abstracting, surgical utilization, infection control, radiology, pharmacy information, and patient accounting.

Nutrition Assessment and Support Services

Numerous computer applications are used in the hospital's nutritional support services. A broad range of anthropometric, biochemical, clinical, and historical data is gathered in the process of the required comprehensive nutritional assessment involved. The computer can quickly analyze these data so that the nutrition-support team can screen and identify patients at risk, institute therapy, and monitor individual patients closely.[8] Such a computerized screening process can be used for all patients on admission to identify subpopulations at risk for nutritional deficiencies. Then immediate follow-up consultation with a clinical nutritionist/dietitian and the support service can be used for more comprehensive assessment and initiation of appropriate nutritional therapy.

Nutrition Analysis

In addition to various clinical data, nutritive analysis of diets is an important basis for comprehensive nutritional assessment. In the past the tedium of manual calculations prohibited widespread use of analysis of dietary intake in the clinical situation. Now computerized nutrient analysis has changed this situation.[9,10] Primary care clinical dietitians can obtain detailed individual patient nutrient information with speed and relative accuracy and generate reports via data processing. This vital nutritional

Light pen Electronic device (looks like a pen) that gives signals to the computer when its tip is touched to the monitor screen.

Module Subcomponents or sections of a system.

status information can then be used by the nursing staff in developing nursing care plans for that patient. Such rapid practical data processing allows the nutrition practioner to spend more professional time with other nutritional assessment work as well as in personal interaction with the patient. Sometimes, as an accessory tool to the broad hospital computer system, nutritionists use a small inexpensive hand-held pocket-sized programmable calculator to facilitate the task of nutrient analysis.[11] These small instruments can be used for special work on team rounds to quickly estimate nutritional and electrolyte requirements and to match intravenous or enteral requirements with pharmacy availability.

Nutritional Therapy and Care Plans

Computerized medical records provide a basis for the nutrition staff to analyze comparative therapy for various conditions. They can determine nutritional status and nutrient needs. Widespread hospital malnutrition in past years has been well documented. In one such study of 100 patients admitted for acute gastrointestinal problems, results indicated that 83% of these patients received diets inadequate in protein and kilocalories during their hospitalization and that their prescribed diet was inadequate for 46% of the time of the hospital study.[12] Comprehensive clinical data, immediately available through computerized patient care systems, have helped reduce this unnecessary and debilitating malnutrition. The system enables clinical dietitians to work closely with physicians and nurses in monitoring hospital patients at risk and avoiding malnutrition by paying closer attention to nutritional therapies. It also assists in planning patient teaching rounds or diet manual revisions and in conducting needed clinical research.

Business Management of Clinical Practice

Whether in a private clinical practice setting or in a hospital-based setting, the clinical nutritionist also carries responsibility in whole or in part for time and fiscal management of nutrition services. This management includes three major aspects: (1) bookkeeping and accounting systems required for cost accounting, cost effectiveness, and fiscal projections, (2) patient scheduling and census tallies, and (3) patient records and reports.

Community Nutrition

A second area of computer application in nutrition practice is in private and public health care in community settings. As computer technology for processing nutritional data has become more sophisticated during the last two decades, it has been applied increasingly in other community settings providing nutritional care. These settings include outpatient clinics, private practice, and public health. This work involves nutrition counseling, surveys, special projects, and program planning.

Nutrition Counseling

To meet special nutritional therapy needs and client-centered counseling, computer-assisted programs are developed for special clinical problems such as diabetes or hyperlipidemia (see Issues and Answers, pp. 576-577).

In addition to dietary analysis and calculation of individual nutrition prescription, computer-planned menus for these clients can be generated, and ongoing care can be monitored.

Nutrition Surveys and Program Planning

Population surveys provide data to identify nutrition needs and help plan programs to meet these needs. Such surveys are conducted on both national and local levels. With the recent development of an optical scanning process for the computer, survey data may be read rapidly by the Optical Character Reader (OCR).[13] It is now used by public health departments for health surveillance of population groups. The OCR can read pencil marks on survey documents and through a series of computer programs convert these marks into computer language with rapid speed. New applications for dietary data tabulation help in tasks such as developing and revising diet manuals to meet regulations of the Joint Commission of Accreditation of Hospitals (FCAH). Such use of computers frees the nutritionist for other professional responsibilities such as making complex management decisions related to patient care and supervision.

Nutrition Education

A third area of computer application in nutrition practice is nutrition education. This learning process takes place in both formal school settings and general health care agencies.

Impact of Educational Technology

Over the next few decades, society will increasingly rely on the computer to economically collect, distribute, and control massive amounts of information. Scientists call this the "spiral evolution." Because of such rapid technologic change, educators face immense change in the methods they use as well as in the students they teach. Potential users of these new educational technologies include every age from very young children to the elderly, students at every level of formal education, those involved in both industrial and professional training, and adults engaged in nonformal learning activities. In short, everyone in our society will be touched. In the face of this rapid change, some educators voice concern about loss of interpersonal communication in such "programmed" learning.[14] Nonetheless, professors have successfully developed "electronic classrooms" through which they combine educational technologies with constant human communication with students. As educators and students our goal is to anticipate the benefits and consequences of these emerging trends and to plan accordingly. Videodisks, satellites and cable communication, facsimile and slow-scan television, as well as the computer, have vast implications as to how students will be reached and taught.

Trends in Educational Technologies

Four revolutionary trends in computer-based learning have been identified:

1. **Integrated technologies**. Such learning technologies include videodisk, stereophonic units, computer, cable television, and satellite and telephone communications.

2. **Multipurpose communications**. Rich multipurpose communications and information systems exist, such as that at the Massachusetts Institute of Technology's Spacial Data Management System which allows the user to "fly" over an animated information landscape of almost any source or format.
3. **Human interface**. A growing emphasis is being placed on human interactions, with curriculums less dependent on the rigid behavioral or competency-based learning models of the past.
4. **Costs**. Costs are rapidly decreasing with less dependence on expensive classroom equipment for small numbers of students.

Professional Education

Computers combined with other audiovisual instruction techniques are used for self-paced courses in nutrition offered to dietetic, nutrition, nursing, and premedical students. Computer-simulated clinical encounters have been successfully used in a number of clinical nutrition courses. The instructor gets a printout reporting the student's knowledge, responses to inquires concerning the patient, and organization of the clinical encounter, thus enabling the instructor to meet individual student needs. The potential use of computers in nutrition-related education covers four areas: (1) *instruction*—drill, practice, and dialogues, (2) *real-life simulations*, (3) *hypothesis/idea testing*—building process models, and (4) *reduction of computational labor*. Investigators recommend that, at the minimum, students should be exposed to courses dealing with computers and information processing—especially with use of microprocessors—for the wave of the future is in widespread multiuse computers.

Patients/Client Education

Computer-assisted learning is used in a variety of ways in private practice, clinics, and hospitals for patient/client education in health care. In one such application, a microcomputer and a program were used to develop a program in diabetes education that did not require constant surveillance by the health care professional.[15] In addition to such specific programs written by nutritionists to meet special learning needs, a number of general diet and exercise programs are available for use in professional health care services. However, the quality is not uniform, and these require careful evaluation (see box, pp. 570-571).

Consumer Education

In the future, taking advantage of the growing use of home computers and the proliferation of cable television, computers may become a major tool for both food marketing and client nutrition education. Consumers will be able to view the entire product lists of grocery stores on the **monitor**, compare prices, and select the local store offering the lowest total cost of the day. Consumers could place orders from their homes with electronic payment transaction. Computer catalog warehouses would replace current supermarkets. There would be space only for fresh produce, which consumers could inspect personally. The bulk of the store space would be warehouse. Cooperative buying clubs could develop as consumers pool their orders via home computers and benefit from quantity-pur-

Monitor Another name for a computer display screen.

Clinical Application

**How to Select
Home Diet/
Exercise Software**

Program Specific series of
instructions written in a
computer language, defining
a particular process the
computer is to perform.

Amazing! Your client who, a few weeks ago had never heard of
sodium, suddenly is able to tell you the sodium content of yesterday's
food intake as well as the percentage of the RDA for eight essential
nutrients. This reflects on your competence as a nutrition counselor,
of course. Or, it might reflect the glimmer of a computer chip. In
today's rapidly developing personal computer market, an increasing
number of our clients may be asking us for recommendations about
nutrition and fitness software for use with their home computers.
Both needs and costs must be considered.

Programs designed to analyze the nutritive value of meals are
burgeoning in the software circuit. For a price of anywhere from $40
to $1,000, you can analyze your food intake for one or more
nutrients, have them compared to their RDAs, plan a kilocalorie-
controlled diet program, evaluate fad diets, plan exercise programs,
and much more. So, you should expect a growing number of clients
to ask for information on how to evaluate the "off-the-shelf" software
that's available in order to get the best buy. Or you may consider
these same questions in considering software purchases for your own
nutrition practice. Here are a few guiding suggestions you can offer
your clients or use yourself:

- **Ask yourself, "why do I want this program?"** Do I need data that
  is graphed or plotted? Will I be keeping records for a month? A
  year? Longer? Do I want a food cost breakdown or shopping list? Do
  I need a special feature, such as information on complementary
  proteins for a vegetarian diet?
- **Is accuracy important?** A data base of 500 to 800 food items is
  recommended for any real value; 4000-6000 items are necessary
  for the most accuracy possible. Data on name brands as well as
  generics increases accuracy.
- **Is it easy to enter data into the computer?** Some larger programs
  use numbered food codes that the user must look up in an
  accompanying codebook. This is time-consuming, however, and
  too much of a chore to be useful.
- **Does the program monitor the nutrient you are interested in?**
  The number of nutrients isn't a major concern for monitoring a
  special condition, such as coronary heart disease. This case only
  requires data on cholesterol, fats, P:S ratios, and a few other
  nutrients.
- **Is the data provided useful for you?** Some programs only
  indicate an excess and deficiency of a particular nutrient and list
  alternative foods. Programs for professionals may be too extensive
  for clients and only confuse them. Advise clients to ask the
  computer company for a sample printout to make sure they can
  understand it.

Clinical Application—cont'd

- **Can you understand the user's manual**? Advise clients to purchase a general nutrition book as a reference, as the manual and program are developed by programmers, not nutritionists.
- **How flexible should the program be**? More ambitious users may want to combine foods eaten frequently, delete foods that are never eaten in order to add those that are, or even update nutritional values.
- **Is the program "time-tested"**? New programs may have "bugs" that will be worked out in time—after enough customer complaints reach the programmers.
- **Can you afford it**? A high price doesn't always mean quality. Considering the eight factors listed above to evaluate software, your clients may find that the $50 program actually meets their needs better than the one costing ten times more.

References
Freifeld, K., Body management, Personal Computing, **6**(8):60, August, 1983.
Schorin, M., Programs for a healthy practice, PC Magazine, **3**(4):131, March 6, 1984.

---

chase discounts. Reductions of in-store advertising and resultant impulse buying would drastically affect food company marketing programs. "User-friendly" ordering could offer the consumer the advantages of reduced shopping time and product costs. Opportunity for involvement of consumer nutrition education in such programs is vast.

Nutrition Research

A fourth area of computer application in nutrition practice is in nutrition research and writing. This area of work includes both general research of clinical problems encountered in daily practice and formal clinical research projects. Automated diet construction programs can assist research nutritionists through the use of an interactive computer system.[17] Both research accuracy and dietary compliance of subjects in a study can be achieved as tedious tabulation work is done by the computer and foods used are of required quality and quantity. In general, computer-based nutrition research involves selecting and using data bases, developing literature-search strategies, and writing reports.

Data Bases

Data base An organized body of information placed into computers for systematic storage and retrieval; usually deals with a specific topic or project.

More information is available through a computer than in any library in the world. A number of computerized nutrient databanks are available for use in nutrient analysis, surveys, and research projects.[9,17] In addition, a large number of **data bases** exist for searching the scientific literature on any desired topic.[18] A wide range of data bases is available for research on a variety of topics related to human nutrition. These files make available a

DIALOG, located in Palo Alto, California, is one of the largest database producers and also one of the oldest services. It offers over 200 databases for developing specific search strategies.

variety of materials including scientific journal articles, monographs, proceedings of conferences, and many other documents.

Literature-Search Strategies

The proper combinations of search words is sometimes difficult especially for the beginner. Bibliographic and referral data bases can be searched via one or more of the three major information service vendors: DIALOG Information Services, System Development Corporation Search Service, and the Bibliographic Retrieval Service (BRS). Proliferating traditional scientific journals have become increasingly specialized and expensive. Thus the wave of the future may well be electronic journals that will challenge their rivals by speeding scientific reports, as well as work in progress, to their subscribers via computer.

Report Writing

Any writing of scientific reports, or educational materials for professional students as well as the public, is facilitated by the use of word processing. This may be done on a dedicated word processor or by use of word-processing programs with a multiuse microcomputer. Such programs allow for initial drafts to be filed, with the necessary follow-up work of revising, proofreading, and editing accomplished much more quickly. For example, this book was written and prepared for submission to the publisher by using a multipurpose microcomputer and an industry-standard word-processing program (WordStar).

To Sum Up

Computers can do many jobs in handling information in numbers and words to reshape our work, relieve us of tedious labor, and provide greater opportunity to work directly with our patients and clients. What computers cannot do is supply the human factor. We need to learn how to use these revolutionary tools with skill and wisdom in providing sensitive, sound, and humanistic health care.

Computer hardware is rapidly advancing in the development of the microprocessor with the next generation of computers being able to assume an ever-widening range of professional, business, and personal uses. Currently the development of industry-specific software (for example, programs in medicine and nutrition) is still in its infancy. Nutritionists/dietitians with programming skills are beginning to help supply some of these specific needs for management of clinical nutrition practices.

Computer applications in the management of nutritional services have been used mostly in food service to control the sequence of activities involved in food planning, procurement, production, and distribution. Applications in clinical and community nutrition have been more recent. However, these applications are beginning to develop in areas such as business management, patient care, public health, education, research, and writing.

Questions for Review

1. Describe several different types of computer applications for management of clinical nutrition support services for hospitalized patients. What are the roles of the clinical nutritionist? The nurse?
2. How would you use computer technology in doing a nutrition assessment for a hospitalized patient at risk for malnutrition?
3. What are nutrient databanks? How are they used?
4. Describe possible computer applications in nutrition education. Would you like such a learning process? Why or why not?
5. What computer resources are available for nutrition research? How are they used?

References

1. Willard, R.: Computers in dietetics, Diet. Currents **9**(3):7, 1982.

2. Herbert, F.: Without me you're nothing: The essential guide to home computers, New York, 1980, Pocket Books.

3. Levinson, D.: Information, computers, and clinical practice, J. Am. Med. Assoc. **249:**607, 1983.

4. Youngwirth, J.: The evolution of computers in dietetics: a review, J.Am. Diet. Assoc. **82**(1):62, 1983.

5. Tougas, J.; Computer profile: plug determination and basic training into a small business computer for big success in hospital food service, Restaurants and Institutions **90:**164, 1982.

6. Dunphy, M.K., and Bratton, B.D.; A computerized dietary order entry system, J. Am. Diet. Assoc. **82**(1):68, 1983.

7. Edmunds, L.: Computer-assisted nursing care, Am. J. Nurs. **82:**1076, 1982.

8. Davidson, F.: Computer applications in the field of nutritional support, Nutr. Support Serv. **2:**42, 1982.

9. Hoover, L.W.: Computerized nutrient data bases: I. Comparison of nutrient analysis systems, J. Am. Diet. Assoc. **82**(5):501, 1983.

10. Hoover, L.W., and Perloff, B.P.: Computerized nutrient data bases: II. Development of model for appraisal of nutrient data base system capabilities, J. Am. Diet. Assoc. **82**(5):506, 1983.

11. Rich, A.J.: A programmable calculator system for the estimation of nutritional intake of hospital patients, Am. J. Clin. Nurt. **34**(10):2276, 1981.

12. Dean, J.: Use of computerized medical records by dietary staff and student, J. Am. Diet. Assoc. **71**(5):533, 1977.

13. Sawicki, M., and Endres, J.: Energy and nutrient calculations using an Optical Character Reader system, J. Am. Diet. Assoc. **82**(2):135, 1983.

14. Lewis, E.J.: Lack of interpersonal communication in programmed learning, N. Engl. J. Med. **306:**1495, 1982.

15. Cook, G.B.: The microcomputer: an extension of the diabetes educator, The Diab. Educator **7:**12, 1982.

16. Schorin, M.: Programs for a healthy practice, PC Magazine **3**(4):131, 1984.

17. Oexmann, M.J.: Automated diet construction for clinical research, J. Am. Diet. Assoc. **82**(1):72, 1983.

18. Frank, R.C.: Information resources for food and human nutrition, J. Am. Diet. Assoc. **80**(4):344, 1982.

Further Readings

Bryant, O., and others, Computerized surveillance of diabetic patient/health care delivery system interfaces, Diab. Care, **1:**144, 1980.
　and
Suitor, C.W., Suitor, R.F., and Adelman, M.O.: Planning high-carbohydrate, high-fiber diets with a microcomputer, J. Am. Diet. Assoc. **82**(3):279, 1983.
　and
Wheeler, M.L., and Wheeler, L.A.: Computer-planned menus for patients with diabetes mellitus, Diab. Care **3:**663, 1980.

These three articles describe clinical applications of computer programs in care of persons with diabetes. They provide for interactive use with clients to determine therapy needs, construct specific diet prescriptions, design personal food plans, and monitor responses.

Danford, D.E.: Computer applications to medical nutrition problems, J. Parent. Enter. Nutr. **5**:441, 1981.

and

Giacoia, G.P., Warden, L.K., and Canfield, B.G.: Computerized total parenteral nutrition formulas for newborn infants, Am. J. Hosp. Pharm. **37**:22, 1980.

These two articles describe clinical applications in medical-nutritional problems, especially in assessment of nutritional needs and calculation of indicated TPN formulas.

Hoover, L.W.: Computerized nutrient data bases: I. Comparison of nutrient analysis systems, II. (Hoover, L.W., and Perloff, B.P.) Development of model for appraisal of nutrient data base system capabilities, J. Am. Diet. Assoc. **82**(5):501, 1983.

This series of articles describes the sources of possible error in computer nutrient analysis and presents a model for detecting and reducing these errors. The need for standardizing nutrient data bases is indicated.

Witschi, J., and others: Analysis of dietary data: an interactive computer method for storage and retrieval, J. Am. Diet. Assoc. **78**(6):609, 1981.

The authors describe their simplified nutrient data base and interactive retrieval method, used initially in hyperlipidemia counseling. The program eliminates the chore of coding and can be used directly with clients during interviewing.

Issues and Answers

Broadening Computer Applications in Nutrition

Mention computer applications in the field of nutrition and the first area that comes to mind is usually food service. This is an accepted widespread area of use. Here computers are used to facilitate cost breakdowns, calculate the payroll, monitor expenses and inventory, etc.

More recently, however, in other areas of nutrition practice, computer applications in human services are also proving their broad effectiveness. Some of the most valuable uses of computers in nutrition practice today are in patient care. Some of the areas in which this technology has been applied successfully include the following:

Nutrient Ratios in Menu Planning
Nutritionists using microcomputers in one New England medical center reported the use of a computer program that facilitated adjustments in the amount of carbohydrate and fiber to improve patient blood sugar control, reduce serum cholesterol or triglycerides, and improve satiety, while at the same time matching the individual's food preferences. The program uses the average composition of carbohydrate, protein, fat, and dietary fiber in each food exchange group and the kcal/g of carbohydrate, protein, and fat. It incorporates minimum and maximum number of servings allowed for each food exchange group, has flexibility, and achieves the desired fraction of each nutritional factor in the diet.

Nutritional Evaluation
A team of surgical researchers report the use of a computer program to determine the nutritional needs of critically burned patients and evaluate the adequacy of nutritional therapy provided. This program monitors intake of kcal, protein, fat, carbohydrate, most minerals and vitamins; route of feeding (nasogastric tube, intravenous, or oral); percentage of predicted nutrient requirement consumed; nitrogen : kcal ratio; nitrogen balance; percentage of weight change. The program can produce summaries for entry into patient charts or produce graphs that research dietitians use to instruct patients and clarify their progress.

Nutritional Research
Another medical research team uses a program that can delete foods from a menu and change the quantity requested or the nutrient goals, in order to design complex research diets in which several nutrients must be calculated with complete accuracy. This combination of flexibility and accuracy is also helpful to dietitians on metabolic wards, where there must be a careful accounting of specific nutrient levels provided and consumed.

Nutritional Counseling
When funds were cut for one university's nutrition information services, the campus computer took over. Senior dietetic studens

Issues and Answers—cont'd

responded to questions and comments submitted via computer by students or staff from any of the 150 terminals on campus. Questions could be submitted anonymously, or users could read previous questions and responses without having to submit their own questions. This flexibility allowed health care workers in Student Health Services to provide information on clinical nutrition in their own facility without formal instruction.

Continuing Education

Computers are used for continuing education as a means of filing key journal articles to be referred to when special problems arise. Computers are also used interactively to enhance continuing education by practice, evaluating procedures, identifying problems, and emphasizing self-assessment of skill and knowledge.

By adapting available nutrition data bases into carefully written programs, nutritionists can save time spent making critical calculations and have usable data available within seconds to evaluate needs and even help patients learn. The precious time that is saved could be invested in reaching a greater segment of the public about sound nutrition and its role in health promotion.

References

Cotugua, N., Corrozi, A.M., and Berrang, C.: Computerized nutrition counseling in a coordinated undergraduate program, J. Am. Diet. Assoc. **82**(2):182, 1983.

McLaurin, N.K., and others: Computergenerated graphic evaluation of nutritional status in critically injured patients, J. Am. Diet. Assoc. **82**(1):49, 1983.

Oexmann, M.J.: Automated diet contruction for clinical research, J. Am. Diet. Assoc. **82**(1):72, 1983.

Suitor, C.W., Suitor, R.F., and Adelman, M.D.: Planning high-carbohydrate, high-fiber diets with a microcomputer, J. Am. Diet. Assoc. **2**(3):279, 1983.

Appendixes

Nutritive Values of the Edible Part of Foods

Foods, Approximate Measures, Units, and Weight		(g)	Water (%)	Food Energy (cal)	Protein (g)	Fat (g)	Saturated (total) (g)	Oleic (g)	Linol (g)
							Nutrients in Indicated Quantity		
								Fatty Acids	
									Unsaturated

Foods, Approximate Measures, Units, and Weight		(g)	Water (%)	Food Energy (cal)	Protein (g)	Fat (g)	Saturated (total) (g)	Oleic (g)	Linol (g)
Dairy Products (Cheese, Cream, Imitation Cream, Milk; Related Products)									
Cheese:									
Natural:									
Blue	1 oz	28	42	100	6	8	5.3	1.9	
Camembert (3 wedges per 4 oz container)	1 wedge	38	52	115	8	9	5.8	2.2	
Cheddar:									
Cut pieces	1 oz	28	37	115	7	9	6.1	2.1	
	1 cu in	17.2	37	70	4	6	3.7	1.3	
Shredded	1 cup	113	37	455	28	37	24.2	8.5	
Cottage (curd not pressed down):									
Creamed (cottage cheese, 4% fat):									
Large curd	1 cup	225	79	235	28	10	6.4	2.4	
Small curd	1 cup	210	79	220	26	9	6.0	2.2	
Low fat (2%)	1 cup	226	79	205	31	4	2.8	1.0	
Low fat (1%)	1 cup	226	82	165	28	2	1.5	.5	
Uncreamed (cottage cheese dry curd, less than ½% fat)	1 cup	145	80	125	25	1	.4	.1	Tr
Cream	1 oz	28	54	100	2	10	6.2	2.4	
Mozzarella, made with—									
Whole milk	1 oz	28	48	90	6	7	4.4	1.7	
Part skim milk	1 oz	28	49	80	8	5	3.1	1.2	
Parmesan, grated:									
Cup, not pressed down	1 cup	100	18	455	42	30	19.1	7.7	
Tablespoon	1 tbsp	5	18	25	2	2	1.0	.4	Tr
Ounce	1 oz	28	18	130	12	9	5.4	2.2	
Provolone	1 oz	28	41	100	7	8	4.8	1.7	
Ricotta, made with—									
Whole milk	1 cup	246	72	430	28	32	20.4	7.1	
Part skim milk	1 cup	246	74	340	28	19	12.1	4.7	
Romano	1 oz	28	31	110	9	8	—	—	
Swiss	1 oz	28	37	105	8	8	5.0	1.7	
Pasteurized process cheese:									
American	1 oz	28	39	105	6	9	5.6	2.1	
Swiss	1 oz	28	42	95	7	7	4.5	1.7	
Pasteurized process cheese food, American	1 oz	28	43	95	6	7	4.4	1.7	
Pasteurized process cheese spread, American	1 oz	28	48	80	5	6	3.8	1.5	
Cream, sweet:									
Half-and-half (cream and milk)	1 cup	242	81	315	7	28	17.3	7.0	
	1 tbsp	15	81	20	Tr	2	1.1	.4	Tr
Light, coffee, or table	1 cup	240	74	470	6	46	28.8	11.7	1
	1 tbsp	15	74	30	Tr	3	1.8	.7	
Whipping, unwhipped (volume about double when whipped):									
Light	1 cup	239	64	700	5	74	46.2	18.3	1
	1 tbsp	15	64	45	Tr	5	2.9	1.1	
Heavy	1 cup	238	58	820	5	88	54.8	22.2	2
	1 tbsp	15	58	80	Tr	6	3.5	1.4	
Whipped topping (pressurized)	1 cup	60	61	155	2	13	8.3	3.4	
	1 tbsp	3	61	10	Tr	1	.4	.2	Tr
Cream, sour	1 cup	230	71	495	7	48	30.0	12.1	1
	1 tbsp	12	71	25	Tr	3	1.6	.6	

From Adams, C.F., and Richardson, M.: Nutritive value of foods, Home and Garden Bulletin No. 72, U.S. Department of Agriculture, Washington, D.C., 1981, U.S. Government Prir Office.
Blanks indicate no data available.
Tr, Trace.
For notes, see end of table.

Nutrients in Indicated Quantity

rbohydrate (g)	Calcium (mg)	Phosphorus (mg)	Iron (mg)	Potassium (mg)	Vitamin A Value (IU)	Thiamin (mg)	Riboflavin (mg)	Niacin (mg)	Ascorbic Acid (mg)
1	150	110	.1	73	200	.01	.11	.3	0
Tr	147	132	.1	71	350	.01	.19	.2	0
Tr	204	145	.2	28	300	.01	.11	Tr	0
Tr	124	88	.1	17	180	Tr	.06	Tr	0
1	815	579	.8	111	1200	.03	.42	.1	0
6	135	297	.3	190	370	.05	.37	.3	Tr
6	126	277	.3	177	340	.04	.34	.3	Tr
8	155	340	.4	217	160	.05	.42	.3	Tr
6	138	302	.3	193	80	.05	.37	.3	Tr
3	46	151	.3	47	40	.04	.21	.2	0
1	23	30	.3	34	400	Tr	.06	Tr	0
1	163	117	.1	21	260	Tr	.08	Tr	0
1	207	149	.1	27	180	.01	.10	Tr	0
4	1376	807	1.0	107	700	.05	.39	.3	0
Tr	69	40	Tr	5	40	Tr	.02	Tr	0
1	390	229	.3	30	200	.01	.11	.1	0
1	214	141	.1	39	230	.01	.09	Tr	0
7	509	389	.9	257	1210	.03	.48	.3	0
13	669	449	1.1	308	1060	.05	.46	.2	0
1	302	215	—	—	160	—	.11	Tr	0
1	272	171	Tr	31	240	.01	.10	Tr	0
Tr	174	211	.1	46	340	.01	.10	Tr	0
1	219	216	.2	61	230	Tr	.08	Tr	0
2	163	130	.2	79	260	.01	.13	Tr	0
2	159	202	.1	69	220	.01	.12	Tr	0
10	254	230	.2	314	260	.08	.36	.2	2
1	16	14	Tr	19	20	.01	.02	Tr	Tr
9	231	192	.1	292	1730	.08	.36	.1	2
1	14	12	Tr	18	110	Tr	.02	Tr	Tr
7	166	146	.1	231	2690	.06	.30	.1	1
Tr	10	9	Tr	15	170	Tr	.02	Tr	Tr
7	154	149	.1	179	3500	.05	.26	.1	1
Tr	10	9	Tr	11	220	Tr	.02	Tr	Tr
7	61	54	Tr	88	550	.02	.04	Tr	0
Tr	3	3	Tr	4	30	Tr	Tr	Tr	0
10	268	195	.1	331	1820	.08	.34	.2	2
1	14	10	Tr	17	90	Tr	.02	Tr	Tr

| | | | | | | | Fatty Acids | | |
| | | | | | | | | Unsaturated | |
Foods, Approximate Measures, Units, and Weight		(g)	Water (%)	Food Energy (cal)	Protein (g)	Fat (g)	Saturated (total) (g)	Oleic (g)	Linole (g)
Cream products, imitation (made with vegetable fat):									
Sweet:									
Creamers:									
Liquid (frozen)	1 cup	245	77	335	2	24	22.8	.3	Tr
	1 tbsp	15	77	20	Tr	1	1.4	Tr	0
Powdered	1 cup	94	2	515	5	33	30.6	.9	Tr
	1 tsp	2	2	10	Tr	1	.7	Tr	0
Whipped topping:									
Frozen	1 cup	75	50	240	1	19	16.3	1.0	.2
	1 tbsp	4	50	15	Tr	1	.9	.1	Tr
Powdered, made with whole milk	1 cup	80	67	150	3	10	8.5	.6	.
	1 tbsp	4	67	10	Tr	Tr	.4	Tr	Tr
Pressurized	1 tbsp	4	60	10	Tr	1	.8	.1	Tr
Sour dressing (imitation sour cream) made with	1 cup	235	75	415	8	39	31.2	4.4	1.
nonfat dry milk	1 tbsp	12	75	20	Tr	2	1.6	.2	
Milk:									
Fluid:									
Whole (3.3% fat)	1 cup	244	88	150	8	8	5.1	2.1	.2
Lowfat (2%):									
No milk solids added	1 cup	244	89	120	8	5	2.9	1.2	.
Lowfat (1%)									
No milk solids added	1 cup	244	90	100	8	3	1.6	.7	.1
Nonfat (skim):									
No milk solids added	1 cup	245	91	85	8	Tr	.3	.1	Tr
Buttermilk	1 cup	245	90	100	8	2	1.3	.5	Tr
Canned:									
Evaporated, unsweetened:									
Whole milk	1 cup	252	74	340	17	19	11.6	5.3	0.
Skim milk	1 cup	255	79	200	19	1	.3	.1	Tr
Sweetened, condensed	1 cup	306	27	980	24	27	16.8	6.7	.
Dried:									
Buttermilk	1 cup	120	3	465	41	7	4.3	1.7	.2
Nonfat instant:									
Envelope, net wt, 3.2 oz[5]	1 envelope	91	4	325	32	1	.4	.1	Tr
Cup[7]	1 cup	68	4	245	24	Tr	.3	.1	Tr
Milk beverages:									
Chocolate milk (commercial):									
Regular	1 cup	250	82	210	8	8	5.3	2.2	.2
Lowfat (2%)	1 cup	250	84	180	8	5	3.1	1.3	.
Lowfat (1%)	1 cup	250	85	160	8	3	1.5	.7	.
Eggnog (commercial)	1 cup	254	74	340	10	19	11.3	5.0	.6
Malted milk, home-prepared with 1 cup of whole milk and 2 to 3 heaping tsp of malted milk powder (about ¾ oz):									
Chocolate	1 cup of milk plus ¾ oz of powder	265	81	235	9	9	5.5	—	—
Natural	1 cup of milk plus ¾ oz of powder	265	81	235	11	10	6.0	—	—
Shakes, thick:[8]									
Chocolate, container, net wt, 10.6 oz	1 container	300	72	355	9	8	5.0	2.0	.
Vanilla, container, net wt, 11 oz	1 container	313	74	350	12	9	5.9	2.4	.
Milk desserts, frozen:									
Ice cream:									
Regular (about 11% fat):									
Hardened	½ gal	1064	61	2155	38	115	71.3	28.8	2.6
	1 cup	133	61	270	5	14	8.9	3.6	.
	3 fl oz container	50	61	100	2	5	3.4	1.4	.
Soft serve (frozen custard)	1 cup	173	60	375	7	23	13.5	5.9	.6
Rich (about 16% fat), hardened	½ gal	1188	59	2805	33	190	118.3	47.8	4.3
	1 cup	148	59	350	4	24	14.7	6.0	.5
Ice milk:									
Hardened (about 4.3% fat)	½ gal	1048	69	1470	41	45	28.1	11.3	1.0
	1 cup	131	69	185	5	6	3.5	1.4	.
Soft serve (about 2.6% fat)	1 cup	175	70	225	8	5	2.9	1.2	0.
Sherbet (about 2% fat)	½ gal	1542	66	2160	17	31	19.0	7.7	.
	1 cup	193	66	270	2	4	2.4	1.0	.

For notes, see end of table.

Nutrients in Indicated Quantity

Carbohydrate (g)	Calcium (mg)	Phosphorus (mg)	Iron (mg)	Potassium (mg)	Vitamin A Value (IU)	Thiamin (mg)	Riboflavin (mg)	Niacin (mg)	Ascorbic Acid (mg)
28	23	157	.1	467	220[1]	0	0	0	0
2	1	10	Tr	29	10[1]	0	0	0	0
52	21	397	.1	763	190[1]	0	.16[1]	0	0
1	Tr	8	Tr	16	Tr[1]	0	Tr[1]	0	0
17	5	6	.1	14	650[1]	0	0	0	0
1	Tr	Tr	Tr	1	30[1]	0	0	0	0
13	72	69	Tr	121	290[1]	.02	.09	Tr	1
1	4	3	Tr	6	10[1]	Tr	Tr	Tr	Tr
1	Tr	1	Tr	1	20[1]	0	0	0	0
11	266	205	.1	380	20[1]	.09	.38	.2	2
1	14	10	Tr	19	Tr	.01	.02	Tr	Tr
11	291	228	.1	370	310[2]	.09	.40	.2	2
12	297	232	.1	377	500	.10	.40	.2	2
12	300	235	.1	381	500	.10	.41	.2	2
12	302	247	.1	406	500	.09	.34	.2	2
12	285	219	.1	371	80[3]	.08	.38	.1	2
25	657	510	.5	764	610[3]	.12	.80	.5	5
29	738	497	.7	845	1000[4]	.11	.79	.4	3
166	868	775	.6	1136	1000[3]	.28	1.27	.6	8
59	1421	1119	.4	1910	260[3]	.47	1.90	1.1	7
47	1120	896	.3	1552	2160[6]	.38	1.59	.8	5
35	837	670	.2	1160	1610[6]	.28	1.19	.6	4
26	280	251	.6	417	300[3]	.09	.41	.3	2
26	284	254	.6	422	500	.10	.42	.3	2
26	287	257	.6	426	500	.10	.40	.2	2
34	330	278	.5	420	890	.09	.48	.3	4
29	304	265	.5	500	330	.14	.43	.7	2
27	347	307	.3	529	380	.20	.54	1.3	2
63	396	378	.9	672	260	.14	.67	.4	0
56	457	361	.3	572	360	.09	.61	.5	0
254	1406	1075	1.0	2052	4340	.42	2.63	1.1	6
32	176	134	.1	257	540	.05	.33	.1	1
12	66	51	Tr	96	200	.02	.12	.1	Tr
38	236	199	.4	338	790	.08	.45	.2	1
256	1213	927	.8	1771	7200	.36	2.27	.9	5
32	151	115	.1	221	900	.04	.28	.1	1
232	1409	1035	1.5	2117	1710	.61	2.78	.9	6
29	176	129	.1	265	210	.08	.35	.1	1
38	274	202	.3	412	180	.12	.54	.2	1
469	827	594	2.5	1585	1480	.26	.71	1.0	31
59	103	74	.3	198	190	.03	.09	.1	4

Foods, Approximate Measures, Units, and Weight		(g)	Water (%)	Food Energy (cal)	Protein (g)	Fat (g)	Nutrients in Indicated Quantity		
							Fatty Acids		
							Saturated (total) (g)	Unsaturated	
								Oleic (g)	Linol (g)
Milk desserts, other:									
Custard, baked	1 cup	265	77	305	14	15	6.8	5.4	
Puddings:									
From home recipe:									
Starch base:									
Chocolate	1 cup	260	66	385	8	12	7.6	3.3	
Vanilla (blancmange)	1 cup	255	76	285	9	10	6.2	2.5	
Tapioca cream	1 cup	165	72	220	8	8	4.1	2.5	
From mix (chocolate) and milk:									
Regular (cooked)	1 cup	260	70	320	9	8	4.3	2.6	
Instant	1 cup	260	69	325	8	7	3.6	2.2	
Yogurt:									
With added milk solids:									
Made with lowfat milk:									
Fruit-flavored[9]	1 container, net wt 8 oz	227	75	230	10	3	1.8	.6	
Plain	1 container, net wt 8 oz	227	85	145	12	4	2.3	.8	
Made with nonfat milk	1 container, net wt 8 oz	227	85	125	13	Tr	.3	.1	Tr
Without added milk solids:									
Made with whole milk	1 container, net wt 8 oz	227	88	140	8	7	4.8	1.7	
Eggs									
Eggs, large (24 oz per dozen):									
Raw:									
Whole, without shell	1 egg	50	75	80	6	6	1.7	2.0	
White	1 white	33	88	15	3	Tr	0	0	0
Yolk	1 yolk	17	49	65	3	6	1.7	2.1	
Cooked:									
Fried in butter	1 egg	46	72	85	5	6	2.4	2.2	
Hard-cooked, shell removed	1 egg	50	75	80	6	6	1.7	2.0	
Poached	1 egg	50	74	80	6	6	1.7	2.0	
Scrambled (milk added) in butter; also omelet	1 egg	64	76	95	6	7	2.8	2.3	
Fats, Oils; Related Products									
Butter:									
Regular (1 brick or 4 sticks per lb):									
Stick (½ cup)	1 stick	113	16	815	1	92	57.3	23.1	2
Tablespoon (about ⅛ stick)	1 tbsp	14	16	100	Tr	12	7.2	2.9	
Pat (1-in square, ⅓ in high; 90 per lb)	1 pat	5	16	35	Tr	4	2.5	1.0	
Whipped (6 sticks or two 8 oz containers per lb)									
Stick (½ cup)	1 stick	76	16	540	1	61	38.2	15.4	1
Tablespoon (about ⅛ stick)	1 tbsp	9	16	65	Tr	8	4.7	1.9	
Pat (1¼ in square, ⅓ in high; 120 per lb)	1 pat	4	16	25	Tr	3	1.9	.8	
Fats, cooking (vegetable shortenings)	1 cup	200	0	1770	0	200	48.8	88.2	48
	1 tbsp	13	0	110	0	13	3.2	5.7	3
Lard	1 tbsp	13	0	115	0	13	5.1	5.3	1
Margarine:									
Regular (1 brick or 4 sticks per lb):									
Stick (½ cup)	1 stick	113	16	815	1	92	16.7	42.9	24
Tablespoon (about ⅛ stick)	1 tbsp	14	16	100	Tr	12	2.1	5.3	3
Pat (1-in square, ⅓ in high; 90 per lb)	1 pat	5	16	35	Tr	4	.7	1.9	1
Soft, two 8 oz containers per lb	1 container	227	16	1635	1	184	32.5	71.5	65
	1 tbsp	14	16	100	Tr	12	2.0	4.5	4
Whipped (6 sticks per lb):									
Stick (½ cup)	1 stick	76	16	545	Tr	61	11.2	28.7	16
Tablespoon (about ⅛ stick)	1 tbsp	9	16	70	Tr	8	1.4	3.6	2
Oils, salad or cooking:									
Corn	1 cup	218	0	1925	0	218	27.7	53.6	125
	1 tbsp	14	0	120	0	14	1.7	3.3	7
Olive	1 cup	216	0	1910	0	216	30.7	154.4	17
	1 tbsp	14	0	120	0	14	1.9	9.7	1
Peanut	1 cup	216	0	1910	0	216	37.4	98.5	67
	1 tbsp	14	0	120	0	14	2.3	6.2	4
Safflower	1 cup	218	0	1925	0	218	20.5	25.9	159
	1 tbsp	14	0	120	0	14	1.3	1.6	10
Soybean oil, hydrogenated	1 cup	218	0	1925	0	218	31.8	93.1	75
(partially hardened)	1 tbsp	14	0	120	0	14	2.0	5.8	4

For notes, see end of table.

Nutrients In Indicated Quantity

bohydrate (g)	Calcium (mg)	Phosphorus (mg)	Iron (mg)	Potassium (mg)	Vitamin A Value (IU)	Thiamin (mg)	Riboflavin (mg)	Niacin (mg)	Ascorbic Acid (mg)
29	297	310	1.1	387	930	.11	.50	.3	1
67	250	255	1.3	445	390	.05	.36	.3	1
41	298	232	Tr	352	410	.08	.41	.3	2
28	173	180	.7	223	480	.07	.30	.2	2
59	265	247	.8	354	340	.05	.39	.3	2
63	374	237	1.3	335	340	.08	.39	.3	2
42	343	269	.2	439	120[10]	.08	.40	.2	1
16	415	326	.2	531	150[10]	.10	.49	.3	2
17	452	355	.2	579	20[10]	.11	.53	.3	2
11	274	215	.1	351	280	.07	.32	.2	1
1	28	90	1.0	65	260	.04	.15	Tr	0
Tr	4	4	Tr	45	0	Tr	.09	Tr	0
Tr	26	86	.9	15	310	.04	.07	Tr	0
1	26	80	.9	58	290	.03	.13	Tr	0
1	28	90	1.0	65	260	.04	.14	Tr	0
1	28	90	1.0	65	260	.04	.13	Tr	0
1	47	97	.9	85	310	.04	.16	Tr	0
Tr	27	26	.2	29	3470[11]	.01	.04	Tr	0
Tr	3	3	Tr	4	430[11]	Tr	Tr	Tr	0
Tr	1	1	Tr	1	150[11]	Tr	Tr	Tr	0
Tr	18	17	.1	20	2310[11]	Tr	.03	Tr	0
Tr	2	2	Tr	2	290[11]	Tr	Tr	Tr	0
Tr	1	1	Tr	1	120[11]	0	Tr	Tr	0
0	0	0	0	0	—	0	0	0	0
0	0	0	0	0	—	0	0	0	0
0	0	0	0	0	0	0	0	0	0
Tr	27	26	.2	29	3750[12]	.01	.04	Tr	0
Tr	3	3	Tr	4	470[12]	Tr	Tr	Tr	0
Tr	1	1	Tr	1	170[12]	Tr	Tr	Tr	0
Tr	53	53	.4	59	7500[12]	.01	.08	.1	0
Tr	3	3	Tr	4	470[12]	Tr	Tr	Tr	0
Tr	18	17	.1	20	2500[12]	Tr	.03	Tr	0
Tr	2	2	Tr	2	310[12]	Tr	Tr	Tr	0
0	0	0	0	0	—	0	0	0	0
0	0	0	0	0	—	0	0	0	0
0	0	0	0	0	—	0	0	0	0
0	0	0	0	0	—	0	0	0	0
0	0	0	0	0	—	0	0	0	0
0	0	0	0	0	—	0	0	0	0
0	0	0	0	0	—	0	0	0	0
0	0	0	0	0	—	0	0	0	0
0	0	0	0	0	—	0	0	0	0
0	0	0	0	0	—	0	0	0	0

Foods, Approximate Measures, Units, and Weight		(g)	Water (%)	Food Energy (cal)	Protein (g)	Fat (g)	Saturated (total) (g)	Unsaturated Oleic (g)	Lino (g)
Soybean-cottonseed oil blend,	1 cup	218	0	1925	0	218	38.2	63.0	99
hydrogenated	1 tbsp	14	0	120	0	14	2.4	3.9	6
Salad dressings:									
Commercial:									
Blue cheese:									
Regular	1 tbsp	15	32	75	1	8	1.6	1.7	3
Low calorie (5 cal per tsp)	1 tbsp	16	84	10	Tr	1	.5	.3	Tr
French:									
Regular	1 tbsp	16	39	65	Tr	6	1.1	1.3	3
Low calorie (5 cal per tsp)	1 tbsp	16	77	15	Tr	1	.1	.1	
Italian:									
Regular	1 tbsp	15	28	85	Tr	9	1.6	1.9	4
Low calorie (2 cal per tsp)	1 tbsp	15	90	10	Tr	1	.1	.1	
Mayonnaise	1 tbsp	14	15	100	Tr	11	2.0	2.4	5
Mayonnaise type:									
Regular	1 tbsp	15	41	65	Tr	6	1.1	1.4	3
Low calorie (8 cal per tsp)	1 tbsp	16	81	20	Tr	2	.4	.4	1
Tartar sauce, regular	1 tbsp	14	34	75	Tr	8	1.5	1.8	4
Thousand Island:									
Regular	1 tbsp	16	32	80	Tr	8	1.4	1.7	4
Low calorie (10 cal per tsp)	1 tbsp	15	68	25	Tr	2	.4	.4	1
From home recipe:									
Cooked type[13]	1 tbsp	16	68	25	1	2	.5	.6	
Fish, Shellfish, Meat, Poultry, Related Products									
Fish and shellfish:									
Bluefish, baked with butter or margarine	3 oz	85	68	135	22	4	—	—	—
Clams:									
Raw, meat only	3 oz	85	82	65	11	1	—	—	—
Canned, solids and liquid	3 oz	85	86	45	7	1	.2	Tr	T
Crabmeat (white or king), canned, not pressed down	1 cup	135	77	135	24	3	.6	0.4	0
Fish sticks, breaded, cooked, frozen (stick, 4 × 1 × ½ in)	1 fish stick or 1 oz	28	66	50	5	3	—	—	
Haddock, breaded, fried[14]	3 oz	85	66	140	17	5	1.4	2.2	1
Ocean perch, breaded, fried[14]	1 fillet	85	59	195	16	11	2.7	4.4	2
Oysters, raw, meat only (13-19 medium Selects)	1 cup	240	85	160	20	4	1.3	.2	
Salmon, pink, canned, solids and liquid	3 oz	85	71	120	17	5	.9	.8	
Sardines, Atlantic, canned in oil, drained solids	3 oz	85	62	175	20	9	3.0	2.5	
Scallops, frozen, breaded, fried, reheated	6 scallops	90	60	175	16	8	—	—	—
Shad, baked with butter or margarine, bacon	3 oz	85	64	170	20	10	—	—	
Shrimp:									
Canned meat	3 oz	85	70	100	21	1	.1	.1	T
French fried[16]	3 oz	85	57	190	17	9	2.3	3.7	2
Tuna, canned in oil, drained solids	3 oz	85	61	170	24	7	1.7	1.7	
Tuna salad[17]	1 cup	205	70	350	30	22	4.3	6.3	
Meat and meat products:									
Bacon (20 slices per lb, raw), broiled or fried, crisp	2 slices	15	8	85	4	8	2.5	3.7	
Beef, cooked:[18]									
Cuts braised, simmered, or pot roasted:									
Lean and fat (piece, 2½ × 2½ × ¾ in)	3 oz	85	53	245	23	16	6.8	6.5	
Lean only from item directly above	2.5 oz	72	62	140	22	5	2.1	1.8	
Ground beef, broiled:									
Lean with 10% fat	3 oz or patty 3 × ⅝ in	85	60	185	23	10	4.0	3.9	
Lean with 21% fat	2.9 oz or patty 3 × ⅝ in	82	54	235	20	17	7.0	6.7	
Roast, oven cooked, no liquid added:									
Relatively fat, such as rib:									
Lean and fat (2 pieces, 4⅛ × 2¼ × ¼ in)	3 oz	85	40	375	17	33	14.0	13.6	
Lean only	1.8 oz	51	57	125	14	7	3.0	2.5	
Relatively lean, such as heel of round:									
Lean and fat (2 pieces, 4⅛ × 2¼ × ¼ in)	3 oz	85	62	165	25	7	2.8	2.7	
Lean only	2.8 oz	78	65	125	24	3	1.2	1.0	

For notes, see end of table.

Nutrients in Indicated Quantity

rbohydrate (g)	Calcium (mg)	Phosphorus (mg)	Iron (mg)	Potassium (mg)	Vitamin A Value (IU)	Thiamin (mg)	Riboflavin (mg)	Niacin (mg)	Ascorbic Acid (mg)
0	0	0	0	0	—	0	0	0	0
0	0	0	0	0	—	0	0	0	0
1	12	11	Tr	6	30	Tr	.02	Tr	Tr
1	10	8	Tr	5	30	Tr	.01	Tr	Tr
3	2	2	.1	13	—	—	—	—	—
2	2	2	.1	13	—	—	—	—	—
1	2	1	Tr	2	Tr	Tr	Tr	Tr	—
Tr	Tr	1	Tr	2	Tr	Tr	Tr	Tr	—
Tr	3	4	.1	5	40	Tr	.01	Tr	—
2	2	4	Tr	1	30	Tr	Tr	Tr	—
2	3	4	Tr	1	40	Tr	Tr	Tr	—
1	3	4	.1	11	30	Tr	Tr	Tr	Tr
2	2	3	.1	18	50	Tr	Tr	Tr	Tr
2	2	3	.1	17	50	Tr	Tr	Tr	Tr
2	14	15	.1	19	80	.01	.03	Tr	Tr
0	25	244	.6	—	40	.09	.08	1.6	—
2	59	138	5.2	154	90	.08	.15	1.1	8
2	47	116	3.5	119	—	.01	.09	.9	—
1	61	246	1.1	149	—	.11	.11	2.6	—
2	3	47	.1	—	0	.01	.02	.5	—
5	34	210	1.0	296	—	.03	.06	2.7	2
6	28	192	1.1	242	—	.10	.10	1.6	—
8	226	343	13.2	290	740	.34	.43	6.0	—
0	167[15]	243	.7	307	60	.03	.16	6.8	—
0	372	424	2.5	502	190	.02	.17	4.6	—
9	—	—	—	—	—	—	—	—	—
0	20	266	.5	320	30	.11	.22	7.3	—
1	98	224	2.6	104	50	.01	.03	1.5	—
9	61	162	1.7	195	—	.03	.07	2.3	—
0	7	199	1.6	—	70	.04	.10	10.1	—
7	41	291	2.7	—	590	.08	.23	10.3	2
Tr	2	34	.5	35	0	.08	.05	.8	—
0	10	114	2.9	184	30	.04	.18	3.6	—
0	10	108	2.7	176	10	.04	.17	3.3	—
0	10	196	3.0	261	20	.08	.20	5.1	—
0	9	159	2.6	221	30	.07	.17	4.4	—
0	8	158	2.2	189	70	.05	.13	3.1	—
0	6	131	1.8	161	10	.04	.11	2.6	—
0	11	208	3.2	279	10	.06	.19	4.5	—
0	10	199	3.0	268	Tr	.06	.18	4.3	—

Foods, Approximate Measures, Units, and Weight		(g)	Water (%)	Food Energy (cal)	Protein (g)	Fat (g)	Saturated (total) (g)	Oleic (g)	Linole (g)
							Fatty Acids		
							Saturated	**Unsaturated**	
Steak:									
Relatively fat-sirloin, broiled:									
Lean and fat (piece, 2½ × 2½ × ¾ in)	3 oz	85	44	330	20	27	11.3	11.1	
Lean only	2.0 oz	56	59	115	18	4	1.8	1.6	
Relatively lean-round, braised:									
Lean and fat (piece, 4⅛ × 2¼ × ½ in)	3 oz	85	55	220	24	13	5.5	5.2	
Lean only	2.4 oz	68	61	130	21	4	1.7	1.5	
Beef, canned:									
Corned beef	3 oz	85	59	185	22	10	4.9	4.5	
Corned beef hash	1 cup	220	67	400	19	25	11.9	10.9	
Beef, dried, chipped	2½ oz jar	71	48	145	24	4	2.1	2.0	
Beef and vegetable stew	1 cup	245	82	220	16	11	4.9	4.5	
Beef potpie (home recipe), baked (piece, ⅓ of 9-in diameter pie)[19]	1 piece	210	55	515	21	30	7.9	12.8	6.
Chili con carne with beans, canned	1 cup	255	72	340	19	16	7.5	6.8	
Chop suey with beef and pork (home recipe)	1 cup	250	75	300	26	17	8.5	6.2	
Heart, beef, lean, braised	3 oz	85	61	160	27	5	1.5	1.1	
Lamb, cooked:									
Chop, rib (cut 3 per lb with bone), broiled:									
Lean and fat	3.1 oz	89	43	360	18	32	14.8	12.1	1.
Lean only	2 oz	57	60	120	16	6	2.5	2.1	
Leg, roasted:									
Lean and fat (2 pieces, 4⅛ × 2¼ × ¼ in)	3 oz	85	54	235	22	16	7.3	6.0	
Lean only	2.5 oz	71	62	130	20	5	2.1	1.8	
Shoulder, roasted:									
Lean and fat (3 pieces, 2½ × 2½ × ¼ in)	3 oz	85	50	285	18	23	10.8	8.8	
Lean only	2.3 oz	64	61	130	17	6	3.6	2.3	
Liver, beef, fried (slice, 6½ × 2⅜ × ⅜ in)[20]	3 oz	85	56	195	22	9	2.5	3.5	
Pork, cured, cooked:									
Ham, light cure, lean and fat, roasted (2 pieces, 4⅛ × 2¼ × ¼ in)[22]	3 oz	85	54	245	18	19	6.8	7.9	1.
Luncheon meat:									
Boiled ham, slice (8 per 8 oz pkg)	1 oz	28	59	65	5	5	1.7	2.0	
Canned, spiced or unspiced:									
Slice, approx. 3 × 2 × ½ in	1 slice	60	55	175	9	15	5.4	6.7	1.
Pork, fresh, cooked:[18]									
Chop, loin (cut 3 per lb with bone), broiled:									
Lean and fat	2.7 oz	78	42	305	19	25	8.9	10.4	2.
Lean only	2 oz	56	53	150	17	9	3.1	3.6	
Roast, oven cooked, no liquid added:									
Lean and fat (piece, 2½ × 2½ × ¾ in)	3 oz	85	46	310	21	24	8.7	10.2	2.
Lean only	2.4 oz	68	55	175	20	10	3.5	4.1	
Shoulder cut, simmered:									
Lean and fat (3 pieces, 2½ × 2½ × ¼ in)	3 oz	85	46	320	20	26	9.3	10.9	2.
Lean only	2.2 oz	63	60	135	18	6	2.2	2.6	
Sausages (see also Luncheon meat):									
Bologna, slice (8 per 8 oz pkg)	1 slice	28	56	85	3	8	3.0	3.4	
Braunschweiger, slice (6 per 6 oz pkg)	1 slice	28	53	90	4	8	2.6	3.4	
Brown and serve (10-11 per 8 oz pkg), browned	1 link	17	40	70	3	6	2.3	2.8	
Deviled ham, canned	1 tbsp	13	51	45	2	4	1.5	1.8	
Frankfurter (8 per 1 lb pkg), cooked (reheated)	1 frankfurter	56	57	170	7	15	5.6	6.5	1.
Meat, potted (beef, chicken, turkey), canned	1 tbsp	13	61	30	2	2	—	—	—
Pork link (16 per 1 lb pkg), cooked	1 link	13	35	60	2	6	2.1	2.4	
Salami:									
Dry type, slice (12 per 4 oz pkg)	1 slice	10	30	45	2	4	1.6	1.6	
Cooked type, slice (8 per 8 oz pkg)	1 slice	28	51	90	5	7	3.1	3.0	
Vienna sausage (7 per 4 oz can)	1 sausage	16	63	40	2	3	1.2	1.4	
Veal, medium fat, cooked, bone removed:									
Cutlet (4⅛ × 2¼ × ½ in), braised or broiled	3 oz	85	60	185	23	9	4.0	3.4	
Rib (2 pieces, 4⅛ × 2¼ × ¼ in), roasted	3 oz	85	55	230	23	14	6.1	5.1	
Poultry and poultry products:									
Chicken, cooked:									
Breast, fried, bones removed, ½ breast (3.3 oz with bones)[23]	2.8 oz	79	58	160	26	5	1.4	1.8	1.
Drumstick, fried, bones removed (2 oz with bones)[23]	1.3 oz	38	55	90	12	4	1.1	1.3	
Half broiler, broiled, bones removed (10.4 oz with bones)	6.2 oz	176	71	240	42	7	2.2	2.5	1.

For notes, see end of table.

Nutrients in Indicated Quantity

bohydrate (g)	Calcium (mg)	Phosphorus (mg)	Iron (mg)	Potassium (mg)	Vitamin A Value (IU)	Thiamin (mg)	Riboflavin (mg)	Niacin (mg)	Ascorbic Acid (mg)
0	9	162	2.5	220	50	.05	.15	4.0	—
0	7	146	2.2	202	10	.05	.14	3.6	—
0	10	213	3.0	272	20	.07	.19	4.8	—
0	9	182	2.5	238	10	.05	.16	4.1	—
0	17	90	3.7	—	—	.01	.20	2.9	—
24	29	147	4.4	440	—	.02	.20	4.6	—
0	14	287	3.6	142	—	.05	.23	2.7	0
15	29	184	2.9	613	2400	.15	.17	4.7	17
39	29	149	3.8	334	1720	.30	.30	5.5	6
31	82	321	4.3	594	150	.08	.18	3.3	—
13	60	248	4.8	425	600	.28	.38	5.0	33
1	5	154	5.0	197	20	.21	1.04	6.5	1
0	8	139	1.0	200	—	.11	.19	4.1	—
0	6	121	1.1	174	—	.09	.15	3.4	—
0	9	177	1.4	241	—	.13	.23	4.7	—
0	9	169	1.4	227	—	.12	.21	4.4	—
0	9	146	1.0	206	—	.11	.20	4.0	—
0	8	140	1.0	193	—	.10	.18	3.7	—
5	9	405	7.5	323	45,390[21]	.22	3.56	14.0	23
0	8	146	2.2	199	0	.40	.15	3.1	—
0	3	47	.8	—	0	.12	.04	.7	—
1	5	65	1.3	133	0	.19	.13	1.8	—
0	9	209	2.7	216	0	.75	.22	4.5	—
0	7	181	2.2	192	0	.63	.18	3.8	—
0	9	218	2.7	233	0	.78	.22	4.8	—
0	9	211	2.6	224	0	.73	.21	4.4	—
0	9	118	2.6	158	0	.46	.21	4.1	—
0	8	111	2.3	146	0	.42	.19	3.7	—
Tr	2	36	.5	65	—	.05	.06	.7	—
1	3	69	1.7	—	1850	.05	.41	2.3	—
Tr	—	—	—	—	—	—	—	—	—
0	1	12	.3	—	0	.02	.01	.2	—
1	3	57	.8	—	—	.08	.11	1.4	—
0	—	—	—	—	—	Tr	.03	.2	—
Tr	1	21	.3	35	0	.10	.04	.5	—
Tr	1	28	.4	—	—	.04	.03	.5	—
Tr	3	57	.7	—	—	.07	.07	1.2	—
Tr	1	24	.3	—	—	.01	.02	.4	—
0	9	196	2.7	258	—	.06	.21	4.6	—
0	10	211	2.9	259	—	.11	.26	6.6	—
1	9	218	1.3	—	70	.04	.17	11.6	—
Tr	6	89	.9	—	50	.03	.15	2.7	—
0	16	355	3.0	483	160	.09	.34	15.5	—

Foods, Approximate Measures, Units, and Weight		(g)	Water (%)	Food Energy (cal)	Protein (g)	Fat (g)	Saturated (total) (g)	Oleic (g)	Linol. (g)
Chicken, canned, boneless	3 oz	85	65	170	18	10	3.2	3.8	2
Chicken a la king, cooked (home recipe)	1 cup	245	68	470	27	34	12.7	14.3	3
Chicken and noodles, cooked (home recipe)	1 cup	240	71	365	22	18	5.9	7.1	3
Chicken chow mein:									
Canned	1 cup	250	89	95	7	Tr	—	—	—
From home recipe	1 cup	250	78	255	31	10	2.4	3.4	3
Chicken potpie (home recipe), baked, piece (⅓ of 9-in diameter pie)[19]	1 piece	232	57	545	23	31	11.3	10.9	5
Turkey, roasted, flesh without skin:									
Dark meat, piece, 2½ × 1⅝ × ¼ in	4 pieces	85	61	175	26	7	2.1	1.5	1
Light meat, piece, 4 × 2 × ¼ in	2 pieces	85	62	150	28	3	.9	.6	
Light and dark meat:									
Chopped or diced	1 cup	140	61	265	44	9	2.5	1.7	1
Pieces (1 slice white meat, 4 × 2 × ¼ in with 2 slices dark meat, 2½ × 1⅝ × ¼ in)	3 pieces	85	61	160	27	5	1.5	1.0	1
Fruits and Fruit Products									
Apples, raw, unpeeled, without cores:									
2¾-in diameter (about 3 per lb with cores)	1 apple	138	84	80	Tr	1	—	—	—
3¼-in diameter (about 2 per lb with cores)	1 apple	212	84	125	Tr	1	—	—	—
Applejuice, bottled or canned[24]	1 cup	248	88	120	Tr	Tr	—	—	—
Applesauce, canned:									
Sweetened	1 cup	255	76	230	1	Tr	—	—	—
Unsweetened	1 cup	244	89	100	Tr	Tr	—	—	—
Apricots:									
Raw, without pits (about 12 per lb with pits)	3 apricots	107	85	55	1	Tr	—	—	—
Canned in heavy syrup (halves and syrup)	1 cup	258	77	220	2	Tr	—	—	—
Dried:									
Uncooked (28 large or 37 medium halves per cup)	1 cup	130	25	340	7	1	—	—	—
Cooked, unsweetened, fruit and liquid	1 cup	250	76	215	4	1	—	—	—
Apricot nectar, canned	1 cup	251	85	145	1	Tr	—	—	—
Avocados, raw, whole, without skins and seeds:									
California, mid- and late-winter (with skin and seed, 3⅛-in diameter; wt 10 oz)	1 avocado	216	74	370	5	37	5.5	22.0	3
Florida, late summer and fall (with skin and seed, 3⅝-in diameter; wt 1 lb)	1 avocado	304	78	390	4	33	6.7	15.7	5
Banana without peel (about 2.6 per lb with peel)	1 banana	119	76	100	1	Tr	—	—	—
Banana flakes	1 tbsp	6	3	20	Tr	Tr	—	—	—
Blackberries, raw	1 cup	144	85	85	2	1	—	—	—
Blueberries, raw	1 cup	145	83	90	1	1	—	—	—
Cantaloupe; see muskmelons									
Cherries:									
Sour (tart), red, pitted, canned, water pack	1 cup	244	88	105	2	Tr	—	—	—
Sweet, raw, without pits and stems	10 cherries	68	80	45	1	Tr	—	—	—
Cranberry juice cocktail, bottled, sweetened	1 cup	253	83	165	Tr	Tr	—	—	—
Cranberry sauce, sweetened, canned, strained	1 cup	277	62	405	Tr	1	—	—	—
Dates:									
Whole, without pits	10 dates	80	23	220	2	Tr	—	—	—
Chopped	1 cup	178	23	490	4	1	—	—	—
Fruit cocktail, canned, in heavy syrup	1 cup	255	80	195	1	Tr	—	—	—
Grapefruit:									
Raw, medium, 3¾-in diameter (about 1 lb 1 oz):									
Pink or red	½ grapefruit with peel[28]	241	89	50	1	Tr	—	—	—
White	½ grapefruit with peel[28]	241	89	45	1	Tr	—	—	—
Canned, sections with syrup	1 cup	254	81	180	2	Tr	—	—	—
Grapefruit juice:									
Raw, pink, red, or white	1 cup	246	90	95	1	Tr	—	—	—
Canned, white:									
Unsweetened	1 cup	247	89	100	1	Tr	—	—	—
Sweetened	1 cup	250	86	135	1	Tr	—	—	—
Frozen, concentrate, unsweetened:									
Undiluted, 6 fl oz can	1 can	207	62	300	4	1	—	—	—
Diluted with 3 parts water by volume	1 cup	247	89	100	1	Tr	—	—	—
Dehydrated crystals, prepared with water (1 lb yields about 1 gal)	1 cup	247	90	100	1	Tr	—	—	—

For notes, see end of table.

Nutrients in Indicated Quantity

arbohydrate (g)	Calcium (mg)	Phosphorus (mg)	Iron (mg)	Potassium (mg)	Vitamin A Value (IU)	Thiamin (mg)	Riboflavin (mg)	Niacin (mg)	Ascorbic Acid (mg)
0	18	210	1.3	117	200	.03	.11	3.7	3
12	127	358	2.5	404	1130	.10	.42	5.4	12
26	26	247	2.2	149	430	.05	.17	4.3	Tr
18	45	85	1.3	418	150	.05	.10	1.0	13
10	58	293	2.5	473	280	.08	.23	4.3	10
42	70	232	3.0	343	3090	.34	.31	5.5	5
0	—	—	2.0	338	—	.03	.20	3.6	—
0	—	—	1.0	349	—	.04	.12	9.4	—
0	11	351	2.5	514	—	.07	.25	10.8	—
0	7	213	1.5	312	—	.04	.15	6.5	—
20	10	14	.4	152	120	.04	.03	.1	6
31	15	21	.6	233	190	.06	.04	.2	8
30	15	22	1.5	250	—	.02	.05	.2	2[25]
61	10	13	1.3	166	100	.05	.03	.1	3[25]
26	10	12	1.2	190	100	.05	.02	.1	2[25]
14	18	25	.5	301	2890	.03	.04	.6	11
57	28	39	.8	604	4490	.05	.05	1.0	10
86	87	140	7.2	1273	14,170	.01	.21	4.3	16
54	55	88	4.5	795	7500	.01	.13	2.5	8
37	23	30	.5	379	2380	.03	.03	.5	36[26]
13	22	91	1.3	1303	630	.24	.43	3.5	30
27	30	128	1.8	1836	880	.33	.61	4.9	43
26	10	31	.8	440	230	.06	.07	.8	12
5	2	6	.2	92	50	.01	.01	.2	Tr
19	46	27	1.3	245	290	.04	.06	.6	30
22	22	19	1.5	117	150	.04	.09	.7	20
26	37	32	.7	317	1660	.07	.05	.5	12
12	15	13	.3	129	70	.03	.04	.3	7
42	13	8	.8	25	Tr	.03	.03	.1	81
104	17	11	.6	83	60	.03	.03	.1	6
58	47	50	2.4	518	40	.07	.08	1.8	0
130	105	112	5.3	1153	90	.16	.18	3.9	0
50	23	31	1.0	411	360	.05	.03	1.0	5
13	20	20	.5	166	540	.05	.02	.2	44
12	19	19	.5	159	10	.05	.02	.2	44
45	33	36	.8	343	30	.08	.05	.5	76
23	22	37	.5	399	([29])	.10	.05	.5	93
24	20	35	1.0	400	20	.07	.05	.5	84
32	20	35	1.0	405	30	.08	.05	.5	78
72	70	124	.8	1250	60	.29	.12	1.4	286
24	25	42	.2	420	20	.10	.04	.5	96
24	22	40	.2	412	20	.10	.05	.5	91

								Fatty Acids		
									Unsaturated	
				Food			Saturated			
		Water	Energy	Protein	Fat	(total)	Oleic	Linole
Foods, Approximate Measures, Units, and Weight		(g)	(%)	(cal)	(g)	(g)	(g)	(g)	(g)
Grapes, European type (adherent skin), raw:									
Thompson seedless	10 grapes	50	81	35	Tr	Tr	—	—	—
Tokay and Emperor, seeded types	10 grapes[30]	60	81	40	Tr	Tr	—	—	—
Grapejuice:									
Canned or bottled	1 cup	253	83	165	1	Tr	—	—	—
Frozen concentrate, sweetened:									
Undiluted, 6 fl oz can	1 can	216	53	395	1	Tr	—	—	—
Diluted with 3 parts water by volume	1 cup	250	86	135	1	Tr	—	—	—
Grape drink, canned	1 cup	250	86	135	Tr	Tr	—	—	—
Lemon, raw, size 165, without peel and seeds (about 4 per lb with peels and seeds)	1 lemon	74	90	20	1	Tr	—	—	—
Lemon juice:									
Raw	1 cup	244	91	60	1	Tr	—	—	—
Canned, or bottled, unsweetened	1 cup	244	92	55	1	Tr	—	—	—
Frozen, single strength, unsweetened, 6 fl oz can	1 can	183	92	40	1	Tr	—	—	—
Lemonade concentrate, frozen:									
Undiluted, 6 fl oz can	1 can	219	49	425	Tr	Tr	—	—	—
Diluted with 4⅓ parts water by volume	1 cup	248	89	105	Tr	Tr	—	—	—
Limeade concentrate, frozen:									
Undiluted, 6 fl oz can	1 can	218	50	410	Tr	Tr	—	—	—
Diluted with 4⅓ parts water by volume	1 cup	247	89	100	Tr	Tr	—	—	—
Limejuice:									
Raw	1 cup	246	90	65	1	Tr	—	—	—
Canned, unsweetened	1 cup	246	90	65	1	Tr	—	—	—
Muskmelons, raw, with rind, without seed cavity:									
Cantaloupe, orange-fleshed (with rind and seed cavity, 5-in diameter, 2⅓ lb)	½ melon with rind[33]	477	91	80	2	Tr	—	—	—
Honeydew (with rind and seed cavity, 6½-in diameter, 5¼ lb)	⅒ melon with rind[33]	226	91	50	1	Tr	—	—	—
Oranges, all commercial varieties, raw:									
Whole, 2⅝-in diameter, without peel and seeds (about 2½ per lb with peel and seeds)	1 orange	131	86	65	1	Tr	—	—	—
Sections without membranes	1 cup	180	86	90	2	Tr	—	—	—
Orange juice:									
Raw, all varieties	1 cup	248	88	110	2	Tr	—	—	—
Canned, unsweetened	1 cup	249	87	120	2	Tr	—	—	—
Frozen concentrate:									
Undiluted, 6 fl oz can	1 can	213	55	360	5	Tr	—	—	—
Diluted with 3 parts water by volume	1 cup	249	87	120	2	Tr	—	—	—
Dehydrated crystals, prepared with water (1 lb yields about 1 gal)	1 cup	248	88	115	1	Tr	—	—	—
Orange and grapefruit juice:									
Frozen concentrate:									
Undiluted, 6 fl oz can	1 can	210	59	330	4	1	—	—	—
Diluted with 3 parts water by volume	1 cup	248	88	110	1	Tr	—	—	—
Papayas, raw, ½-in cubes	1 cup	140	89	55	1	Tr	—	—	—
Peaches:									
Raw:									
Whole, 2½-in diameter, peeled, pitted (about 4 per lb with peels and pits)	1 peach	100	89	40	1	Tr	—	—	—
Sliced	1 cup	170	89	65	1	Tr	—	—	—
Canned, yellow-fleshed, solids and liquid (halves or slices):									
Syrup pack	1 cup	256	79	200	1	Tr	—	—	—
Water pack	1 cup	244	91	75	1	Tr	—	—	—
Dried:									
Uncooked	1 cup	160	25	420	5	1	—	—	—
Cooked, unsweetened, halves and juice	1 cup	250	77	205	3	1	—	—	—
Frozen, sliced, sweetened:									
10-oz container	1 container	284	77	250	1	Tr	—	—	—
Cup	1 cup	250	77	220	1	Tr	—	—	—
Pears:									
Raw, with skin, cored:									
Bartlett, 2½-in diameter (about 2½ per lb with cores and stems)	1 pear	164	83	100	1	1	—	—	—
Bosc, 2½-in diameter (about 3 per lb with cores and stems)	1 pear	141	83	85	1	1	—	—	—

For notes, see end of table.

Nutrients in Indicated Quantity

Carbohydrate (g)	Calcium (mg)	Phosphorus (mg)	Iron (mg)	Potassium (mg)	Vitamin A Value (IU)	Thiamin (mg)	Riboflavin (mg)	Niacin (mg)	Ascorbic Acid (mg)
9	6	10	.2	87	50	.03	.02	.2	2
10	7	11	.2	99	60	.03	.02	.2	2
42	28	30	.8	293	—	.10	.05	.5	Tr[25]
100	22	32	.9	255	40	.13	.22	1.5	32[31]
33	8	10	.3	85	10	.05	.08	.5	10[31]
35	8	10	.3	88	—	.03[32]	.03[32]	.3	([32])
6	19	12	.4	102	10	.03	01	.1	39
20	17	24	.5	344	50	07	02	.2	112
19	17	24	.5	344	50	07	02	.2	102
13	13	16	.5	258	40	.05	02	.2	81
112	9	13	.4	153	40	.05	.06	.7	66
28	2	3	.1	40	10	.01	.02	.2	17
108	11	13	.2	129	Tr	.02	.02	.2	26
27	3	3	Tr	32	Tr	Tr	Tr	Tr	6
22	22	27	.5	256	20	.05	.02	.2	79
22	22	27	.5	256	20	.05	.02	.2	52
20	38	44	1.1	682	9240	.11	.08	1.6	90
11	21	24	.6	374	60	.06	.04	.9	34
16	54	26	.5	263	260	.13	.05	.5	66
22	74	36	.7	360	360	.18	.07	.7	90
26	27	42	.5	496	500	.22	.07	1.0	124
28	25	45	1.0	496	500	.17	.05	.7	100
87	75	126	.9	1500	1620	.68	.11	2.8	360
29	25	42	.2	503	540	.23	.03	.9	120
27	25	40	.5	518	500	.20	.07	1.0	109
78	61	99	.8	1308	800	.48	.06	2.3	302
26	20	32	.2	439	270	.15	.02	.7	102
14	28	22	.4	328	2450	.06	.06	.4	78
10	9	19	.5	202	1330[34]	.02	.05	1.0	7
16	15	32	.9	343	2260[34]	.03	.09	1.7	12
51	10	31	.8	333	1100	.03	.05	1.5	8
20	10	32	.7	334	1100	.02	.07	1.5	7
109	77	187	9.6	1520	6240	.02	.30	8.5	29
54	38	93	4.8	743	3050	.01	.15	3.8	5
64	11	37	1.4	352	1850	.03	.11	2.0	116[35]
57	10	33	1.3	310	1630	.03	.10	1.8	103[35]
25	13	18	.5	213	30	.03	.07	.2	7
22	11	16	.4	83	30	.03	.06	.1	6

					Nutrients in Indicated Quantity				
							Fatty Acids		
							Saturated (total) (g)	Unsaturated	
								Oleic (g)	Linoleic (g)
Foods, Approximate Measures, Units, and Weight		(g)	Water (%)	Food Energy (cal)	Protein (g)	Fat (g)			
D'Anjou, 3-in diameter (about 2 per lb with cores and stems)	1 pear	200	83	120	1	1	—	—	—
Canned, solids and liquid, syrup pack, heavy (halves or slices)	1 cup	255	80	195	1	1	—	—	—
Pineapple:									
Raw, diced	1 cup	155	85	80	1	Tr	—	—	—
Canned, heavy syrup pack, solids and liquid:									
Crushed, chunks, tidbits	1 cup	255	80	190	1	Tr	—	—	—
Slices and liquid:									
Large	1 slice; 2¼ tbsp liquid	105	80	80	Tr	Tr	—	—	—
Medium	1 slice; 1¼ tbsp liquid	58	80	45	Tr	Tr	—	—	—
Pineapple juice, unsweetened, canned	1 cup	250	86	140	1	Tr	—	—	—
Plums:									
Raw, without pits:									
Japanese and hybrid (2⅛-in diameter, about 6½ per lb with pits)	1 plum	66	87	30	Tr	Tr	—	—	—
Prune-type (1½-in diameter, about 15 per lb with pits)	1 plum	28	79	20	Tr	Tr	—	—	—
Canned, heavy syrup pack (Italian prunes), with pits and liquid:									
Cup	1 cup[36]	272	77	215	1	Tr	—	—	—
Portion	3 plums; 2¾ tbsp liquid[36]	140	77	110	1	Tr	—	—	—
Prunes, dried, "softenized," with pits:									
Uncooked	4 extra large or 5 large prunes[36]	49	28	110	1	Tr	—	—	—
Cooked, unsweetened, all sizes, fruit and liquid	1 cup[36]	250	66	255	2	1	—	—	—
Prune juice, canned or bottled	1 cup	256	80	195	1	Tr	—	—	—
Raisins, seedless:									
Cup, not pressed down	1 cup	145	18	420	4	Tr	—	—	—
Packet, ½ oz (1½ tbsp)	1 packet	14	18	40	Tr	Tr	—	—	—
Raspberries, red:									
Raw, capped, whole	1 cup	123	84	70	1	1	—	—	—
Frozen, sweetened, 10 oz container	1 container	284	74	280	2	1	—	—	—
Rhubarb, cooked, added sugar:									
From raw	1 cup	270	63	380	1	Tr	—	—	—
From frozen, sweetened	1 cup	270	63	385	1	1	—	—	—
Strawberries:									
Raw, whole berries, capped	1 cup	149	90	55	1	1	—	—	—
Frozen, sweetened:									
Sliced, 10 oz container	1 container	284	71	310	1	1	—	—	—
Whole, 1 lb container (about 1¾ cups)	1 container	454	76	415	2	1	—	—	—
Tangerine, raw, 2⅜-in diameter, size 176, without peel (about 4 per lb with peels and seeds)	1 tangerine	86	87	40	1	Tr	—	—	—
Tangerine juice, canned, sweetened	1 cup	249	87	125	1	Tr	—	—	—
Watermelon, raw, 4 × 8 in wedge with rind and seeds (1/16 of 32⅔ lb melon, 10 × 16 in)	1 wedge with rind and seeds	926	93	110	2	1	—	—	—
Grain Products									
Bagel, 3-in diameter:									
Egg	1 bagel	55	32	165	6	2	.5	.9	.8
Water	1 bagel	55	29	165	6	1	.2	.4	.6
Barley, pearled, light, uncooked	1 cup	200	11	700	16	2	.3	.2	.8
Biscuits, baking powder, 2-in diameter (enriched flour, vegetable shortening):									
From home recipe	1 biscuit	28	27	105	2	5	1.2	2.0	1.2
From mix	1 biscuit	28	29	90	2	3	.6	1.1	.7
Breadcrumbs (enriched)[38]:									
Dry, grated	1 cup	100	7	390	13	5	1.0	1.6	1.4
Soft; see White bread									
Breads:									
Boston brown bread, canned, slice, 3¼ × ½ in[38]	1 slice	45	45	95	2	1	.1	.2	.2
Cracked-wheat bread (¾ enriched wheat flour, ¼ cracked wheat)[38]·									
Slice (18 per loaf)	1 slice	25	35	65	2	1	.1	.2	.2
French or Vienna bread, enriched[38]									
Slice:									
French (5 × 2½ × 1 in)	1 slice	35	31	100	3	1	.2	.4	.4

For notes, see end of table.

Nutrients in Indicated Quantity

arbohydrate (g)	Calcium (mg)	Phosphorus (mg)	Iron (mg)	Potassium (mg)	Vitamin A Value (IU)	Thiamin (mg)	Riboflavin (mg)	Niacin (mg)	Ascorbic Acid (mg)
31	16	22	.6	260	40	.04	.08	.2	8
50	13	18	.5	214	10	.03	.05	.3	3
21	26	12	.8	226	110	.14	.05	.3	26
49	28	13	.8	245	130	.20	.05	.5	18
20	12	5	.3	101	50	.08	.02	.2	7
11	6	3	.2	56	30	.05	.01	.1	4
34	38	23	.8	373	130	.13	.05	.5	80[27]
8	8	12	.3	112	160	.02	.02	.3	4
6	3	5	.1	48	80	.01	.01	.1	1
56	23	26	2.3	367	3130	.05	.05	1.0	5
29	12	13	1.2	189	1610	.03	.03	.5	3
29	22	34	1.7	298	690	.04	.07	.7	1
67	51	79	3.8	695	1590	.07	.15	1.5	2
49	36	51	1.8	602	—	.03	.03	1.0	5
112	90	146	5.1	1106	30	.16	.12	.7	1
11	9	14	.5	107	Tr	.02	.01	.1	Tr
17	27	27	1.1	207	160	.04	.11	1.1	31
70	37	48	1.7	284	200	.06	.17	1.7	60
97	211	41	1.6	548	220	.05	.14	.8	16
98	211	32	1.9	475	190	.05	.11	.5	16
13	31	31	1.5	244	90	.04	.10	.9	88
79	40	48	2.0	318	90	.06	.17	1.4	151
107	59	73	2.7	472	140	.09	.27	2.3	249
10	34	15	.3	108	360	.05	.02	.1	27
30	44	35	.5	440	1040	.15	.05	.2	54
27	30	43	2.1	426	2510	.13	.13	.9	30
28	9	43	1.2	41	30	.14	.10	1.2	0
30	8	41	1.2	42	0	.15	.11	1.4	0
158	32	378	4.0	320	0	.24	.10	6.2	0
13	34	49	.4	33	Tr	.08	.08	.7	Tr
15	19	65	.6	32	Tr	.09	.08	.8	Tr
73	122	141	3.6	152	Tr	.35	.35	4.8	Tr
21	41	72	.9	131	0[39]	.06	.04	.7	0
13	22	32	.5	34	Tr	.08	.06	.8	Tr
19	15	30	.8	32	Tr	.14	.08	1.2	Tr

| | | | | | | | | Fatty Acids | | |
| | | | | | | | | | Unsaturated | |
Foods, Approximate Measures, Units, and Weight		(g)	Water (%)	Food Energy (cal)	Protein (g)	Fat (g)	Saturated (total) (g)	Oleic (g)	Linolei (g)
Vienna (4¾ × 4 × ½ in)	1 slice	25	31	75	2	1	.2	.3	.3
Italian bread enriched:									
Slice, 4½ × 3¼ × ¾ in	1 slice	30	32	85	3	Tr	Tr	Tr	.1
Raisin bread, enriched[38]:									
Slice (18 per loaf)	1 slice	25	35	65	2	1	.2	.3	.2
Rye bread:									
American, light (⅔ enriched wheat flour, ⅓ rye flour):									
Slice (4¾ × 3¾ × ⁷⁄₁₆ in)	1 slice	25	36	60	2	Tr	Tr	Tr	.1
Pumpernickel (⅔ rye flour, ⅓ enriched wheat flour):									
Slice (5 × 4 × ⅜ in)	1 slice	32	34	80	3	Tr	.1	Tr	.2
White bread, enriched[38]:									
Soft-crumb type[38]:									
Slice (18 per loaf)	1 slice	25	36	70	2	1	.2	.3	.3
Slice, toasted	1 slice	22	25	70	2	1	.2	.3	.3
Slice (22 per loaf)	1 slice	20	36	55	2	1	.2	.2	.2
Slice, toasted	1 slice	17	25	55	2	1	.2	.2	.2
Slice (24 per loaf)	1 slice	28	36	75	2	1	.2	.3	.3
Slice, toasted	1 slice	24	25	75	2	1	.2	.3	.3
Slice (28 per loaf)	1 slice	24	36	65	2	1	.2	.3	.2
Slice, toasted	1 slice	21	25	65	2	1	.2	.3	.2
Cubes	1 cup	30	36	80	3	1	.2	.3	.3
Crumbs	1 cup	45	36	120	4	1	.3	.5	.5
Firm-crumb type[38]:									
Slice (20 per loaf)	1 slice	23	35	65	2	1	.2	.3	.3
Slice, toasted	1 slice	20	24	65	2	1	.2	.3	.3
Slice (34 per loaf)	1 slice	27	35	75	2	1	.2	.3	.3
Slice, toasted	1 slice	23	24	75	2	1	.2	.3	.3
Whole-wheat bread:									
Soft-crumb type:									
Slice (16 per loaf)	1 slice	28	36	65	3	1	.1	.2	.2
Slice, toasted	1 slice	24	24	65	3	1	.1	.2	.2
Firm-crumb type:									
Slice (18 per loaf)	1 slice	25	36	60	3	1	.1	.2	.3
Slice, toasted	1 slice	21	24	60	3	1	.1	.2	.3
Breakfast cereals:									
Hot type, cooked:									
Corn (hominy) grits, degermed:									
Enriched	1 cup	245	87	125	3	Tr	Tr	Tr	.1
Unenriched	1 cup	245	87	125	3	Tr	Tr	Tr	.1
Farina, quick-cooking, enriched	1 cup	245	89	105	3	Tr	Tr	Tr	.1
Oatmeal or rolled oats	1 cup	240	87	130	5	2	.4	.8	.9
Wheat, rolled	1 cup	240	80	180	5	1	—	—	—
Wheat, whole-meal	1 cup	245	88	110	4	1	—	—	—
Ready-to-eat:									
Bran flakes (40% bran), added sugar, salt, iron, vitamins	1 cup	35	3	105	4	1	—	—	—
Bran flakes with raisins, added sugar, salt, iron, vitamins	1 cup	50	7	145	4	1	—	—	—
Corn flakes:									
Plain, added sugar, salt, iron, vitamins	1 cup	25	4	95	2	Tr	—	—	—
Sugar-coated, added salt, iron, vitamins	1 cup	40	2	155	2	Tr	—	—	—
Corn, oat flour, puffed, added sugar, salt, iron, vitamins	1 cup	20	4	80	2	1	—	—	—
Corn, shredded, added sugar, salt, iron, thiamin, niacin	1 cup	25	3	95	2	Tr	—	—	—
Oats, puffed, added sugar, salt, minerals, vitamins	1 cup	25	3	100	3	1	—	—	—
Rice, puffed:									
Plain, added iron, thiamin, niacin	1 cup	15	4	60	1	Tr	—	—	—
Presweetened, added salt, iron, vitamins	1 cup	28	3	115	1	0	—	—	—
Wheat flakes, added sugar, salt, iron, vitamins	1 cup	30	4	105	3	Tr	—	—	—
Wheat, puffed:									
Plain, added iron, thiamin, niacin	1 cup	15	3	55	2	Tr	—	—	—
Presweetened, added salt, iron, vitamins	1 cup	38	3	140	3	Tr	—	—	—

Nutrients in Indicated Quantity

For notes, see end of table.

Nutrients in Indicated Quantity

arbohydrate (g)	Calcium (mg)	Phosphorus (mg)	Iron (mg)	Potassium (mg)	Vitamin A Value (IU)	Thiamin (mg)	Riboflavin (mg)	Niacin (mg)	Ascorbic Acid (mg)
14	11	21	.6	23	Tr	.10	.06	.8	Tr
17	5	23	.7	22	0	.12	.07	1.0	0
13	18	22	.6	58	Tr	.09	.06	.6	Tr
13	19	37	.5	36	0	.07	.05	.7	0
17	27	73	.8	145	0	.09	.07	.6	0
13	21	24	.6	26	Tr	.10	.06	.8	Tr
13	21	24	.6	26	Tr	.08	.06	.8	Tr
10	17	19	.5	21	Tr	.08	.05	.7	Tr
10	17	19	.5	21	Tr	.06	.05	.7	Tr
14	24	27	.7	29	Tr	.11	.07	.9	Tr
14	24	27	.7	29	Tr	.09	.07	.9	Tr
12	20	23	.6	25	Tr	.10	.06	.8	Tr
12	20	23	.6	25	Tr	.08	.06	.8	Tr
15	25	29	.8	32	Tr	.12	.07	1.0	Tr
23	38	44	1.1	47	Tr	.18	.11	1.5	Tr
12	22	23	.6	28	Tr	.09	.06	.8	Tr
12	22	23	.6	28	Tr	.07	.06	.8	Tr
14	26	28	.7	33	Tr	.11	.06	.9	Tr
14	26	28	.7	33	Tr	.09	.06	.9	Tr
14	24	71	.8	72	Tr	.09	.03	.8	Tr
14	24	71	.8	72	Tr	.07	.03	.8	Tr
12	25	57	.8	68	Tr	.06	.03	.7	Tr
12	25	27	.8	68	Tr	.05	.03	.7	Tr
27	2	25	.7	27	Tr[40]	.10	.07	1.0	0
27	2	25	.2	27	Tr[40]	.05	.02	.5	0
22	147	113[41]	([42])	25	0	.12	.07	1.0	0
23	22	137	1.4	146	0	.19	.05	.2	0
41	19	182	1.7	202	0	.17	.07	2.2	0
23	17	127	1.2	118	0	.15	.05	1.5	0
28	19	125	5.6	137	1540	.46	.52	6.2	0
40	28	146	7.9	154	2200[43]	([44])	([44])	([44])	0
21	([44])	9	([44])	30	([44])	([44])	([44])	([44])	13[45]
37	1	10	([44])	27	1760	.53	.60	7.1	21[45]
16	4	18	5.7	—	880	.26	.30	3.5	11
22	1	10	.6	—	0	.33	.05	4.4	13
19	44	102	4.0	—	1100	.33	.38	4.4	13
13	3	14	.3	15	0	.07	.01	.7	0
26	3	14	([44])	43	1240[45]	([44])	([44])	([44])	15[45]
24	12	83	4.8	81	1320	.40	.45	5.3	16
12	4	48	.6	51	0	.08	.03	1.2	0
33	7	52	([44])	63	1680	.50	.57	6.7	20[45]

Foods, Approximate Measures, Units, and Weight		(g)	Water (%)	Food Energy (cal)	Protein (g)	Fat (g)	Saturated (total) (g)	Oleic (g)	Linole (g)
							Fatty Acids		
								Unsaturated	
Wheat, shredded, plain	1 oblong biscuit or ½ cup spoon-size biscuits	25	7	90	2	1	—	—	—
Wheat germ, without salt and sugar, toasted	1 tbsp	6	4	25	2	1	—	—	—
Buckwheat flour, light, sifted	1 cup	98	12	340	6	1	.2	.4	.4
Bulgur, canned, seasoned	1 cup	135	56	245	8	4	—	—	—
Cake icings; see Sugars and sweets									
Cakes made from cake mixes with enriched flour[46]:									
Angelfood:									
Piece, 1/12 of cake	1 piece	53	34	135	3	Tr	—	—	—
Coffeecake:									
Piece, 1/6 of cake	1 piece	72	30	230	5	7	2.0	2.7	1.5
Cupcakes, made with egg, milk, 2½-in diameter:									
Without icing	1 cupcake	25	26	90	1	3	.8	1.2	.7
With chocolate icing	1 cupcake	36	22	130	2	5	2.0	1.6	.6
Devil's food with chocolate icing:									
Piece, 1/16 of cake	1 piece	69	24	235	3	8	3.1	2.8	1.1
Cupcake, 2½-in diameter	1 cupcake	35	24	120	2	4	1.6	1.4	.5
Gingerbread:									
Piece, 1/9 of cake	1 piece	63	37	175	2	4	1.1	1.8	1.1
White, 2 layer with chocolate icing:									
Piece, 1/16 of cake	1 piece	71	21	250	3	8	2.0	2.9	1.2
Yellow, 2 layer with chocolate icing:									
Piece, 1/16 of cake	1 piece	69	26	235	3	8	3.0	3.0	1.3
Cakes made from home recipes using enriched flour[47]:									
Boston cream pie with custard filling:									
Whole cake (8-in diameter)	1 cake	825	35	2490	41	78	23.0	30.1	15.2
Piece, 1/12 of cake	1 piece	69	35	210	3	6	1.9	2.5	1.3
Fruitcake, dark:									
Slice, 1/30 of loaf	1 slice	15	18	55	1	2	.5	1.1	.5
Plain, sheet cake:									
Without icing:									
Whole cake (9-in sq)	1 cake	777	25	2830	35	108	29.5	44.4	23.9
Piece, 1/9 of cake	1 piece	86	25	315	4	12	3.3	4.9	2.6
With uncooked white icing:									
Piece, 1/9 of cake	1 piece	121	21	445	4	14	4.7	5.5	2.7
Pound[49]:									
Loaf, 8½ × 3½ × 3¼ in	1 loaf	565	16	2725	31	170	42.9	73.1	39.6
Slice, 1/17 of loaf	1 slice	33	16	160	2	10	2.5	4.3	2.3
Spongecake:									
Whole cake (9¾-in diameter tube cake)	1 cake	790	32	2345	60	45	13.1	15.8	5.7
Piece, 1/12 of cake	1 piece	66	32	195	5	4	1.1	1.3	.5
Cookies made with enriched flour[50,51]:									
Brownies with nuts:									
Home-prepared, 1¾ × 1¾ × 7/8 in:									
From home recipe	1 brownie	20	10	95	1	6	1.5	3.0	1.2
From commercial recipe	1 brownie	20	11	85	1	4	.9	1.4	1.3
Frozen, with chocolate icing, 1½ × 1¾ × 7/8 in[52]	1 brownie	25	13	105	1	5	2.0	2.2	.7
Chocolate chip:									
Commercial, 2¼-in diameter, 3/8 in thick	4 cookies	42	3	200	2	9	2.8	2.9	2.2
From home recipe, 2 1/3-in diameter	4 cookies	40	3	205	2	12	3.5	4.5	2.9
Fig bars, square (1 5/8 × 1 5/8 × 3/8 in) or rectangular (1½ × 1¾ × ½ in)	4 cookies	56	14	200	2	3	.8	1.2	.7
Gingersnaps, 2-in diameter, ¼ in thick	4 cookies	28	3	90	2	2	.7	1.0	.6
Macaroons, 2¾-in diameter, ¼ in thick	2 cookies	38	4	180	2	9	—	—	—
Oatmeal with raisins, 2 5/8-in diameter, ¼ in thick	4 cookies	52	3	235	3	8	2.0	3.3	2.0
Plain, prepared from commercial chilled dough, 2½-in diameter, ¼ in thick	4 cookies	48	5	240	2	12	3.0	5.2	2.9
Sandwich type (chocolate or vanilla), 1¾-in diameter, 3/8 in thick	4 cookies	40	2	200	2	9	2.2	3.9	2.2
Vanilla wafers, 1¾-in diameter, ¼ in thick	10 cookies	40	3	185	2	6	—	—	—

For notes, see end of table.

Nutrients in Indicated Quantity

arbohydrate (g)	Calcium (mg)	Phosphorus (mg)	Iron (mg)	Potassium (mg)	Vitamin A Value (IU)	Thiamin (mg)	Riboflavin (mg)	Niacin (mg)	Ascorbic Acid (mg)
20	11	97	.9	87	0	.06	.03	1.1	0
3	3	70	.5	57	10	.11	.05	.3	1
78	11	86	1.0	314	0	.08	.04	.4	0
44	27	263	1.9	151	0	.08	.05	4.1	0
32	50	63	.2	32	0	.03	.08	.3	0
38	44	125	1.2	78	120	.14	.15	1.3	Tr
14	40	59	.3	21	40	.05	.05	.4	Tr
21	47	71	.4	42	60	.05	.06	.4	Tr
40	41	72	1.0	90	100	.07	.10	.6	Tr
20	21	37	.5	46	50	.03	.05	.3	Tr
32	57	63	.9	173	Tr	.09	.11	.8	Tr
45	70	127	.7	82	40	.09	.11	.8	Tr
40	63	126	.8	75	100	.08	.10	.7	Tr
412	553	833	8.2	734[48]	1730	1.04	1.27	9.6	2
34	46	70	.7	61[48]	140	.09	.11	.8	Tr
9	11	17	.4	74	20	.02	.02	.2	Tr
434	497	793	8.5	614[48]	1320	1.21	1.40	10.2	2
48	55	88	.9	68[48]	150	.13	.15	1.1	Tr
77	61	91	.8	74	240	.14	.16	1.1	Tr
273	107	418	7.9	345	1410	.90	.99	7.3	0
16	6	24	.5	20	80	.05	.06	.4	0
427	237	885	13.4	687	3560	1.10	1.64	7.4	0
36	20	74	1.1	57	300	.09	.14	.6	Tr
10	8	30	.4	38	40	.04	.03	.2	Tr
13	9	27	.4	34	20	.03	.02	.2	Tr
15	10	31	.4	44	50	.03	.03	.2	Tr
29	16	48	1.0	56	50	.10	.17	.9	Tr
24	14	40	.8	47	40	.06	.06	.5	Tr
42	44	34	1.0	111	60	.04	.14	.9	Tr
22	20	13	.7	129	20	.08	.06	.7	0
25	10	32	.3	176	0	.02	.06	.2	0
38	11	53	1.4	192	30	.15	.10	1.0	Tr
31	17	35	.6	23	30	.10	.08	.9	0
28	10	96	.7	15	0	.06	.10	.7	0
30	16	25	.6	29	50	.10	.09	.8	0

							Fatty Acids		
							Saturated	Unsaturated	
Foods, Approximate Measures, Units, and Weight		(g)	Water (%)	Food Energy (cal)	Protein (g)	Fat (g)	(total) (g)	Oleic (g)	Linolei (g)
Cornmeal									
Whole-ground, unbolted, dry form	1 cup	122	12	435	11	5	.5	1.0	2.5
Bolted (nearly whole-grain), dry form	1 cup	122	12	440	11	4	.5	.9	2.1
Degermed, enriched:									
Dry form	1 cup	138	12	500	11	2	.2	.4	.9
Cooked	1 cup	240	88	120	3	Tr	Tr	.1	.2
Degermed, unenriched:									
Dry form	1 cup	138	12	500	11	2	.2	.4	.9
Cooked	1 cup	240	88	120	3	Tr	Tr	.1	.2
Crackers[38]:									
Graham, plain, 2½-in square	2 crackers	14	6	55	1	1	.3	.5	.3
Rye wafers, whole-grain, 1⅞ × 3½ in	2 wafers	13	6	45	2	Tr	—	—	—
Saltines, made with enriched flour	4 crackers or 1 packet	11	4	50	1	1	.3	.5	.4
Danish pastry (enriched flour), plain without fruit or nuts[54]:									
Round piece, about 4¼-in diameter × 1 in	1 pastry	65	22	275	5	15	4.7	6.1	3.2
Ounce	1 oz	28	22	120	2	7	2.0	2.7	1.4
Doughnuts, made with enriched flour[38]:									
Cake type, plain, 2½-in diameter, 1 in high	1 doughnut	25	24	100	1	5	1.2	2.0	1.1
Yeast-leavened, glazed, 3¾-in diameter, 1¼ in high	1 doughnut	50	26	205	3	11	3.3	5.8	3.3
Macaroni, enriched, cooked (cut lengths, elbows, shells):									
Firm stage (hot)	1 cup	130	64	190	7	1	—	—	—
Tender stage:									
Cold macaroni	1 cup	105	73	115	4	Tr	—	—	—
Hot macaroni	1 cup	140	73	155	5	1	—	—	—
Macaroni (enriched) and cheese[55]:									
Canned	1 cup	240	80	230	9	10	4.2	3.1	1.4
From home recipe (served hot)[56]	1 cup	200	58	430	17	22	8.9	8.8	2.9
Muffins made with enriched flour[38]:									
From home recipe:									
Blueberry, 2⅜-in diameter, 1½ in high	1 muffin	40	39	110	3	4	1.1	1.4	.7
Bran	1 muffin	40	35	105	3	4	1.2	1.4	.8
Corn (enriched degermed cornmeal and flour), 2⅜-in diameter, 1½ in high	1 muffin	40	33	125	3	4	1.2	1.6	.9
Plain, 3-in diameter, 1½ in high	1 muffin	40	38	120	3	4	1.0	1.7	1.0
From mix, egg, milk:									
Corn, 2⅜-in diameter, 1½ in high[58]	1 muffin	40	30	130	3	4	1.2	1.7	.9
Noodles (egg noodles), enriched, cooked	1 cup	160	71	200	7	2	—	—	—
Noodles, chow mein, canned	1 cup	45	1	220	6	11	—	—	—
Pancakes (4-in diameter)[38]:									
Buckwheat, made from mix (with buckwheat and enriched flour), egg and milk added	1 cake	27	58	55	2	2	.8	.9	.4
Plain:									
Made from home recipe using enriched flour	1 cake	27	50	60	2	2	.5	.8	.5
Made from mix with enriched flour, egg and milk added	1 cake	27	51	60	2	2	.7	.7	.3
Pies, piecrust made with enriched flour, vegetable shortening (9-in diameter):									
Apple:									
Sector, ⅐ of pie	1 sector	135	48	345	3	15	3.9	6.4	3.6
Banana cream:									
Sector, ⅐ of pie	1 sector	130	54	285	6	12	3.8	4.7	2.3
Blueberry:									
Sector, ⅐ of pie	1 sector	135	51	325	3	15	3.5	6.2	3.6
Cherry:									
Sector, ⅐ of pie	1 sector	135	47	350	4	15	4.0	6.4	3.6
Custard:									
Sector, ⅐ of pie	1 sector	130	58	285	8	14	4.8	5.5	2.5
Lemon meringue:									
Sector, ⅐ of pie	1 sector	120	47	305	4	12	3.7	4.8	2.3
Mince:									
Sector, ⅐ of pie	1 sector	135	43	365	3	16	4.0	6.6	3.6
Peach:									
Sector, ⅐ of pie	1 sector	135	48	345	3	14	3.5	6.2	3.6
Pecan:									
Sector, ⅐ of pie	1 sector	118	20	495	6	27	4.0	14.4	6.3
Pumpkin:									
Sector, ⅐ of pie	1 sector	130	59	275	5	15	5.4	5.4	2.4

For notes, see end of table.

Nutrients in Indicated Quantity

arbohydrate (g)	Calcium (mg)	Phosphorus (mg)	Iron (mg)	Potassium (mg)	Vitamin A Value (IU)	Thiamin (mg)	Riboflavin (mg)	Niacin (mg)	Ascorbic Acid (mg)
90	24	312	2.9	346	620[53]	.46	.13	2.4	0
91	21	272	2.2	303	590[53]	.37	.10	2.3	0
108	8	137	4.0	166	610[53]	.61	.36	4.8	0
26	2	34	1.0	38	140[53]	.14	.10	1.2	0
108	8	137	1.5	166	610[53]	.19	.07	1.4	0
26	2	34	.5	38	140[53]	.05	.02	.2	0
10	6	21	.5	55	0	.02	.08	.5	0
10	7	50	.5	78	0	.04	.03	.2	0
8	2	10	.5	13	0	.05	.05	.4	0
30	33	71	1.2	73	200	.18	.19	1.7	Tr
13	14	31	.5	32	90	.08	.08	.7	Tr
13	10	48	.4	23	20	.05	.05	.4	Tr
22	16	33	.6	34	25	.10	.10	.8	0
39	14	85	1.4	103	0	.23	.13	1.8	0
24	8	53	.9	64	0	.15	.08	1.2	0
32	11	70	1.3	85	0	.20	.11	1.5	0
26	199	182	1.0	139	260	.12	.24	1.0	Tr
40	362	322	1.8	240	860	.20	.40	1.8	Tr
17	34	53	.6	46	90	.09	.10	.7	Tr
17	57	162	1.5	172	90	.07	.10	1.7	Tr
19	42	68	7	54	120[57]	.10	.10	.7	Tr
17	42	60	.6	50	40	.09	.12	.9	Tr
20	96	152	.6	44	100[57]	.08	.09	.7	Tr
37	16	94	1.4	70	110	.22	.13	1.9	0
26	—	—	—	—	—	—	—	—	—
6	59	91	.4	66	60	.04	.05	.2	Tr
9	27	38	.4	33	30	.06	.07	.5	Tr
9	58	70	.3	42	70	.04	.06	.2	Tr
51	11	30	.9	108	40	.15	.11	1.3	2
40	86	107	1.0	264	330	.11	.22	1.0	1
47	15	31	1.4	88	40	.15	.11	1.4	4
52	19	34	.9	142	590	.16	.12	1.4	Tr
30	125	147	1.2	178	300	.11	.27	.8	0
45	17	59	1.0	60	200	.09	.12	.7	4
56	38	51	1.9	240	Tr	.14	.12	1.4	1
52	14	39	1.2	201	990	.15	.14	2.0	4
61	55	122	3.7	145	190	.26	.14	1.0	Tr
32	66	90	1.0	208	3210	.11	.18	1.0	Tr

Foods, Approximate Measures, Units, and Weight		(g)	Water (%)	Food Energy (cal)	Protein (g)	Fat (g)	Saturated (total) (g)	Oleic (g)	Linolei (g)
								Fatty Acids	
								Unsaturated	
Piecrust (home recipe) made with enriched flour and vegetable shortening, baked	1 pie shell, 9-in diameter	180	15	900	11	60	14.8	26.1	14.9
Pizza (cheese) baked, 4¾-in sector; ⅛ of 12-in diameter pie[19]	1 sector	60	45	145	6	4	1.7	1.5	0.6
Popcorn, popped:									
Plain, large kernel	1 cup	6	4	25	1	Tr	Tr	.1	.2
With oil (coconut) and salt added, large kernel	1 cup	9	3	40	1	2	1.5	.2	.2
Sugar coated	1 cup	35	4	135	2	1	.5	.2	.4
Pretzels, made with enriched flour:									
Dutch, twisted, 2¾ × 2⅝ in	1 pretzel	16	5	60	2	1	—	—	—
Thin, twisted, 3¼ × 2¼ × ¼ in	10 pretzels	60	5	235	6	3	—	—	—
Stick, 2¼ in long	10 pretzels	3	5	10	Tr	Tr	—	—	—
Rice, white, enriched:									
Instant, ready-to-serve, hot	1 cup	165	73	180	4	Tr	Tr	Tr	Tr
Long grain:									
Raw	1 cup	185	12	670	12	1	.2	.2	.2
Cooked, served hot	1 cup	205	73	225	4	Tr	.1	.1	.1
Parboiled:									
Raw	1 cup	185	10	685	14	1	.2	.1	.2
Cooked, served hot	1 cup	175	73	185	4	Tr	.1	.1	.1
Rolls, enriched:									
Commercial:									
Brown-and-serve (12 per 12-oz pkg), browned	1 roll	26	27	85	2	2	.4	.7	.5
Cloverleaf or pan, 2½-in diameter, 2 in high	1 roll	28	31	85	2	2	.4	.6	.4
Frankfurter and hamburger (8 per 11½-oz pkg)	1 roll	40	31	120	3	2	.5	.8	.6
Hard, 3¾-in diameter, 2 in high	1 roll	50	25	155	5	2	.4	.6	.5
Hoagie or submarine, 11½ × 3 × 2½ in	1 roll	135	31	390	12	4	.9	1.4	1.4
From home recipe:									
Cloverleaf, 2½-in diameter, 2 in high	1 roll	35	26	120	3	3	.8	1.1	.7
Spaghetti, enriched, cooked:									
Firm stage, "al dente," served hot	1 cup	130	64	190	7	1	—	—	—
Tender stage, served hot	1 cup	140	73	155	5	1	—	—	—
Spaghetti (enriched) in tomato sauce with cheese:									
From home recipe	1 cup	250	77	260	9	9	2.0	5.4	.7
Canned	1 cup	250	80	190	6	2	.5	.3	.4
Spaghetti (enriched) with meat balls and tomato sauce:									
From home recipe	1 cup	248	70	330	19	12	3.3	6.3	.9
Canned	1 cup	250	78	260	12	10	2.2	3.3	3.9
Toaster pastries	1 pastry	50	12	200	3	6	—	—	—
Waffles, made with enriched flour, 7-in diameter[38]:									
From home recipe	1 waffle	75	41	210	7	7	2.3	2.8	1.4
From mix, egg and milk added	1 waffle	75	42	205	7	8	2.8	2.9	1.2
Wheat flours:									
All-purpose or family flour, enriched:									
Sifted, spooned	1 cup	115	12	420	12	1	.2	.1	0.5
Unsifted, spooned	1 cup	125	12	455	13	1	.2	.1	.5
Cake or pastry flour, enriched, sifted, spooned	1 cup	96	12	350	7	1	.1	.1	.3
Self-rising, enriched, unsifted, spooned	1 cup	125	12	440	12	1	.2	.1	.5
Whole-wheat, from hard wheats, stirred	1 cup	120	12	400	16	2	.4	.2	1.0
Legumes (Dry), Nuts, Seeds; Related Products									
Almonds, shelled:									
Chopped (about 130 almonds)	1 cup	130	5	775	24	70	5.6	47.7	12.8
Slivered, not pressed down (about 115 almonds)	1 cup	115	5	690	21	62	5.0	42.2	11.3
Beans, dry:									
Common varieties as Great Northern, navy, and others:									
Cooked, drained:									
Great Northern	1 cup	180	69	210	14	1	—	—	—
Pea (navy)	1 cup	190	69	225	15	1	—	—	—
Canned, solids and liquid:									
White with:									
Frankfurters (sliced)	1 cup	255	71	365	19	18	—	—	—
Pork and tomato sauce	1 cup	255	71	310	16	7	2.4	2.8	.6
Pork and sweet sauce	1 cup	255	66	385	16	12	4.3	5.0	1.1
Red kidney	1 cup	255	76	230	15	1	—	—	—

For notes, see end of table.

Nutrients in Indicated Quantity

arbohydrate (g)	Calcium (mg)	Phosphorus (mg)	Iron (mg)	Potassium (mg)	Vitamin A Value (IU)	Thiamin (mg)	Riboflavin (mg)	Niacin (mg)	Ascorbic Acid (mg)
79	25	90	3.1	89	0	.47	.40	5.0	0
22	86	89	1.1	67	230	.16	.18	1.6	4
5	1	17	.2	—	—	—	.01	.1	0
5	1	19	.2	—	—	—	.01	.2	0
30	2	47	.5	—	—	—	.02	.4	0
12	4	21	.2	21	0	.05	.04	.7	0
46	13	79	.9	78	0	.20	.15	2.5	0
2	1	4	Tr	4	0	.01	.01	.1	0
40	5	31	1.3	—	0	.21	(^{59})	1.7	0
149	44	174	5.4	170	0	.81	.06	6.5	0
50	21	57	1.8	57	0	.23	.02	2.1	0
150	111	370	5.4	278	0	.81	.07	6.5	0
41	33	100	1.4	75	0	.19	.02	2.1	0
14	20	23	.5	25	Tr	.10	.06	.9	Tr
15	21	24	.5	27	Tr	.11	.07	.9	Tr
21	30	34	.8	38	Tr	.16	.10	1.3	Tr
30	24	46	1.2	49	Tr	.20	.12	1.7	Tr
75	58	115	3.0	122	Tr	.54	.32	4.5	Tr
20	16	36	.7	41	30	.12	.12	1.2	Tr
39	14	85	1.4	103	0	.23	.13	1.8	0
32	11	70	1.3	85	0	.20	.11	1.5	0
37	80	135	2.3	408	1080	.25	.18	2.3	13
39	40	88	2.8	303	930	.35	.28	4.5	10
39	124	236	3.7	665	1590	.25	.30	4.0	22
29	53	113	3.3	245	1000	.15	.18	2.3	5
36	54^{60}	67^{60}	1.9	74^{60}	500	.16	.17	2.1	(^{60})
28	85	130	1.3	109	250	.17	.23	1.4	Tr
27	179	257	1.0	146	170	.14	.22	.9	Tr
88	18	100	3.3	109	0	0.74	0.46	6.1	0
95	20	109	3.6	119	0	.80	.50	6.6	0
76	16	70	2.8	91	0	.61	.38	5.1	0
93	331	583	3.6	—	0	.80	.50	6.6	0
85	49	446	4.0	444	0	.66	.14	5.2	0
25	304	655	6.1	1005	0	.31	1.20	4.6	Tr
22	269	580	5.4	889	0	.28	1.06	4.0	Tr
38	90	266	4.9	749	0	.25	.13	1.3	0
40	95	281	5.1	790	0	.27	.13	1.3	0
32	94	303	4.8	668	330	.18	.15	3.3	Tr
48	138	235	4.6	536	330	.20	.08	1.5	5
54	161	291	5.9	—	—	.15	.10	1.3	—
42	74	278	4.6	673	10	.13	.10	1.5	—

				Food			Fatty Acids		
							Saturated	Unsaturated	
Foods, Approximate Measures, Units, and Weight		(g)	Water (%)	Energy (cal)	Protein (g)	Fat (g)	(total) (g)	Oleic (g)	Linole (g)
Lima, cooked, drained	1 cup	190	64	260	16	1	—	—	—
Blackeye peas, dry, cooked (with residual cooking liquid)	1 cup	250	80	190	13	1	—	—	—
Brazil nuts, shelled (6-8 large kernels)	1 oz	28	5	185	4	19	4.8	6.2	7.1
Cashew nuts, roasted in oil	1 cup	140	5	785	24	64	12.9	36.8	10.2
Coconut meat, fresh:									
Piece, about 2 × 2 × ½ in	1 piece	45	51	155	2	16	14.0	.9	.3
Shredded or grated, not pressed down	1 cup.	80	51	275	3	28	24.8	1.6	.5
Filberts (hazelnuts), chopped (about 60 kernels)	1 cup	115	6	730	14	72	5.1	55.2	7.3
Lentils, whole, cooked	1 cup	200	72	210	16	Tr	—	—	—
Peanuts, roasted in oil, salted (whole, halves, chopped)	1 cup	144	2	840	37	72	13.7	33.0	20.7
Peanut butter	1 tbsp	16	2	95	4	8	1.5	3.7	2.3
Peas, split, dry, cooked	1 cup	200	70	230	16	1	—	—	—
Pecans, chopped or pieces (about 120 large halves)	1 cup	118	3	810	11	84	7.2	50.5	20.0
Pumpkin and squash kernels, dry, hulled	1 cup	140	4	775	41	65	11.8	23.5	27.5
Sunflower seeds, dry, hulled	1 cup	145	5	810	35	69	8.2	13.7	43.2
Walnuts:									
Black:									
Chopped or broken kernels	1 cup	125	3	785	26	74	6.3	13.3	45.7
Ground (finely)	1 cup	80	3	500	16	47	4.0	8.5	29.2
Persian or English, chopped (about 60 halves)	1 cup	120	4	780	18	77	8.4	11.8	42.2
Sugars and Sweets									
Cake icings:									
Boiled, white:									
Plain	1 cup	94	18	295	1	0	0	0	—
With coconut	1 cup	166	15	605	3	13	11.0	.9	Tr
Uncooked:									
Chocolate made with milk and butter	1 cup	275	14	1035	9	38	23.4	11.7	1.0
Creamy fudge from mix and water	1 cup	245	15	830	7	16	5.1	6.7	3.1
White	1 cup	319	11	1200	2	21	12.7	5.1	.5
Candy:									
Caramels, plain or chocolate	1 oz	28	8	115	1	3	1.6	1.1	.1
Chocolate:									
Milk, plain	1 oz	28	1	145	2	9	5.5	3.0	.3
Semisweet, small pieces (60 per oz)	1 cup or 6-oz pkg	170	1	860	7	61	36.2	19.8	1.7
Chocolate-coated peanuts	1 oz	28	1	160	5	12	4.0	4.7	2.1
Fondant, uncoated (mints, candy corn, other)	1 oz	28	8	105	Tr	1	.1	.3	.1
Fudge, chocolate, plain	1 oz	28	8	115	1	3	1.3	1.4	.6
Gum drops	1 oz	28	12	100	Tr	Tr	—	—	—
Hard	1 oz	28	1	110	0	Tr	—	—	—
Marshmallows	1 oz	28	17	90	1	Tr	—	—	—
Chocolate-flavored beverage powders (about 4 heaping tsp per oz):									
With nonfat dry milk	1 oz	28	2	100	5	1	.5	.3	Tr
Without milk	1 oz	28	1	100	1	1	.4	.2	Tr
Honey, strained or extracted	1 tbsp	21	17	65	Tr	0	0	0	0
Jams and preserves	1 tbsp	20	29	55	Tr	Tr	—	—	—
	1 packet	14	29	40	Tr	Tr	—	—	—
Jellies	1 tbsp	18	29	50	Tr	Tr	—	—	—
	1 packet	14	29	40	Tr	Tr	—	—	—
Syrups:									
Chocolate-flavored syrup or topping:									
Thin type	1 fl oz or 2 tbsp	38	32	90	1	1	.5	.3	Tr
Fudge type	1 fl oz or 2 tbsp	38	25	125	2	5	3.1	1.6	.1
Molasses, cane:									
Light (first extraction)	1 tbsp	20	24	50	—	—	—	—	—
Blackstrap (third extraction)	1 tbsp	20	24	45	—	—	—	—	—
Sorghum	1 tbsp	21	23	55	—	—	—	—	—
Table blends, chiefly corn, light and dark	1 tbsp	21	24	60	0	0	0	0	0
Sugars:									
Brown, pressed down	1 cup	220	2	820	0	0	0	0	0
White:									
Granulated	1 cup	200	1	770	0	0	0	0	0
	1 tbsp	12	1	45	0	0	0	0	0
	1 packet	6	1	23	0	0	0	0	0
Powdered, sifted, spooned into cup	1 cup	100	1	385	0	0	0	0	0

For notes, see end of table.

Nutrients in Indicated Quantity

Carbohydrate (g)	Calcium (mg)	Phosphorus (mg)	Iron (mg)	Potassium (mg)	Vitamin A Value (IU)	Thiamin (mg)	Riboflavin (mg)	Niacin (mg)	Ascorbic Acid (mg)
49	55	293	5.9	1163	—	.25	.11	1.3	—
35	43	238	3.3	573	30	.40	.10	1.0	—
3	53	196	1.0	203	Tr	.27	.03	.5	—
41	53	522	5.3	650	140	.60	.35	2.5	—
4	6	43	.8	115	0	.02	.01	.2	1
8	10	76	1.4	205	0	.04	.02	.4	2
19	240	388	3.9	810	—	.53	—	1.0	Tr
39	50	238	4.2	498	40	.14	.12	1.2	0
27	107	577	3.0	971	—	.46	.19	24.8	0
3	9	61	.3	100	—	.02	.02	2.4	0
42	22	178	3.4	592	80	.30	.18	1.8	—
17	86	341	2.8	712	150	1.01	.15	1.1	2
21	71	1602	15.7	1386	100	.34	.27	3.4	—
29	174	1214	10.3	1334	70	2.84	.33	7.8	—
19	Tr	713	7.5	575	380	.28	.14	.9	—
12	Tr	456	4.8	368	240	.18	.09	.6	—
19	119	456	3.7	540	40	.40	.16	1.1	2
75	2	2	Tr	17	0	Tr	0.03	Tr	0
124	10	50	.8	277	0	.02	.07	.3	0
185	165	305	3.3	536	580	.06	.28	.6	1
183	96	218	2.7	238	Tr	.05	.20	.7	Tr
260	48	38	Tr	57	860	Tr	.06	Tr	Tr
22	42	35	.4	54	Tr	.01	.05	.1	Tr
16	65	65	.3	109	80	.02	.10	.1	Tr
97	51	255	4.4	553	30	.02	.14	.9	0
11	33	84	.4	143	Tr	.10	.05	2.1	Tr
25	4	2	.3	1	0	Tr	Tr	Tr	0
21	22	24	.3	42	Tr	.01	.03	.1	Tr
25	2	Tr	.1	1	0	0	Tr	Tr	0
28	6	2	.5	1	0	0	0	0	0
23	5	2	.5	2	0	0	Tr	Tr	0
20	167	155	.5	227	10	.04	.21	.2	1
25	9	48	.6	142	—	.01	.03	.1	0
17	1	1	.1	11	0	Tr	.01	.1	Tr
14	4	2	.2	18	Tr	Tr	.01	Tr	Tr
10	3	1	.1	12	Tr	Tr	Tr	Tr	Tr
13	4	1	.3	14	Tr	Tr	.01	Tr	1
10	3	1	.2	11	Tr	Tr	Tr	Tr	1
24	6	35	.6	106	Tr	.01	.03	.2	0
20	48	60	.5	107	60	.02	.08	.2	Tr
13	33	9	.9	183	—	.01	.01	Tr	—
11	137	17	3.2	585	—	.02	.04	.4	—
14	35	5	2.6	—	—	—	.02	Tr	—
15	9	3	.8	1	0	0	0	0	0
212	187	42	7.5	757	0	.02	.7	.4	0
199	0	0	.2	6	0	0	0	0	0
12	0	0	Tr	Tr	0	0	0	0	0
6	0	0	Tr	Tr	0	0	0	0	0
100	0	0	.1	3	0	0	0	0	0

Foods, Approximate Measures, Units, and Weight		(g)	Water (%)	Food Energy (cal)	Protein (g)	Fat (g)	Nutrients in Indicated Quantity		
							Fatty Acids		
							Saturated (total) (g)	Unsaturated	
								Oleic (g)	Linolei (g)
Vegetable and Vegetable Products									
Asparagus, green:									
Cooked, drained:									
Cuts and tips, 1½- to 2-in lengths:									
From raw	1 cup	145	94	30	3	Tr	—	—	—
From frozen	1 cup	180	93	40	6	Tr	—	—	—
Spears, ½-in diameter at base:									
From raw	4 spears	60	94	10	1	Tr	—	—	—
From frozen	4 spears	60	92	15	2	Tr	—	—	—
Canned, spears, ½-in diameter at base	4 spears	80	93	15	2	Tr	—	—	—
Beans:									
Lima, immature seeds, frozen, cooked, drained:									
Thick-seeded types (Fordhooks)	1 cup	170	74	170	10	Tr	—	—	—
Thin-seeded types (baby limas)	1 cup	180	69	210	13	Tr	—	—	—
Snap:									
Green:									
Cooked, drained:									
From raw (cuts and French style)	1 cup	125	92	30	2	Tr	—	—	—
From frozen:									
Cuts	1 cup	135	92	35	2	Tr	—	—	—
French style	1 cup	130	92	35	2	Tr	—	—	—
Canned, drained solids (cuts)	1 cup	135	92	30	2	Tr	—	—	—
Yellow or wax:									
Cooked, drained:									
From raw (cuts and French style)	1 cup	125	93	30	2	Tr	—	—	—
From frozen (cuts)	1 cup	135	92	35	2	Tr	—	—	—
Canned, drained solids (cuts)	1 cup	135	92	30	2	Tr	—	—	—
Beans, mature. See Beans, dry and Blackeye peas, dry.									
Bean sprouts (mung):									
Raw	1 cup	105	89	35	4	Tr	—	—	—
Cooked, drained	1 cup	125	91	35	4	Tr	—	—	—
Beets:									
Cooked, drained, peeled:									
Whole beets, 2-in diameter	2 beets	100	91	30	1	Tr	—	—	—
Diced or sliced	1 cup	170	91	55	2	Tr	—	—	—
Canned, drained solids:									
Whole beets, small	1 cup	160	89	60	2	Tr	—	—	—
Diced or sliced	1 cup	170	89	65	2	Tr	—	—	—
Beet greens, leaves and stems, cooked, drained	1 cup	145	94	25	2	Tr	—	—	—
Blackeye peas, immature seeds, cooked and drained:									
From raw	1 cup	165	72	180	13	1	—	—	—
From frozen	1 cup	170	66	220	15	1	—	—	—
Broccoli, cooked, drained:									
From raw:									
Stalk, medium size	1 stalk	180	91	45	6	1	—	—	—
Stalks cut into ½-in pieces	1 cup	155	91	40	5	Tr	—	—	—
From frozen:									
Stalk, 4½ to 5 in long	1 stalk	30	91	10	1	Tr	—	—	—
Chopped	1 cup	185	92	50	5	1	—	—	—
Brussels sprouts, cooked, drained:									
From raw, 7-8 sprouts (1¼- to 1½-in diameter)	1 cup	155	88	55	7	1	—	—	—
From frozen	1 cup	155	89	50	5	Tr	—	—	—
Cabbage:									
Common varieties:									
Raw:									
Coarsely shredded or sliced	1 cup	70	92	15	1	Tr	—	—	—
Finely shredded or chopped	1 cup	90	92	20	1	Tr	—	—	—
Cooked, drained	1 cup	145	94	30	2	Tr	—	—	—
Red, raw, coarsely shredded or sliced	1 cup	70	90	20	1	Tr	—	—	—
Savoy, raw, coarsely shredded or sliced	1 cup	70	92	15	2	Tr	—	—	—
Cabbage, celery (also called pe-tsai or wongbok), raw, 1-in pieces	1 cup	75	95	10	1	Tr	—	—	—
Cabbage, white mustard (also called bokchoy or pakchoy), cooked, drained	1 cup	170	95	25	2	Tr	—	—	—
Carrots:									
Raw, without crowns and tips, scraped:									
Whole, 7½ × 1⅛ in, or strips, 2½ to 3 in long	1 carrot or 18 strips	72	88	30	1	Tr	—	—	—

For notes, see end of table.

Nutrients in Indicated Quantity

Carbohydrate (g)	Calcium (mg)	Phosphorus (mg)	Iron (mg)	Potassium (mg)	Vitamin A Value (IU)	Thiamin (mg)	Riboflavin (mg)	Niacin (mg)	Ascorbic Acid (mg)
5	30	73	.9	265	1310	.23	.26	2.0	38
6	40	115	2.2	396	1530	.25	.23	1.8	41
2	13	30	.4	110	540	.10	.11	.8	16
2	13	40	.7	143	470	.10	.08	.7	16
3	15	42	1.5	133	640	.05	.08	.6	12
32	34	153	2.9	724	390	.12	.09	1.7	29
40	63	227	4.7	709	400	.16	.09	2.2	22
7	63	45	.8	189	680	.09	.11	.6	15
8	54	43	.9	205	780	.09	.12	.5	7
8	49	39	1.2	177	690	.08	.10	.4	9
7	61	34	2.0	128	630	.04	.07	.4	5
6	63	46	.8	189	290	.09	.11	.6	16
8	47	42	.9	221	140	.09	.11	.5	8
7	61	34	2.0	128	140	.04	.07	.4	7
7	20	67	1.4	234	20	.14	.14	.8	20
7	21	60	1.1	195	30	.11	.13	.9	8
7	14	23	.5	208	20	.03	.04	.3	6
12	24	39	.9	354	30	.05	.07	.5	10
14	30	29	1.1	267	30	.02	.05	.2	5
15	32	31	1.2	284	30	.02	.05	.2	5
5	144	36	2.8	481	7400	.10	.22	.4	22
30	40	241	3.5	625	580	.50	.18	2.3	28
40	43	286	4.8	573	290	.68	.19	2.4	15
8	158	112	1.4	481	4500	.16	.36	1.4	162
7	136	96	1.2	414	3880	.14	.31	1.2	140
1	12	17	.2	66	570	.02	.03	.2	22
9	100	104	1.3	392	4810	.11	.22	.9	105
10	50	112	1.7	423	810	.12	.22	1.2	135
10	33	95	1.2	457	880	.12	.16	.9	126
4	34	20	.3	163	90	.04	.04	.2	33
5	44	26	.4	210	120	.05	.05	.3	42
6	64	29	.4	236	190	.06	.06	.4	48
5	29	25	.6	188	30	.06	.04	.3	43
3	47	38	.6	188	140	.04	.06	.2	39
2	32	30	.5	190	110	.04	.03	.5	19
4	252	56	1.0	364	5270	.07	.14	1.2	26
7	27	26	.5	246	7930	.04	.04	.4	6

Foods, Approximate Measures, Units, and Weight		(g)	Water (%)	Food Energy (cal)	Protein (g)	Fat (g)	Saturated (total) (g)	Oleic (g)	Linolei (g)
								Fatty Acids	
								Unsaturated	
Grated	1 cup	110	88	45	1	Tr	—	—	—
Cooked (crosswise cuts), drained	1 cup	155	91	50	1	Tr	—	—	—
Canned:									
Sliced, drained solids	1 cup	155	91	45	1	Tr	—	—	—
Strained or junior (baby food)	1 oz (1¾ to 2 tbsp)	28	92	10	Tr	Tr	—	—	—
Cauliflower:									
Raw, chopped	1 cup	115	91	31	3	Tr	—	—	—
Cooked, drained:									
From raw (flower buds)	1 cup	125	93	30	3	Tr	—	—	—
From frozen (flowerets)	1 cup	180	94	30	3	Tr	—	—	—
Celery, Pascal type, raw:									
Stalk, large outer, 8 × 1½ in, at rood end	1 stalk	40	94	5	Tr	Tr	—	—	—
Pieces, diced	1 cup	120	94	20	1	Tr	—	—	—
Collards, cooked, drained:									
From raw (leaves without stems)	1 cup	190	90	65	7	1	—	—	—
From frozen (chopped)	1 cup	170	90	50	5	1	—	—	—
Corn, sweet:									
Cooked, drained:									
From raw, ear 5 × 1¾ in	1 ear[61]	140	74	70	2	1	—	—	—
From frozen:									
Ear, 5 in long	1 ear[61]	229	73	120	4	1	—	—	—
Kernels	1 cup	165	77	130	5	1	—	—	—
Canned:									
Cream style	1 cup	256	76	210	5	2	—	—	—
Whole kernel:									
Vacuum pack	1 cup	210	76	175	5	1	—	—	—
Wet pack, drained solids	1 cup	165	76	140	4	1	—	—	—
Cowpeas; see Blackeye peas									
Cucumber slices, ⅛ in thick (large, 2⅛-in diameter; small, 1¾-in diameter):									
With peel	6 large or 8 small slices	28	95	5	Tr	Tr	—	—	—
Without peel	6½ large or 9 small pieces	28	96	5	Tr	Tr	—	—	—
Dandelion greens, cooked, drained	1 cup	105	90	35	2	1	—	—	—
Endive, curly (including escarole), raw, small pieces	1 cup	50	93	10	1	Tr	—	—	—
Kale, cooked, drained:									
From raw (leaves without stems and midribs)	1 cup	110	88	45	5	1	—	—	—
From frozen (leaf style)	1 cup	130	91	40	4	1	—	—	—
Lettuce, raw:									
Butterhead, as Boston types:									
Head, 5-in diameter	1 head[63]	220	95	25	2	Tr	—	—	—
Leaves	1 outer or 2 inner or 3 heart leaves	15	95	Tr	Tr	Tr	—	—	—
Crisphead, as Iceberg:									
Head, 6-in diameter	1 head[64]	567	96	70	5	1	—	—	—
Wedge, ¼ of head	1 wedge	135	96	20	1	Tr	—	—	—
Pieces, chopped or shredded	1 cup	55	96	5	Tr	Tr	—	—	—
Looseleaf (bunching varieties including romaine or cos), chopped or shredded pieces	1 cup	55	94	10	1	Tr	—	—	—
Mushrooms, raw, sliced or chopped	1 cup	70	90	20	2	Tr	—	—	—
Mustard greens, without stems and midribs, cooked, drained	1 cup	140	93	30	3	1	—	—	—
Okra pods, 3 × ⅝ in, cooked	10 pods	106	91	30	2	Tr	—	—	—
Onions:									
Mature:									
Raw:									
Chopped	1 cup	170	89	65	3	Tr	—	—	—
Sliced	1 cup	115	89	45	2	Tr	—	—	—
Cooked (whole or sliced), drained	1 cup	210	92	60	3	Tr	—	—	—
Young green, bulb (⅜-in diameter) and white portion of top	6 onions	30	88	15	Tr	Tr	—	—	—
Parsley, raw, chopped	1 tbsp	4	85	Tr	Tr	Tr	—	—	—
Parsnips, cooked (diced or 2-in lengths)	1 cup	155	82	100	2	1	—	—	—
Peas, green:									
Canned:									
Whole, drained solids	1 cup	170	77	150	8	1	—	—	—
Strained (baby food)	1 oz (1¾ to 2 tbsp)	28	86	15	1	Tr	—	—	—
Frozen, cooked, drained	1 cup	160	82	110	8	Tr	—	—	—

For notes, see end of table.

Nutrients in Indicated Quantity

rbohydrate (g)	Calcium (mg)	Phosphorus (mg)	Iron (mg)	Potassium (mg)	Vitamin A Value (IU)	Thiamin (mg)	Riboflavin (mg)	Niacin (mg)	Ascorbic Acid (mg)
11	41	40	.8	375	12,100	.07	.06	.7	9
11	51	48	.9	344	16,280	.08	.08	.8	9
10	47	34	1.1	186	23,250	.03	.05	.6	3
2	7	6	.1	51	3690	.01	.01	.1	1
6	29	64	1.3	339	70	.13	.12	.8	90
5	26	53	.9	258	80	.11	.10	.8	69
6	31	68	.9	373	50	.07	.09	.7	74
2	16	11	.1	136	110	01	.01	.1	4
5	47	34	.4	409	320	.04	.04	.4	11
10	357	99	1.5	498	14,820	.21	.38	2.3	144
10	299	87	1.7	401	11,560	.10	.24	1.0	56
16	2	69	.5	151	310[62]	.09	.08	1.1	7
27	4	121	1.0	291	440[62]	.18	.10	2.1	9
31	5	120	1.3	304	580[62]	.15	.10	2.5	8
51	8	143	1.5	248	840[62]	.08	.13	2.6	13
43	6	153	1.1	204	740[62]	.06	.13	2.3	11
33	8	81	.8	160	580[62]	.05	.08	1.5	7
1	7	8	.3	45	70	.01	.01	.1	3
1	5	5	.1	45	Tr	.01	.01	.1	3
7	147	44	1.9	244	12,290	.14	.17	—	19
2	41	27	.9	147	1650	.04	.07	.3	5
7	206	64	1.8	243	9130	.11	.20	1.8	102
7	157	62	1.3	251	10,660	.08	.20	.9	49
4	57	42	3.3	430	1580	.10	.10	.5	13
Tr	5	4	.3	40	150	.01	.01	Tr	1
16	108	118	2.7	943	1780	.32	.32	1.6	32
4	27	30	.7	236	450	.08	.08	.4	8
2	11	12	.3	96	180	.03	.03	.2	3
2	37	14	.8	145	1050	.03	.04	.2	10
3	4	81	.6	290	Tr	.07	.32	2.9	2
6	193	45	2.5	308	8120	.11	.20	.8	67
6	98	43	.5	184	520	.14	.19	1.0	21
15	46	61	.9	267	Tr[65]	.05	.07	.3	17
10	31	41	.6	181	Tr[65]	.03	.05	.2	12
14	50	61	8	231	Tr[65]	.06	.06	.4	15
3	12	12	.2	69	Tr[65]	.02	.01	.1	8
Tr	7	2	.2	25	300	Tr	.01	Tr	6
23	70	96	.9	587	50	.11	.12	.2	16
29	44	129	3.2	163	1170	.15	.10	1.4	14
3	3	18	.3	28	140	.02	.03	.3	3
19	30	138	3.0	216	960	.43	.14	2.7	21

				Nutrients in Indicated Quantity					
								Fatty Acids	
									Unsaturated
				Food			Saturated		
			Water	Energy	Protein	Fat	(total)	Oleic	Linole
Foods, Approximate Measures, Units, and Weight		(g)	(%)	(cal)	(g)	(g)	(g)	(g)	(g)
Peppers, hot, red, without seeds, dried (ground chili powder, added seasonings)	1 tsp	2	9	5	Tr	Tr	—	—	—
Peppers, sweet (about 5 per lb, whole), stem and seeds removed:									
Raw	1 pod	74	93	15	1	Tr	—	—	—
Cooked, boiled, drained	1 pod	73	95	15	1	Tr	—	—	—
Potatoes, cooked:									
Baked, peeled after baking (about 2 per lb, raw)	1 potato	156	75	145	4	Tr	—	—	—
Boiled (about 3 per lb, raw):									
Peeled after boiling	1 potato	137	80	105	3	Tr	—	—	—
Peeled before boiling	1 potato	135	83	90	3	Tr	—	—	—
French-fried, strip, 2 to 3½ in long:									
Prepared from raw	10 strips	50	45	135	2	7	1.7	1.2	3.
Frozen, oven heated	10 strips	50	53	110	2	4	1.1	.8	2.
Hashed brown, prepared from frozen	1 cup	155	56	345	3	18	4.6	3.2	9.
Mashed, prepared from:									
Raw:									
Milk added	1 cup	210	83	135	4	2	.7	.4	Tr
Milk and butter added	1 cup	210	80	195	4	9	5.6	2.3	0.
Dehydrated flakes (without milk), water, milk, butter, and salt added	1 cup	210	79	195	4	7	3.6	2.1	.
Potato chips, 1¾ × 2½-in oval cross section	10 chips	20	2	115	1	8	2.1	1.4	4.
Potato salad, made with cooked salad dressing	1 cup	250	76	250	7	7	2.0	2.7	1.
Pumpkin, canned	1 cup	245	90	80	2	1	—	—	—
Radishes, raw (prepackaged) stem ends, rootlets cut off	4 radishes	18	95	5	Tr	Tr	—	—	—
Sauerkraut, canned, solids and liquid	1 cup	235	93	40	2	Tr	—	—	—
Southern peas; see Blackeye peas									
Spinach:									
Raw, chopped	1 cup	55	91	15	2	Tr	—	—	—
Cooked, drained:									
From raw	1 cup	180	92	40	5	1	—	—	—
From frozen:									
Chopped	1 cup	205	92	45	6	1	—	—	—
Leaf	1 cup	190	92	45	6	1	—	—	—
Canned, drained solids	1 cup	205	91	50	6	1	—	—	—
Squash, cooked:									
Summer (all varieties), diced, drained	1 cup	210	96	30	2	Tr	—	—	—
Winter (all varieties), baked, mashed	1 cup	205	81	130	4	1	—	—	—
Sweet potatoes:									
Cooked (raw, 5 × 2 in; about 2½ per lb):									
Baked in skin, peeled	1 potato	114	64	160	2	1	—	—	—
Broiled in skin, peeled	1 potato	151	71	170	3	1	—	—	—
Candied, 2½ × 2-in piece	1 piece	105	60	175	1	3	2.0	.8	.
Canned:									
Solid pack (mashed)	1 cup	255	72	275	5	1	—	—	—
Vacuum pack, piece 2¾ × 1 in	1 piece	40	72	45	1	Tr	—	—	—
Tomatoes:									
Raw, 2⅗-in diameter (3 per 12 oz pkg)	1 tomato[66]	135	94	25	1	Tr	—	—	—
Canned, solids and liquid	1 cup	241	94	50	2	Tr	—	—	—
Tomato catsup	1 cup	273	69	290	5	1	—	—	—
	1 tbsp	15	69	15	Tr	Tr	—	—	—
Tomato juice, canned:									
Cup	1 cup	243	94	45	2	Tr	—	—	—
Glass (6 fl oz)	1 glass	182	94	35	2	Tr	—	—	—
Turnips, cooked, diced	1 cup	155	35	35	1	Tr	—	—	—
Turnip greens, cooked, drained:									
From raw (leaves and stems)	1 cup	145	94	30	3	Tr	—	—	—
From frozen (chopped)	1 cup	165	93	40	4	Tr	—	—	—
Vegetables, mixed, frozen, cooked	1 cup	182	83	115	6	1	—	—	—
Miscellaneous Items									
Baking powders for home use:									
Sodium aluminum sulfate:									
With monocalcium phosphate monohydrate	1 tsp	3.0	2	5	Tr	Tr	0	0	0
With monocalcium phosphate monohydrate, calcium sulfate	1 tsp	2.9	1	5	Tr	Tr	0	0	0
Straight phosphate	1 tsp	3.8	2	5	Tr	Tr	0	0	0
Low sodium	1 tsp	4.3	2	5	Tr	Tr	0	0	0
Barbecue sauce	1 cup	250	81	230	4	17	2.2	4.3	10.

For notes, see end of table.

Nutrients in Indicated Quantity

rbohydrate (g)	Calcium (mg)	Phosphorus (mg)	Iron (mg)	Potassium (mg)	Vitamin A Value (IU)	Thiamin (mg)	Riboflavin (mg)	Niacin (mg)	Ascorbic Acid (mg)
1	5	4	.3	20	1300	Tr	.02	.2	Tr
4	7	16	.5	157	310	.06	.06	.4	94
3	7	12	.4	109	310	.05	.05	.4	70
33	14	101	1.1	782	Tr	.15	.07	2.7	31
23	10	72	.8	556	Tr	.12	.05	2.0	22
20	8	57	.7	385	Tr	.12	.05	1.6	22
18	8	56	.7	427	Tr	.07	.04	1.6	11
17	5	43	.9	326	Tr	.07	.01	1.3	11
45	28	78	1.9	439	Tr	.11	.03	1.6	12
27	50	103	.8	548	40	.17	.11	2.1	21
26	50	101	.8	525	360	.17	.11	2.1	19
30	65	99	.6	601	270	.08	.08	1.9	11
10	8	28	.4	226	Tr	.04	.01	1.0	3
41	80	160	1.5	798	350	.20	.18	2.8	28
19	61	64	1.0	588	15,680	.07	.12	1.5	12
1	5	6	.2	58	Tr	.01	.01	.1	5
9	85	42	1.2	329	120	.07	.09	.5	33
2	51	28	1.7	259	4460	.06	.11	.3	28
6	167	68	4.0	583	14,580	.13	.25	.9	50
8	232	90	4.3	683	16,200	.14	.31	.8	39
7	200	84	4.8	688	15,390	.15	.27	1.0	53
7	242	53	5.3	513	16,400	.04	.25	.6	29
7	53	53	.8	296	820	.11	.17	1.7	21
32	57	98	1.6	945	8610	.10	.27	1.4	27
37	46	66	1.0	342	9230	.10	.08	.8	25
40	48	71	1.1	367	11,940	.14	.09	.9	26
36	39	45	.9	200	6620	.06	.04	.4	11
63	64	105	2.0	510	19,890	.13	.10	1.5	36
10	10	16	.3	80	3120	.02	.02	.2	6
6	16	33	.6	300	1110	.07	.05	.9	28[67]
10	14[68]	46	1.2	523	2170	.12	.07	1.7	41
69	60	137	2.2	991	3820	.25	.19	4.4	41
4	3	8	.1	54	210	.01	.01	.2	2
10	17	44	2.2	552	1940	.12	.07	1.9	39
8	13	33	1.6	413	1460	.09	.05	1.5	29
8	54	34	.6	291	Tr	.06	.08	.5	34
5	252	49	1.5	—	8270	.15	.33	.7	68
6	195	64	2.6	246	11,390	.08	.15	.7	31
24	46	115	2.4	348	9010	.22	.13	2.0	15
1	58	87	—	5	0	0	0	0	0
1	183	45	—	—	0	0	0	0	0
	239	359	—	6	0	0	0	0	0
2	207	314	—	471	0	0	0	0	0
20	53	50	2.0	435	900	.03	.03	.8	13

Foods, Approximate Measures, Units, and Weight		(g)	Water (%)	Food Energy (cal)	Protein (g)	Fat (g)	Saturated (total) (g)	Oleic (g)	Linole (g)
							Fatty Acids		
								Unsaturated	
Beverages, alcoholic:									
Beer	12 fl oz	360	92	150	1	0	0	0	0
Gin, rum, vodka, whisky:									
80 proof	1½ fl oz jigger	42	67	95	—	—	0	0	0
86 proof	1½ fl oz jigger	42	64	105	—	—	0	0	0
90 proof	1½ fl oz jigger	42	62	110	—	—	0	0	0
Wines:									
Dessert	3½ fl oz glass	103	77	140	Tr	0	0	0	0
Table	3½ fl oz glass	102	86	85	Tr	0	0	0	0
Beverages, carbonated, sweetened, nonalcoholic:									
Carbonated water	12 fl oz	366	92	115	0	0	0	0	0
Cola type	12 fl oz	369	90	145	0	0	0	0	0
Fruit-flavored sodas and Tom Collins mixer	12 fl oz	372	88	170	0	0	0	0	0
Ginger ale	12 fl oz	366	92	115	0	0	0	0	0
Root beer	12 fl oz	370	90	150	0	0	0	0	0
Chili powder; see Peppers, hot, red									
Chocolate:									
Bitter or baking	1 oz	28	2	145	3	15	8.9	4.9	
Semisweet; see Candy, chocolate									
Gelatin, dry	1 7 g envelope	7	13	25	6	Tr	0	0	0
Gelatin dessert prepared with gelatin dessert powder and water	1 cup	240	84	140	4	0	0	0	0
Mustard, prepared, yellow	1 tsp or individual serving pouch or cup	5	80	5	Tr	Tr	—	—	
Olives, pickled, canned:									
Green	4 medium or 3 extra large or 2 giant[69]	16	78	15	Tr	2	.2	1.2	
Ripe, Mission	3 small or 2 large[69]	10	73	15	Tr	2	.2	1.2	
Pickles, cucumber:									
Dill, medium, whole, 3¾ in long, 1¼-in diameter	1 pickle	65	93	5	Tr	Tr	—	—	
Fresh-pack, slices 1½-in diameter, ¼ in thick	2 slices	15	79	10	Tr	Tr	—	—	
Sweet gherkin, small, whole, about 2½ in long, ¾-in diameter	1 pickle	15	61	20	Tr	Tr	—	—	
Relish, finely chopped, sweet	1 tbsp	15	63	20	Tr	Tr	—	—	
Popsicle, 3 fl oz size	1 popsicle	95	80	70	0	0	0	0	0
Soups:									
Canned, condensed:									
Prepared with equal volume of milk:									
Cream of chicken	1 cup	245	85	180	7	10	4.2	3.6	1.
Cream of mushroom	1 cup	245	83	215	7	14	5.4	2.9	4.
Tomato	1 cup	250	84	175	7	7	3.4	1.7	1.
Prepared with equal volume of water:									
Bean with pork	1 cup	250	84	170	8	6	1.2	1.8	2.
Beef broth, bouillon, consomme	1 cup	240	96	30	5	0	0	0	0
Beef noodle	1 cup	240	93	65	4	3	.6	.7	
Clam chowder, Manhattan type (with tomatoes, without milk)	1 cup	245	92	80	2	3	.5	.4	1
Cream of chicken	1 cup	240	92	95	3	6	1.6	2.3	1.
Cream of mushroom	1 cup	240	90	135	2	10	2.6	1.7	4.
Minestrone	1 cup	245	90	105	5	3	.7	.9	1.
Split pea	1 cup	245	85	145	9	3	1.1	1.2	
Tomato	1 cup	245	91	90	2	3	.5	.5	1.
Vegetable beef	1 cup	245	92	80	5	2	—	—	—
Vegetarian	1 cup	245	92	80	2	2	—	—	—
Dehydrated:									
Bouillon cube, ½ in	1 cube	4	4	5	1	Tr	—	—	—
Mixes:									
Unprepared:									
Onion	1½ oz pkg	43	3	150	6	5	1.1	2.3	1.
Prepared with water:									
Chicken noodle	1 cup	240	95	55	2	1	—	—	—
Onion	1 cup	240	96	35	1	1	—	—	—
Tomato vegetable with noodles	1 cup	240	93	65	1	1	—	—	—
Vinegar, cider	1 tbsp	15	94	Tr	Tr	0	0	0	0
White sauce, medium, with enriched flour	1 cup	250	73	405	10	31	19.3	7.8	
Yeast:									
Baker's dry, active	1 pkg	7	5	20	3	Tr	—	—	—
Brewer's, dry	1 tbsp	8	5	25	3	Tr	—	—	—

For notes, see end of table.

Nutrients in Indicated Quantity

rbohydrate (g)	Calcium (mg)	Phosphorus (mg)	Iron (mg)	Potassium (mg)	Vitamin A Value (IU)	Thiamin (mg)	Riboflavin (mg)	Niacin (mg)	Ascorbic Acid (mg)
14	18	108	Tr	90	—	.01	.11	2.2	—
Tr	—	—	—	1	—	—	—	—	—
Tr	—	—	—	1	—	—	—	—	—
Tr	—	—	—	1	—	—	—	—	—
8	8	—	—	77	—	.01	.02	.2	—
4	9	10	.4	94	—	Tr	.01	.1	—
29	—	—	—	—	0	0	0	0	0
37	—	—	—	—	0	0	0	0	0
45	—	—	—	—	0	0	0	0	0
29	—	—	—	0	0	0	0	0	0
39	—	—	—	0	0	0	0	0	0
8	22	109	1.9	235	20	.01	.07	.4	0
0	—	—	—	—	—	—	—	—	—
34	—	—	—	—	—	—	—	—	—
Tr	4	4	.1	7	—	—	—	—	—
Tr	8	2	.2	7	40	—	—	—	—
Tr	9	1	.1	2	10	Tr	Tr	—	—
1	17	14	.7	130	70	Tr	.01	Tr	4
3	5	4	.3	—	20	Tr	Tr	Tr	1
5	2	2	.2	—	10	Tr	Tr	Tr	1
5	3	2	.1	—	—	—	—	—	—
18	0	—	Tr	—	0	0	0	0	0
15	172	152	0.5	260	610	0.05	0.27	0.7	2
16	191	169	.5	279	250	.05	.34	.7	1
23	168	155	.8	418	1200	.10	.25	1.3	15
22	63	128	2.3	395	650	.13	.08	1.0	3
3	Tr	31	.5	130	Tr	Tr	.02	1.2	—
7	7	48	1.0	77	50	.05	.07	1.0	Tr
12	34	47	1.0	184	880	.02	.02	1.0	—
8	24	34	.5	79	410	.02	.05	.5	Tr
10	41	50	.5	98	70	.02	.12	.7	Tr
14	37	59	1.0	314	2350	.07	.05	1.0	—
21	29	149	1.5	270	440	.25	.15	1.5	1
16	15	34	.7	230	1000	.05	.05	1.2	12
10	12	49	.7	162	2700	.05	.05	1.0	—
13	20	39	1.0	172	2940	.05	.05	1.0	—
Tr	—	—	—	4	—	—	—	—	—
23	42	49	.6	238	30	.05	.03	.3	6
8	7	19	.2	19	50	.07	.05	.5	Tr
6	10	12	.2	58	Tr	Tr	Tr	Tr	2
12	7	19	.2	29	480	.05	.02	.5	5
1	1	1	.1	15	—	—	—	—	—
22	288	233	.5	348	1150	.12	.43	.7	2
3	3	90	1.1	140	Tr	.16	.38	2.6	Tr
3	17[70]	140	1.4	152	Tr	1.25	.34	3.0	Tr

Footnotes to accompany pp. A-1 to A-35.

[1]Vitamin A value is largely from beta-carotene used for coloring. Riboflavin value for powdered sweet creamers applies to products with added riboflavin.

[2]Applies to product without added vitamin A. With added vitamin A, value is 500 IU.

[3]Applies to product without vitamin A added.

[4]Applies to product with added vitamin A. Without added vitamin A, value is 20 IU.

[5]Yields 1 qt of fluid milk when reconstituted according to package directions.

[6]Applies to product with added vitamin A.

[7]Weight applies to product with label claim of 1⅓ cups equal 3.2 oz.

[8]Applies to products made from thick shake mixes and that do not contain added ice cream. Products made from milk shake mixes are higher in fat and usually contain added cream.

[9]Content of fat, vitamin A, and carbohydrate varies. Consult the label when precise values are needed for special diets.

[10]Applies to product made with milk containing no added vitamin A.

[11]Based on year-round average.

[12]Based on average vitamin A content of fortified margarine. Federal specifications for fortified margarine require a minimum of 15,000 IU of vitamin A per pound.

[13]Fatty acid values apply to product made with regular-type margarine.

[14]Dipped in egg, milk or water, and breadcrumbs; fried in vegetable shortening.

[15]If bones are discarded, value for calcium will be greatly reduced.

[16]Dipped in egg, breadcrumbs, and flour or batter.

[17]Prepared with tuna, celery, salad dressing (mayonnaise type), pickle, onion, and egg.

[18]Outer layer of fat on the cut was removed to within approximately ½ in of the lean. Deposits of fat within the cut were not removed.

[19]Crust made with vegetable shortening and enriched flour.

[20]Regular-type margarine used.

[21]Value varies widely.

[22]About one fourth of the outer layer of fat on the cut was removed. Deposits of fat within the cut were not removed.

[23]Vegetable shortening used.

[24]Also applies to pasteurized apple cider.

[25]Applies to product without added ascorbic acid. For value of product with added ascorbic acid, refer to label.

[26]Based on product with label claim of 45% of U.S. RDA in 6 fl oz.

[27]Based on product with label claim of 100% of U.S. RDA in 6 fl oz.

[28]Weight includes peel and membranes between sections. Without these parts, the weight of the edible portion is 123 g for ½ pink or red grapefruit and 118 g for ½ white grapefruit.

[29]For white-fleshed varieties, value is about 20 IU per cup; for red-fleshed varieties, 1080 IU.

[30]Weight includes seeds. Without seeds, weight of the edible portion is 57 g.

[31]Applies to product without added ascorbic acid. With added ascorbic acid, based on claim that 6 fl oz of reconstituted juice contains 45% or 50% of the U.S. RDA, value in milligrams is 108 or 120 for a 6 fl oz can (undiluted, frozen concentrate grape juice), 36 or 40 for 1 cup of diluted juice (diluted frozen concentrate grape juice).

[32]For products with added thiamin and riboflavin but without added ascorbic acid, values in milligrams would be .60 for thiamin, .80 for riboflavin, and Tr for ascorbic acid. For products with only ascorbic acid added, value varies with the brand. Consult the label.

[33]Weight includes rind. Without rind, the weight of the edible portion is 272 g for cantaloup and 149 g for honeydew melon.

[34]Represents yellow-fleshed varieties. For white-fleshed varieties, value is 50 IU for 1 peach, 90 IU for 1 cup of slices.

[35]Value represents products with added ascorbic acid. For products without added ascorbic acid, value in milligrams is 116 for a 10 oz container, 103 for 1 cup.

[36]Weight includes pits. After removal of the pits, the weight of the edible portion is 258 g for 1 cup plums in heavy syrup, 133 g for 3 plums in heavy syrup, 43 g for 4 dried prunes, and 213 g for 1 cup cooked, unsweetened prunes.

[37]Weight includes rind and seeds. Without rind and seeds, weight of the edible portion is 426 g.

[38]Made with vegetable shortening.

[39]Applies to product made with white cornmeal. With yellow cornmeal, value is 30 IU.

[40]Applies to white varieties. For yellow varieties, value is 150 IU.

[41]Applies to products that do not contain disodium phosphate. If disodium phosphate is an ingredient, value is 162 mg.

[42]Value may range from less than 1 mg to about 8 mg, depending on the brand. Consult the label.

[43]Applies to product with added nutrient. Without added nutrient, value is trace.

[44]Value varies with the brand. Consult the label.

[45]Applies to product with added nutrient. Without added nutrient, value is trace.

[46]Excepting angelfood cake, cakes were made from mixes containing vegetable shortening; icings, with butter.

[47]Excepting spongecake, vegetable shortening used for cake portion; butter, for icing. If butter or margarine used for cake portion, vitamin A values would be higher.

[48]Applies to product made with a sodium aluminum-sulfate type of baking power. With a low-sodium type of baking powder containing potassium, value would be about twice the amount shown.

[49]Equal weights of flour, sugar, eggs, and vegetable shortening.

[50]Products are commercial unless otherwise specified.

[51]Made with enriched flour and vegetable shortening except for macaroons, which do not contain flour or shortening.

[52]Icing made with butter.

[53]Applies to yellow varieties; white varieties contain only a trace.

[54]Contains vegetable shortening and butter.

[55]Made with corn oil.

[56]Made with regular margarine.

[57]Applies to product made with yellow cornmeal.

[58]Made with enriched degermed cornmeal and enriched flour.

[59]Product may or may not be enriched with riboflavin. Consult the label.

[60]Value varies with the brand. Consult the label.

[61]Weight includes cob. Without cob, weight is 77 g for 1 ear cooked, drained sweet corn, 126 g for 1 frozen 5-in ear.

[62]Based on yellow varieties. For white varieties, value is trace.

[63]Weight includes refuse of outer leaves and core. Without these parts, weight is 163 g.

[64]Weight includes core. Without core, weight is 539 g.

[65]Value based on white-fleshed varieties. For yellow-fleshed varieties, value in IU is 70 for 1 cup chopped raw onions, 50 for 1 cup sliced raw onions, and 80 for 1 cup cooked onions.

[66]Weight inclues cores and stem ends. Without these parts, weight is 123 g.

[67]Based on year-round average. For tomatoes marketed from November through May, value is about 12 mg; from June through October, 32 mg.

[68]Applies to product without calcium salts added. Value for products with calcium salts added may be as much as 63 mg for whole tomatoes, 241 mg for cut forms.

[69]Weight includes pits. Without pits, weight is 13 g for 4 medium (or 3 extra large or 2 giant) green pickled olives, 9 g for 3 small (or 2 large) ripe pickled olives.

[70]Value may vary from 6 to 60 mg.

B

Cholesterol Content of Foods

Item	Amount of Cholesterol in		Refuse from Item as Purchased (%)
	100 g Edible Portion[1] (mg)	Edible Portion of 450 g (1 lb) as Purchased (mg)	
Beef, raw			
With bone[2]	70	270	15
Without bone[2]	70	320	0
Brains, raw	>2000	>9000	0
Butter	250	1135	0
Cavier or fish roe	>300	>1300	0
Cheese			
Cheddar	100	455	0
Cottage, creamed	15	70	0
Cream	120	545	0
Other (25%-30% fat)	85	385	0
Cheese spread	65	295	0
Chicken, flesh only, raw	60	—	0
Crab			
In shell[2]	125	270	52
Meat only[2]	125	565	0
Egg, whole	550	2200	12
Egg white	0	0	0
Egg yolk			
Fresh	1500	6800	0
Frozen	1280	5800	0
Dried	2950	13,380	0
Fish			
Steak[2]	70	265	16
Fillet[2]	70	320	0
Heart, raw	150	680	0
Ice cream	45	205	0
Kidney, raw	375	1700	0
Lamb, raw			
With bone[2]	70	265	16
Without bone[2]	70	320	0
Lard and other animal fat	95	430	0
Liver, raw	300	1360	0
Lobster			
Whole[2]	200	235	74
Meat only[2]	200	900	0
Margarine			
All vegetable fat	0	0	0
Two-thirds animal fat, one-third vegetable fat	65	295	0
Milk			
Fluid, whole	11	50	0

From Watt, B.K., and Merrill, A.L.: Composition of foods—raw, processed, prepared, U.S. Department of Agriculture, Agriculture Handbook No. 8, Dec. 1963.

[1]Data apply to 100 g of edible portion of the item, although it may be purchased with the refuse indicated and described or implied in the first column.

[2]Items that have the same chemical composition for the edible portion but differ in the amount of refuse.

| Item | Amount of Cholesterol in | | Refuse from Item as Purchased (%) |
	100 g Edible Portion[1] (mg)	Edible Portion of 450 g (1 lb) as Purchased (mg)	
Dried, whole	85	385	0
Fluid, skim	3	15	0
Mutton			
With bone[2]	65	250	16
Without bone[2]	65	295	0
Oysters			
In shell[2]	>200	>90	90
Meat only[2]	>200	>900	0
Pork			
With bone[2]	70	260	18
Without bone[2]	70	320	0
Shrimp			
In shell[2]	125	390	31
Flesh only[2]	125	565	0
Sweetbreads (thymus)	250	1135	0
Veal			
With bone[2]	90	320	21
Without bone[2]	90	410	0

C

Dietary Fiber in Selected Plant Foods

Food	Amount	Weight (g)	Total Dietary Fiber (g)	Noncellulose Polysaccharides (g)	Cellulose (g)	Lignin (g)
Apple	1 med					
Flesh		138	1.96	1.29	0.66	0.01
Skin		100	3.71	2.21	1.01	0.49
Banana	1 small	119	2.08	1.33	0.44	0.31
Beans						
Baked	1 cup	255	18.53	14.45	3.59	0.48
Green, cooked	1 cup	125	4.19	2.31	1.61	0.26
Bread						
White	1 slice	25	0.68	0.50	0.18	Trace
Whole meal	1 slice	25	2.13	1.49	0.33	0.31
Broccoli, cooked	1 cup	155	6.36	4.53	1.78	0.05
Brussels sprouts, cooked	1 cup	155	4.43	3.08	1.24	0.11
Cabbage, cooked	1 cup	145	4.10	2.55	1.00	0.55
Carrots, cooked	1 cup	155	5.74	3.44	2.29	Trace
Cauliflower, cooked	1 cup	125	2.25	0.84	1.41	Trace
Cereals						
All-Bran	1 oz	30	8.01	5.35	1.80	0.86

Adapted from Southgate, D.A.T., and others: A guide to calculating intakes of dietary fiber, J. Hum. Nutr. **30**:303, 1976.

Food	Amount	Weight (g)	Total Dietary Fiber (g)	Noncellulose Polysaccharides (g)	Cellulose (g)	Lignin (g)
Corn Flakes	1 cup	25	2.75	1.82	0.61	0.33
Grapenuts	¼ cup	30	2.10	1.54	0.38	0.17
Puffed Wheat	1 cup	15	2.31	1.55	0.39	0.37
Rice Krispies	1 cup	30	1.34	1.04	0.23	0.07
Shredded Wheat	1 biscuit	25	3.07	2.20	0.66	0.21
Special K	1 cup	30	1.64	1.10	0.22	0.32
Cherries	10 cherries	68	0.84	0.63	0.17	0.05
Cookies						
Ginger	4 snaps	28	0.56	0.41	0.08	0.07
Oatmeal	4 cookies	52	2.08	1.64	0.21	0.22
Plain	4 cookies	48	0.80	0.68	0.05	0.06
Corn	1 cup	165	7.82	7.11	0.51	0.20
Canned	1 cup	165	9.39	8.20	1.06	0.13
Flour						
Bran	1 cup	100	44.00	32.70	8.05	3.23
White	1 cup	115	3.62	2.90	0.69	0.03
Whole meal	1 cup	120	11.41	7.50	2.95	0.96
Grapefruit	½ cup	100	0.44	0.34	0.04	0.06
Jam, strawberry	1 tbsp	20	0.22	0.17	0.02	0.03
Lettuce	⅙ head	100	1.53	0.47	1.06	Trace
Marmalade, orange	1 tbsp	20	0.14	0.13	0.01	Trace
Onions, raw, sliced	1 cup	100	2.10	1.55	0.55	Trace
Orange	1 cup	200	0.58	0.44	0.08	0.06
Parsnips, raw, diced	1 cup	100	4.90	3.77	1.13	Trace
Peanuts	1 oz	30	2.79	1.92	0.51	0.36
Peanut butter	1 tbsp	16	1.21	0.90	0.31	Trace
Peach, flesh and skin	1 med	100	2.28	1.46	0.20	0.62
Pear	1 med					
Flesh		164	4.00	2.16	1.10	0.74
Skin		100	8.59	3.72	2.18	2.67
Peas, canned	1 cup	170	13.35	8.84	3.91	0.60
Peas, raw or frozen	1 cup	100	7.75	5.48	2.09	0.18
Plums	1 plum	66	1.00	0.65	0.15	0.20
Potato, raw	1 med	135	4.73	3.36	1.38	Trace
Raisins	1 oz	30	1.32	0.72	0.25	0.35
Strawberries	1 cup	149	2.65	1.39	1.04	0.22
Tomato						
Raw	1 med	135	1.89	0.88	0.61	0.41
Canned, drained	1 cup	240	2.04	1.08	0.89	0.07
Turnips, raw	1 med	100	2.20	1.50	0.70	Trace

D

Sodium and Potassium Content of Foods, 100 g, Edible Portion

Food and Description	Sodium (mg)	Potassium (mg)
Almonds		
Dried	4	773
Roasted and salted	198	773
Apples		
Raw, pared	1	110
Frozen, sliced, sweetened	14	68
Apple juice, canned or bottled	1	101
Applesauce, canned, sweetened	2	65
Apricots		
Raw	1	281
Canned, syrup pack, light	1	239
Dried, sulfured, cooked, fruit, and liquid	8	318
Asparagus		
Cooked spears, boiled, drained	1	183
Canned spears, green		
Regular pack, solids and liquid	236[1]	166
Special dietary pack (low sodium), solids and liquid	3	166
Frozen		
Cuts and tips, cooked, boiled, drained	1	220
Spears, cooked, boiled, drained	1	238
Avocados, raw, all commercial varieties	4	604
Bacon, cured, cooked, broiled or fried, drained	1021	236
Bacon, Canadian, cooked, broiled or fried, drained	2555	432
Bananas, raw, common	1	370
Bass, black sea, raw	68	256
Beans, common, mature seeds, dry		
White		
Cooked	7	416
Canned, solids and liquid, with pork and tomato sauce	463	210
Red, cooked	3	340
Beans, lima		
Immature seeds		
Cooked, boiled, drained	1	422
Canned		
Regular pack, solids and liquid	236[1]	222
Special dietary pack (low sodium), solids and liquid	4	222
Frozen, thin-seeded types, commonly called baby limas, cooked, boiled, drained	129	394
Mature seeds, dry, cooked	2	612
Beans, mung, sprouted seeds, cooked, boiled, drained	4	156
Beans, snap		
Green		
Cooked, boiled, drained	4	151
Canned		
Regular pack, solids and liquid	236[1]	95

Numbers in parentheses denote values inputed, usually from another form of the food or from a similar food. Dashes denote lack of reliable data for a constituent believed to be present in measurable amount. Values are selected from Watt, B.K., and Merrill, A.L.: Composition of foods—raw, processed, prepared, U.S. Department of Agriculture, Agriculture Handbook No. 8, Dec. 1963.
For notes, see end of table.

Food and Description	Sodium (mg)	Potassium (mg)
Special dietary pack (low sodium), solids and liquid	2	95
Frozen, cut, cooked, boiled, drained	1	152
Yellow or wax		
Cooked, boiled, drained	3	151
Canned		
Regular pack, solids and liquid	236[1]	95
Special dietary pack (low sodium), solids and liquid	2	95
Frozen, cut, cooked, boiled, drained	1	164
Beef		
Retail cuts, trimmed to retail level		
Round	60	370
Rump	60	370
Hamburger, regular ground, cooked	47	450
Beef, corned, boneless		
Cooked, medium fat	1740	150
Canned corned-beef hash (with potato)	540	200
Beef, dried, cooked, creamed	716	153
Beef potpie, commercial, frozen, unheated	366	93
Beets, common, red		
Canned		
Regular pack, solids and liquid	236[1]	167
Special dietary pack (low sodium), solids and liquid	46	167
Beet greens, common, cooked, boiled, drained	76	332
Biscuits, baking powder, made with enriched flour	626	117
Blackberries, including dewberries, boysenberries, and young-berries, raw	1	170
Blueberries		
Raw	1	81
Frozen, not thawed, sweetened	1	66
Bouillon cubes or powder	24,000	100
Bran, added sugar and malt extract	1060	1070
Bran flakes (40% bran), added thiamine	925	—
Bran flakes with raisins, added thiamine	800	—
Breads		
Cracked wheat	529	134
French or Vienna, enriched	580	90
Italian, enriched	585	74
Raisin	365	233
Rye, American (⅓ rye, ⅔ clear flour)	557	145
White, enriched, made with 3%-4% nonfat dry milk	507	105
Whole wheat, made with 2% nonfat dry milk	527	273
Bread stuffing mix and stuffings prepared from mix, dry form	1331	172
Broccoli		
Cooked spears, boiled, drained	10	267
Frozen, spears, cooked, boiled, drained	12	220
Brussels sprouts, frozen, cooked, boiled, drained	14	295
Buffalo fish, raw	52	293
Bulgur (parboiled wheat), canned, made from hard red winter wheat		
Unseasoned[2]	599	87
Seasoned[3]	460	112
Butter[4]	987	23
Buttermilk, fluid, cultured (made from skim milk)	130	140
Cabbage		
Common varieties (Danish, domestic, and pointed types)		
Raw	20	233
Cooked, boiled until tender, drained, shredded, cooked in small amount of water	14	163

For notes, see end of table.

Food and Description	Sodium (mg)	Potassium (mg)
Red, raw	26	268
Cakes		
Baked from home recipes		
Angle food	283	88
Fruit cake, made with enriched flour, dark	158	496
Gingerbread, made with enriched flour	237	454
Plain cake or cupcake, without icing	300	79
Pound, modified	178	78
Frozen, commercial, devil's food, with chocolate icing	420	119
Candy		
Caramels, plain or chocolate	226	192
Chocolate, sweet	33	269
Chocolate coated, chocolate fudge	228	193
Gum drops, starch jelly pieces	35	5
Hard	32	4
Marshmallows	39	6
Peanut bars	10	448
Carrots		
Raw	47	341
Canned		
Regular pack, solids and liquid	236[1]	120
Special dietary pack (low sodium), solids and liquid	39	120
Cashew nuts	15[5]	464
Cauliflower		
Cooked, boiled, drained	9	206
Frozen, cooked, boiled, drained	10	207
Celery, all, including green and yellow varieties		
Raw	126	341
Cooked, boiled, drained	88	239
Chard, Swiss, cooked, boiled, drained	86	321
Cheeses		
Natural cheeses		
Cheddar (domestic type, commonly called American)	700	82
Cottage (large or small curd)		
Creamed	229	85
Uncreamed	290	72
Cream	250	74
Parmesan	734	149
Swiss (domestic)	710	104
Pasteurized process cheese, American	1136[6]	80
Pasteurized process cheese spread, American	1625[6]	240
Cherries		
Raw, sweet	2	191
Canned		
Sour, red, solids and liquid, water pack	2	130
Sweet, solids and liquid, syrup pack, light	1	128
Frozen, not thawed, sweetened	2	130
Chicken, all classes		
Light meat without skin, cooked, roasted	64	411
Dark meat without skin, cooked, roasted	86	321
Chicken potpie, commercial, frozen, unheated	411	153
Chili con carne, canned, with beans	531	233
Clams, raw		
Soft, meat only	36	235
Hard or round, meat only	205	311
Cocoa and chocolate-flavored beverage powders		
Cocoa powder with nonfat dry milk	525	800
Mix for hot chocolate	382	605

Food and Description	Sodium (mg)	Potassium (mg)
Cocoa, dry powder, high-fat or breakfast		
Plain	6	1522
Processed with alkali	717	651
Coconut meat, fresh	23	256
Cod		
Cooked, broiled	110	407
Dehydrated, lightly salted	8100	160
Coffee, instant, water-soluble solids		
Dry powder	72	3256
Beverage	1	36
Coleslaw, made with French dressing (commercial)	268	205
Collards, cooked, boiled, drained, leaves, including stems, cooked in small amount of water	25	234
Cookies		
Assorted, packaged, commercial	365	67
Butter, thin, rich	418	60
Gingersnaps	571	462
Molasses	386	138
Oatmeal with raisins	162	370
Sandwich type	483	38
Vanilla wafer	252	72
Corn, sweet		
Cooked, boiled, drained, white and yellow, kernels, cut off cob before cooking	Trace	165
Canned		
Regular pack, cream style, white and yellow, solids and liquid	236[1]	(97)
Special dietary pack (low sodium), cream style, white and yellow, solids and liquid	2	(97)
Frozen, kernels cut off cob, cooked, boiled, drained	1	184
Corn grits, degermed, enriched, dry form	1	80
Corn products used mainly as ready-to-eat breakfast cereals		
Corn flakes, added nutrients	1005	120
Corn, puffed, added nutrients	1060	—
Corn, rice, and wheat flakes, mixed, added nutrients	950	—
Cornbread, baked from home recipes, southern style, made with degermed cornmeal, enriched	591	157
Cornmeal, white or yellow, degermed, enriched, dry form	1	120
Cornstarch	Trace	Trace
Cowpeas, including blackeye peas		
Immature seeds, canned, solids and liquid	236[1]	352
Young pods, with seeds, cooked, boiled, drained	3	196
Crab, canned	1000	110
Crackers		
Butter	1092	113
Graham, plain	670	384
Saltines	(1100)	(120)
Sandwich type, peanut-cheese	992	226
Soda	1100	120
Cream, fluid, light, coffee, or table, 20% fat	43	122
Cream substitutes, dried, containing cream, skim milk (calcium reduced), and lactose	575	—
Cucumbers, raw, pared	6	160
Custard, baked	79	146
Doughnuts, cake type	501	90
Duck, domesticated, raw, flesh only	74	285

For notes, see end of table.

Food and Description	Sodium (mg)	Potassium (mg)
Eggs, chicken		
Raw		
Whole, fresh and frozen	122	129
Whites, fresh and frozen	146	139
Yolks, fresh	52	98
Eggplant, cooked, boiled, drained	1	150
Farina		
Enriched		
Regular		
Dry form	2	83
Cooked	144	9
Quick-cooking, cooked	165	10
Instant-cooking, cooked	188	13
Nonenriched, regular, dry form	2	83
Flatfishes (flounders, soles, sand dabs), raw	78	342
Fruit cocktail, canned, solids and liquid, water pack, with or without artificial sweetener	5	168
Garlic, cloves, raw	19	529
Grapefruit		
Raw, pulp, pink, red, white, all varieties	1	135
Canned, juice, sweetened	1	162
Grapes, raw, American type (slip skin), such as Concord, Delaware, Niagara, Catawba, and Scuppernong	3	158
Haddock, cooked, fried	177	348
Halibut, Atlantic and Pacific, cooked, broiled	134	525
Ice cream and frozen custard, regular, approximately 10% fat	63[7]	181
Ice cream cones	232	244
Ice milk	68[7]	195
Jams and preserves	12	88
Kale, cooked, boiled, drained, leaves including stems	43	221
Lamb, retail cuts	70	290
Lettuce, raw crisphead varieties such as Iceberg, New York, and Great Lakes strains	9	175
Liver, beef, cooked, fried	184	380
Lobster, northern, canned or cooked	210	180
Macaroni, unenriched, dry form	2	197
Margarine[8]	987	23
Milk, cow		
Fluid (pasteurized and raw)		
Whole, 3.7% fat	50	144
Skim	52	145
Canned, evaporated (unsweetened)	118	303
Dry, skim (nonfat solids), regular	532	1745
Malted		
Dry powder	440	720
Beverage	91	200
Chocolate drink, fluid, commercial		
Made with skim milk	46	142
Made with whole (3.5% fat) milk	47	146
Molasses, cane		
First extraction or light	15	917
Third extraction or blackstrap	96	2927
Muskmelons, raw, cantaloupes, other netted varieties	12	251
Mustard greens, cooked, boiled, drained	18	220
Nectarines, raw	6	294
New Zealand spinach, cooked, boiled, drained	92	463

Food and Description	Sodium (mg)	Potassium (mg)
Noodles, egg noodles, enriched, cooked	2	44
Oat products used mainly as hot breakfast cereals, oatmeal or rolled oats		
Dry form	2	352
Cooked	218	61
Oat products used mainly as ready-to-eat breakfast cereals, with or without corn, puffed, added nutrients	1267	—
Okra		
Raw	3	249
Cooked, boiled, drained	2	174
Olives, pickled; canned or bottled		
Green	2400	55
Ripe, Ascolano (extra large, mammoth, giant jumbo)	813	34
Ripe, salt-cured, oil-coated, Greek style	3288	—
Onions, mature (dry), raw	10	157
Onions, young green (bunching varieties), raw, bulb and entire top	5	231
Oranges, raw, peeled fruit, all commercial varieties	1	200
Orange juice		
Raw, all commercial varieties	1	200
Canned, unsweetened	1	199
Frozen concentrate, unsweetened, diluted with 3 parts water, by volume	1	186
Oysters		
Raw, meat only, Eastern	73	121
Cooked, fried	206	203
Frozen, solids and liquid	380	210
Parsnips, cooked, boiled, drained	8	379
Peaches		
Raw	1	202
Canned, solids and liquid, water pack, with or without artificial sweetener	2	137
Frozen, sliced, sweetened, not thawed	2	124
Peanuts		
Roasted with skins	5	701
Roasted and salted	418	674
Peanut butters made with small amounts of added fat, salt	607	670
Pears		
Raw, including skin	2	130
Canned, solids and liquid, syrup pack, light	1	85
Peas, green, immature		
Cooked, boiled, drained	1	196
Canned, Alaska (early or June peas)		
Regular pack, solids and liquid	236[1]	96
Special dietary pack (low sodium), solids and liquid	3	96
Frozen, cooked, boiled, drained	115	135
Pecans	Trace	603
Peppers, sweet, garden varieties, immature, green, raw	13	213
Perch, yellow, raw	68	230
Pickles, cucumber, dill	1428	200
Piecrust or plain pastry, made with enriched flour, baked	611	50
Pineapple		
Raw	1	146
Frozen chunks, sweetened, not thawed	2	100
Pizza, with cheese, from home recipe, baked		
With cheese topping	702	130
With sausage topping	729	168

For notes, see end of table.

Food and Description	Sodium (mg)	Potassium (mg)
Plate dinners, frozen, commercial, unheated		
Beef pot roast, whole oven-browned potatoes, peas, corn	259	244
Chicken, fried; mashed potatoes; mixed vegetables (carrots, peas, corn, beans)	344	112
Meat loaf with tomato sauce, mashed potatoes, peas	393	115
Turkey, sliced; mashed potatoes; peas	400	176
Plums		
Raw, Damson	2	299
Canned, solids and liquid, purple (Italian prunes), syrup pack, light	1	145
Popcorn, popped		
Plain	(3)	—
Oil and salt added	1940	—
Pork, fresh, retail cuts, trimmed to retail level, loin	65	390
Pork, cured, canned ham, contents of can	(1100)	(340)
Potatoes		
Cooked, boiled in skin	3[9]	407
Dehydrated mashed, flakes without milk		
Dry form	89	1600
Prepared, water, milk, table fat added	231	286
Pretzels	1680[10]	130
Prunes, dried, "softenized," cooked (fruit and liquid), with added sugar	3	262
Pudding mixes and puddings made from mixes, with starch base		
With milk, cooked	129	136
With milk, without cooking	124	129
Pumpkin, canned	2	240
Raspberries		
Canned, solids and liquid, water pack, with or without artificial sweetener, red	1	114
Frozen, red, sweetened, not thawed	1	100
Rice		
Brown		
Raw	9	214
Cooked	282	70
White (fully milled or polished), enriched, common commercial varieties, all types		
Raw	5	92
Cooked	374	28
Rice products used mainly as ready-to-eat breakfast cereals		
Rice flakes, added nutrients	987	180
Rice, puffed; added nutrients, without salt	2	100
Rice, puffed or open-popped, presweetened, honey and added nutrients	706	—
Roe, cooked, baked or broiled, cod and shad[11]	73	132
Rolls and buns, commercial, ready-to-serve		
Danish pastry	366	112
Hard rolls, enriched	625	97
Plain (pan rolls), enriched	506	95
Sweet rolls	389	124
Rusk	246	161
Rutabagas, cooked, boiled, drained	4	167
Rye, flour, medium	(1)	203
Rye wafers, whole grain	882	600

Food and Description	Sodium (mg)	Potassium (mg)
Salad dressings, commercial[12]		
Blue and Roquefort cheese		
Regular	1094	37
Special dietary (low calorie), low fat (approx. 5 kcal/tsp)	1108	34
French		
Regular	1370	79
Special dietary (low calorie), low fat (approx. 5 kcal/tsp)	787	79
Mayonnaise	597	34
Thousand Island		
Regular	700	113
Special dietary (low calorie, approx. 10 kcal/tsp)	700	113
Salmon, coho (silver)		
Raw	48[13]	421
Canned, solids and liquid	351[14]	339
Salt pork, raw	1212	42
Salt sticks, regular type	1674	92
Sandwich spread (with chopped pickle)		
Regular	626	92
Special dietary (low calorie, approx. 5 kcal/tsp)	626	92
Sardines, Atlantic, canned in oil, drained solids	823	590
Sardines, Pacific, in tomato sauce, solids and liquid	400	320
Sauerkraut, canned, solids and liquid	747[15]	140
Sausage, cold cuts, and luncheon meats		
Bologna, all samples	1300	230
Frankfurters, raw, all samples	1100	220
Luncheon meat, pork, cured ham or shoulder, chopped, spiced or unspiced, canned	1234	222
Pork sausage, links or bulk, cooked	958	269
Scallops, bay and sea, cooked, steamed	265	476
Soups, commercial, canned		
Beef broth, bouillon, and consomme, prepared with equal volume of water	326	54
Chicken noodle, prepared with equal volume of water	408	23
Tomato		
Prepared with equal volume of water	396	94
Prepared with equal volume of milk	422	167
Vegetable beef, prepared with equal volume of water	427	66
Soy sauce	7325	366
Spaghetti, enriched, cooked, tender stage	1	61
Spinach		
Cooked, boiled, drained	50	324
Canned		
Regular pack, drained solids	236[1]	250
Special dietary pack (low sodium), solids and liquid	34	250
Frozen, chopped, cooked, boiled, drained	52	333
Squash, summer, all varieties, cooked, boiled, drained	1	141
Strawberries		
Raw	1	164
Frozen, sweetened, not thawed, sliced	1	112
Sweet potatoes		
Cooked, all, baked in skin	12	300
Canned, liquid pack, solids and liquid, regular pack in syrup	48	(120)
Dehydrated flakes, prepared with water	45	140
Tangerines, raw (Dancy variety)	2	126
Tea, instant (water-soluble solids), carbohydrate added		
Dry powder	—	4530
Beverage	—	25

For notes, see end of table.

Food and Description	Sodium (mg)	Potassium (mg)
Tomatoes, ripe		
Raw	3	244
Canned, solids and liquid, regular pack	130	217
Tomato catsup, bottled	1042[16]	363
Regular pack	200	227
Special dietary pack (low sodium)	3	227
Tomato puree, canned		
Regular pack	399	426
Special dietary pack (low sodium)	6	426
Tuna, canned		
In oil, solids and liquid	800	301
In water, solids and liquid	41[17]	279[17]
Turkey, all classes		
Light meat, cooked, roasted	82	411
Dark meat, cooked, roasted	99	398
Turkey potpie, commercial, frozen, unheated	369	114
Turnips, cooked, boiled, drained	34	188
Turnip greens, leaves, including stems		
Canned, solids and liquid	236[1]	243
Frozen, cooked, boiled, drained	17	149
Veal, retail cuts, untrimmed	80	500
Waffles, frozen, made with enriched flour	644	158
Walnuts		
Black	3	460
Persian or English	2	450
Watermelon, raw	1	100
Wheat flours		
Whole (from hard wheats)	3	370
Patent		
All-purpose or family flour, enriched	2	95
Self-rising flour, enriched (anhydrous monocalcium phosphate used as a baking acid)[18]	1079	—[19]
Yogurt, made from whole milk	47	132

[1]Estimated average based on addition of salt in the amount of 0.6% of the finished product.

[2]Processed, partially debranned, whole-kernel wheat with salt added.

[3]Processed, partially debranned, whole-kernel wheat with chicken fat, chicken stock base, dehydrated onion flakes, salt, monosodium glutamate, and herbs.

[4]Values apply to salted butter. Unsalted butter contains less than 10 mg of either sodium or potassium per 100 g. Value for vitamin A is the year-round average.

[5]Applies to unsalted nuts. For salted nuts, value is approximately 200 mg per 100 g.

[6]Values for phosphorus and sodium are based on use of 1.5% anhydrous disodium phosphate as the emulsifying agent. If emulsifying agent does not contain either phosphorus (P) or sodium (Na), the content of these two nutrients in milligrams per 100 g is as follows:

	P	Na
American process cheese	444	650
Swiss process cheese	540	681
American cheese food	427	—
American cheese spread	548	1139

[7]Value for product without added salt.

[8]Values apply to salted margarine. Unsalted margarine contains less than 10 mg/100 g of either sodium or potassium. Vitamin A value based on the minimum required to meet federal specifications for margarine with vitamin A added, 15,000 IUA/lb.

[9]Applies to product without added salt. If salt is added, an estimated average value for sodium is 236 mg/100 g.

[10]Sodium content is variable. For example, very thin pretzel sticks contain about twice the average amount listed.

[11]Prepared with butter or margarine, lemon juice or vinegar.

[12]Values apply to products containing salt. For those without salt, sodium content is low, ranging from less than 10 to 50 mg/100 g; the amount usually is indicated on the label.

Continued.

Footnotes to table, pp. A-41 to A-49, cont'd.

[13]Sample dipped in brine contained 215 mg sodium/100 g.

[14]For product canned without added salt, value is approximately the same as for raw salmon.

[15]Values for sauerkraut and sauerkraut juice are based on salt content of 1.9% and 2.0%, respectively, in the finished products. The amounts in some samples may vary significantly from this estimate.

[16]Applies to regular pack. For special dietary pack (low sodium), values range from 5-35 mg/100 g.

[17]One sample with salt added contained 875 mg of sodium/100 g and 275 mg of potassium.

[18]The acid ingredient most commonly used in self-rising flour. When sodium acid pyrophosphate in combination with either anhydrous monocalcium phosphate or calcium carbonate is used, the value for calcium is approximately 120 mg/100 g; for phosphorus, 540 mg; for sodium, 1360 mg.

[19]90 mg of potassium/100 g contributed by flour. Small quantities of additional potassium may be provided by other ingredients.

E

Sodium Levels in Mineral Waters

Sodium Levels	Beverage (8 fl oz)
Low (less than 5 mg)	Black Mountain spring water Bel-Air mineral water Perrier Poland Springs sparkling water Sheffield's O_2 sparkling spring water
Moderate-low (30-60 mg)	Calistoga mineral water Canada Dry club soda Napa Valley springs mineral water Schweppes club soda
Moderate-high (100-110 mg)	Calso water
High (more than 400 mg)	Lady Lee club soda

Adapted from Sodium in mineral waters—8 fluid ounce servings, American Heart Association, Alameda County Chapter, Oakland, Calif., Feb. 1981.

F

Sodium Levels in Popular Soft Drinks

Regular	Sugar-Free
Less than 20 mg/12 fl oz	
Aspen, Bubble-Up, Canada Dry ginger ale, Canada Dry tonic water, Orange Crush, Pepsi, Schweppes ginger ale, Schweppes tonic water, Shasta cola, Squirt	
20-40 mg/12 fl oz	
Canada Dry collins mix, Coca-Cola, Dr. Pepper, Fanta (orange, grape, root beer), Mountain Dew, Mr. Pibb, Seven-Up, Shasta (all flavors except cola, strawberry, lemon-lime), Sunkist, Teem	Sugar-free Dr. Pepper, Diet Shasta grape, Diet Squirt
40-60 mg/12 fl oz	
Fanta ginger ale, Schweppes bitter lemon, Shasta (lemon-lime, strawberry), Sprite	Fresca, Sugar-free Mr. Pibb, Pepsi Light, Diet Seven-Up, Diet Shasta (all flavors except grape), Tab, Tab-Strawberry
60-80 mg/12 fl oz	
	Diet-Rite Cola, Diet Pepsi, Sugar-free Sprite, Tab (black cherry, ginger ale, grape, lemon-lime, orange, root beer)
80-100 mg/12 fl oz	
	Sugar-free Bubble-Up, Diet Mug Root Beer, Diet Sunkist

Adapted from Sodium in soft drinks—12 fl oz servings, American Heart Association, Alameda County Chapter, Oakland, Calif., Feb. 1981.

G

Nutritional Analyses of Fast Foods

	Wt (g)	Energy (kcal)	PRO (g)	CHO (g)	Fat (g)	Chol (mg)	Vitamins A (IU)	B_1 (mg)	B_2 (mg)	Nia. (mg)	B_6 (mg)	B_{12} (μg)	C (mg)	D (IU)
Arby's														
Roast Beef	140	350	22	32	15	45	X	0.30	0.34	5	—	—	X	—
Beef and Cheese	168	450	27	36	22	55	X	0.38	0.43	6	—	—	X	—
Super Roast Beef	263	620	30	61	28	85	X	0.53	0.43	7	—	—	X	—
Junior Roast Beef	74	220	12	21	9	35	X	0.15	0.17	3	—	—	X	—
Ham & Cheese	154	380	23	33	17	60	X	0.75	0.34	5	—	—	X	—
Turkey Deluxe	236	510	28	46	24	70	X	0.45	0.34	8	—	—	X	—
Club Sandwich	252	560	30	43	30	100	X	0.68	0.43	7	—	—	X	—

From Consumer Affairs, Arby's, Inc, Atlanta, Ga. Nutritional analysis by Technological Resources, Camden, N.J.

	Wt (g)	Energy (kcal)	PRO (g)	CHO (g)	Fat (g)	Chol (mg)	A (IU)	B_1 (mg)	B_2 (mg)	Nia. (mg)	B_6 (mg)	B_{12} (μg)	C (mg)	D (IU)
Burger Chef														
Hamburger	91	244	11	29	9	27	114	0.17	0.16	2.7	0.16	0.26	1.2	—
Cheeseburger	104	290	14	29	13	39	267	0.18	0.21	2.8	0.17	0.36	1.2	—
Double Cheeseburger	145	420	24	30	22	77	431	0.20	0.32	4.4	0.31	0.73	1.2	—
Fish Filet	179	547	21	46	31	43	400	0.23	0.22	2.7	0.04	0.10	1.0	—
Super Shef Sandwich	252	563	29	44	30	105	754	0.31	0.40	6.0	0.45	0.87	9.3	—
Big Shef Sandwich	186	569	23	38	36	81	279	0.26	0.31	4.7	0.31	0.63	1.0	—
TOP Shef Sandwich	138	661	41	36	38	134	273	0.35	0.47	8.1	0.56	1.16	0	—
Funmeal Feast	—	545	15	55	30	27	123	0.25	0.21	4.6	0.16	0.26	12.8	—
Rancher Platter*	316	640	32	33	42	106	1750*	0.29	0.38	8.6	0.61	1.01	23.5	—
Mariner Platter*	373	734	29	78	34	35	2069*	0.34	0.23	5.2	0.09	0.56	23.5	—
French Fries, small	68	250	2	20	19	0	0	0.07	0.04	1.7	—	0	11.5	—
French Fries, large	85	351	3	28	26	0	0	0.10	0.06	2.4	—	0	16.2	—
Vanilla Shake (12 oz)	336	380	13	60	10	40	387	0.10	0.66	0.5	0.1	1.77	0	—
Chocolate Shake (12 oz)	336	403	10	72	9	36	292	0.16	0.76	0.4	0.1	1.07	0	—
Hot Chocolate	—	198	8	23	8	30	288	0.93	0.39	0.3	0.1	0.79	2.1	—

From Burger Chef Systems, Inc, Indianapolis, Ind. Nutritional analysis from *Handbook No. 8.* Washington; U.S. Dept of Agriculture.
*Includes salad.

	Wt (g)	Energy (kcal)	PRO (g)	CHO (g)	Fat (g)	Chol (mg)	A (IU)	B_1 (mg)	B_2 (mg)	Nia. (mg)	B_6 (mg)	B_{12} (μg)	C (mg)	D (IU)
Burger King*														
Hamburger	110	290	15 (25%*)	29	13	—	tr	10%	10%	10%	—	—	tr	—
Cheeseburger	124	350	18 (30%)	30	17	—	tr	8%	10%	10%	—	—	tr	—
Double Cheeseburger	179	530	30 (50%)	32	31	—	tr	10%	10%	20%	—	—	tr	—
Whopper	261	630	26 (40%)	50	36	—	tr	4%	15%	20%	—	—	tr	—
Whopper w/Ch	289	740	32 (50%)	52	45	—	tr	8%	20%	15%	—	—	tr	—
Double Beef Whopper	337	850	44 (70%)	52	52	—	tr	6%	25%	30%	—	—	tr	—
Double Beef Whopper w/Ch	365	950	50 (80%)	54	60	—	tr	6%	25%	30%	—	—	tr	—
Whopper Jr.	144	370	15 (25%)	31	20	—	tr	15%	10%	15%	—	—	tr	—
Whopper Jr. w/Ch	158	420	18 (30%)	32	25	—	tr	15%	10%	15%	—	—	tr	—
Bacon Double Cheeseburger	202	600	35 (50%)	36	35	—	8%	20%	25%	35%	—	—	2%	—
Whaler	—	540	24 (35%)	57	24	—	tr	15%	10%	10%	—	—	tr	—
Whaler w/Ch	—	590	26 (40%)	58	28	—	4%	15%	15%	10%	—	—	tr	—
Chicken Sandwich	—	690	26 (40%)	26	42	—	4%	20%	15%	50%	—	—	2%	—
Veal Parmagiana	—	600	28 (45%)	65	25	—	20%	25%	30%	35%	—	—	10%	—
Regular Fries	68	210	3 (4%)	25	11	—	tr	4%	tr	4%	—	—	4%	—
Regular Onion Rings	76	270	3 (4%)	29	16	—	tr	4%	tr	tr	—	—	tr	—
Apple Pie	85	240	2 (4%)	32	12	—	tr	tr	2%	tr	—	—	tr	—
Chocolate Shake	282	340	8 (10%)	57	10	—	tr	8%	15%	tr	—	—	tr	—
Vanilla Shake	282	340	8 (10%)	52	11	—	tr	10%	20%	tr	—	—	tr	—

From Burger King Corp., Miami, Fla. Nutritional analysis by Raltech Scientific Services, Inc. (formerly WARF), Madison, Wis., and Campbell Labs, Camden, N.J.
*NOTE: Analyses for vitamins and minerals shown with percent signs indicate percent U.S. RDA.

From Young, E.A.: Update: nutritional analysis of fast foods, Public Health Currents, 1981, Reprinted with permission of Ross Laboratories, Columbus, Ohio 43216.
See Burger King section for that restaurant's source for nutritional analysis.
Dashes indicate no data available; X, less than 2% U.S. RDA; tr, trace.
NOTE: Older Pizza Hut data are invalid because of reformulation of the products.

Minerals								Moisture (g)	Crude Fiber (g)
Ca (mg)	Cu (mg)	Fe (mg)	K (mg)	Mg (mg)	P (mg)	Na (mg)	Zn (mg)		
80	—	3.6	—	—	—	880	—	—	—
200	—	4.5	—	—	—	1220	—	—	—
100	—	5.4	—	—	—	1420	—	—	—
40	—	1.8	—	—	—	530	—	—	—
200	—	2.7	—	—	—	1350	—	—	—
80	—	2.7	—	—	—	1220	—	—	—
200	—	3.6	—	—	—	1610	—	—	—
45	0.08	2.0	208	9	106	—	1.6	41	0.2
132	0.08	2.2	218	9	202	—	1.9	46	0.2
223	0.10	3.2	360	15	355	—	3.6	67	0.2
145	0.04	2.2	271	19	302	—	1.2	72	0.4
205	0.21	4.5	578	25	377	—	4.5	143	0.5
152	0.05	3.6	382	14	280	—	3.4	80	0.3
194	0.13	5.4	612	26	445	—	5.9	91	0.1
61	0.24	2.8	688	26	183	—	1.6	70	0.8
66	0.38	5.3	1237	53	326	—	5.6	209	1.3
63	0.32	3.3	996	49	397	—	1.2	195	1.8
9	0.16	0.7	473	16	62	—	<0.1	29	0.6
13	0.23	0.9	661	22	86	—	<0.1	40	0.9
497	—	0.3	622	40	392	—	1.3	—	—
449	—	1.1	762	54	429	—	1.6	—	—
271	0.09	0.7	436	50	245	—	1.1	—	—
tr	6%	15%	240	6%	10%	525	10%	—	—
4%	6%	15%	230	6%	15%	730	15%	—	—
8%	6%	15%	360	10%	30%	990	30%	—	—
4%	6%	15%	520	10%	25%	990	15%	—	—
15%	6%	15%	590	10%	35%	1435	20%	—	—
2%	6%	25%	760	10%	40%	1080	40%	—	—
15%	6%	20%	730	15%	50%	1535	45%	—	—
tr	2%	10%	280	6%	10%	560	15%	—	—
8%	2%	10%	270	8%	20%	785	15%	—	—
25%	—	25%	540	—	45%	985	—	—	—
8%	—	15%	150	—	25%	745	—	—	—
20%	—	15%	160	—	35%	885	—	—	—
6%	—	10%	340	—	20%	775	—	—	—
30%	—	25%	340	—	35%	1130	—	—	—
tr	tr	2%	380	6%	tr	230	tr	—	—
8%	2%	2%	140	2%	6%	450	tr	—	—
tr	tr	2%	50	tr	tr	335	tr	—	—
25%	4%	tr	340	10%	25%	280	6%	—	—
30%	tr	tr	210	4%	10%	320	4%	—	—

	Wt (g)	Energy (kcal)	PRO (g)	CHO (g)	Fat (g)	Chol (mg)	Vitamins							
							A (IU)	B$_1$ (mg)	B$_2$ (mg)	Nia. (mg)	B$_6$ (mg)	B$_{12}$ (μg)	C (mg)	D (IU)
Church's Fried Chicken														
White Chicken Portion	100	327	21	10	23	—	160	0.10	0.18	7.2	—	—	0.7	—
Dark Chicken Portion	100	305	22	7	21	—	140	0.10	0.27	5.3	—	—	1.0	—
From Church's Fried Chicken, San Antonio, Tex. Nutritional analysis by Medallion Laboratories, Minneapolis, Minn.														
Dairy Queen														
Frozen Dessert	113	180	5	27	6	20	100	0.09	0.17	X	—	0.6	X	—
DQ Cone, small	71	110	3	18	3	10	100	0.03	0.14	X	—	0.4	X	X
DQ Cone, regular	142	230	6	35	7	20	300	0.09	0.26	X	—	0.6	X	X
DQ Cone, large	213	340	10	52	10	30	400	0.15	0.43	X	—	1.2	X	8
DQ Dip Cone, small	78	150	3	20	7	10	100	0.03	0.17	X	—	0.4	X	X
DQ Dip Cone, regular	156	300	7	40	13	20	300	0.09	0.34	X	—	0.6	X	X
DQ Dip Cone, large	234	450	10	58	20	30	400	0.12	0.51	X	—	0.9	X	8
DQ Sundae, small	106	170	4	30	4	15	100	0.03	0.17	X	—	0.5	X	X
DQ Sundae, regular	177	290	6	51	7	20	300	0.06	0.26	X	—	0.6	X	X
DQ Sundae, large	248	400	9	71	9	30	400	0.09	0.43	0.4	—	1.2	X	8
DQ Malt, small	241	340	10	51	11	30	400	0.06	0.34	0.4	—	1.2	2.4	60
DQ Malt, regular	418	600	15	89	20	50	750	0.12	0.60	0.8	—	1.8	3.6	100
DQ Malt, large	588	840	22	125	28	70	750	0.15	0.85	1.2	—	2.4	6	140
DQ Float	397	330	6	59	8	20	100	0.12	0.17	X	—	0.6	X	X
DQ Banana Split	383	540	10	91	15	30	750	0.60	0.60	0.8	—	0.9	18	X
DQ Parfait	284	460	10	81	11	30	400	0.12	0.43	0.4	—	1.2	X	8
DQ Freeze	397	520	11	89	13	35	200	0.15	0.34	X	—	1.2	X	X
Mr. Misty Freeze	411	500	10	87	12	35	200	0.15	0.34	X	—	0.12	X	X
Mr. Misty Float	404	440	6	85	8	2C	100	0.12	0.17	X	—	0.6	X	X
"Dilly" Bar	85	240	4	22	15	10	100	0.06	0.17	X	—	0.5	X	X
DQ Sandwich	60	140	3	24	4	10	100	0.03	0.14	0.4	—	0.2	X	X
Mr. Misty Kiss	89	70	0	17	0	0	X	X	X	X	—	X	X	X
Brazier Cheese Dog	113	330	15	24	19	—	—	—	0.18	3.3	0.07	1.22	—	23
Brazier Chili Dog	128	330	13	25	20	—	—	0.15	0.23	3.9	0.17	1.29	11.0	20
Brazier Dog	99	273	11	23	15	—	—	0.12	0.15	2.6	0.08	1.05	11.0	23
Fish Sandwich	170	400	20	41	17	—	tr	0.15	0.26	3.0	0.16	1.20	tr	40
Fish Sandwich w/Ch	177	440	24	39	21	—	100	0.15	0.26	3.0	0.16	1.50	tr	40
Super Brazier Dog	182	518	20	41	30	—	tr	0.42	0.44	7.0	0.17	2.09	14.0	44
Super Brazier Dog w/Ch	203	593	26	43	36	—	—	0.43	0.48	8.1	0.18	2.34	14.0	44
Super Brazier Chili Dog	210	555	23	42	33	—	—	0.42	0.48	8.8	0.27	2.67	18.0	32
Brazier Fries, small	71	200	2	25	10	—	tr	0.06	tr	0.8	0.16	—	3.6	16
Brazier Fries, large	113	320	3	40	16	—	tr	0.09	0.03	1.2	0.30	—	4.8	24
Brazier Onion Rings	85	300	6	33	17	—	tr	0.09	tr	0.4	0.08	—	2.4	8
From International Dairy Queen, Inc., Minneapolis, Minn. Nutritional analysis by Raltech Scientific Services, Inc. (formerly WARF), Madison, Wis. (Nutritional analysis														
Jack-in-the-Box														
Hamburger	97	263	13	29	11	26	49	0.27	0.18	5.6	0.11	0.73	1.1	20
Cheeseburger	109	310	16	28	15	32	338	0.27	0.21	5.4	0.12	0.87	<1.1	20
Jumbo Jack Hamburger	246	551	28	45	29	80	246	0.47	0.34	11.6	0.30	2.68	3.7	42
Jumbo Jack Hamburger w/Ch	272	628	32	45	35	110	734	0.52	0.38	11.3	0.31	3.05	4.9	41
Regular Taco	83	189	8	15	11	22	356	0.07	0.08	1.8	0.14	0.5^l	<0.9	6
Super Taco	146	285	12	20	17	37	599	0.10	0.12	2.8	0.22	0.77	1.6	9
Moby Jack Sandwich	141	455	17	38	26	56	240	0.30	0.21	4.5	0.12	1.1	1.4	24
Breakfast Jack Sandwich	121	301	18	28	13	182	442	0.41	0.47	5.1	0.14	1.1	3.4	51
French Fries	80	270	3	31	15	13	—	0.12	0.02	1.9	0.22	0.17	3.7	<1
Onion Rings	85	351	5	32	23	24	—	0.24	0.12	3.1	0.07	0.26	<1.2	<1
Apple Turnover	119	411	4	45	24	17	—	0.23	0.12	2.5	0.03	0.17	<1.2	1
Vanilla Shake*	317	317	10	57	6	26	—	0.16	0.38	0.5	0.20	1.36	<3.2	41
Strawberry Shake*	328	323	11	55	7	26	—	0.16	0.46	0.6	0.15	1.25	<3.3	43
Chocolate Shake*	322	325	11	55	7	26	—	0.16	0.64	0.6	0.19	1.55	<3.2	45
Vanilla Shake	314	342	10	54	9	36	440	0.16	0.47	0.5	0.18	1.1	3.5	44
Strawberry Shake	328	380	11	63	10	33	426	0.16	0.62	0.5	0.18	0.92	<3.3	30
Chocolate Shake	317	365	11	59	10	35	380	0.16	0.60	0.6	0.18	0.98	<3.2	38

| | | Minerals | | | | | | Moisture | Crude Fiber |
Ca (mg)	Cu (mg)	Fe (mg)	K (mg)	Mg (mg)	P (mg)	Na (mg)	Zn (mg)	(g)	(g)
94	—	1.00	186	—	—	498	—	45	0.10
15	—	1.3	206	—	—	475	—	48	0.20
150	—	X	—	—	100	—	—	—	—
100	—	X	—	—	60	—	—	—	—
200	—	X	—	—	150	—	—	—	—
300	—	X	—	—	200	—	—	—	—
100	—	X	—	—	80	—	—	—	—
200	—	0.4	—	—	150	—	—	—	—
300	—	0.4	—	—	200	—	—	—	—
100	—	0.7	—	—	100	—	—	—	—
200	—	1.1	—	—	150	—	—	—	—
300	—	1.8	—	—	250	—	—	—	—
300	—	1.8	—	—	200	—	—	—	—
500	—	3.6	—	—	400	—	—	—	—
600	—	5.4	—	—	600	—	—	—	—
200	—	X	—	—	200	—	—	—	—
350	—	1.8	—	—	250	—	—	—	—
300	—	1.8	—	—	250	—	—	—	—
300	—	X	—	—	250	—	—	—	—
300	—	X	—	—	200	—	—	—	—
200	—	X	—	—	200	—	—	—	—
100	—	0.4	—	—	100	—	—	—	—
60	—	0.4	—	—	60	—	—	—	—
X	—	X	—	—	X	—	—	—	—
168	0.08	1.6	—	24	182	—	1.9	—	—
86	0.13	2.0	—	38	139	939	1.8	—	—
75	0.79	1.5	—	21	104	868	1.4	—	—
60	0.08	1.1	—	24	200	—	0.3	—	—
150	0.08	0.4	—	24	250	—	0.3	—	—
158	0.18	4.3	—	37	195	1552	2.8	—	—
297	0.18	4.4	—	42	312	1986	3.5	—	—
158	0.21	4.0	—	48	231	1640	2.8	—	—
tr	0.04	0.4	—	16	100	—	tr	—	—
tr	0.08	0.4	—	24	150	—	0.3	—	—
20	0.08	0.4	—	16	60	—	0.3	—	—
not applicable in the state of Texas.)									
82	0.10	2.3	165	20	115	566	1.8	43	0.2
172	0.10	2.6	177	22	194	877	2.3	47	0.2
134	0.22	4.5	492	44	261	1134	4.2	139	0.7
273	0.24	4.6	499	49	411	1666	4.8	153	0.8
116	0.11	1.2	264	36	150	460	1.3	47	0.6
196	0.18	1.9	415	53	235	968	2.1	92	1.0
167	0.08	1.7	246	30	263	837	1.1	57	0.1
177	0.11	2.5	190	24	310	1037	1.8	59	0.1
19	0.10	0.7	423	27	88	128	0.3	29	0.6
26	0.07	1.4	109	16	69	318	0.4	24	0.3
11	0.06	1.4	69	10	33	352	0.2	45	0.2
349	0.06	0.2	599	38	312	229	1.0	243	0.3
371	0.10	0.6	613	40	328	241	1.1	253	0.3
348	0.13	0.7	676	53	328	270	1.1	247	0.3
349	0.06	0.4	536	48	318	263	1.0	238	0.3
351	0.07	0.3	556	47	316	268	1.0	242	0.3
350	0.16	1.2	633	57	332	294	1.2	235	0.3

	Wt (g)	Energy (kcal)	PRO (g)	CHO (g)	Fat (g)	Chol (mg)	Vitamins							
							A (IU)	B₁ (mg)	B₂ (mg)	Nia. (mg)	B₆ (mg)	B₁₂ (µg)	C (mg)	D (IU)

	Wt (g)	Energy (kcal)	PRO (g)	CHO (g)	Fat (g)	Chol (mg)	A (IU)	B_1 (mg)	B_2 (mg)	Nia. (mg)	B_6 (mg)	B_{12} (µg)	C (mg)	D (IU)
Ham & Cheese Omelette	174	425	21	32	23	355	766	0.45	0.70	3.0	0.18	1.44	<1.7	64
Double Cheese Omelette	166	423	19	30	25	370	797	0.33	0.68	2.5	0.14	1.33	1.7	61
Ranchero Style Omelette	196	414	20	33	23	343	853	0.33	0.74	2.6	0.18	1.51	<2.0	78
French Toast	180	537	15	54	29	115	522	0.56	0.30	4.4	0.47	1.62	9.2	22
Pancakes	232	626	16	79	27	87	488	0.63	0.44	4.6	0.19	0.56	<26.2	23
Scrambled Eggs	267	719	26	55	44	259	694	0.69	0.56	5.2	0.34	1.31	<12.8	80

*Special formula for shakes sold in California, Arizona, Texas and Washington. From Jack-in-the-Box, Foodmaker, Inc. San Diego, Calif. Nutritional analysis by Raltech

Kentucky Fried Chicken

	Wt (g)	Energy (kcal)	PRO (g)	CHO (g)	Fat (g)	Chol (mg)	A (IU)	B_1 (mg)	B_2 (mg)	Nia. (mg)	B_6 (mg)	B_{12} (µg)	C (mg)	D (IU)
Original Recipe Dinner														
Wing & Rib	322	603	30	48	32	133	25.5	0.22	0.19	10.0	—	—	36.6	—
Wing & Thigh	341	661	33	48	38	172	25.5	0.24	0.27	8.4	—	—	36.6	—
Drum & Thigh	346	643	35	46	35	180	25.5	0.25	0.32	8.5	—	—	36.6	—
Extra Crispy Dinner*														
Wing & Rib	349	755	33	60	43	132	25.5	0.31	0.29	10.4	—	—	36.6	—
Wing & Thigh	371	812	36	58	48	176	25.5	0.31	0.35	10.3	—	—	36.6	—
Drum & Thigh	376	765	38	55	44	183	25.5	0.32	0.38	10.4	—	—	36.6	—
Mashed Potatoes	85	64	2	12	1	0	<18	<0.01	0.02	0.8	—	—	4.9	—
Gravy	14	23	0	1	2	0	<3	0.00	0.01	0.1	—	—	<0.2	—
Cole Slaw	91	122	1	13	8	7	—	—	—	—	—	—	—	
Rolls	21	61	2	11	1	1	<5	0.10	0.04	1.0	—	—	0.3	—
Corn (5.5-in ear)	135	169	5	31	3	X	162	0.12	0.07	1.2	—	—	2.6	—

*Includes two pieces of chicken, mashed potato and gravy, cole slaw, and roll. From Kentucky Fried Chicken, Inc. Louisville, Ky. Nutritional analysis by Raltech Scientific

Long John Silver's

	Wt (g)	Energy (kcal)	PRO (g)	CHO (g)	Fat (g)	Chol (mg)	A (IU)	B_1 (mg)	B_2 (mg)	Nia. (mg)	B_6 (mg)	B_{12} (µg)	C (mg)	D (IU)
Fish w/Batter (2 pc)	136	366	22	21	22	—	—	—	—	—	—	—	—	—
Fish w/Batter (3 pc)	207	549	32	32	32	—	—	—	—	—	—	—	—	—
Treasure Chest	143	506	30	32	33	—	—	—	—	—	—	—	—	—
Chicken Planks (4 pc)	166	457	27	35	23	—	—	—	—	—	—	—	—	—
Peg Legs w/Batter (5 pc)	125	350	22	26	28	—	—	—	—	—	—	—	—	—
Ocean Scallops (6 pc)	120	283	11	30	13	—	—	—	—	—	—	—	—	—
Shrimp w/Batter (6 pc)	88	268	8	30	13	—	—	—	—	—	—	—	—	—
Breaded Oysters (6 pc)	156	441	13	53	19	—	—	—	—	—	—	—	—	—
Breaded Clams	142	617	18	61	34	—	—	—	—	—	—	—	—	—
Fish Sandwich	193	337	22	49	31	—	—	—	—	—	—	—	—	—
French Fryes	85	288	4	33	16	—	—	—	—	—	—	—	—	—
Cole Slaw	113	138	1	16	8	—	—	—	—	—	—	—	—	—
Corn on the Cob (1 ear)	150	176	5	29	4	—	—	—	—	—	—	—	—	—
Hushpuppies (3)	45	153	3	20	7	—	—	—	—	—	—	—	—	—
Clam Chowder (8 oz)	170	107	5	15	3	—	—	—	—	—	—	—	—	—

From Long John Silver's Food Shoppes, Lexington, Ky. Nutritional analysis by L.V. Packett, PhD., The Department of Nutrition and Food Science, University of Kentucky.

McDonald's

	Wt (g)	Energy (kcal)	PRO (g)	CHO (g)	Fat (g)	Chol (mg)	A (IU)	B_1 (mg)	B_2 (mg)	Nia. (mg)	B_6 (mg)	B_{12} (µg)	C (mg)	D (IU)
Egg McMuffin	138	327	19	31	15	229	97	0.47	0.44	3.8	0.21	0.75	<1.4	46
English Muffin, Buttered	63	186	5	30	5	13	164	0.28	0.49	2.6	0.04	0.02	0.8	14
Hotcakes w/Butter & Syrup	214	500	8	94	10	47	257	0.26	0.36	2.3	0.12	0.19	4.7	5
Sausage (Pork)	53	206	9	tr	19	43	<32	0.27	0.11	2.1	0.18	0.53	0.5	31
Scrambled Eggs	98	180	13	3	13	349	652	0.08	0.47	0.2	0.19	0.93	1.2	65
Hashbrown Potatoes	55	125	2	14	7	7	<14	0.06	<0.01	0.8	0.13	0.01	4.1	<1
Big Mac	204	563	26	41	33	86	530	0.39	0.37	6.5	0.27	1.8	2.2	33
Cheeseburger	115	307	15	30	14	37	345	0.25	0.23	3.8	0.12	0.91	1.6	13
Hamburger	102	255	12	30	10	25	82	0.25	0.18	4.0	0.12	0.81	1.7	12
Quarter Pounder	166	424	24	33	22	67	133	0.32	0.28	6.5	0.27	1.88	<1.7	23
Quarter Pounder w/Ch	194	524	30	32	31	96	660	0.31	0.37	7.4	0.23	2.15	2.7	25
Filet-O-Fish	139	432	14	37	25	47	42	0.26	0.20	2.6	0.10	0.82	<1.4	25
Regular Fries	68	220	3	26	12	9	<17	0.12	0.02	2.3	0.22	<0.03	12.5	<1
Apple Pie	85	253	2	29	14	12	<34	0.02	0.02	0.2	0.02	<0.04	<0.8	2
Cherry Pie	88	260	2	32	14	13	114	0.03	0.02	0.4	0.02	<0.02	<0.8	<2
McDonaldland Cookies	67	308	4	49	11	10	<27	0.23	0.23	2.9	0.03	0.03	0.9	10
Chocolate Shake	291	383	10	66	9	30	349	0.12	0.44	0.5	0.13	1.16	<2.9	44
Strawberry Shake	290	362	9	62	9	32	377	0.12	0.44	0.4	0.14	1.16	4.1	32
Vanilla Shake	291	352	9	60	8	31	349	0.12	0.70	0.3	0.12	1.19	3.2	26

		Minerals							Crude
Ca (mg)	Cu (mg)	Fe (mg)	K (mg)	Mg (mg)	P (mg)	Na (mg)	Zn (mg)	Moisture (g)	Fiber (g)
260	0.14	4.0	237	29	397	975	2.3	94	0.2
276	0.13	3.6	208	26	370	899	2.1	88	0.2
278	0.14	3.8	260	29	372	1098	2.0	117	0.4
119	0.11	3.0	194	27	256	1130	1.8	78	0.9
105	0.12	2.8	237	36	633	1670	1.9	104	0.7
257	0.24	5.0	635	55	483	1110	3.0	137	1.3

Scientific Services, Inc. (formerly WARF), Madison, Wis.

—	—	—	—	—	—	—	—	—	—
—	—	—	—	—	—	—	—	—	—
—	—	—	—	—	—	—	—	—	—
—	—	—	—	—	—	—	—	—	—
—	—	—	—	—	—	—	—	—	—
—	—	—	—	—	—	—	—	—	—
—	—	—	—	—	—	—	—	—	—
—	—	—	—	—	—	—	—	—	—
—	—	—	—	—	—	—	—	—	—
—	—	—	—	—	—	—	—	—	—

Services, Inc. (formerly WARF). Madison, Wis.

—	—	—	—	—	—	—	—	—	—
—	—	—	—	—	—	—	—	—	—
—	—	—	—	—	—	—	—	—	—
—	—	—	—	—	—	—	—	—	—
—	—	—	—	—	—	—	—	—	—
—	—	—	—	—	—	—	—	—	—
—	—	—	—	—	—	—	—	—	—
—	—	—	—	—	—	—	—	—	—
—	—	—	—	—	—	—	—	—	—
—	—	—	—	—	—	—	—	—	—
—	—	—	—	—	—	—	—	—	—
—	—	—	—	—	—	—	—	—	—
—	—	—	—	—	—	—	—	—	—
—	—	—	—	—	—	—	—	—	—
—	—	—	—	—	—	—	—	—	—

226	0.12	2.9	168	26	322	885	1.9	70.7	0.1
117	0.69	1.5	71	13	74	318	0.5	21.7	0.1
103	0.11	2.2	187	28	501	1070	0.7	97.8	0.2
16	0.05	0.8	127	9	95	615	1.5	22.9	0.1
61	0.06	2.5	135	13	264	205	1.7	68.1	<0.1
5	0.04	0.4	247	13	67	325	0.2	30.9	0.3
157	0.18	4.0	237	38	314	1010	4.7	100.4	0.6
132	0.11	2.4	156	23	205	767	2.6	108.4	0.2
51	0.10	2.3	142	19	126	520	2.1	48.0	0.3
63	0.17	4.1	322	37	249	735	5.1	83.7	0.7
219	0.18	4.3	341	41	382	1236	5.7	96.0	0.8
93	0.10	1.7	150	27	229	781	0.9	59.5	0.1
9	0.03	0.6	564	27	101	109	0.3	25.4	0.5
14	0.05	0.6	39	6	27	398	0.2	38.3	0.3
12	0.06	0.6	35	7	27	427	0.2	38.9	0.1
12	0.07	1.5	52	11	74	358	0.3	2.2	0.1
320	0.19	0.8	580	49	335	300	1.4	203.0	0.3
322	0.07	0.2	423	31	313	207	1.2	207.9	<0.3
329	0.09	0.2	422	31	314	201	1.2	211.3	<0.3

	Wt (g)	Energy (kcal)	PRO (g)	CHO (g)	Fat (g)	Chol (mg)	Vitamins A (IU)	B$_1$ (mg)	B$_2$ (mg)	Nia. (mg)	B$_6$ (mg)	B$_{12}$ (μg)	C (mg)	D (IU)
Hot Fudge Sundae	164	310	7	46	11	18	230	0.07	0.31	1.1	0.13	0.7	2.5	16
Caramel Sundae	165	328	7	53	10	26	279	0.07	0.31	1.0	0.05	0.6	3.6	14
Strawberry Sundae	164	289	7	46	9	20	230	0.07	0.30	1.0	0.05	0.6	2.8	16

From McDonald's Corporation, Oak Brook, Ill. Nutritional analysis by Raltech Scientific Services, Inc. (formerly WARF), Madison, Wis.

Taco Bell

	Wt (g)	Energy (kcal)	PRO (g)	CHO (g)	Fat (g)	Chol (mg)	A (IU)	B$_1$ (mg)	B$_2$ (mg)	Nia. (mg)	B$_6$ (mg)	B$_{12}$ (μg)	C (mg)	D (IU)
Bean Burrito	166	343	11	48	12	—	1657	0.37	0.22	2.2	—	—	15.2	—
Beef Burrito	184	466	30	37	21	—	1675	0.30	0.39	7.0	—	—	15.2	—
Beefy Tostada	184	291	19	21	15	—	3450	0.16	0.27	3.3	—	—	12.7	—
Bellbeefer	123	221	15	23	7	—	2961	0.15	0.20	3.7	—	—	10.0	—
Bellbeefer w/Ch	137	278	19	23	12	—	3146	0.16	0.27	3.7	—	—	10.0	—
Burrito Supreme	225	457	21	43	22	—	3462	0.33	0.35	4.7	—	—	16.0	—
Combination Burrito	175	404	21	43	16	—	1666	0.34	0.31	4.6	—	—	15.2	—
Enchirito	207	454	25	42	21	—	1178	0.31	0.37	4.7	—	—	9.5	—
Pintos'N Cheese	158	168	11	21	5	—	3123	0.26	0.16	0.9	—	—	9.3	—
Taco	83	186	15	14	8	—	120	0.09	0.16	2.9	—	—	0.2	—
Tostada	138	179	9	25	6	—	3152	0.18	0.15	0.8	—	—	9.7	—

From (menu item portions) San Antonio, Tex.: Taco Bell Co., July 1976; Adams C.F.: Nutritive value of American foods in common units, in *Handbook No. 456.* H.N., eds.: Food values of portions commonly used, ed. 12, Philadelphia, 1975, J.B. Lippincott Co.; Valley Baptist Medical Center. Food Service Department: Descriptions

Wendy's

	Wt (g)	Energy (kcal)	PRO (g)	CHO (g)	Fat (g)	Chol (mg)	A (IU)	B$_1$ (mg)	B$_2$ (mg)	Nia. (mg)	B$_6$ (mg)	B$_{12}$ (μg)	C (mg)	D (IU)
Single Hamburger	200	470	26	34	26	70	94	0.24	0.36	5.8	—	—	0.6	—
Double Hamburger	285	670	44	34	40	125	128	0.43	0.54	10.6	—	—	1.5	—
Triple Hamburger	360	850	65	33	51	205	220	0.47	0.68	14.7	—	—	2.0	—
Single w/Ch	240	580	33	34	34	90	221	0.38	0.43	6.3	—	—	0.7	—
Double w/Ch	325	800	50	41	48	155	439	0.49	0.75	11.4	—	—	2.3	—
Triple w/Ch	400	1040	72	35	68	225	472	0.80	0.84	15.1	—	—	3.4	—
Chili	250	230	19	21	8	25	1188	0.22	0.25	3.4	—	—	2.9	—
French Fries	120	330	5	41	16	5	40	0.14	0.07	3.0	—	—	6.4	—
Frosty	250	390	9	54	16	45	355	0.20	0.60	X	O	X	0.7	—

From Wendy's International, Inc. Dublin, Ohio. Nutritional analysis by Medallion Laboratories, Minneapolis, Minn.

	Wt (g)	Energy (kcal)	PRO (g)	CHO (g)	Fat (g)	Chol (mg)	Vitamins A (IU)	B$_1$ (mg)	B$_2$ (mg)	Nia. (mg)	B$_6$ (mg)	B$_{12}$ (μg)	C (mg)	D (IU)
Beverages														
Coffee*	180	2	tr	tr	tr	—	0	0	tr	0.5	—	—	0	—
Tea*	180	2	tr	—	tr	—	0	0	0.04	0.1	—	—	1	—
Orange Juice	183	82	1	20	tr	—	366	0.17	0.02	0.6	—	—	82.4	—
Chocolate Milk	250	213	9	28	9	—	330	0.08	0.40	0.3	—	—	3.0	—
Skim Milk	245	88	9	13	tr	—	10	0.09	0.44	0.2	—	—	2.0	—
Whole Milk	244	159	9	12	9	27	342	0.07	0.41	0.2	—	—	2.4	100
Coca-Cola	246	96	0	24	0	—	—	—	—	—	—	—	—	—
Fanta Ginger Ale	244	84	0	21	0	—	—	—	—	—	—	—	—	—
Fanta Grape	247	114	0	29	0	—	—	—	—	—	—	—	—	—
Fanta Orange	248	117	0	30	0	—	—	—	—	—	—	—	—	—
Fanta Root Beer	246	103	0	27	0	—	—	—	—	—	—	—	—	—
Mr. Pibb	245	95	0	25	0	—	—	—	—	—	—	—	—	—
Mr. Pibb w/o Sugar	236	1	0	tr	0	—	—	—	—	—	—	—	—	—
Sprite	245	95	0	24	0	—	—	—	—	—	—	—	—	—
Sprite w/o Sugar	236	3	0	0	0	—	—	—	—	—	—	—	—	—
Tab	236	tr	0	tr	0	—	—	—	—	—	—	—	—	—
Fresca	236	2	0	0	0	—	—	—	—	—	—	—	—	—

From Adams, C.F.: Nutritive value of American foods in common units, in *Handbook No. 456.* Washington: U.S.D.A. Agricultural Research *American Hospital Formulary Service,* Washington, D.C., American Society of Hospital Pharmacists, Section 28:20, March 1978.
*6 oz serving; all other data are for 8 oz serving.
†Caffeine content depends on strength of beverage.
‡Value when bottling water with average sodium content (12 mg/8 oz) is used.

Ca (mg)	Cu (mg)	Fe (mg)	K (mg)	Mg (mg)	P (mg)	Na (mg)	Zn (mg)	Moisture (g)	Crude Fiber (g)
				Minerals					
215	0.13	0.6	410	35	236	175	1.0	97.9	0.2
200	0.09	0.2	338	30	230	195	0.9	93.2	<0.2
174	0.11	0.4	290	28	80	96	0.8	101.0	0.2
98	—	2.8	235	—	173	272	—	—	—
83	—	4.6	320	—	288	327	—	—	—
208	—	3.4	277	—	265	138	—	—	—
40	—	2.6	183	—	140	231	—	—	—
147	—	2.7	195	—	208	330	—	—	—
121	—	3.8	350	—	245	367	—	—	—
91	—	3.7	278	—	230	300	—	—	—
259	—	3.8	491	—	338	1175	—	—	—
150	—	2.3	307	—	210	102	—	—	—
120	—	2.5	143	—	175	79	—	—	—
191	—	2.3	172	—	186	101	—	—	—

Washington USDA. Agricultural Research Service. November 1975; Church, E.F., and Church, of Mexican-American Foods. Fort Atkinson, Wis., NASCO.

Ca	Cu	Fe	K	Mg	P	Na	Zn	Moisture	Crude Fiber
84	—	5.3	—	—	239	774	4.8	110.6	0.8
138	—	8.2	—	—	364	980	8.4	162.1	1.1
104	—	10.7	—	—	525	1217	13.5	204.6	1.4
228	—	5.4	—	—	315	1085	5.5	133.4	1.0
177	—	10.2	—	—	489	1414	10.1	179.2	1.3
371	—	10.9	—	—	712	1848	14.3	216.4	1.6
83	—	4.4	—	—	168	1065	3.7	195.9	2.3
16	—	1.2	—	—	196	112	0.5	54.9	1.2
270	—	0.9	—	—	278	247	1.0	169.8	0.0

Ca (mg)	Cu (mg)	Fe (mg)	K (mg)	Mg (mg)	P (mg)	Na (mg)	Zn (mg)	Caffeine (mg)	Sacchar. (mg)
				Minerals					
4	—	0.2	65	—	7	2	—	100†	0
5	—	0.2	—	—	4	—	—	40†	0
17	—	0.2	340	18	29	2	—	0	0
278	—	0.5	365	—	235	118	—	—	0
296	—	0.1	355	—	233	127	—	—	0
188	—	tr	351	32	227	122	—	—	0
—	—	—	—	—	40	20‡	—	28	0
—	—	—	—	—	0	30‡	—	0	0
—	—	—	—	—	0	21‡	—	0	0
—	—	—	—	—	0	21‡	—	0	0
—	—	—	—	—	0	23‡	—	0	0
—	—	—	—	—	29	23‡	—	27	0
—	—	—	—	—	28	37‡	—	38	76
—	—	—	—	—	0	42‡	—	0	0
—	—	—	—	—	0	42‡	—	0	57
—	—	—	—	—	30	30‡	—	30	74
—	—	—	—	—	0	38	—	0	54

Service, November 1975; The Coca-Cola Company, Atlanta, Ga., Jan. 1977;

H

Food Guide:
Exchange Lists for Meal Planning

The *exchange system of dietary control*, developed by professional organizations such as the American Dietetic Association, is based on a simple grouping of common foods according to generally equivalent nutritional values. This system may be used for any situation requiring caloric and food value control.

The foods are divided into six basic groups (some with subgroups), called the "exchange groups" (pp. 402-403). Each food item within a group or subgroup contains approximately the same food value as any other food item in that group, allowing for exchange within groups, thus providing for variety in food choices as well as food value control. Hence the term *food exchanges* is used to refer to food choices or servings. The total number of exchanges per day depends on individual nutritional needs, based on normal nutritional standards. Although there is some variation in the composition of foods within the exchange groups, for simplicity the following values for carbohydrate, protein fat, and calories are used.

Food	Approximate Measure	Carbohydrate (g)	Protein (g)	Fat (g)	Calories
Milk exchanges	1 cup				
A (nonfat)		12	8	—	80
B (low fat)		12	8	5	125
C (full fat)		12	8	10	170
Vegetable exchanges	½ cup	5	2	—	25
Fruit exchanges	Varies	10	—	—	40
Bread exchanges	1 slice	15	2	—	70
Meat exchanges	28 g (1 oz)				
A (lean)		—	7	3	55
B (medium fat)		—	7	6	78
C (high fat)		—	7	8	100
Fat exchanges	1 tsp				
A (unsaturated)		—	—	5	45
B (monounsaturated)		—	—	5	45
C (saturated)		—	—	5	45

List 1: Milk exchanges (Cream portion of whole milk equals two fat exchanges. Hence 1 cup whole milk equals 1 cup skim milk plus two fat exchanges.)

Group A (nonfat)	
Skim or nonfat milk	1 cup
Buttermilk	1 cup
Canned, evaporated skim milk	½ cup
Powdered, nonfat dry milk (before adding liquid)	⅓ cup
Yogurt made from skim milk (plain, unflavored)	1 cup
Group B (low fat)	
Low-fat milk (2% butterfat)	1 cup
Yogurt made from low-fat milk (plain, unflavored)	1 cup

Food	Approximate Measure	Carbohydrate (g)	Protein (g)	Fat (g)	Calories
Group C (full fat)					
Whole milk	1 cup				
Canned, evaporated whole milk	½ cup				
Powdered, whole dry milk (before adding liquid)	⅓ cup				
Yogurt made from whole milk (plain, unflavored)	1 cup				

List 2: Vegetable exchanges (As served plain, without fat, seasoning, or dressing. Any fat used is taken from the fat exchange allowance.)

(One exchange equals ½ cup)

Artichoke	Green pepper, chili pepper	Pimientos
Asparagus	Greens	Rhubarb
Bok choy, gai choy	Beet	Rutabagas
Bamboo shoots	Chard	Sauerkraut
Bean sprouts	Collards	String beans: green, yellow, wax
Beets	Dandelion	Summer squash
Broccoli	Kale	Tomato juice
Brussels sprouts	Mustard	Tomatoes
Cabbage	Spinach	Turnips
Carrots	Turnip	Vegetable juice, mixed
Cauliflower	Mushrooms	Zucchini
Celery	Okra	
Cucumber	Onions	
Eggplant		

Vegetables for use as desired: chicory, Chinese cabbage, endive, escarole, lettuce, parsley, radishes, and watercress. For starchy vegetables, see List 4.

List 3: Fruit exchanges (Unsweetened: fresh, frozen, canned, cooked. One exchange is the portion indicated by the fruit.)

Berries			*Other fruits*	
Blackberries	½ cup		Apple	1 small
Blueberries	½ cup		Apple cider	⅓ cup
Raspberries	½ cup		Apple juice	⅓ cup
Strawberries	¾ cup		Applesauce	½ cup
Citrus fruits			Apricots	2 medium
Grapefruit	½ small		Banana	½ small
Grapefruit juice	½ cup		Cherries	10 large, 17 small
Orange	1 small		Fig	1 large
Orange juice	½ cup		Fruit cocktail	½ cup
Tangerine	1 medium		Grape juice	¼ cup
Melons			Grapes	10 medium
Cantaloupe	¼ medium		Kiwi fruit	1 medium
Honeydew	⅛ medium		Mango	½ small
Watermelon	1 cup diced (approx. ½ center slice)		Nectarine	1 small
			Papaya	⅓ medium, ½ small
Dried fruits			Peach	1 medium
Apricots	4 halves		Pear	1 medium
Dates	2 medium		Persimmon	1 medium
Figs	1 medium		Pineapple	½ cup; 1 round center slice
Peaches	2 halves			
Pears	2 halves		Pineapple juice	⅓ cup
Prunes	2 medium		Plums	2 medium
Raisins	2 tbsp		Prune juice	¼ cup
			Prunes, fresh	2 medium

Food	Approximate Measure	Carbohydrate (g)	Protein (g)	Fat (g)	Calories

List 4: Bread exchanges (Equivalent portions indicated by each item.)

Bread

Food	Approximate Measure
Bagel	½
Bread (loaf, average size slice)	1 slice
French	
Italian	
Pumpernickel	
Raisin	
Rye	
White	
Whole wheat	
Bread crumbs, dried	3 tbsp
English muffin	½
Hamburger bun	½
Roll, frankfurter	1
Roll, plain	1 small
Tortilla (6 inches diameter)	1

Cereal

Food	Approximate Measure
Bulgur, cooked	½ cup
Cereal, cooked	½
Cereal, dry (ready-to-eat, unsweetened)	
Bran flakes	½ cup
Grape nuts	¼ cup
Other (flake, puff)	¾ cup
Cornmeal, dry	2 tbsp
Flour	2½ tbsp
Grits, cooked	½ cup
Pasta, cooked (spaghetti, noodles, macaroni)	½ cup
Popcorn (popped, no fat)	1½ cup
Rice, cooked	½ cup
Wheat germ, plain	3 tbsp

Crackers

Food	Approximate Measure
Arrowroot	3
Graham, 2½-in square	2
Matzoth, 4 × 6 in	1
Oyster crackers	20
Pretzels, 3⅛ × ⅛ in	25
Round butter type crackers	6
Rye wafers, 2 × 3½ in	3
Saltines	5
Soda crackers, 2½-in square	3

Dried beans, peas, lentils

Food	Approximate Measure
Beans, peas, lentils (dried and cooked)	⅓ cup
Baked beans, no pork	¼ cup

Starchy vegetables

Food	Approximate Measure
Corn	⅓ cup
Corn on the cob (6-in ear)	½ ear
Lima beans	½ cup
Parsnips	½ cup
Peas, green	½ cup
Potato, white	1 small
Potato, white mashed	½ cup
Pumpkin	1 cup
Sweet potato	½ small; ⅓ cup
Winter squash (acorn, butternut, banana)	½ cup
Yam	½ small; ⅓ cup

Prepared foods

Food	Approximate Measure
Angel food cake (1½-in cube or small slice)	1 slice
Biscuit, 2-in diameter (omit 1 fat exchange)	1
Chips, potato or corn (omit 2 fat exchanges)	15
Corn muffin, 2-in diameter (omit 1 fat exchange)	1
Cornbread, 2 × 2 × 1¼ in (omit 1 fat exchange)	1 square
Crepe, 6-in diameter (omit 1 fat exchange)	1
Ice milk, ½ cup scoop (omit 1 fat exchange)	1 scoop
Muffin, plain, 2-in diameter (omit 1 fat exchange)	1
Pancakes, 4-in diameter (omit 1 fat exchange)	1
Potatoes, french fried (length 2-3 in; omit 1 fat exchange)	8 pieces
Sherbet, fruit ice, ½-cup scoop	1 scoop
Waffle, 4-in diameter (omit 1 fat exchange)	1

Food	Approximate Measure	Carbohydrate (g)	Protein (g)	Fat (g)	Calories
List 5: Meat exchanges					
Group A (lean)					
I. Lean meats, less tissue fat					
Fish (any fresh or frozen)	28 g (1 oz)				
Canned salmon, tuna, mackerel	¼ cup				
Sardines, drained	3				
Shellfish					
Clams, oysters, scallops	5				
Crab, lobster	¼ cup				
Poultry (no skin)	28 g				
Chicken, turkey, cornish hen, guinea hen, pheasant					
Veal (any lean trimmed cut)	28 g				
II. Lean meats, more tissue fat					
Beef	28 g				
Very lean young beef; chipped beef; lean cuts of chuck, flank steak, tender loin, plate ribs and skirt steak, round (top, bottom), rump, spare ribs, tripe					
Lamb	28 g				
Lean cuts: leg, rib, sirloin, loin (roast, chops), shank, shoulder					
Pork	28 g				
Lean cuts of leg (rump, center shank), ham (smoked center cut)					
III. Cheese	28 g				
Cottage cheese	¼ cup				
Dry curd					
Low fat, partially re-creamed					
Other cheeses	28 g				
Less than 5% butterfat; partially skim milk					
Group B (medium fat)					
Beef	28 g				
Ground (15% fat), corned beef (canned)					
Pork	28 g				
Loin (roast, chops), shoulder arm (picnic), shoulder blade, Boston butt, Canadian bacon, boiled ham					
Cheese	28 g				
Mozzarella, ricotta, Swiss, Jack, farmer's cheese, Neufchâtel					
Parmesan	3 tbsp				
Cottage cheese, re-creamed	¼ cup				
Cholesterol foods					
Egg	1				
Organ meats	28 g				
Liver, kidney, sweetbreads, heart					
Shrimp	5 large				
Other					
Peanut butter (omit 2 fat exchanges)	2 tbsp				
Tofu	98 g (3½ oz)				
Group C (high fat)					
Beef	28 g				
Brisket (fresh or corned), ground (20% or more fat)					
Lamb breast	28 g				
Pork	28 g				
Spare ribs, back ribs, ground pork, sausage, country style ham, deviled ham					
Cheese, cheddar types	28 g				
Cold cuts	1 slice				
Frankfurter	1 small				
Poultry	28 g				
Capon duck, goose					

Food	Approximate Measure	Carbohydrate (g)	Protein (g)	Fat (g)	Calories
List 6: Fat exchanges					
Group A (polyunsaturated plant fats)					
Margarine,* soft (stick or tub)	1 tsp				
Mocha mix (cream substitute)	2 tbsp				
Salad dressings*					
French	1 tbsp				
Italian	1 tbsp				
Mayonnaise	1 tsp				
Seeds (sunflower, sesame, pumpkin)	1 tbsp				
Vegetable oils (safflower, corn, soy, cottonseed, sesame)	1 tsp				
Walnuts	4-5 halves				
Group B (monounsaturated plant fats)					
Avocado	⅛				
Nuts					
Almonds	10 whole				
Peanuts	20 whole				
Pecans	2 whole				
Olives	5 small				
Vegetable oils (olive, peanut)	1 tsp				
Group C (saturated animal fats)					
Butter	1 tsp				
Cheese spreads	1 tbsp				
Cream					
Half & Half (10% cream)	2 tbsp				
Light (20% cream)	2 tbsp				
Heavy (40% cream)	1 tbsp				
Sour (light)	2 tbsp				
Cream cheese	1 tbsp				
Pork fat					
Bacon crisp	1 strip				
Bacon fat	1 tsp				
Lard	1 tsp				
Salt pork	¾-in cube				

Miscellaneous foods allowed as desired (negligible carbohydrate, protein, fat)

Artificial sweeteners, as permitted	Gelatin, plain or D-Zerta
Bouillon, broth, clear fat free	Herbs and spices
Catsup, mustard, horseradish, meat sauce	Lemon, lime
Coffee, tea	Pickles, dill and sour
Cranberries, cranberry juice (unsweetened)	Salt and pepper
Garlic	Vinegar

*Made with safflower, corn, soy, cottonseed oil.

I

Calculation Aids and Conversion Tables

More than 185 years ago a group of French scientists set up the metric system of weights and measures. Today, with refinements over years of use, it is called the "Systeme International" (SI). In 1975 our American Congress passed the Metric Conversion Act, which provides for conversion of our customary British/American system to the simpler metric system used by the rest of the world. We are now in the midst of this conversion, as evidenced by distance signs along highways and labels on many packaged foods in supermarkets. Here are a few conversion factors to help you make these transitions in your necessary calculations.

Metric System of Measurement

Like our money system, this is a simple decimal system based on units of 10. It is uniform and used internationally.

Weight units: 1 kilogram (kg) = 1000 grams (gm or g)

1 g = 1000 milligrams (mg)

1 mg = 1000 micrograms (mcg or μg)

Length units: 1 meter (m) = 100 centimeters (cm)

1000 meters = 1 kilometer (km)

Volume units: 1 liter (L) = 1000 millimeters (ml)

1 milliliter = 1 cubic centimeter (cc)

Temperature units: Celsius (C) scale, based on 100 equal units between 0° C (freezing point of water) and 100° C (boiling point of water); this scale is used entirely in all scientific work.

Energy units: Kilocalorie (kcal) = Amount of energy required to raise

1 kg water 1° C

Kilojoule (kJ) = Amount of energy required to move

1 kg mass 1 m by a force of 1 newton

1 kcal = 4.184 kJ

In 1970 the American Institute of Nutrition's Committee on Nomenclature recommended that the term *kilojoule* (kJ) replace the kilocalorie (kcal). This change is gradually coming about.

British/American System of Measurement

Our customary system is a confusion of units with no uniform relationships. It is not a decimal system, but rather a jumbled collection of different units collected in usage and language over time. It is used mainly in America.

Weight units: 1 pound (lb) = 16 ounces (oz)

Length units: 1 foot (ft) = 12 inches (in)

1 yard (yd) = 3 feet (ft)

Volume units: 3 teaspoons (tsp) = 1 tablespoon (tbsp)

16 tbsp = 1 cup

1 cup = 8 fluid ounces (fl oz)

4 cups = 1 quart (qt)

5 cups = 1 imperial quart (qt), Canada

Approximate Metric
Conversions

When You Know	Multiply by	To Find
Weight		
Ounces	28	Grams
Pounds	0.45	Kilograms
Length		
Inches	2.5	Centimeters
Feet	30	Centimeters
Yards	0.9	Meters
Miles	1.6	Kilometers
Volume		
Teaspoons	5	Millimeters
Tablespoons	15	Millimeters
Fluid ounces	30	Millimeters
Cups	0.24	Liters
Pints	0.47	Liters
Quarts	0.95	Liters
Temperature		
Fahrenheit temperature	5/9 (after subtracting 32)	Celsius temperature

British/American System of Measurement, cont'd

Temperature units: Fahrenheit (F) scale, based on 180 equals units between 32° F (freezing point of water) and 212° F (boiling point of water) at standard atmospheric pressure

Conversions between Measurement Systems

Weight: 1 oz = 28.35 g (usually used as 28 or 30 g)
2.2 lb = 1 kg

Length: 1 in = 2.54 cm
1 ft = 30.48 cm
39.37 in = 1 m

Volume: 1.06 qt = 1 L
0.85 imperial qt = 1 L (Canada)

Temperature:

Boiling point of water	100° C	212° F
Body temperature	37° C	98.6° F
Freezing point of water	0° C	32° F

Interconversion formulas:

$$\text{Fahrenheit temperature (°F)} = \tfrac{9}{5}° \text{ C} + 32$$
$$\text{Celsius temperature (°C)} = \tfrac{5}{9} \text{ (°F} - 32)$$

Retinol Equivalents

The following definitions and equivalences that are internationally agreed on provide a basis for calculating retinol equivalent conversions.

Definitions International units (IU) and retinol equivalents (RE) are defined as follows:

$$1 \text{ IU} = 0.3 \ \mu g \text{ retinol } (0.0003 \text{ mg})$$
$$1 \text{ IU} = 0.6 \ \mu g \text{ beta-carotene } (0.0006 \text{ mg})$$
$$1 \text{ RE} = 6 \ \mu g \text{ retinol}$$
$$1 \text{ RE} = 6 \ \mu g \text{ beta-carotene}$$
$$1 \text{ RE} = 12 \ \mu g \text{ other provitamin A carotenoids}$$
$$1 \text{ RE} = 3.33 \text{ IU retinol}$$
$$1 \text{ RE} = 10 \text{ IU beta-carotene}$$

Conversion formulas On the basis of weight beta-carotene is ½ as active as retinol; on the basis of structure the other provitamin carotenoids are ¼ as active as retinol. In addition, retinol is more completely absorbed in the intestine, whereas the provitamin carotenoids are much less well utilized, with an average absorption of about ⅓. Therefore in overall activity beta-carotene is ⅙ as active as retinol, and the other carotenoids are ¹⁄₁₂ as active. These differences in utilization provide the basis for the 1:6:12 relationship shown in the equivalences given and in the following formulas for calculating retinol equivalents from values of vitamin A, beta-carotene, and other active carotenoids, expressed either as international units or micrograms:

If retinol and beta-carotene are given in micrograms:
Micrograms of retinol + (Micrograms of beta-carotene ÷ 6) = RE
If both are given as IU:
International units of retinol ÷ 3.33) + (International units of beta-carotene ÷ 10) = RE
If beta-carotene and other carotenoids are given in micrograms:
(Micrograms of beta-carotene ÷ 6) + (Micrograms of other carotenoids ÷ 12) = RE

Glossary

Pronunciation Key

ə	banana, collect
'ə, ˌə	humdrum
ə̄	as in one pronunciation used by r-droppers for **bi**rd (alternative \əi\)
ə̇	two-value symbol equivalent to the unstressed variants \ə\, \i\, as in ha**bit**, du**ch**ess (\'habə̇t\ = \'habət, -bit\)
ə	immediately preceding \l\, \n\, \m\, \ŋ\, as in bat**tle**, mit**ten**, and in one pronunciation of cap **and** bells \-ᵊam-\, lock **and** key \-ᵊŋ-\; immediately following \l\, \m\, \r\, as in one pronunciation of French tab**le**, pris**me**, tit**re**
əi	as in one pronunciation used by r-droppers for **bi**rd (alternative \ə̄\)
ər	op**er**ation; stressed, as in **bi**rd as pronounced by speakers who do not drop r; stressed and with centered period after the \r\, as in one pronunciation of **bur**ry (alternative \ə̄r\) and in one pronunciation of **hur**ry (alternative \ə·r\); stressed and with centered period between \ə\ and \r\, as in one pronunciation of **hur**ry (alternative \ər·\)
a	mat, map
ā	day, fade, date, aorta
ä	bother, cot; most American speakers have the same vowel in father, cart
ȧ	father as pronounced by speakers who do not rhyme it with bother; farther and cart as pronounced by r-droppers
aa	bad, bag, fan as often pronounced in an area having New York City and Washington, D.C., on its perimeter; in an emphatic syllable, as before a pause, often \aaə\
ai	as in some pronunciations of bag, bang, pass
aủ	now, loud, some pronunciations of talcum
b	baby, rib
ch	chin, nature \'nāchə(r)\ (actually, this sound is \t\ + \sh\)
d	elder, undone
d·	as in the usual American pronunciation of latter, ladder
e	bet, bed
'ē, ˌē	beat, nosebleed, evenly, sleepy
ē	as in one pronunciation of evenly, sleepy, envious, igneous (alternative \i\)
ee	(in transcriptions of foreign words only) indicates a vowel with the quality of e in bet but long, not the sound of ee in sleep: en arrière \äⁿ nȧryeer\
eủ	as in one pronunciation of elk, helm
f	fifty, cuff
g	go, big
h	hat, ahead
hw	whale as pronounced by those who do not have the same pronunciation for both whale and wall
i	tip, one pronunciation of banish (alternative unstressed \ē\), one pronunciation of habit (alternative \ə\; see ə̇)
ī	site, side, buy (actually, this sound is \ä\ + \i\, or \ȧ\ + \i\)
iủ	as in one pronunciation of milk, film
\	slant line used in pairs to mark the beginning and end of a transcription: \'pen\
'	mark preceding a syllable with primary (strongest) stress: \'penmənˌship\
ˌ	mark preceding a syllable with secondary (next-strongest) stress: \'penmənˌship\
ᵎ	combined marks preceding a syllable whose stress varies between primary and secondary: backbone \'=ˌ=\
_	inferior minus sign canceling a stress in the same position in a preceding pronunciation or emphasizing that a following syllable is without stress: optimism \'äptəˌmizəm\, optimist \-_məst\
·	mark of syllable division inserted in a sequence of sounds that can have more than one syllable division: nitrate \'nī·ˌtrāt\
(), (	indicate that what is symbolized between or after is present in some utterances but not in others: factory \'fakt(ə)rē\, bar \'bär, 'bȧ(r\
j	job, gem, edge, procedure \prə'sējə(r)\ (actually, this sound is \d\ + \zh\)
k	kin, cook, ache
ḵ	as in one pronunciation of loch (alternative \k\), as in German ich-laut
l	lily, pool
m	murmur, dim, nymph
n	no, own
ŋ	sing \'siŋ\, singer \'siŋə(r)\, finger \'fiŋgə(r)\, ink \'iŋk\

ō	bone, snow, beau; one pronunciation of glory
ȯ	saw, all, saurian; one pronunciation of horrid
œ	French bœuf, German Hölle
œ̄	French feu, German Höhle
ȯi	coin, destroy, strawy, sawing
o͞o	(in transcriptions of foreign words only) indicates a vowel with the quality of o in bone but longer, not the sound of oo in food: comte \koont\
p	pepper, lip
r	rarity, one pronunciation of tar
s	source, less
sh	with nothing between, as in shy, mission, machine, special (actually, this is a single sound, not two); with a stress mark between, two sounds as in death's-head \'deths,hed\
t	tie, attack; one pronunciation of latter (alternative \d·\
th	with nothing between, as in thin, either (actually, this is a single sound, not two); with a stress mark between, two sounds as in knighthood \'nīt,hu̇d\
<u>th</u>	then, either (actually, this is a single sound, not two)
ü	rule, fool, youth, union \'yünyən\, few \'fyü\

u̇	pull, wood, curable \'kyu̇rəbəl\
ᴜe	German füllen, hübsch
ᴜ̄e	French rue, German, fühlen
v	vivid, give
w	we, away
y	yard, cue \'kyü\, union \'yünyən\
ʸ	(in transcriptions of foreign words only) indicates that during the articulation of the sound represented by the preceding character the tip of the tongue has substantially the position it has for the articulation of the first sound of yard, as in French digne\dēnʸ\
yü	youth, union, cue, few
yu̇	curable
z	zone, raise
zh	with nothing between, as in vision, azure \'azhə(r)\ (actually, this is a single sound, not two); with a stress mark between, two sounds as in rosehill \'rōz,hil\
|	facilitates the placement of a variant pronunciation: flightily\'flīd·ᵊlē, -īt\, ᵊ\i, ǝi-\

Absorption \əb'sȯrpshən\ (L. ab, away; sorbere, to suck in) Process by which digested food materials pass through the epithelial cells of the alimentary canal (mainly of the small intestine) into the blood or lymph.

Acetone \'asə,tōn\ (acetic, sour; ketone) A by-product of the breakdown of fats for energy. It builds up when the body's glycogen stores are depleted, which happens when carbohydrate is not available for fuel. High urine levels are one sign of poor diabetes control.

Acetylation \ə,se·ᵊl'āshən\ Key reaction in cell metabolism, introduction of the monovalent acetyl group (—CH_3CO) into an organic compound.

Acetyl-CoA \ə'sēd·ᵊl\ (acetylcoenzyme A) (L. acetum, vinegar; Gr. hyle, matter; Gr. en, in; Gr. zyme, leaven) Chief precursor of lipids, an important intermediate in the Krebs' cycle; formed by an acetyl group attaching itself to coenzyme A during the oxidation of amino acids, fatty acids, or pyruvate.

Achlorhydria \,ā,klȯr'hīdrēə\ (Gr. a-, without; chlorohydria, excess gastric hydrochloric acid) Lack of hydrochloric acid (HCl) secretion in the stomach.

Acid \'asəd\ (L. acidus, sour) Substance that neutralizes base substances by donating H ions. Acids are essentially ionized hydrogen donors—in solution they provide H ions.

Acidosis \,asə'dōsəs\ Disturbance in acid-base balance in which there is a reduction of the alkali reserve. Acidosis may be caused by an accumulation of acids, as in diabetic acidosis, or by an excess loss of bicarbonate, as in renal disease.

Acinus \'asənəs\ pl. acini (L. acinus, grape) Groups of secretory cells in glands such as the salivary glands, the pancreas, and the liver. These organized clusters of cells are called acini because their shape resembles that of a bunch of grapes. Their secretions of enzymes and bile feed into the ducts that empty into the gastrointestinal lumen.

Actin \'aktən\ Myofibril protein that acts with myosin to cause the contraction and relaxation of muscle.

Active transport \aktiv tranz'pō(ə)rt\ Movement of solutes in solution (for example, products of digestion such as glucose) across a membrane against the usual opposing forces. Such movement requires energy, which is supplied by the cell. Sometimes an additional transporting substance is required, such as sodium, for absorbing glucose.

Acute renal failure \ə'kyüt 'rēnᵊl 'fālyə(r)\ Total shutdown of renal function; requires emergency treatment.

Adenocarcinoma \,adᵊn(,)o,kärsᵊn'ōmə\ Cancer derived from glandular tissue or in which tumor cells form recognizable glandular structures; may be classified according to predominant pattern of cell arrangement.

Adenosine triphosphate (ATP) \ə'denə,sēn (')trī'fä,sfāt\ A compound of adenosine (a nucleotide containing adenine and ribose) that has three phosphoric acid groups. ATP is a high-energy phosphate compound important in energy exchange for cellular activity. The splitting off of the terminal phosphate bond (PO_4) of ATP to produce adenosine diphosphate (ADP) releases bound energy and transfers it to free energy available for body work. The reforming of ATP in cell oxidation again stores energy in high-energy phosphate bonds for use as needed. They may be considered to act as biologic storage batteries that can be charged and discharged according to conditions in the cell.

Adipose \'adə,pōs\ (L. *adeps*, fat; *adiposus*, fatty) Fat present in cells of adipose—fatty—tissue.

Adrenergic \,adrə'nərjik\ Activated by or secreting adrenal hormones such as epinephrine or similar acting substances; characteristic of such substances.

Adult beriberi \ə'dəlt'berē'berē\ Typically occurs in young adults in reaction to added physiologic stress such as pregnancy or lactation.

Aerobic \'a(ə)'rōbik\ (Gr., L., *aer*, air or gas) Requiring oxygen to proceed.

Ageism \'ā(,)jizəm\ Discrimination on the basis of age, usually applying to older persons.

Aldosterone \al'dästə,rōn\ Potent hormone of the cortex of the adrenal glands, which acts on the distal renal tubule to cause reabsorption of sodium in an ion exchange with potassium. The aldosterone mechanism is essentially a sodium-conserving mechanism but indirectly also conserves water since water absorption follows the sodium reabsorption.

Alkalosis \,alkə'lōsəs\ Disturbance in acid-base balance in which there is a reduction of the acid partner in the buffer system or an increase in the base. In either case, the necessary 20:1 ratio between base and acid is upset by an increase in the relative amount of base.

Alpha-lipoprotein (HDL) \'alfə ,līpə'prō,tēn\ High-density lipoprotein that carries cholesterol to the liver to be excreted.

Alpha-tocopherol equivalent (αTE) \,alfə tə'käfə,rȯl ə'kwiv(ə)lənt\ Standard unit of measurement (in mg) for designating vitamin E requirements, since potencies of the other members of the vitamin E group vary; a change from the former measure of international units (IU) for greater precision and clarity.

Alveolus \al'vē'ə-ləs\ *pl.* alveoli (L., *alveus*, hollow) Small, dilated, saclike structures in the lungs; point of oxygen and carbon dioxide gas exchange during respiration.

Alzheimer's disease \'älts,hīmə(r)z də'zēz\ Named for a German neurologist, Alois Alzheimer; a form of senile dementia that may occur in middle as well as in old age.

Ameloblasts \'amələ,blast\ (Old Fr. *amel*, enamel; Gr. *blastos*, germ) Special epithelial cells surrounding tooth buds in gum tissue that form cup-shaped organs for producing the enamel structure of the developing teeth. Insufficient vitamin A causes faulty production of ameloblasts, and it therefore impairs the soundness of the tooth structure.

Amino acid \ə'mē(,)nō 'asəd\ These compounds form the structural units of protein. Out of a total of 20 or more, 10 are considered dietary essentials, indispensable to life (see *essential amino acid*). The term *amino* represents the presence of the NH_2 group—a base. The various food proteins, when digested, yield their specific constituent amino acids. These amino acids are then available for use by the cells as the cells synthesize specific tissue proteins.

Amphoteric \,amfə'terik\ (Gr. *amphoteros*, both) Having properties of both an acid and a base and therefore able to function as either. Amino acids have this dual chemical nature because of their structure—they contain both an acid (carboxyl, COOH) and a base (amino, NH_2) group.

Ampulla \am-pu'ə\ (L., "a jug") Flasklike dilation (stretched part) of a tubular structure.

Amylose \'amə,lōs\ (Gr. *amylon*, starch; *-ose*, sugar) Simple single sugar; a carbohydrate containing a single saccharide (sugar) unit.

Amylopectin \,amə(,)lō'pektən\ (Gr. *amylon*, starch; *pektos*, congealed) Polysaccharide, the insoluble part of starch, forms a paste with hot water and thickens during cooking.

Amyotropic lateral sclerosis \,ā,mīə'trōpik 'lad·ərəl sklə'rōsəs\ Muscular weakness and atrophy in the arm and hands caused by damage to motor neurons. Deterioration continues without remission.

Anabolism \ə'nabə,lizəm\ (Gr. *anabole*, a building up) Constructive metabolic processes that build up the body substances; the synthesis in living organisms of more complex substances from simpler ones. Anabolism *uses* energy; available energy generated by catabolic processes is taken up in forming the chemical bonds that unite the components of the increasingly complex molecules as they are developed in the anabolic processes. Anabolism is the opposite of catabolism.

Anachronism \ə'nakrə,nizəm\ (Gr. *anachronismos*, a wrong time reference) Thing placed or occurring out of its proper time; an obsolete or archaic form.

Anaerobic \,anə'rōbik\ (*an*, negative; Gr. *aer*, air) Not requiring oxygen to function.

Analog \'anəl,ȯg\ (or *analogue*) (Gr. *analogos*, due ratio, proportionate) In chemistry, a compound having a similar structure to that of another but differing in a particular component.

Analysis \ənəl'əsis\ (Gr. *ana*, so much of each; *lysis*, dissolve) Study of phenomena—things, events, etc.—by separating them into their component parts.

Anemia \ə'nēmēə\ Blood condition characterized by decrease in number of circulating red blood cells, hemoglobin, or both.

Anergy \'a,nərjē\ (*an* negative + G. *ergon*, work) Abnormal diminished reaction or sensitivity to specific antigens; often occurs in debilitated malnourished persons. A measure of degree of function of body's immune system.

Angina pectoris \an'jīnə 'pektərəs\ Chest pain, usually radiating down the arm, with a feeling of suffocation; caused most often by lack of oxygen to the heart muscle (myocardium), sometimes precipitated by effort or excitement.

Angiotensin \ˌanjēōtensin\ (Gr. *angeion*, vessel; L. *tensio*, stretching, pressure) Pressor substance produced in the body by interaction of the enzyme renin, produced by the renal cortex, and a serum globulin fraction, angiotensinogen, produced by the liver. Successive products are formed by the interaction—angiotensin I and II. Angiotensin II is the active pressure substance that increases arterial muscle tone and triggers the production of aldosterone by the adrenal gland. Angiotensin I and II therefore are key products in the cycle of the aldosterone mechanism.

Anion \'aˌnīən\ an ion that carries a negative electric charge.

Anorexia nervosa \ˌanō'reksēə (')ner'vōsə\ (Gr. "want of appetite"; *nervosa*, nervous) Psychologic condition manifested by a refusal to eat to achieve a thin—usually abnormally thin—appearance.

Antagonist \an·'tagə, nəst\ A substance that counteracts the action of another substance. The antagonist prevents the normal action because its molecular structure is so like that of the first substance that it *almost* fits into the first substance's position in a metabolic process. It gets in the way and prevents the reaction from taking place.

Anthropometry \ˌanˌ(t)thrə'pämətrē\ Science of measuring size, weight, and proportions of the human body.

Antibody \'antəˌbädē\ Animal protein made up of a specific sequence of amino acids that is designed to interact with a specific *antigen* during an allergic response or to prevent infection.

Antidiuretic hormone (ADH) \ˌanˌtəˌdiyəˌred·ik 'hȯr'mōn\ Secreted by the posterior pituitary gland in response to body stress. It acts on the renal tubules, chiefly the distal tubule, to cause reabsorption of water. The ADH mechanism is the body's primary water-conserving mechanism and is therefore essential to life; see also *vasopressin*.

Antigen \'antəjən\ (*antibody* + Gr. *gennan*, to produce) Any substance that stimulates the production of an antibody specifically designed to interact with it. Examples of antibodies include toxins, bacteria, and foreign proteins.

Antinutrient \ˌantə'n(y)ütrēənt\ (Gr. *anti-*, against) Substance acting to block normal use of a nutrient.

Antioxidant \ˌan(ˌ)tī'äksadənt\ A substance added to a product to delay or prevent its breakdown by oxygen.

Anuria \ə'n(y)ùrēa\ (*an*, negative + Gr. *ouron*, urine + -ia) Complete lack of urine secretion by the kidneys; also known as *anuresis*.

Apo- \ˌapō'\ (Gr. *apo*, from) Prefix implying separation or derivation.

Apoferritin \ˌapə'ferət'n\ (Gr. *apo*, away, separation; L. *ferr*, iron) Protein base in intestinal mucosa cells, which will bind with iron (from food) to form ferritin, the storage form of iron.

Apoprotein \ˌapō'protein\ Protein part of a compound, as of a lipoprotein. For example, apoprotein C II, an apoprotein of HDL and VLDL that functions to activate the enzyme lipoprotein lipase.

Ariboflavinosis \ˌˌāˌrībəˌflāvə'nōsəs\ Group of clinical manifestations of riboflavin deficiency.

Arteriosclerosis \ärˌtirēə(ˌ)ōskləˈrōsəs\ (*artery* + Gr. *skleros*, hard) Group of cardiovascular diseases, the major one of which is atherosclerosis: characterized by a thickening of the arterial walls and their loss of elasticity.

Ascites \ə'sīd·ēz\ (Gr. *askites*, from; *askos*, bag) Outflow and accumulation of fluid in the abdominal cavity; also known as *abdominal* or *peritoneal dropsy*.

Asterixis \astərixəs\ (*a*, negative + Gr. *sterixis*, a fixed position) Motor disturbance marked by a temporary lapse of an assumed position; result of a sustained contraction in a group of muscles.

Atheroma \ˌathə'rōmə\ Characteristic lesion of atherosclerosis; tumor-type growths on inside lining of blood vessels, composed of lipid material (largely cholesterol) and cellular debris.

Atherosclerosis \ˌathə(ˌ)rōsklō'rōsəs\ (Gr. *athere*, gruel, *sklerosis*, hardness) Condition in which yellowish plaques (atheromas) are deposited within the medium and large arteries.

Atrophy \'a·trəfē\ (Gr. *atrophia*) Wasting away; reduced size of a cell, tissue, or organ.

Azotemia \ˌazə'tēmēə\ (Gr. *a*, without; *zoe*, life) Term meaning nitrogen, referring to an excess of urea and other nitrogenous substances in the blood.

Bacteriuria \(ˌ)bakˌtirē'yùrēa\ (*bacteria* + Gr. *ouron*, urine + -ia) Presence of bacteria in the urine.

Basal ganglion \'bāsəlˌganglēon\ *pl.* ganglia (basal = base; Gr. *ganglion*, knot) Group of nerve cells found deep in the cerebral hemispheres of the brain and in the upper brainstem.

Basal metabolic rate (BMR) \'bāsəl med·əˌbälik 'rāt\ Rate of internal chemical activity of resting tissue.

Basal metabolism \'bāsəl mə'tabəˌlizəm\ (Gr. *basis*, base; *metabole*, change) The amount of energy needed by the body for maintenance of life when the person is at digestive, physical, and emotional rest. The amount of oxygen consumed at rest is used as a measure of the basal energy requirements and is expressed as kilocalories per square meter of body surface per hour. This basal metabolic rate (BMR) is reported as the percent of variation in the person above or below the normal number of kilocalories required for a person of like height, weight, and sex.

Base \'bās\ Chemical substance that is capable of neutralizing acid by accepting hydrogen ions from the acid. A synonymous term is *alkali*.

Base bicarbonate \,bās (')bī'kärbə,nāt\ "Base" in this term refers to *any* base that might be combined with bicarbonate. In the main buffer system of the human body, this base is sodium bicarbonate.

Beikost \'bīkȯst\ (Ger.) Solid and semisolid baby foods.

Benign \bə'nīn\ Not malignant or recurring.

Beriberi \'berē'berē\ (Singhalese "I cannot, I cannot") A disease of the peripheral nerves caused by a deficiency of thiamin (vitamin B_1). It is characterized by pain (neuritis) and paralysis of the extremities, cardiovascular changes and edema. Beriberi is common in the Orient, where diets consist largely of milled rice with little protein.

Bile \'bīl\ (L. *bilis*) Greenish yellow to golden brown alkaline fluid secreted by the liver and concentrated in the gallbladder, made of bile salts, cholesterol, phospholipid, bilirubin diglucuronide, and electrolytes. Bile salts are essential in the digestion and absorption of fat in the small intestine.

Binary digit (bit) \'bīnərē 'dijət\ Smallest unit of computer information; several bits make up a letter, number, or word. Eight bits = one byte.

Bioavailability \bī(,)ōə'vālə'biləd·ē\ Degree to which the amount of a nutrient ingested actually gets absorbed and is available to the body.

Bioflavonoid \'bīō'flāvə,nȯid\ (L. *flavus*, yellow) Compounds that are widely distributed in nature as pigments in flowers, fruits, tree barks, vegetables, and grains. They have been found to have little nutritional value, and thus are not considered essential nutrients.

Biologic activity \'bīə'läjik ak'tivəd·ē\ Degree of effect in an organism of a specific vitamin; a means of measuring required amount of a vitamin to prevent a deficiency.

Blastocyst \'blastō,sist\ (Gr. *blastos*, bud, sprout; *kystis*, bag, bladder) Early developmental stage of the embryo; consists of a single layer of cells surrounding a central area.

Blood urea nitrogen (BUN) \'blod yə'rēə 'nī·trəjən\ Blood test used to identify any disorder in kidney function.

Body composition \'bädē ,kämpə'zishən\ Determined by how much of the body weight is fat, and how much is lean body mass.

Bolus \'bōləs\ (Gr. *bolos*, lump) Rounded mass of food that is ready to be swallowed.

Bone compartment \'bōn kəm'pärtmənt\ Body's total content of skeletal tissue. The bone compartment contains 99% of the body's total metabolic calcium pool.

Bowman's capsule \'bōmənz 'kapsəl\ (after Sir William Bowman, British physician, 1816-1892) Cupped membrane surrounding the glomerulus; site of cell-free filtrate formation.

Bradykinin \'brādə'kīnən\ (Gr. *bradys*, slow; *kinein*, to move) Kinin (member of a group of endogenous peptides that cause vasodilation, increase blood pressure, and induce contraction of smooth muscle) formed from kallidin II by the action of the enzyme kallikrein. It is a very powerful vasodilator; increases capillary permeability, constricts smooth muscle, and stimulates pain receptors.

Brittle diabetes \'brid·ᵊl ,dīə'bēd·ēz\ A form of type I diabetes, which is difficult to control and is sensitive to hypoglycemia and acidosis.

Brunner's glands \'br'unə(r)z 'gland\ Mucus-secreting glands in the duodenum that provide mucus to protect the mucosa from irritation and erosion by the strongly acid gastric juices entering from the stomach. Emotional tension and stress inhibit these mucous secretions—a primary factor in duodenal ulcer formation.

Buffer \'bəfə(r)\ Mixture of acidic and alkaline components that, when added to a solution, is able to protect the solution against wide variations in its pH, even when strong acids and bases are added to it. If an acid is added, the alkaline partner reacts with it to counteract its acidic effect. If a base is added, the acid partner reacts with it to counteract its alkalizing effect. A solution to which a buffer has been added is called a buffered solution.

Buffer capacity \'bəfə(r) kə'pasəd·ē\ Substance capable of serving as a buffer to excess acid or base materials entering the body.

Bulimia \byü'limēə\ (Gr. *bous*, ox; *limos*, hunger) Abnormal increase in the sensation of hunger; a clinical gorge-purge syndrome associated with anorexia nervosa.

Byte \'bīt\ Group of adjacent *bits* forming a specific part of a binary word. One byte = eight bits.

Cachexia \ka'keksēə\ (Gr. *kakos*, bad; *hexis*, habit; + -ia) A specific profound effect caused by a disturbance in glucose metabolism usually seen in cancer patients; general poor health and malnutrition usually indicated by an emaciated appearance.

Calcium to phosphorus ratio (Ca:P) \'kalsēəm 'fäsf(a)rəs 'rā,shō\ Inverse ratio affecting the absorption rate of each mineral. The *dietary ratio* of 1:1 is ideal for periods of rapid growth, 1:1.5 for normal adult functions. The normal *serum ratio* for adults is 40 (10 mg/dl calcium × 4 mg/dl calcium phosphorus); for children it is 50 (10 mg/dl × 5 mg/dl phosphorus).

Calcitonin \,kalsə'tōnən\ Quick-acting hormone secreted

by the C cells of the parathyroids in response to hypercalcemia; acts to induce hypocalcemia.

Calculus \'kalkyələs\ *pl.* calculi (L. "pebble") Any abnormal accretion within the body of material that forms a "stone." Calculi are usually composed of mineral salts.

Callus \'kaləs\ (L. *kalus*) Unorganized meshwork of newly grown, woven bone developed on pattern of original fibrin clot (formed after fracture) and normally replaced by hard adult bone.

Calorie \'kal(ə)rē\ (L. *calor*, heat) A measure of heat. The *energy* required to do the work of the body is measured as the amount of *heat* produced by the body's work. The energy value of food is expressed as the number of kilocalories a specified portion of that food will yield when oxidized, either in the body or on being burned. Physicists use several different standard calories in investigative work. The calorie commonly used in metabolic studies and dietetic studies is the large calorie or kilocalorie (kcal), which is the amount of heat required to raise 1 kg of water 1° C.

Calorimetry \,kalə'rimə·trē\ (L. *calor* heat; Gr. *metron*, measure) The measurement of heat loss. An instrument for measuring heat output of the body or the energy value of foods is called a calorimeter.

Cancer \'kan(t)sə(r)\ (L. "crab") Cellular tumor whose natural course is fatal. Unlike benign tumor cells, cancer growths are invasive and spread easily.

Candidiasis \,kandə'dīəsəs\ Superficial fungus infection (genus, *Candida*) of moist parts of the body; infection of oral mucous membranes is called *thrush*.

Capillary fluid shift mechanism \'kapə,lerē 'flüəd 'shift 'mekə·nizəm\ Process that controls the movement of water and small molecules in solution (electrolytes, nutrients) between the blood in the capillary and the surrounding interstitial area. Filtration of water and solutes out of the capillary at the arteriole end and reabsorption at the venule end are accomplished by shifts in balance between the intracapillary hydrostatic blood pressure and the colloidal osmotic pressure exerted by the plasma proteins.

Carbonic acid \'kärbənik ásəd\ Acid partner in the carbonic acid–base bicarbonate buffer system in the body.

Carboxypeptidase \(,)kär,bäksē'peptə,dās\ Pancreatic enzyme that acts in protein digestion in the small intestine; it breaks the peptide bond of terminal amino acids having a free carboxyl (COOH) group.

Carcinoma \,kärs°n'ōmə\ (Gr. *karkinos*, crab) Tumor, usually malignant, arising from epithelial tissue.

Cardiac arrhythmia \'kärdē,ak ā'rithmēə\ Irregular heart beat. Often caused by nutritional or hormonal imbalances that affect the heart muscle's ability to contract.

Cardiac output \'kärdē,ak 'aùt,pùt\ (Gr. *kardia*, heart) Volume of blood propelled from the heart with each contraction; also called *stroke volume*.

Cardiac rate \'kärdē,ak 'rāt\ Number of heart beats per minute; pulse rate.

Carpodedal spasm \,kärpə,ped°l 'spasəm\ (Gr. *karpos*, L. *capus*, wrist; L. *pedalis*, foot) tonic contracture of the hands and feet.

Catabolism \kə'tabə,lizəm\ (Gr. *katabole*, a throwing down) The breaking-down phase of metabolism, the opposite of anabolism. Catabolism includes all the processes in which complex substances are progressively broken down into simpler ones. Catabolism usually involves the release of energy. Together, anabolism and catabolism constitute metabolism, which is the coordinated operation of anabolic and catabolic processes into a dynamic balance of energy and substance.

Catatonia \'kad·ə'tōnēə\ (Gr. *kata*, down; *tonos*, tension) Type of schizophrenia characterized either by excessive or violent actions or generalized inhibition.

Catecholamine \,kad·ə¦kōlə¦mēn\ (*catechol*, aromatic chemical substance; *amine*, organic compound containing nitrogen) Group of compounds having similar effects to those of the sympathetic nervous system; includes dopamine, norepinephrine, and epinephrine.

Cathode ray tube (CRT) \ka,thōd'rā 't(y)üb\ Term applied to a computer terminal or monitor screen; uses a vacuum tube that projects a beam of electrons onto a sensitized screen at one end. Common example is a television screen.

Cation \'kad·,īən\ Ion that carries a positive electric charge.

Celiac disease \'sēlē,ak də'zēz\ Malabsorption syndrome brought on by eating gluten-rich foods (wheat, rye, barley, oats). Characterized by steatorrhea, distention, flatulence, weight loss, and malnutrition resulting from poor absorption associated with damage to the mucosal villi; may be a hereditary condition.

Cellular immunity \'selyələr à'myünəd·ē\ Specific, acquired immunity in which the role of the T lymphocytes predominates.

Cerebrovascular accident (CVA) \sə'rēbrō'vaskyələ(r) 'aksədənt\ Stroke; brain tissue damage caused by reduced blood flow from arterial blockage or breakage; may result in *hemiplegia, hemiparesis,* or *hemianopsia.*

Ceruloplasmin \sə'rülōplazmən\ Plasma protein containing copper-forming ferroxidase, an enzyme that oxidizes iron in preparation for its absorption.

Cheilosis \kī'lōsəs\ Swelling and reddening of the lips. Chapped appearance. Fissures at corners of the mouth.

Chelate \'kē,lāt\ (Gr. *chele*, claw) Chemical compound capable of grasping and incorporating a metallic ion into its molecular structure. By binding the metal, the chelate removes it from a tissue or from the circulating blood.

Chelating agent \'kē,kātiŋ 'ājənt\ (Gr. *chele,* claw) Substance that combines with a metal, firmly binding it; chemotherapeutic use for metal poisoning.

Chemical bonding \'kemȧkəl 'bändiŋ\ Mutual attachment of various chemical elements to form chemical compounds. The chemical bonds that hold the elements of a compound together consist of stored potential energy. When the compound is broken up into parts, free energy is released to do the body's work.

Chemotherapy \'kēmō'therapē\ Treatment of disease with chemicals that destroy unhealthy tissue.

Chief cells \'chēf 'sels\ Special cells in the lining of the tubular gastric glands that secrete pepsinogen. Previously formed pepsin and hydrochloric acid in the stomach convert the inactive pepsinogen to the active enzyme pepsin, which begins the breakdown of protein to polypeptides.

Chloride-bicarbonate shift mechanism \'klōr,id (')bī'kärbə,nāt 'shift 'mekə,nizəm\ Exchange of bicarbonate for chloride. In red blood cells, it provides constant bicarbonate buffering for the rapidly forming carbonic acid from water and carbon dioxide ($H_2O + CO_2$).

Cholecystitis \'kōlə,si'stīd·əs\ (Gr. *chole,* bile, gall; *kystis,* bladder) Inflammation of the gallbladder.

Cholecystokinin \'kōlə,sistə,kīnən\ (Gr. *chole,* bile or gall; *kystis,* bladder, *kinein,* to move) A hormone that is secreted by the mucosa of the duodenum in response to the presence of fat. The cholecystokinin causes the gallbladder to contract. This contraction propels bile into the duodenum, where it is needed to emulsify the fat. The fat is thus prepared for digestion and absorption.

Cholecystokinin mechanism \'kōlə,sistə'kīnən meka,nizom\ Hormone secreted by mucosa of upper intestine that stimulates contraction of the gallbladder.

Cholelithiasis \,kōlələ'thīəsəs\ (Gr. *chole,* bile, gall; *lithos,* stone) Formation of gallstones.

Cholera \'kälərə\ Acute infectious disease characterized by severe diarrhea, acidosis, vomiting, muscle cramps, and prostration; associated with drinking contaminated water.

Cholestasis \'kōlə'stāsəs\ (Gr. *chole,* bile; *stasis,* stoppage) Suppression or stoppage of the bile flow.

Cholesterol \kə'lestər,röl\ A fat-related compound, a sterol ($C_{27}H_{45}OH$). It is a normal constituent of bile and a principal constituent of gallstones. In body metabolism cholesterol is important as a precursor of various steroid hormones such as sex hormones and adrenal corticoids. Cholesterol is synthesized by the liver. It is widely distributed in nature, especially in animal tissue such as glandular meats and egg yolk.

Cholestyramine \'kə,lestirəmīn\ Drug that prevents cholesterol absorption by binding it in the gut.

Chorion frondosum \'kōrē,än frän'dōsəm\ Fetal portion of the placenta. About 2 weeks after implantation occurs, villi develop at this site.

Chylomicron \,kīlə'mī,krän\ (Gr. *chylos,* chyle; *mikros,* small) Particle of fat—lipoprotein—appearing in the lymph and blood after a meal rich in fat. These particles are composed largely of triglycerides with lesser amounts of phospholipids, cholesterol, cholesterol esters, and protein. About 2 to 3 hours after a fat meal, the chylomicrons cause lactescense (milkiness) in the blood plasma; this is termed *alimentary lipemia.*

Chyme \'kīm\ (Gr. *chymos,* juice) Semifluid food mass in gastrointestinal tract following gastric digestion.

Chymotrypsin \,kīmə'tripsən\ A protein-splitting (proteolytic) enzyme produced by the pancreas that acts in the intestine. Together with trypsin, it reduces proteins to shorter chain polypeptides and dipeptides.

Cis \,sis\ (L., "on the same side") Having certain atoms or radicals in a chemical structure on the same side.

Cisterna chyli \sī'stərnə ¦kīlē\ Cistern or receptacle of the chyle is a dilated sac at the origin of the thoracic duct, which is the common truck that receives all the lymphatic vessels. The cisterna chyli lies in the abdomen between the second lumbar vertebra and the aorta. It receives the lymph from the intestinal trunk, the right and left lumbar lymphatic trunks, and two descending lymphatic trunks. The chyle, after passing through the cisterna chyli, is carried upward into the chest through the thoracic duct and empties into the venous blood at the point where the left subclavian vein joins the left internal jugular vein.

Clinical ecology \'klinəkəl ē'käləjē\ Term used to indicate study and treatment of allergy and similar problems by attention to multiple environmental agents.

Coenzyme \(')kō'en,zīm\ (L. *co,* together; Gr. *en,* in; *zyme,* leaven). Enzyme activators required by some enzymes to produce their reactions. Coenzymes are diffusible, heat-stable substances of low molecular weight that combine with inactive proteins called apoenzymes. Each such combination of apoenzyme and coenzyme forms an active compound or a complete enzyme called a holoenzyme. A number of the B vitamins function as coenzymes in the energy-producing pathways in cell metabolism.

Collagen disease \'käləjən dəzēz\ Connective tissue diseases such as rheumatoid arthritis, scleroderma, lupus erythematosus, and others.

Colloid \'kä,lȯid\ (Gr. *kollodes,* glutinous) Glutinous, gluelike; a dispersion of matter throughout a medium.

Colloidal osmotic pressure (COP) \kə'lȯidᵊl (')äz¦mäd·ik 'preshə(r)\ Pressure produced by the protein molecules in the plasma and in the cell. Because proteins are large molecules, they do not pass through the separating membranes of the capillary cells. Thus they remain in their respective compartments, exerting a constant osmotic pull that protects vital plasma and cell fluid volumes in these compartments.

Compactin \'käm,paktin\ Drug that prevents cholesterol production in the liver by inhibiting enzyme activity.

Compartment \kəm'pärtmənt\ The collective quantity of material in a given type of tissue space in the body. For example, in speaking of body water, the physiologist calls all the water in the body that is outside of cells the extracellular fluid compartment (ECF); all the body water inside of cells is the intracellular fluid compartment (ICF).

Complete protein \kəm'plēt 'prō,tēn\ A protein that contains the essential amino acids in quantities sufficient for maintenance of the body and for a normal rate of growth. Such proteins are said to have a high biologic value. Eggs, milk, cheese, and meat are complete protein foods.

Complement \'kämpləmənt\ Enzymatic protein that combines with the antigen-antibody complex, separating them when the antigen is an intact cell.

Concept \'kän,sept\ (L. *cum,* with *capere,* to seize) Combined ideas forming a whole.

Coronary \'kórə,nerē\ Referring to the arteries that carry nutrients and oxygen to the heart muscle.

Cortex \'kór,teks\ Outer layer; the renal cortex contains the glomeruli and tubules.

Corticosteroid \¦kórd·ə,kō,sti(ə),róid\ Steroid (hormonal substance) secreted by the adrenal cortex to influence the metabolism of nutrients, electrolytes, and water. Clinically they are given to reduce, among other things, inflammation, as in inflammatory bowel disease such as Crohn's disease or ulcerative colitis.

Costochondral \¦kästə'kändrəl\ (L. *costa,* rib) Regarding a rib and its associated cartilage.

Creatinine \'krē¦atinēn\ End product of the breakdown of body tissue; found in muscles and blood and excreted in urine. High levels indicate abnormally high catabolism of body proteins and possibly inadequate intake of carbohydrate and fat, which have a protein-sparing effect.

Cruciferous vegetables \(')krü¦sif(ə)rəs 'vejtəbəls\ Belonging to the botanical family *Cruciferae* or *Brassicaceae,* whose members have crosslike, four-petaled flowers; broccoli, cabbage, brussels sprouts, and cauliflower.

Crypts of Lieberkühn \'kripts -əv 'lēbə(r),k(y)ün\ (Gr. *Kryptein,* to hide) Tubular glands of the intestine that secrete intestinal juice. These special secretory organs open between the bases of the villi. Their walls are lined with special cells that secrete digestive enzymes, water, and electrolytes.

Cystinuria \,sistə'n(y)ùrēə\ (*cystine* + *uria,* from Gr. *ouron,* urine) Condition caused by a rare hereditary defect, characterized by excessive urinary excretion of cystine (a sulfur-containing amino acid). Cystine crystals often accumulate and form small, smooth, yellow kidney stones (cystine renal calculi).

Cystitis \si'stīd·əs\ (Gr. *kystis, kystides,* sac or bladder) Inflammation of the bladder; can be caused by allergy, bacteria, gonorrhea, and other conditions; often characterized by frequent voiding and burning. Untreated, it may lead to stone formation.

Dalton \'dólt°n\ (John Dalton, English physicist and chemist, 1766-1844; founder of the atomic theory) Unit of measuring mass, $\frac{1}{12}$ the mass of carbon-12, equal to 1.657×10^{-24}g; also called atomic mass unit.

Data base \'dād·e 'bās\ An organized body of information placed into computers for systematic storage and retrieval; usually deals with a specific topic or project.

Deamination \(¦)dē,amə'nāshən\ Removal of amino group (NH_2) from amino acid.

Decarboxylation \(¦)dē(,)kär,bäksə'lāshən\ Key reaction in cell metabolism; the removal of the carboxyl group (—COOH).

Decidua basalis \də'sijəwə 'bāsələs\ (L. *deciduus,* falling off) Maternal portion of the placenta.

Decubitus ulcer \də'kyübəd·əs 'əlsə(r)\ Bed sore.

Dehiscence \də'his°n(t)s\ (L. *dehiscere,* to gape) Splitting open, separation of the layers of a surgical wound.

Dehydration \(,)dē,hī,drāshən\ (L. *de,* away; Gr. *hydor,* water) Excessive water loss from body tissues.

Delirium \də'lirēəm\ (L. *de,* away; *lira,* furrow or track, that is, "off the track") Mental disturbance characterized by hallucinations, delusions, physical restlessness, and being incoherent; a sign of toxicity.

Delirium tremens \də'lirēəm 'trēmənz\ (L. *de-,* negative connotation; *lira,* furrow or track, that is, "off the track"; *tremere,* to shake) Mental disturbance marked by delirium with trembling and great excitment.

Delusion \də'lüzhən\ (L. *delusio; de,* front + *ludus,* a game) False personal belief that is firmly held, despite strong evidence to the contrary.

Dementia \də'menchə\ (L. *dementia,* mad) Reduction in intellectual function.

Deoxyribonucleic acid (DNA) \(,)dē¦äksē¦rïbō¦n(y)ü klēik'asəd\ Complex, double-chain protein of high molecular weight, which is the nucleic acid found in the chromosomes of the cell nucleus. It is the chemical basis of heredity and the carrier of genetic information for specific protein synthesis. DNA is composed of four nitrogenous bases (two purines, adenine and guanine, and two pyrimidines, thymine and cytosine), a sugar (deoxyribose), and phosphoric acid. A similar single-chain nucleic acid, ribonucleic acid (RNA), in which the sugar is ribose, also functions with DNA in protein synthesis in the cell.

Depression \də'preshən\ (L. *de,* down + *premare,* to press) Psychiatric syndrome characterized by feelings of dejection or guilt, slowed psychomotor activity, insomnia, weight loss, delusions, and so on.

Diabetes insipidus \,dīə'bēd·'ēz in'sipədəs\ Condition that shares some of the symptoms of diabetes mellitus: large urine output, great thirst and, sometimes, a large appetite. But these are symptoms of a specific injury, not a collection of metabolic disorders. The impaired pituitary gland produces less antidiuretic hormone, a substance that normally helps the kidneys retain water.

Dialysis \dī'aləsəs\ (Gr. *dia,* through + *lysis,* separate) Separating substances in solution by taking advantage of the different rates at which they pass through a semipermeable membrane.

Diastolic \,dīə¦stälik\ (Gr. *diastole,* expansion) Referring to the heart's period of dilation; the "relaxation" phase of the heartbeat.

Diffusion \də'fyüzhən\ (L. *diffundere,* to spread or to pour forth) Processes by which particles in solution spread throughout the solution and across separating membranes from the place of highest solute concentration to all surrounding spaces of lesser solute concentration.

Digestion \də'jes(h)chən\ (L. *dis,* apart + *genere,* to carry; *digerere,* to separate, arrange, dissolve, digest) Process by which food is broken down chemically in the gastrointestinal tract through the action of secretions containing specific enzymes. Digestion separates complex food structures into their simpler parts, which are the chemicals needed by the body to sustain life.

1,25-Dihydroxycholecalciferol \1,25 ¦dī,hī¦dräksē,kōlə,kal'sifə,ról\ The physiologically active hormone form of "vitamin" D.

Disability \¦disə'biləd·ē\ Mental or physical impairment that prevents the individual from performing one or more gainful activities; no longer considered synonymous with *handicap,* which implies serious disadvantage or hopelessness.

Disaccharide \(')dī'sakə,rīd\ Class of compound sugars composed of two molecules of monosaccharide. The three common members are sucrose (table sugar), lactose (milk sugar), and maltose (grain sugar).

Disk drive \'disk 'drīv\ The electromechanical device that houses and spins the information-carrying disks (floppy or hard), transferring the data from the disk to the working memory of the computer.

Disulfiram \dī'səlfə,ram\ White to off-white crystalline powder antioxidant; inhibits oxidation of the acetaldehyde metabolized from alcohol. It is used in treatment of alcoholism, producing extremely uncomfortable symptoms when alcohol is ingested following oral administration of the drug.

Diuresis \,dīyə'rēsəs\ (Gr. *diourein,* to urinate) Increased urination.

Diuretic \¦dīyə¦red·ik\ (Gr. *diouretikos,* promoting urine) Increasing urine excretion; an agent that promotes urine excretion.

Diverticulitis \,dīvə(r),tikyə'līd·əs\ Inflammation of "pockets" of tissue (diverticuli) in the lining of the mucous membrane in the colon.

"Dumping" syndrome \'dəmpiŋ 'sin,drōm\ Number of physical problems (nausea, vomiting, sweating, palpitations, syncope, diarrhea, and so on) that develop when stomach contents are emptied at an abnormally fast rate; occurs when part of the stomach or intestinal tract is removed.

Dynamic \(')dī¦namik\ Pertaining to change. A dynamic process is one that is constantly changing.

Dysgeusia \dəsgüsiə\ (Gr. *dys,* disordered, abnormal; *geusis,* taste) Altered sense of taste.

Dysphagia \dəs¦fāzh(ē)ə\ (Gr. *dys,* bad, painful, difficult; *phagein,* to eat) Difficulty swallowing.

Dyspnea \'dis(p)nēə\ (Gr. *dyspnoia,* difficulty in breathing) Labored, difficult breathing.

Ecchymosis \,ekə'mōsəs\ *pl.* ecchymoses (Gr. *ekchymosis*) Bruiselike hemorrhagic spot in the skin or mucous membranes.

Ecology \ē'käləjē\ (Gr. *oikos,* house) Relations between organisms and their environments.

Eclampsia \e'klampsēə\ (Gr. *eklampein,* to shine forth) Advanced pregnancy-induced hypertension (PIH) manifested by convulsions.

Ectoderm \'ektə,dərm\ (Gr. *ektos,* article; *derma,* skin) Layer of embryonic tissue from which the nails, skin glands, nervous system, external sensory organs, and mucous membrane of the mouth are formed.

Eczema \÷ig'zēmə, 'eksəmə\ Inflammation of the skin, characterized by redness, itching, crusting, and eventually scaling or pigmentation.

Edema \ə'dēmə\ (Gr. *oidema,* swelling) Large abnormal amounts of fluid filling the intercellular tissue spaces; may be either localized or systemic.

Educate \'ejə,kāt\ (L. *educatus,* from *educere,* to lead forth; from *e,* out + *ducere,* to lead) To develop and cultivate by systematic instruction.

Electrolyte \ə'lektrə,līt\ (Gr. *electron,* amber [which emits electricity if it is rubbed]; *lytos,* soluble) Chemical compound, which in solution dissociates by releasing ions. (An ion is an atomic particle that carries a positive or a negative electric charge.) The process of dissociating into ions is termed *ionization.*

Electroneutrality \ə'lektrə'n(y)ütrələdē\ Condition of a solution of charged particles in which there are equal numbers of positive and negative ions, a balanced neutral state.

Elemental formula \\'elə¦mənt°l 'förmyələ'\ Formula whose components cannot be broken down into simpler parts.

Embolus \'embələs\ Circulating blood clot that may lodge in a blood vessel, causing an embolism.

Emulsifier \ə'məlsə,fī(a)r\ An agent that breaks down large fat globules to smaller, uniformly distributed particles. This action is accomplished in the intestine chiefly by the bile acids, which lower surface tension of the fat particles. Emulsification greatly increases the surface area of fat, facilitating contact with fat-digesting enzymes.

Encephalopathy \ən,sefə'läpəthē\ Any degenerative disease of the brain.

Endarteritis \¦end,ärd·ə'rīd·əs\ (end-; Gr. *arteria,* artery; -itis) Inflammation of the inner lining of an artery.

Endoderm \'en(,)dō,dərm\ (Gr. *endo,* inside; *derma,* skin) The layer of embryonic tissue from which the epithelium of the respiratory and digestive tract, as well as bladder and urethra, are formed.

Endogenous \(')en¦däjənəs\ (Gr. *endon,* within; *gennan,* to produce) Developing within an organism.

Endometrium \(')en¦dō'mē·trēəm\ (Gr. *endon,* within; *metra,* uterus) The inner lining of the uterus.

Endorphin \'en'dörfən\ (*endo*genous + mor*phine*) Group of polypeptides in the brain that raise the threshold for pain.

Energy \'enə(r)jē\ (Gr. *en,* in or with +*ergon,* work) The capacity of a system for doing work; available power. Energy is manifest in various forms—motion, position, light, heat, and sound. Energy is interchangeable among these various forms and is constantly being transformed and transferred among them.

Enkephalin \en'kefələn\ Type of endorphin made up of five amino acids that raise the threshold of pain and might also serve as a neurotransmitter; it is found in nerve endings in brain tissue, spinal cord, and gastrointestinal tract.

Enteritis \,entə'rīd·əs\ Inflammation of the intestine.

Enterogastrone \,entərō'ga,strōn'\ Hormone produced by glands in the duodenal mucosa that counteracts excessive gastric activity by inhibiting acid and pepsin secretion and gastric motility.

Enterotoxin \¦entərō'täksən\ Substance, usually proteinaceous, that has toxic effect on the cells of the intestinal lining.

Enzyme \'en,zīm\ (Gr. *en,* in; *zyme,* leaven) Various complex proteins produced by living cells, which act independently of these cells. Enzymes are capable of producing certain chemical changes in other substances without themselves being changed in the process. Their action is therefore that of a catalyst. Digestive enzymes of the gastrointestinal secretions act on food substances to break them down into simpler compounds and greatly accelerate the speed of these chemical reactions. An enzyme is usually named according to the substance (substrate) on which it acts and has the common suffix *-ase;* sucrase is the specific enzyme for sucrose and breaks it down to glucose and fructose.

Epidemiology \,epə,dēmē'äləjē\ Branch of medicine dealing with the study of various factors that determine the frequency and distribution of disease in given populations.

Epilepsy \'epə,lepsē\ (Gr. *epilepsia,* a seizing) Transient disturbances of brain function resulting in loss of consciousness, which may be accompanied by convulsive seizures.

Epiphyses \ə'pifəsəs\ Parts of a long bone separated from the main body of the bone by a layer of cartilage.

Ergogenic \¦ərgə¦jenik\ (Gr. *ergon,* work; *gennan,* to produce) Tendency to increase work output.

Erythema \,erə'thēmə\ (Gr. *erythema,* flush on the skin) Redness of the skin produced by congestion of the capillaries: results from a variety of causes, one of which can be radiant heat, or burns.

Essential amino acid \ə'senchəl ə'mē(,)nō 'asəd\ An amino acid that is indispensable to life and growth and that the body cannot manufacture; it must be supplied in the diet. Eight amino acids are essential: threonine, leucine, isoleucine, valine, lysine, methionine, phenylalanine, and tryptophan.

Essential fatty acid (EFA) \ə'senchəl 'fad·ē 'asəd\ A fatty acid that is (1) necessary for body metabolism or function and (2) cannot be manufactured by the body and must therefore be supplied in the diet. The major essential fatty acid is linoleic acid ($C_{17}H_{31}COOH$). It is found principally in vegetable oils. The other fatty acids usually classified as essential are linolenic acid and arachidonic acid.

Essential hypertension \ə'senchəl 'hīpə(r)tenchən\ High blood pressure of unknown cause.

Ester \'estə(r)\ A compound produced by the reaction between an acid and an alcohol with elimination of a molecule of water. This process is called esterification. For example, a triglyceride is a glycerol ester. Cholesterol esters are formed in the mucosal cells by combination with fatty acids, largely linoleic acid.

Exudate \'eksə,dāt\ (L. *exsudare,* to sweat out) Material that escapes from blood vessels and is deposited in tissues or tissue surfaces; characterized by a high content of protein, cells, or other cellular solid matter.

Exudative enteropathy \ig'züdəd·iv ,entə'räpəthē\ Any inflammatory intestinal disease accompanied by cellular components (fluid, debris) escaping the blood vessels to be deposited in or near tissue.

Extravasate \ik'stravə,sāt\ (L. *extra,* outside of, beyond, in addition; *vas,* vessel) Escape or discharge from a vessel into the surrounding tissue (for example, blood leakage forming a bruise).

Familial hypercholesterolemia \fə'milyəl ˌhīpə(r)kə, les-tə(ˌ)rō'lēmēə\ Presence of defective LDL receptors, resulting in an increase in LDL-cholesterol levels.

Fatty acid \'fad·ē 'asəd\ The structural components of fats.

Febrile \'febrəl\ (L. *febrilis*) Condition characterized by fever.

Feedback mechanism \'fēd,bak 'mekə,nizəm\ Mechanism that regulates production and secretion by an endocrine gland (A_g) of its hormone (A_h), which stimulates another endocrine gland (T_g; the *target gland*) to produce its hormone (T_h). As sufficient T_h is produced, blood levels of T_h signal A_g to stop secreting A_h.

Ferritin \'ferət°n\ Protein-iron compound in which iron is stored in tissues; the storage form of iron in the body.

Fetal hydrops \'fēd·°l 'hīdräps\ (Gr. *hydor*, water) Extensive edema of the entire fetus associated with severe anemia.

Fetor hepaticus \'fēd·ə(r) hə'padikəs\ Breath odor resembling the smell of fecal material; a characteristic of liver disease.

Fibrinogen \fī'brinəjən\ Fraction of human plasma given via transfusion to increase coagulation of the blood.

File \'fīl\ Body of related information recorded on a computer disk.

Filtration \fil·'trāshən\ (Medieval L. *filtrum*, felt used to strain liquids) Passage of a fluid through a semipermeable membrane (a membrane that permits passage of water and small solutes but not large molecules) as a result of a difference in pressures on the two sides of the membrane. For example, the net filtration pressure in the capillaries is the difference between the outward-pushing hydrostatic force of the blood pressure and the opposing inward-pulling force of the colloidal osmotic pressure exerted by the plasma proteins retained in the capillary.

Fistula \'fis(h)chələ\ (L. *fistula*, pipe) Abnormal passage, usually between two internal organs, or leading from an internal organ to the surface of the body.

Flavin mononucleotide (FMN) \'flāvən ˌmänō'n(y)üklēə,tīd\ A riboflavin phosphate compound that acts as a coenzyme in the deamination of certain amino acids.

Flavin-adenine dinucleotide (FAD) \'flāvən 'ad°n,ēn (')dī'n(y)üklēə,tīd\ A riboflavin enzyme that operates in many reactions affecting amino acids, glucose, and fatty acids.

Flavoprotein \ˈflā(ˌ)vō'prō,tēn\ The enzymes of which riboflavin is an important constituent (FMN and FAD).

Floppy disk (diskette) \'fläpē 'disk ('dis,ket)\ Thin, flexible, circular mylar disks coated for magnetic recording of information. Comes in either 8-inch or 5¼-inch diameters.

Fluoridation \ˌflúrə'dāshən\ Process by which fluorine is added to a substance. Proper fluoridation of public water supplies in areas where the fluorine content is naturally low has been demonstrated to control the incidence of dental caries.

Fluorometric \'flúrəmetrik\ Of or related to fluorometry, an analytic technique that measures small amounts of a substance by the characteristic wavelength of light it emits while being exposed to various wavelengths of light.

Flushing reaction \'fləshiŋ rē'akshən\ Short-term reaction resulting in redness of neck and face.

Folic acid \'fōlik 'asəd\ The B vitamin discovered as a factor in the control of pernicious anemia. It functions in metabolism as a coenzyme for transferring single carbon units for attachment in many reactions. In this role, folic acid acts as a key substance in cell growth and reproduction by aiding in the formation of nucleoproteins and hemoglobin.

Folinic acid \fō'linik 'asəd\ A derivative of folic acid, which has been used in the treatment of megaloblastic anemia. Vitamin C influences this conversion of folic acid in the liver.

Follicular hyperkeratosis \fə'likyələ(r) ˌhīpə(r),kerə'tōsəs\ A vitamin A deficiency condition in which the skin becomes dry and scaly and small pustules or hardened, pigmented, papular eruptions form around the hair follicles.

"Food jag" \'füd 'jag\ Colloquial expression referring to repeated use of single foods over a brief time.

Fuel factor \'fyüel 'faktə(r)\ The kilocalorie value (energy potential) of food nutrients; that is, the number of kilocalories 1 g of the nutrient yields when oxidized. The kilocalorie fuel factor for carbohydrate is 4; for protein, 4; and for fat, 9. These basic figures are used in computing diets and energy values of foods.

Gastrectomy \ga'strek tamē\ (Gr. *gaster*, stomach; *ektome*, excision) Surgical removal of all or part of the stomach.

Gastrin \'gastrən\ Hormone secreted by mucosal cells in the antrum of the stomach that stimulates the parietal cells to produce hydrochloric acid. Gastrin is released in response to entry of stimulants, especially coffee, alcohol, and meat extractives, into the stomach. When the gastric pH reaches 2.0, a feedback mechanism cuts off gastrin secretion and prevents excess acid formation.

Gastritis \ga'strīd·əs\ Inflammation of the stomach.

Gavage \gə'väzh\ (Fr. *gavage*, cramming) Forced tube feeding into stomach; superalimentation.

Generativity \'jenə,rā|d·|ivitē\ Active nurturing transmission of culture from one generation to the next.

Geophagia \ˈjēō'fäj(ē)ə\ (Gr. *ge*, earth; *phagein*, to eat) Eating of clay or earth.

Geriatrics \ˌjerēˈaˑtriks\ (Gr. *geron*, old man; *iatrike*, medical treatment) Study and treatment of diseases of old age; a branch of medicine concerned with medical problems associated with old age.

Gerontology \ˌjerənˑˈtäləjē\ (Gr. *geron*, old man; *logos*, study of) Study of the aging process and its phenomena.

Gestation \jeˈstāshən\ (L. *gestatio*, from *gestare*, to bear) The period of embryonic and fetal development from feritilization to birth; pregnancy.

Glomerulonephritis \gläˌmer(y)ə(ˌ)lōnəˈfrīdˑəs\ Inflammation of the capillary glomeruli in the kidney; may result after a streptococcal infection.

Glomerulosclerosis \gläˌmer(y)ə(ˌ)lōsklēˈrōsəs\ (L. *glomerulus*, dim. of *glomus*, ball; *sklerosis*, hardness) Scarring and aging of the renal glomeruli.

Glomerulus \gläˈmer(y)əˌlōs\ (L. diminutive form of *glomus*, ball) Convoluted cluster of blood vessels in the cortex of the kidney at the head of the nephron; site of cell-free filtrate formation.

Glossitis \gläˈsīdˑəs\ (Gr. *glossa*, tongue + *-itis*) Swollen, reddened tongue; riboflavin deficiency symptom.

Glucagon \ˈglükəˌgän\ Hormone produced by the A cells in the islets of Langerhans and secreted when blood sugar levels are low or in response to growth hormone. It stimulates the breakdown of glycogen in the liver and raises blood sugar levels during fasting states to ensure adequate levels for normal nerve and brain function.

Gluconeogenesis \ˌglükōˌnēōˈjenəsəs\ (Gr. *gleukos*, sweetness; *neos*, new; *genesis*, production, generation) Formation of glucose from noncarbohydrate sources (protein or fat).

Glucose tolerance factor (GTF) \ˈglüˌkōs ˈtäl(ə)rən(t)s ˈfaktə(r)\ Chromium compound associated with glucose and lipid metabolism and insulin activity.

Gluten-sensitive enteropathy \ˈglütᵊn ˈsen(t)sədˑiv ˌentəˈräpəthē\ Disorder characterized by the inability to absorb gluten, a protein found in wheat, barley, oats, and rye. The presence of gluten is accompanied by damage to the mucosal villi, which in turn interferes with the absorption of other essential nutrients; commonly found in celiac disease and sprue.

Glycemic index \(ˈ)glīˌsēmik ˈinˌdeks\ Blood sugar response value of a food in relation to that of glucose. It is an expression of the area under the blood glucose response curve for each food stated as the percentage of the area after taking the same amount of carbohydrate as glucose.

Glyceride \ˈglisəˌrīd\ Group name for fats; any of a group of esters obtained from glycerol by the replacement of one, two, or three hydroxyl (OH) groups with a fatty acid. Monoglycerides contain one fatty acid; diglycerides contain two fatty acids; triglycerides contain three fatty acids. Glycerides are the principal constituent of adipose tissue and are found in animal and vegetable fats and oils.

Glycerol \ˈglisəˌròl\ A colorless, odorless, syrupy, sweet liquid; a constituent of fats usually obtained by the hydrolysis of fats. Chemically glycerol is an alcohol; it is esterified with fatty acids to produce fats.

Glycogen \ˈglīkəjən\ (Gr. *glykys*, sweet; *gennan*, to produce) Polysaccharide, the main storage form of carbohydrate, largely stored in the liver and to a lesser extent in muscle tissue.

Glycogenesis \ˌglīkəˈjenəsəs\ Formation of glycogen, the storage form of carbohydrates in animals.

Glycogenolysis \ˌglīkəjəˈnäləsəs\ (*glycogen* + Gr. *lysis*, dissolution) Specific term for conversion of glycogen into glucose in the liver; chemical process of enzymatic hydrolysis or breakdown by which this conversion is accomplished.

Glycolysis \glīˈkäləsəs\ (Gr. *glykys*, sweet; *lysis*, dissolution) Catabolism of carbohydrate (glucose and glycogen) by enzymes with release of energy and production of pyruvic acid or lactic acid.

Glycosuria \ˈglī(ˌ)kōˈs(h)ùrēə\ (Gr. *glykys*, sweet; *ouron*, urine + *-ia*) Abnormally high concentrations of glucose in the urine.

Goblet cell \ˈgäblòt ˈsel\ Special single secretory cells on the mucosal surface that produce mucus. Mucin droplets accumulate in the cell, causing it to swell. The free surface finally ruptures and liberates the mucus. This mucus coats and protects the mucosa.

Goiter \ˈgòidˑə(r)\ (L. *guttur*, throat) Enlargement of the thyroid gland caused by lack of sufficient available iodine to produce the thyroid hormone, thyroxine.

Hallucination \həˌlüsᵊnˈāshən\ (L. *hallucinari*, to wander in the mind, dream) Perception of a stimulus that does not exist in reality.

Handicap \ˈhandēˌkap\ Mental or physical defect, which may or may not be congenital, that prevents the individual from participating in normal life activities; implies disadvantage.

Hard copy \ˈhärd ˈkäpē\ Printed sheets of paper one can hold in hand, as opposed to information only displayed on a monitor screen.

Hardware\ˈhärdˌwa(a)(ə)r\Mechanicalequipmentcomprising a computer system and necessary for its operation.

Hemarthrosis \ˌhēmärˈthrōsəs\ Hemorrhage into joint cavities, causing local heat, painful swelling, and immobility.

Hematuria \ˌhēməˈtùrēə\ (Gr. *hemato*, blood; *ouron*, urine) Presence of blood in the urine.

Heme \ˈhēm\ Iron-containing, nonprotein portion of the hemoglobin.

Hemodialysis \ˌhēmōdīˈaləsəs\ (Gr. *haima*, blood; *dia*, through; *lysis*, separate) Removal of toxic substances from the blood by passing it through a machine that contains a semipermeable membrane and a liquid into which the substances will be diffused; process by which persons with chronic renal failure are kept alive. The machine is often referred to as an "artificial kidney."

Hemoglobin \'hēmə‚glōbən\ (Gr. *haima*, blood; L. *globus*, globe) Protein that gives the color to red blood cells. A conjugated protein composed of an iron-containing pigment called heme and a simple protein, globin. Carries oxygen in the blood; combines with oxygen to form oxyhemoglobin.

Hemopoiesis \‚hēmō‚pói'ēsəs\ (Gr. *haima*, blood; *poiein*, to form) The formation of blood.

Hemosiderin \‚hēmō'sidərən\ (Gr. *haima*, blood; *sideros*, iron) Insoluble iron oxide-protein compound in which iron is stored in the liver if the amount of iron in the blood exceeds the storage capacity of ferritin, for example, during rapid destruction of red blood cells (malaria, hemolytic anemia).

Hepatomegaly \‚hepəd·ō'megəlē\ Enlargement of the liver.

Hexose \'hek‚sōs\ Class of simple sugars (monosaccharides) that contain six carbon atoms ($C_6H_{12}O_6$). The most common members are glucose (dextrose), fructose (levulose), and galactose.

Hiatus \hī'ād·əs\ Opening or gap.

Hierarchy \'hīə‚rärkē\ (Gr. *hieros*, sacred, holy) System of persons or things in a graded order according to held values, functions, or goals.

High-density lipoprotein (HDL) \hī 'den(t)səd·ē ‚līpə'prō‚tēn\ Carries less total lipid and more protein.

Homeostasis \‚hōmēō'stāsis\ (Gr. *homoios*, unchanging or resembling; *stasis*, standing) State of internal stability of a body or an organism.

Hormone \'hȯr‚mōn\ (Gr. *hormaein*, to set in motion, spur on) Various internally secreted substances from the endocrine organs, which are conveyed by the blood to another organ or tissue on which they act to stimulate increased functional activity or secretion. The tissue or substance acted on by a specific hormone is called its target organ or substance. For example, insulin, a hormone secreted by special cells of the pancreas (islets of Langerhans), acts to facilitate glucose metabolism.

Humoral immunity \(h)yümərəl ə'myünəd·ē\ Acquired immunity in which the role of antibodies, produced by B lymphocytes and plasma cells, predominates.

Hydatidiform mole \‚hīdə‚tidəfȯrm 'mōl\ (L. *hydatis*, a drop of water; *moles*, a shapeless mass) An abnormal pregnancy resulting in a cystic mass resembling a bunch of grapes formed by a pathologic ovum in the uterus; a mole pregnancy.

Hydramnios \hī'dramnē‚äs\ (Gr. *hydor*, water; *amnion*, bowl, the membrane containing the fetus) An excess of amniotic fluid.

Hydrochloric acid (HCl) \‚hī(‚)drō'klōrik 'asəd\ Acid secreted by special gastric mucosal cells; provides necessary acid medium for enzyme action in the stomach.

Hydrogenation \‚hīdrəjə'nāshən\ The process of adding hydrogen to unsaturated fats to produce a solid, saturated fat. This process is used to produce vegetable shortening from vegetable oils.

Hydrolysis \hī'dräləsəs\ (Gr. *hydor*, water; *lysis*, dissolution) Process by which a chemical compound is split into other compounds by taking up the elements of water. Common examples are the reactions of digestion, in which the nutrients are split into simpler compounds by the digestive enzymes; that is, the conversion of starch to maltose, of fat to fatty acids and glycerol, and so on.

Hydrophilic \‚hī(‚)drə'filik\ (Gr. *hydor*, water; *philein*, to love) Readily absorbing water; having strong polar groups that readily interact with water; water soluble. Glycerol is hydrophilic.

Hydrophobic \‚hīdrə'fōbik\ (Gr. *hydor*, water; *phobein*, to be frightened by) Not readily absorbing water; lacking polar groups and therefore insoluble in water. Fat is hydrophobic.

Hydrostatic pressure \hī(i)drō‚stadik 'preshə(r)\ Pressure exerted by a liquid on the surfaces of the walls that contain it. Such pressure is equal in the direction of all containing walls. In body fluid balance hydrostatic pressure usually refers to the blood pressure, which, together with the plasma proteins, maintains fluid circulation and volume in the blood vessels.

Hygroscopic \‚hīgrə'skäpik\ (Gr. *hygros*, moist) Taking up and retaining moisture readily.

Hyperemesis gravidarum \‚hīpə(r)'eməsəs ‚gravə'da(a)rəm\ (Gr. *hyper*, over + Gr. *emesis*, vomiting) Severe vomiting that is potentially fatal.

Hyperglycemia \‚hīpə(r)glī'sēmēə\ Elevated blood sugar; above normal levels.

Hyperkalemia \‚hīpə(r)‚kā'lēmēə\ (Gr. *hyper*; L. *Kalium*, potassium; Gr. *haima*, blood) Excessive amounts of potassium (K) in blood plasma.

Hyperkeratosis \‚hīpə(r)‚kerə'tōsəs\ (Gr. *hyper*; *keras*, horn or horny tissue) Overgrowth of the corneous or horny layer of the skin, consisting of keratin.

Hyperkinesis \‚hīpə(r)kə'nēsəs\ (Gr. *hyper*; *kinesis*, motion) Nerve disorder characterized by abnormally high motor activity; may occur in children and interferes with their learning ability; also known as *hyperactivity.*

Hyperlipoproteinemia \‚hīpə(r)‚līpə‚prō‚tē'nēmēə\ Elevation of lipoproteins in the blood.

Hypermotility \‚hīpə(r)mō'tiləd·ē\ Excessive peristaltic activity along the alimentary canal.

Hypernatremia \‚hīpə(r)nətrēmēə\ (Gr. *hyper*; L. *natrium*, sodium; Gr. *haima*, blood) Abnormally high levels of sodium in the blood.

Hyperoxaluria \‚hīpə(r)äksəl'yurēə\ (Gr. *hyper* + *oxa-*

late + uria) Excretion of high levels of oxalate in the urine. Oxalates, found in several vegetables (spinach, tomatoes, rhubarb) combine with calcium to form urinary stones.

Hyperparathyroidism \,hīpə(r),parə'thī,ŕoid,izəm\ (Gr. *hyper + parathyroid + ism*) Greater-than-normal levels of activity by the parathyroid glands, which regulate calcium and phosphorus. High calcium levels increase the chances of developing calcium-containing urinary calculi.

Hyperphagia \,hīpə(r)'fājēə\ (Gr. *hyper; phagein,* to eat) Eating more than necessary for optimal body function.

Hyperphosphatemia \'hīpə(r)fäsfətēmēə\ High serum phosphorus levels.

Hypertriglyceridemia \'hīpə(r),trī¦glisə,rī'dēmēə\ Elevated blood level of triglycerides.

Hypertonic dehydration \'hīpə(r)'tänik (,)dē,hī 'drāshən\ Loss of water from the cell as a result of hypertonicity (excess solutes, thus greater osmotic pressure) of the surrounding extracellular fluid.

Hypochloremic alkalosis \'hīpōklōrēmik ,alkəlōsəs\ Excessive loss of gastric secretion (hydrochloric acid).

Hypocupremia \,hī(,)pō,k(y)ü'prēmēə\ Low serum copper level.

Hypogeusia \hī(,)pōgyüzh(ē)\ Impaired taste associated with zinc deficiency.

Hypoglycemia \'hī(,)pōglī'sēmēə\ Low blood sugar; below normal levels.

Hypokalemia \,hī(,)pō,kā'lēmēə\ Low potassium levels in the blood.

Hypophosphatemia \,hī(,)pō,fäsfə'tēmēə\ Low serum phosphorus levels.

Hypoplasia \,hī(,)pō'plāzh(ē)ə\ (Gr. *hypo,* under; *plasis,* formation) Incomplete organ; underdevelopment of an organ.

Hypophagia \,hī(,)pō'fājēə\ (Gr. *hypo; phagein,* to eat) Eating less than necessary for optimal health.

Hyposmia \,hī(,)pozmēə\ Impaired smell acuity associated with zinc deficiency.

Hypotonic dehydration \'hī(,)pō'tänik (,)dē,hī 'drāshən\ Increase of water in the cell (cellular edema) at the expense of extracellular fluid, resulting from hypotonicity (decreased solutes, thus diminished osmotic pressure) of the extracellular fluid surrounding the cell. A dangerous shrinking of the extracellular fluid (especially blood) volume follows.

Hypovolemia \,hī(,)pō,vä'lēmēə\ (Gr. *hypo;* volume; *haima,* blood) Abnormal reduction in volume of circulatory plasma.

Iatrogenic \ī¦a·trō¦jenik\ (Gr. *iatros,* physician; *gennan,* to produce) Illness induced by medical treatment.

Idiopathic \¦idēə¦pathik\ Of unknown cause.

Immunocompetence \ə'myüno'kämpəd·ən(t)s\ Ability to produce antibodies in response to an antigen.

Incomplete protein \¦inkəm'plēt 'prō,tēn\ Food protein lacking a sufficient amount of one or more of the essential amino acids.

Indole \'in,dōl\ Compound produced in the intestines by the decomposition of tryptophan; obtained from indigo and coal tar.

Infantile beriberi \'infən·tīl ¦berē'berē\ Occurs in the first year of life. Symptoms: convulsions, respiratory difficulties, gastrointestinal disorders; terminal symptoms: cyanosis, dyspnea, tachycardia.

Infarct \'in,färkt\ Death of tissue caused by a loss of blood flow to that area, usually caused by a thrombus (clot) clogging the artery feeding the area.

Insulin \'in(t)sələn\ (L. *insula,* island) Hormone formed in the B cells of the pancreas. It is secreted when blood glucose and amino acid levels rise and assists their entry into the cells. It also promotes glycogenesis and conversion of glucose into fat and inhibits lipolysis and gluconeogenesis (protein breakdown). Commercial insulin is manufactured from pigs and cows; new "artificial" human insulin products have recently been made available.

Intermittent claudication \¦intə(r)¦mit³nt ,klòdə' kāshən\ Leg pain induced by walking that is relieved by rest.

Intervillous space \¦intə(r)'viləs 'spās\ (L. *inter-,* between; *villus,* tuft of hair) Spaces situated between villi, small vascular protrusions.

Intermediate-density lipoprotein (IDL) \¦intə(r)¦ mēdēət'den'(t)səd·ē ,līpə'prō,tēn\ Approximately 30% cholesterol; carries triglycerides to body cells.

Intrinsic factor \(')in·¦trinzik 'faktə(r)\ (L. *intrinsecus,* on the inside) Substance situated entirely within a part of the body; common term for component of the gastric secretions, a mucoprotein, also called Castle's factor, necessary for the absorption of cyanocobalamin (vitamin B_{12}).

Intima \'intəmə\ (L.) Innermost layer of a blood vessel.

Intramural nerve plexus \¦in·trə'myürəl 'nərv 'pleksəs\ (L. *intra,* within; *murus,* wall; *plexus,* a braid) Network of interwoven nerve structures within a particular organ. The action of smooth muscle layers comprising the gastrointestinal wall is controlled by such a network of nerve fibers.

Ion \'īən\ (Gr. *ion,* to wander) Molecular constituent of one or more atoms that is a free-wandering particle in solution. An ion carries a positive or negative electric charge. Ions carrying negative charges are called anions; those carrying positive charges are called cations.

Ionized free calcium (Ca^{++}) \'īənizd frē 'kalsēəm\ Free, diffusible form of calcium in the blood and other body fluids. Makes up a very small amount of the total body calcium (1%); the remaining 99% of the total body calcium is deposited as calcium salts in bone tissue.

Ischemia \ə'skēmēə\ (Gr. *ischein*, to suppress; *haima*, blood) Deficiency of blood to a body part resulting from constriction or actual obstruction of a blood vessel.

Isomer \ˌīsōmə(r)\ (Gr. *isos*, equal; *meros*, part) The possession by two or more distinct compounds of the same molecular formula, each molecule possessing an identical number of atoms of each element but in different arrangement.

Isotonic \ˌīsoˌtänik\ (Gr. *isos*, equal; *tonos*, tone, tension) Having the same tension or pressure. Two given solutions are isotonic if they have the same osmotic pressure and therefore balance each other. For example, the law of isotonicity operates between the gastrointestinal fluids and the surrounding extracellular fluid. Shifts of water and electrolytes in and out of the gastrointestinal lumen are controlled to maintain this state of isotonicity.

Isotope \'īsōˌtōp\ (Gr. *isos*, equal; *topos*, place) Element that has the same number of protons (atomic number) as another element but a different number of neutrons (atomic mass).

Joule \jül\ A measure of energy; 1 kcal = 4.184 kJ.

Kallikrein \kaləˈkrēən\ Any member of a group of peptide enzymes of the subgroup serine proteinases present in blood plasma and various glands, such as the pancreas and salivary gland. Major action is to liberate polypeptides called *kinins* (bradykinin and kallidin).

Keratinization \ˌkerəd·ənəˈzāshən\ (Gr. *keras, kerat,* horn) A process occurring in vitamin A deficiency states in which the epithelial cells either slough off or become dry and flattened, then gradually harden and form rough horny scales. This process may occur in the cornea, the respiratory tract, the gastrointestinal tract, the genitourinary tract, or the skin.

Keratomalacia \ˌkerəd·ōməˈlās(h)ēə\ Softening of the cornea.

Ketone \'kēˌtōn\ Intermediate fat metabolite; large class of organic compounds that contain the carbonyl group C=O, where the carbon atom is jointed to two other carbon atoms.

Keto acid \'kēd·(ˌ)ō 'asəd\ Amino acid residue after deamination. The glycogenic keto acids are used to form carbohydrates. The ketogenic keto acids are used to form fats.

Ketoacidosis \'kēd·(ˌ)ōasadōsəs\ Abnormally high concentration of ketone bodies (ketones) in body tissues and fluids; a complication of diabetes mellitus and starvation.

Kilobyte (K) \'kē(ˌ)lōbīt\ 1,024 bytes, or characters, of memory storage. Thus 4 K = 4,096 bytes of memory and 64 K = 65,536 bytes of memory.

Kinetic \kəˈned·ik\ (Gr. *kinesis*, movement) Regarding or producing motion.

Kinin \'kīnən\ Any of a group of endogenous peptides that cause vasodilation, increase vascular permeability, reduce blood pressure, and induce contraction of smooth muscle.

Koilonychia \ˌkȯilōˈnikēə\ (Gr. *koilos*, hollow; *onyx*, nail) Spoon-shaped fingernails.

Kwashiorkor \ˌkwäshēˈȯrkər\ (Gold Coast, Africa, "displaced child") Disease syndrome produced by severe protein deficiency.

Kyphosis \kīˈfōsəs\ (Gr. *hyphos*, a hump) Increased, abnormal convexity of the upper part of the spine; hunchback.

Lactated Ringer's solution \'laktātəd 'rˌŋə(r)s sə 'lüshən\ Sterile solution of calcium chloride, potassium chloride, sodium chloride, and sodium lactate in water given to replenish fluid and electrolytes; named for Sydney Ringer (1835-1910), an English physiologist.

Lactic acid \'laktik 'asəd\ (L. *lactis*, milk) Produced by anaerobic glycolysis in the muscles during exertion; can be converted to glucose by the liver.

Lactoflavin \'lak(ˌ)tōˈflāvən\ The form in which riboflavin occurs in milk.

Lacuna \ləˈk(y)ünə\ A hollow space (pl. lacunae).

Lean body mass (LBM) \'lēn 'bädē 'mas\ All component parts of the body, excluding neutral storage lipid; the entire fat-free mass.

Lecithin \'lesəthən\ (Gr. *lekithos*, egg yolk) A yellow-brown fatty substance of the group called phospholipids. It occurs in animal and plant tissues and egg yolk. It is composed of units of choline, phosphoric acid, fatty acids, and glycerol. Commercial forms of lecithin, obtained chiefly from soybeans, corn, and egg yolk, are used in candies, foods, cosmetics, and inks. Lecithin plays an important role in the metabolism of fat in the liver. It provides an effective lipotropic factor, choline, which prevents the accumulation of abnormal quantities of fat.

Lecithin-cholesterol acyltransferase (LCAT) \'lesəthən kōˈləˈsterˌrȯl asiltranzfərās\ Enzyme that helps HDLs transport cholesterol.

Lecithinase \'lesəthənās\ Enzyme acting on lecithin. Suffix *-ase* indicates an enzyme. Word to which it is attached indicates substrate material on which it acts.

Lethargy \'lethə(r)jē\ Drowsiness; indifference.

Light pen \'līt 'pen\ Electronic device (looks like a pen) that gives signals to the computer by touching its tip to the monitor screen.

Linoleic acid \ˌlinəˈlēik àsəd\ (L. *linum*, flax; *oleum*, oil) Essential fatty acid, preferred fuel for the heart muscle.

Lipase \'līˌpās\ (Gr. *lipos*, fat; *-ase*, the suffix for enzyme) Any of a class of enzymes that break down fats. A small quantity of gastric lipase (lipase secreted by the gastric mucosa) acts on emulsified fats of cream and egg yolk. The major digestive lipase is pancreatic lipase, which acts on fats in the small intestine. Enteric lipase acts within the mucosal cells, and lipoprotein lipase clears initial transport fats (chylomicrons) from the bloodstream.

Lipid \'lipəd\ (Gr. *lipos,* fat) The group name for organic substances of fatty nature. The lipids include fats, oils, waxes, and related compounds.

Lipogenesis \,līpə'jenəsəs\ (Gr. *lipos,* fat; *genesis,* formation) Conversion of carbohydrates and protein into body fat; occurs when excessive amounts of these nutrients are consumed.

Lipolysis \lī'päləsəs\ (Gr. *lipos,* fat; *lysis,* dissolution) Breakdown of fat into its component fatty acids and glycerol.

Lipoprotein \,līpə'prō,tēn\ Noncovalent complexes of fat with protein. The lipoproteins probably function as major carriers of lipids in the plasma, since most of the plasma fat is associated with them. Such a combination makes possible the transport of fatty substances in a predominantly aqueous medium such as plasma.

Lipoprotein lipase \,lipə'prō,tēn 'lī,pās\ Enzyme that helps remove triglycerides from chylomicrons.

Log on \'lȯg (¦)ȯn\ To be admitted to a data base or large computer system by the use of a personal code or password for security.

Low-density lipoprotein (LDL) \'lō 'den(t)səd·ē ,līpə'prō,tēn\ Carries at least 66% of the total amount of cholesterol in plasma.

Luminal segmentation \'lümənᵊl ,segmən·,tāshən\ Formation of divisions, or segments, along the alimentary canal. In diverticulitis, this may occur at the site of diverticula and increase the motility of the gastrointestinal tract, promoting diarrhea.

Macrocytic anemia \,makrō¦sid·ik a'nēmēa\ Anemia characterized by red cells that are larger and paler than normal.

Mainframe computer \'mān¦frām kəm'pyüd·ə(r)\ The largest type of computer system; used by large institutions, research centers, universities, and corporations.

Malignant \mə'lignənt\ (L. *malignans,* acting maliciously) Not improving, worsening; resulting in death.

Malnutrition \¦maln(y)ü·'trishən\ Faulty nutrition resulting from poor diet, malassimilation, or overeating.

Marasmus \mə'raz,məs\ (Gr. *marasmos,* withering) Lack of nutrition manifested by wasting.

Medulla \mə'dələ\ Innermost portion of the kidney; site of the loop of Henle.

Megaloblastic anemia \¦megəlō¦blastik ənēmēə\ (Gr. *mega,* large; *blastos,* embryo) Anemia characterized by formation of large immature red blood cells, deficient carriers of oxygen; caused by deficiency of folic acid and hence faulty synthesis of heme.

Menarche \mə'när(,)kē\ Onset of menstruation.

Mendel, Gregor Johann \'mendəl\ (1822-1884) Austrian monk and naturalist; discovered the natural laws governing direct inheritance by offspring of certain traits or characters from one or the other parent.

Mesoderm \'me¦zə,dərm\ Embryonic tissue from which connective tissue, bone, cartilage, muscle, blood, blood vessels, kidney, gonads, lymph, and other organs are derived.

Metabolism \mə'tabə,lizəm\ (Gr. *metaballein,* to turn about, change, alter) The sum of all chemical changes that take place within an organism by which it maintains itself and produces energy for its functioning. Products of these various reactions are called metabolites. Interrelationships of substances in these processes are called metabolic relationships.

Metabolite \mə'tabə,līt\ (Gr. *metaballein,* to turn about, alter, change) Any substance that forms as a result of the breakdown (catabolism), growth, or maintenance (anabolism) of living tissue.

Metallothionein \'med,ᵊlōthīōnē,ēn\ Copper-binding protein; plasma transport carrier.

Micellar bile-fat complex \(')mī¦selə(r) 'bīl 'fat (')käm¦pleks\ (L. *mica,* crumb, grain; *ella,* diminutive suffix) A micelle is a particle formed by an aggregate of molecules, a microscopic unit of protoplasm. In micellar bile-fat complex the particle is formed by the combination of bile salts with fat substances (fatty acids and glycerides) to achieve the absorption of fat across the intestinal mucosa. Bile salt micelles act as detergents to solubilize lipids for digestion and absorption.

Microcomputer \¦mīkrōkəm'pyüd·ə(r)\ The smallest computers, developed around 1975. Microcomputers today have as much or more computing ability as earlier mainframe computers.

Microcytic hypochromic anemia \¦mīkro¦sid·ik 'hīpō-krōmik ə'nēmēə\ Iron deficiency anemia characterized by small pale red blood cells.

Microprocessor \¦mīkrō'prä,sesə(r)\ Small integrated circuit chip holding all the circuits of the "brains" of a computer.

Microvillus \¦mīkrō'viləs\ (*pl.* microvilli) Minute surface projections that cover the edge of each intestinal villus; they are visible only through the electron microscope. This vast array of microvilli on each villus is called the "brush border." The microvilli add a tremendous surface area for absorption.

Milliequivalent \¦milēə'kwiv(ə)lənt\ Unit of measure used for electrolytes in a solution. It is based on the number of ions (cations and anions) in solution, as determined by their concentration in a given volume, not the weights of the various particles. The term refers to the chemical combining power of the solution and is expressed as the number of milliequivalents per liter (mEq/L).

Minicomputer \\ˌminēkəmˈpyüd·ə(r)\\ Larger than a microcomputer but smaller than a standard mainframe computer, though based on the same system as the mainframe. Main unit ranges in size from that of a desk to a refrigerator.

Mitochondrion \\ˌmīd·əˈkändrēən\\ (Gr. *mitos,* thread; *chondrion,* granule) Cell's "powerhouse," a small, spheric- to rod-shaped organelle located in the cell cytoplasm; principal site of energy generation (ATP synthesis); contains enzymes of Krebs cycle and cell respiration, as well as ribonucleic and deoxyribonucleic acids (RNA and DNA) for synthesis of some proteins.

MODEM \\ˈmō̄ˌdem\\ Contraction of "modulator-demodulator"; device that converts and reconverts data and signals transmitted over telephone lines, allowing computers to "speak" with each other.

Module \\ˈmä(ˌ)jül\\ Subcomponents or sections of a system.

Monitor \\ˈmänəd·ə(r)\\ Another name for computer display screen.

Monoamine \\ˈmä(ˌ)nōōmēn\\ Amine molecule containing one amino group, for example, serotonin, dopamine, norepinephrine.

Monosaccharide \\ˈmä(ˌ)nōˈsakəˌrīd\\ (Gr. *monos,* single; *sakcharon,* sugar) Simple single sugar; a carbohydrate containing a single saccharide (sugar) unit.

Monozygote \\ˈmä(ˌ)nōˈzīˌgōt\\ (Gr. *monos,* single; *zygotos,* yoked together) Single fertilized ovum; may result in identical twins.

Mucus \\ˈmyükəs\\ Viscid fluid secreted by mucous membranes and glands, consisting mainly of mucin (a glycoprotein), inorganic salts, and water. Mucus serves to lubricate and protect the gastrointestinal mucosa and to help move the food mass along the digestive tract.

Multiple-purpose \\məltəpəl ˈpərpəs\\ Computer term used to designate those microcomputers that have multiple applications or task capacities, as compared with single special-purpose instruments.

Myelinated \\ˈmīələˌnād·əd\\ (Gr. *myelos,* marrow) Having a sheath or covering of myelin, a protective lipid membrane, such as that insulating axons of nerve cells.

Myelin sheath \\ˈmīələn ˈshēth\\ Protective lipid membrane covering axon shafts of nerve cells; serves as an electrical insulator and impulse transmittor.

Myocardial infarction (MI) \\ˈmīəˌkärdēəl ənˈfärkshən\\ Death of heart tissue resulting from blockage that prevents the flow of blood to or through its coronary arteries.

Myosin \\ˈmīəsən\\ (Gr. *myo,* muscle) Myofibril protein that acts in conjunction with actin to cause the contraction and relaxation of muscle.

Myofibril \\ˈmīoˈfībrəl\\ (Gr. *myo,* muscle; L. *fibrilla,* very small fiber) Slender thread of muscle; runs parallel to the muscle fiber's long axis.

Myoglobin \\ˈmīəˈglōbən\\ Muscle protein (globin) that contains iron (also called myohemoglobin).

Necrosis \\nəˈkrōsəs\\ (Gr. *nekrosis,* deadness) Cell death.

Neoplasm \\ˈnēəˌplazəm\\ (Gr. *neo,* new; *plasma,* a formation) Any new or abnormal growth; uncontrolled or progressive growth. Also called a tumor.

Nephron \\ˈneˌfrän\\ (Gr. *nephros,* kidney) Structural and functional unit of the kidney. The nephron includes the renal corpuscle (glomerulus), the proximal convoluted tubule, the loop of Henle, the distal convoluted tubule, and the collecting tubule, which empties the urine into the renal medulla. The urine passes into the papilla and then to the pelvis of the kidney. Urine is formed by filtration of blood in the glomerulus and by the selective reabsorption and secretion of solutes by cells that comprise the walls of the renal tubules. There are approximately 1 million nephrons in each kidney.

Nephropathy \\neˈfräpəthē\\ (Gr. *nephros,* kidney; *pathos,* disease) Disease of the nephrons in the kidneys, a complication of diabetes.

Nephrosis \\nəˈfrōsəs\\ Inflammation of the nephron.

Network \\ˈnetˌwərk\\ Interconnected group of computers, terminals, or telephones.

Neuritis \\n(y)üˌrīd·əs\\ Inflammation of nerve tissue, accompanied by pain, paralysis, atrophy, and loss of reflexes.

Neuropathy \\n(y)üˈräpəthē\\ (Gr. *neuron,* nerve; *pathos,* disease) Presence of disease and/or change in function of the peripheral nervous system. Also defined as noninflammatory injury to the peripheral nervous system, a complication of diabetes.

Neurotransmiter \\ˈn(y)ürōtran(t)ˈsmid·ə(r)\\ (Gr. *neuron,* nerve + transmitter) Chemical substances that relay messages through the central nervous system.

Niacin \\ˈnīəsən\\ (nicotinic acid) B vitamin; deficiency produces pellagra. Important niacin compounds (NAD and NADP) function as key coenzymes in glucose oxidation. Niacin's relation to pellagra was discovered by Joseph Goldberger. Meat, peanuts, enriched grains, and legumes are major sources of niacin. The essential amino acid, tryptophan, is a precursor of niacin.

Niacin equivalent (NE) \\ˈnīəsən əˈkwiv(ə)lənt\\ A measure of the total dietary sources of niacin equivalent to 1 mg of niacin. Thus an NE is 1 mg of niacin or 60 mg of tryptophan.

Nicotinamide-adenine dinucleotide (NAD) \\ˌnikəˈtēnaˌmīd ˈadᵊnˌēn (ˈ)dīˈn(y)üklēˌoˌtīd\\ A niacin compound that functions in tissue oxidation to release controlled energy.

Nicotinamide-adenine dinucleotide phosphate (NADP) \\ˌnikəˈtēnaˌmīd ˈadᵊnˌēn(ˈ)dīˈn(y)üklēˌōˌtīd ˈfäˌsfāt\\ A niacin compound with three high-energy phosphate bonds, which acts as a vital coenzyme in the "respiratory chains" of tissue oxidation within the cell; controlled energy is made available by this reaction.

Night blindness \'nīt, blīnnəs\ Inability to see well at night in diminished light; due to faulty operation of eyes' light adjustment mechanism result from lack of required vitamin A.

Nitrogen balance \'nītrəjən 'balən(t)s\ The difference between intake and output of nitrogen in the body. If intake is greater, a positive nitrogen balance exists. If output is greater, a negative nitrogen balance exists. For example, during growth when new tissue protein is being formed, nitrogen is retained for protein synthesis, and a state of positive nitrogen balance prevails.

Nonheme \(¦)nänhēm\ Protein portion of hemoglobin that does not contain the heme.

Nonicteric \(¦)nän(')¦k¦terik\ Hepatic disease without jaundice (icterus).

Nulligravida \¦nələ'gravədə\ (L. *nullus*, none; *gravida*, pregnant) Woman who has never been pregnant.

Obesity \ō'bēsəd·ē\ Excessive adipose tissue, more than required for optimal body function.

Occult bleeding \ə'kəlt 'blēdiŋ\ Such a small blood loss that it can be detected only by a microscope or chemical test.

Oliguria \¸älə'g(y)ůrēə\ (Gr. *oligos*, little; *ouron*, urine) Reduced amount of urine in comparison with fluid intake.

Omega (ω) \ō'megə\ The twenty-fourth and final letter of the Greek alphabet; used in numbering system for fatty acids.

Operating system \'äpə¸ratiŋ 'sistəm\ Program that provides specific commands for operating a computer; helps the computer to operate more easily.

Orthomolecular medicine \¦ȯ(r)thəmə'lekyələ(r) 'med əsən\ (Gr. *ortho*, straight, normal, correct) A controversial practice of medicine aimed at restoring the optimal concentrations and functions at the molecular level of substances (for example, vitamins) normally present in the body.

Osmolarity \¸äzmə'larəd·ē\ Concentration of osmotically active particles in solution.

Osmole \'äz¸mōl\ Standard unit of osmotic pressure; equal to the gram molecular weight of a substance divided by the number of ions or particles into which the substance is dissociated in solution.

Osmosis \äz'mōsəs\ (Gr. *osmos*, a thrusting) Passage of a solvent such as water through a membrane that separates solutions of different concentrations. The water passes through the membrane from the area of lower concentration of solute to that of higher concentration of solute, which tends to equalize the concentrations of the two solutions. The rate of osmosis depends on (1) the difference in osmotic pressures of the two solutions, (2) the permeability of

the membrane, and (3) the electric potential across the membrane.

Osteoblast \'ästēə¸blast\ (Gr. *osteo*, bone; *blastos*, germ) Bone-forming cells.

Osteoclast \'ästēə¸klast\ (Gr. *osteo*, bone; *klan*, to break) Giant, multinuclear cells found in depressions on bone surfaces, which caused resorption of bone tissue and the formation of canals.

Osteodystrophy \¸ästēō'distrəfē\ (Gr. *osteon*, bone; L. *dystrophia*, faulty nutrition) Disease often accompanying renal failure in which calcium is lost from the bones; poor bone formation. Renal osteodystrophy is a result of chronic kidney disease, which may begin in childhood, and can lead to renal dwarfism.

Osteomalacia \¸ästēōmə'lāsh(ē)ə\ Softening of bone caused by impaired mineral uptake; usually resulting from calcium and vitamin D deficiency.

Osteoporosis \¸ästēōpə'rōsəs\ (Gr. *osteon*, bone; *poros*, passage + -osis) Abnormal thinning of bone tissue as a result of calcium loss.

Oxidation \¸äksə'dāshən\ Process of cell metabolism resulting in release of energy; involves reactions in which hydrogen atoms are removed from a molecule of substance (oxidation) and transferred to the acceptor molecule (reduction).

Palliative care \'palē¸ād·iv 'ke(ə)r\ (L. *palliatus*, cloaked) Care that gives relief but no cure.

Pantothenic acid \¸pantə¦thenik 'asəd\ (Gr. *pantothen*, "from all sides" or "in every corner") A B vitamin found widely distributed in nature and occurring throughout the body tissues. Pantothenic acid is an essential constituent of the coenzyme A, which has extensive metabolic responsibility as an activating agent of a number of compounds in many tissues.

Paralytic ileus \¸parə¦lid·ik 'ilēəs\ (Gr. *eileos*, from *eilein*, to roll up) Obstruction of the intestines, resulting from inhibition of bowel motility.

Parathyroid hormone (PH) \¦parə'thī¸rȯid 'hȯr¸mōn\ Hormone of the parathyroid gland, which controls calcium and phosphorus metabolism by stimulating the intestinal mucosa to increase calcium absorption, mobilizing calcium rapidly from bone, and causing renal excretion of phosphate.

Parenchyma \pə'reŋkəmə\ (Gr. "anything poured in bedside") Functional elements of an organ.

Parenteral \pər'entərəl\ Not through the alimentary canal; given by injection through a subcutaneous, intramuscular, intravenous, or other route.

Paresthesia \¦pares'thēzh(ē)ə\ (Gr. *para*, beyond; *aisthesis*, perception) Abnormal sensations, such as prickling, burning, and "crawling" of skin.

Parietal cell \pə'riəd·ᵊl 'sel\ (L. *paries*, wall) Cell of the gastric glands in the fundus of the stomach that produces hydrochloric acid.

Parity \'parəd·ē\ (L. *parere*, to bring forth) (1) Number of children born alive. (2) System of regulating prices of farm commodities, usually by government price supports, to provide farmers with the same purchasing power they had in a selected base period.

Paroxysmal \\ˌparəkˈsizməl\\ Recurring in paroxysms.

Pastoral counseling \\ˈpastərəl ˈkaŭn(t)s(ə)liŋ\\ Counseling services provided by a member of the clergy.

Protein-bound iodine (PBI) test \\ˈprō̄ˌtēn ˈbaŭnd ˈīəˌdīn ˈtest\\ Test used to measure thyroid activity by determining the amount of iodine bound to thyroxine and in transit in the plasma.

Pedal edema \\ˈpedᵊl əˈdēmə\\ Edema in the feet.

Pellagra \\pəˈlāgrə\\ (L. *pelle*, skin; Gr. *agra*, seizure) A deficiency disease caused by a lack of niacin in the diet and an inadequate amount of protein containing the amino acid, tryptophan, a precursor of niacin. Pellagra is characterized by skin lesions that are aggravated by exposure to sunlight and by gastrointestinal, mucosal, neurologic, and mental symptoms. Four *D*s often associated with pellagra are dermatitis, diarrhea, dementia, and death.

Peptide linkage \\ˈpepˌtīd ˈliŋkij\\ The characteristic joining of amino acids to form proteins. Such a chain of amino acids is termed a peptide. Depending on its size, it may be a dipeptide fragment of protein digestion or a large polypeptide.

Pepsin \\ˈpepsən\\ The main gastric enzyme specific for proteins. Pepsin begins breaking large protein molecules into shorter chain polypeptides, proteoses, and peptones. Gastric hydrochloric acid is necessary to activate pepsin.

Periodontal disease \\ˌperēōˈdäntᵊl dəˈzēz\\ Disease, such as inflammation, occurring in tissue surrounding the teeth; facilitates tooth loss.

Peristalsis \\ˈperəˈstȯlsəs\\ (Gr. *peri-*, around; *stalsis*, contraction) Coordinated action of circular and longitudinal muscles of the intestine that produces wavelike motions and propels the food mass forward.

Pernicious anemia \\pə(r)ˈnishəs əˈnēmēə\\ A chronic, macrocytic anemia occurring most commonly in whites after age 40. It is caused by the absence of the intrinsic factor normally present in gastric juice and necessary for the absorption of cobalamin (vitamin B_{12}). Pernicious anemia is controlled by intramuscular injections of cobalamin.

Peroral \\ˈpərˈōrəl\\ (L. *per*, through; *oris*, mouth) Performed or administered through the mouth.

Petechiae \\pəˈtēkēə\\ Pinpoint hemorrhages.

pH Symbol used in chemistry to express the degree of acidity or alkalinity (the concentration of H^+) of a solution. It is mathematically based on the negative logarithm expressed as an exponential power (pH = *p*ower of *H*ydrogen ion concentration). Therefore the acidity of a solution varies inversely with the figure expressing it—the smaller the pH number, the greater the degree of acidity. A neutral solution (pure water) has a pH of 7.0. Solutions with a lower pH are acid; those with a higher pH are alkaline. The blood buffer system maintains the blood at a pH of 7.4.

Phlebothrombosis \\ˌflebōthrämˈbōsəs\\ Presence of a clot in a vein.

Phospholipid \\ˈfäsfōˈlipəd\\ Any of a class of fat-related substances that contain phosphorus, fatty acids, and a nitrogenous base. The phospholipids are essential elements in every cell.

Phosphorylation \\ˌfäsˌfȯrəˈlāshən\\ Combining of glucose with a phosphoric acid radical to produce glucose-6-phosphate as a first step in the cellular oxidation of glucose to produce energy. This reaction is catalyzed by the enzyme glucokinase, the specific hexokinase for this purpose.

Photosynthesis \\ˌfōdˈōˈsin(t)thəsəs\\ (Gr. *photos*, light; *synthesis*, putting together) process by which plants containing chlorophyll are able to manufacture carbohydrate by combining carbon dioxide from the air and water from the soil. Sunlight is used as energy, and chlorophyll is a catalyst. The basic chemical reaction is:

$$6CO_2 + 6H_2O \rightarrow C_6H_{12}O_6 + 6O_2$$

Physiatrist \\ˌfizēˈaˌtrəst\\ Physician who uses physical elements (light, heat, cold, electricity) to diagnose, treat, and prevent disease; specialist in rehabilitation medicine.

Pinocytosis \\ˌpinōsīdōsəs\\ (Gr. *pinein*, to drink; *kytos*, cell) Absorption of both fluid and large molecules (products of digestion, such as fat substances) by engulfing them directly into the cell cytoplasm.

Placenta \\pləˈsentə\\ (L. "a flat cake") Tissue that becomes active during pregnancy, providing a selective exchange of soluble particles in the blood to and from the fetus.

Plaque \\ˈplak\\ Patch or flat area forming on tissue; in coronary heart disease, a buildup of fat and other tissue debris in the inside lining of blood vessels.

Plummer-Vinson syndrome \\ˈpləmə(r) ˈvin(t)sən ˈsinˌdrōm\\ Difficulty in swallowing.

Polycythemia \\ˌpäleˌsīˈthēmēə\\ Condition characterized by an excess of red blood cells with a high concentration of hemoglobin. May be caused by an excess of cobalt (the core of vitamin B_{12}), an essential factor in red blood cell formation.

Polysaccharide \\ˈpäleˈsakəˌrīd\\ Class of complex carbohydrates composed of many monosaccharide units. The common members are starch, dextrins, dietary fiber, and glycogen.

Polyunsaturated \\ˈpäleˈənˈsachəˌrātəd\\ Carbon chain containing more than one double bond.

Portal \\ˈpōrˈdᵊl\\ An entryway, usually referring to the portal circulation of blood through the liver. Blood is brought into the liver by the portal vein and out by the hepatic vein.

Postprandial \(')pōst'prandēəl\ Occurring after dinner or after a meal.

Poverty \'pävə(r)d·ē\ Having little or no money, goods, or means of support; scantiness, insufficiency; meagerness. The 1981 federal government definition of the poverty level was an annual income of less than $9287 for a family of four.

Precipitate \prē'sipə,tāt\ (L. *praecipitare*, to cast down) Solid separated out from a solution or suspension.

Precursor \prē'kərsər\ (L. *praecursor*, a forerunner) Something that precedes; in biology, a substance from which another substance is derived.

Preicteric \prēik¦'terik\ Phase of hepatic disease before jaundice (icterus) appears.

Primary deficiency disease \'primerē də'fishənsē də'zēz\ Disease that results directly from dietary lack of a specific essential nutrient. For example, scurvy results if the diet is deficient in vitamin C; beriberi results if the diet is deficient in thiamin.

Primigravida \¦primə'gravədə\ (L. *prima*, first; *gravida*, pregnant) A woman pregnant for the first time.

Printer \'printə(r)\ Major component of a computer system; prints output from the computer. Two main types are dot-matrix and letter-quality impact (daisy wheel) printers.

Printout \'print,aut\ Hard copy computer output printed on paper.

Proenzyme \(')prō'en,zīm\ An inactive precursor converted to the active enzyme by the action of an acid, another enzyme, or other means. Also called zymogen.

Program \'prō,gram\ Specific series of instructions written in a computer language, defining a particular process the computer is to perform.

Prostaglandin \,prästə'glandən\ A group of naturally occurring long-chain fatty acids having local hormonelike actions of widely diverse forms.

Protein-energy malnutrition \prō,tēn 'enə(r)jē (')maln(y)ü·'trishən\ A state of malnutrition caused by a deficiency of both protein and kilocalories as compared with a protein deficiency in the presence of adequate kilocalories.

Proteinuria \,prō,tē'n(y)ùrēə\ Presence of abnormally high levels of serum protein in the urine.

Prothrombin \(')prō'thrämbən\ (Gr. *pro*, before; *thrombos*, a clot) A protein (globulin) circulating in the plasma, essential to the clotting of blood. Prothrombin is produced by the liver. The process requires the presence of vitamin K.

P/S ratio \P/S 'rā,sho\ Ratio of polyunsaturated to saturated fat (fatty acids) in a diet.

Puerperium \,pyüə(r)'pirēəm\ The period of "confinement" after labor.

Pulmonary edema \'pùlmə,nerē ə'dēmə\ Fluid accumulation in the lungs.

Purpura \'pərpyərə\ (L. "purple") Hemorrhaging into the skin producing the reddish purple discoloration of a bruise.

Pyridoxine (vitamin B₆) \,pirə'däk,sēn\ In its active phosphate form (B₆-PO₄), pyridoxine functions as an important coenzyme in many reactions in the metabolism of amino acids and to a lesser extent in the metabolism of glucose and fatty acids. Clinically, pyridoxine deficiency produces a hypochromic, microcytic anemia and disturbances of the central nervous system.

Pyrosis \pī'rōsəs\ (Gr. "burning") Heartburn.

Pyruvate \pī'rü,vāt\ Metabolic end product of glycolysis, which may then be converted to lactate or acetyl CoA.

Radiation \,rādē'āshən\ (L. *radiatio*) Electromagnetic phenomena that has properties combining both wave and particle functions; spans the entire spectrum from low-frequency radio waves through white light to high-frequency gamma rays.

Radioactive ¹³¹I uptake tests \¦rādē(,)ō'aktiv 'əptāk 'test\ Tests of thyroid function using a radioactive isotope of iodine, ¹³¹I.

Renin \'rēnən\ This word is often mispronounced 'renən. (It may then be confused with *rennin*, an enzyme from a calf's stomach used to sour milk to make cheese or puddings.) Enzyme formed in the renal cortex. In response to blood pressure changes, it is secreted to act on its specific substrate, angiotensinogen, to form angiotensin I and II.

Rennin \'renən\ Milk-curdling enzyme of the gastric juice found in human infants and in young animals such as calves. Do not confuse with *renin*, an important enzyme produced by the kidney that plays a vital role in producing angiotensin, a potent vasoconstrictor and stimulant for release of the hormone aldosterone from the adjacent adrenal glands.

Retinol equivalent (RE) \'retᵊnəl ə'kwiv(ə)lənt\ Measure of vitamin A activity currently adopted by FAO/WHO and U.S. National Research Council's Food and Nutrition Board recommendations for vitamin A, replacing the term IU (international units). The measure accounts for dietary variances in preformed vitamin A (retinol) and its precursor, carotene. One RE (retinol equivalent) equals 3.33 IU or 1 μg retinol.

Retinol-binding protein (RBP) \'retᵊnəl 'bindiŋ 'prō,tēn\ The protein carrier for vitamin A.

Retinopathy \,retᵊn'äpəthē\ (L. *retina*, net or network; Gr. *pathos*, disease) Noninflammatory disease of the retina. In diabetes it is characterized by small hemorrhages from broken arteries, yellow waxy discharge, and retinal detachment.

Riboflavin (vitamin B₂) \,rībə'flāvən\ A yellow-green pigment that contains ribose. Vitamin B₂ is found in milk as lactoflavin and also in leafy green vegetables and organ meats. Riboflavin forms coenzymes (FMN and FAD) important in the metabolism of amino acids, glucose, and fatty acids.

Salmonellosis \,salmə,ne'lōsəs\ Infection caused by *Salmonella* (a genus of microbes), characterized by violent diarrhea, abdominal cramps, painful straining on defecation (tenesmus), and fever.

Saponification \sə,pänə_fə'kāshən\ (L. *sapo*, soap; *facere*, to make) Hydrolysis of fats by alkali to produce soaps.

Sarcoma \sär'kōmə\ (Gr. *sarkoma*, fleshy growth) Tumor, usually malignant, arising from connective tissue.

Satiety \sə'tīəd·ē\ (L. *satis*, sufficient + -*ety*, state or condition) A feeling of fullness or satisfaction as after a meal or quenching one's thirst.

Saturate \'sach(ə)rət\ (L. *saturare*, to fill) To cause to unite with the greatest possible amount of another substance through solution, chemical combination, or the like. A saturated fat, for example, is one in which the component fatty acids are filled with hydrogen atoms. A fatty acid is said to be saturated if all available chemical bonds of its carbon chain are filled with hydrogen. If one bond remains unfilled, it is a monounsaturated fatty acid. If two or more bonds remain unfilled, it is a polyunsaturated fatty acid. Fats of animal sources are more saturated. Fats of plant sources are unsaturated.

Schizophrenia \,skitsə'frēnēə\ (Ger. *schizein*, to cleave, split; *phren*, mind) One of a group of severe emotional disorders characterized by retreat from reality (delusions, hallucinations, or ambivalence) or bizarre or regressive behavior. Usually of psychotic proportions.

Scoliosis \,skōlē'ōsəs\ (Ger. *skoliosis*, curvature) Lateral curvature of the spine.

Scurvy \'skərvē\ A hemorrhagic disease caused by lack of vitamin C. Diffuse tissue bleeding occurs, limbs and joints are painful and swollen, bones thicken due to subperiosteal hemorrhage, ecchymoses (large irregular discolored skin areas due to tissue hemorrhages) form, bones fracture easily, wounds do not heal well, gums are swollen and bleeding, and teeth loosen.

Sebaceous \səbāshəs\ Secreting the fatty lubricating substance sebum.

Seborrheic dermatitis \'sebə¦rēik ,dərmə'tīd·əs\ Reddened skin covered with small, greasy flakes. Hard sebaceous plugs may project from pores on the nose, cheeks, or forehead.

Secondary deficiency disease \'sekən,derē də'fishənsē də'zēz\ Disease that results from the inability of the body to use a specific nutrient properly. Such inability may result from either of two general types of failure: (1) failure to absorb the nutrient from the alimentary tract into the blood or (2) failure to metabolize the nutrient normally after it has been absorbed. For example, the malabsorption syndrome is characterized by failure of absorption of fats through the intestinal wall, so that fat is lost in the stool. Phenylketonuria is the inability of the body to metabolize the essential amino acid phenylalanine, so that phenylalanine is lost in the urine.

Secretin \sə'krēd·ən\ Hormone produced in the mucous membrane of the duodenum in response to the entrance of the acid contents of the stomach into the duodenum. Secretin in turn stimulates the flow of pancreatic juice, providing needed enzymes and the proper alkalinity for their action.

Sepsis \'sepsəs\ (Gr. *sepsis*, decay) Presence in the blood or other tissues of pathogenic microorganisms or their toxins; the condition associated with such presence.

Serotonin \,sirə'tōnən\ (L. *sero*-, serum; *tonos*, normal degree of muscle tension) Vasoconstrictor, central neurotransmitter; produced enzymatically from tryptophan.

Software \'soft,wa(a)(e)r\ Computer programs; so named because they have no electronic circuits or other "hard" ware.

Solute \'säl,yüt\ Dissolved substance; particles in solution.

Somatostatin \¦sōməd·ə¦statᵊn\ (Gr. *somatos*, body; *statin*, at rest, not in motion) Hormone produced by the D cells of the islets of Langerhans and the hypothalamus. It inhibits insulin and glucagon production in the pancreas as needed to maintain normal blood glucose levels.
Sample blood glucose self-monitoring schedule
1. Before breakfast
2. 2 hours after breakfast
3. 2 hours after lunch
4. 2 hours before dinner
5. 2 hours after dinner

Spinal cord injury \'spīnᵊl 'kȯ(ə)rd 'inj(ə)rē\ Partial or complete severing of the spinal cord caused by trauma. Partial severance results in general muscle weakness and sensory motor loss. Complete severance results in total paralysis of muscles that are controlled by nerves leaving the spinal cord *below* the level of injury, especially in paraplegia or quadriplegia.

Splanchnic \'splaŋknik\ (Gr. *splanchnikos*, viscus; L. *splanchnicus*) Pertaining to the large interior organs of the body, especially those located in the abdomen.

Sprue \'sprü\ Alternate term for adult celiac disease, a malabsorption syndrome.

Steatorrhea \stēəd·ə'rēə\ (Gr. *steatos*, fat; *rhoia*, flow) Excessive fat amounts in the feces; often caused by malabsorption syndromes.

Stenosis \stə'nōsəs\ Narrowing or closing of a canal or duct.

Steroid \'sti(ə),rȯid\ Any of a large group of fat-related organic compounds, including sterols, bile acids, sex hormones, hormones of the adrenal cortex, and D vitamins.

Stomatitis \\,stomə'tīd·ə̇s\ (Gr. *stoma*, mouth; -itis) Inflammation of the oral mucosa.

Stria \'strīə\ (*pl.* striae) (L. "furrow, groove") Streaks or lines on stretched skin caused by weakening of the elastic tissue by constant tension.

Stricture \'strikchə(r)\ Constriction, as in the gastrointestinal tract, that causes a partial or complete obstruction.

Struvite stone \'strü,vīt 'stōn\ Urinary stone made up of ammonium magnesium phosphate, a very hard crystal.

Substance P \'səbztən(t)s P\ Peptide composed of 11 amino acids; contracts the intestine and dilates blood vessels; may be a neurotransmitter that helps send pain impulses.

Substrate \'səbz,trāt\ (L. *sub*, under *stratum*, layer) The specific organic substance on which a particular enzyme acts.

Sucrose polyester (SPE) \'sü,krōs 'pälē,estə(r)\ "Artificial" fat, manufactured by substitution of sucrose for glycerol in the fat molecule, and thus not usable as fat by the body.

Sulfhydryl group \,səlf'hīdrəl 'grüp\ The —SH radical that forms high-energy sulfur bonds in chemical compounds. In such compounds sulfur participates in important tissue respiration (oxidation) reactions.

Syncope \'siṇkə(,)pē\ Brief loss of consciousness associated with, among other things, reduced levels of extracellular fluid, as occurs during uncontrolled diarrhea.

Syncytium \sə̇n'sish(ē)əm\ Mass of protoplasm that results when cells merge.

Synergism \'sinər,jizəm\ (Gr. *syn*, with or together; *ergon*, work) The joint action of separate agents in which the total effect of their combined action is greater than the sum of their separate actions.

Synthesis \'sin(t)thəsə̇s\ (Gr. *syn-*, with, together; *thesis*, a stated idea or proposition; hence "a putting together") Study of phenomena or development of concepts or substances by putting together the parts to make a whole.

Systolic \sə̇'stälik\ (Gr. *systole*, contraction) Referring to the heart's period of contraction.

Tachycardia \,takə̇'kärdēə\ Rapid heart rate above normal.

Tardive dyskinesia \'tärdiv ,diskə̇'nēzh(ē)ə\ (Fr. tardy, late; Gr. *dyskinesia*, difficulty of moving) Late-appearing brain lesion impairing voluntary movement; typical involuntary repetitive facial movements, mostly affecting elderly persons, induced chiefly by long-term use of antipsychotic drugs.

Terminal \'tərmən°l\ Computer system component, usually including a keyboard and display screen, through which one can send or receive information.

Tetany \'tet(ə)nē\ Disorder caused by abnormal calcium metabolism. Characterized by severe, intermittent, tonic contractions of the extremities and muscular pain caused by lowered blood calcium levels.

Thiamin (vitamin B₁) \thī'amən\ A major B vitamin; essential for the normal metabolism of carbohydrates and fats. It acts as a coenzyme (TPP and TDP) in key reactions.

Thiamin pyrophosphate (TPP) \thī'amə̇n ¦pīrō'fä,sfāt\ Activating coenzyme form of thiamin; plays a key role in carbohydrate metabolism.

Thrombosis \thräm'bōsə̇s\ Development of a blood clot (thrombus) that lodges in a blood vessel and cuts off the blood supply at that point.

Thyroid-stimulating hormone (TSH) \'thī,roid 'stimyəlātiṇ 'hȯr,mōn\ Hormone secreted by the anterior pituitary gland that regulates uptake of iodine and synthesis of thyroxine by the thyroid gland.

Thyroxine \thī'räk,sēn\ The iodine-containing hormone produced by the thyroid gland.

Tocopherol \tə'käfə,rȯl\ (Gr. *tokos*, childbirth; *pherein*, to bring) Vitamin E; so named because of its association with reproduction in rats.

Total parenteral nutrition (TPN) \'tōd·°l 'pa(a)rənteral n(y)ü-¦trishən\ Feeding of a nutritionally complete solution through a large central vein (see Chapter 22).

Toxemia \täk'sēmēə\ Formerly used term (current official term of American College of Obstetricians and Gynecologists is pregnancy-induced hypertension—PIH); a metabolic disturbance that usually manifests itself in the third trimester with symptoms of hypertension, abnormal edema, and albuminemia. If uncontrolled, leads to a coma or convulsions.

Trans \'tran(t)s\ (L., "through") Having certain atoms or radicals in a chemical structure on opposite sides.

Transamination \(,)tran(t)s,amə'nāshən\ Transfer of the amino group (NH₂) from an amino acid to a carbon residue to form another amino acid. The newly formed compound is classed a nonessential amino acid, since the body can synthesize it and does not depend on the diet to supply it.

Transcobalamin I \\,tranz'kōbōlə¦mēn\ Cobalamin-binding protein carrier for transport in bloodstream.

Transferrin \tranz'ferən\ An iron-binding protein complex, a serum beta-globulin; the transport form of iron in the body.

Transketolation \tranz'kēdolāshən\ Transfer of the first unit two-carbon group from one sugar to another in glucose oxidation.

Transmangamin \tranz'maṇgəmən\ Manganese transport carrier, a compound with a plasma protein beta-globulin.

Transmural \tranz'myùrəl\ (L. *trans*, across, through; *muralis*, from *murus*, wall) Through the wall of an organ; extending through or affecting the entire thickness of the wall of an organ or cavity.

Transpyloric \tranz'pīlȯrik\ Passing through the distal opening of the stomach.

Triglyceride \(')trī'glisə,rīd\ A compound of three

fatty acids esterified to glycerol. A neutral fat, synthesized from carbohydrate, stored in adipose tissue. It releases free fatty acids into the blood on being hydrolyzed by enzymes.

Trophoblast \'träfə,blast\ (Gr. *trope,* nutrition; *blastos,* germ) Ectodermal tissue that attaches the ovum to the wall of the uterus and supplies nutrients to the embryo.

Trypsin \'tripsən\ A protein-splitting (proteolytic) enzyme secreted by the pancreas that acts in the small intestine to reduce proteins to shorter chain polypeptides and dipeptides.

Ultrasound \ˌəltrə'saủnd\ Sound waves at a frequency above that which can be heard by the human ear (20 kilocycles/second); in controlled doses can be used as a therapeutic or diagnostic tool, such as to determine skinfold thickness.

Uremia \yə'rēmēə\ (Gr. *ouron,* urine; *haima,* blood) Presence in the blood of large amounts of by-products of protein metabolism; caused by impaired nephron function leading to the inability to excrete urea and other products. This is a toxic condition characterized by headache, nausea, vomiting, diminished vision, convulsions, or coma.

User-friendly \'yüzə(r) 'frendlē\ Easy to use; self-explanatory; systems that are more tolerant of human error or carelessness.

Vagotomy \vā'gäd·ə_mē\ (L. *vagus,* wandering; Gr. *tome,* a cutting) Interruption of the impulses carried by the vagus nerve(s), resulting in prevention of increased flow or acidity of gastric secretions.

Valence \'vālən(t)s\ (L. *valens,* powerful) Power of an element or a radical to combine with or to replace other elements or radicals. Atoms of various elements combine in definite proportions. The valence number of an element is the number of atoms of hydrogen with which one atom of the element can combine.

Varices \'va(a)rə,sēz\ Enlarged veins.

Vasoactive \ˌvā(ˌ)zōaktiv\ (L. *vas,* vessel) Having an effect on the diameter of blood vessels.

Vasopressin (ADH) \ˌvāzō'presˀn\ Hormone secreted by the posterior pituitary gland in response to body stress, which acts primarily on the distal renal tubule, causing the reabsorption of water. The result is diminished urinary output, thus the term antidiuretic hormone (ADH).

Very low–density lipoprotein (VLDL) \'verē 'lō 'den(t)səd·ē ˌlipə'prō,tēn\ Name derived from its position in electrophoresis, a method of analyzing lipoprotein fractions in the blood.

Villikinin \'viləkinən\ Hormone produced by glands in the upper intestinal mucosa in response to presence of chyme entering the intestine. Villikinin stimulates alternating contractions and extensions of the villi. This motion of the villi constantly agitates the mucosal surface, which stirs and mixes the chyme and exposes additional nutrient material for absorption.

Villous adenoma \'viləs ˌadˀn'ōmə\ (L. *villus,* "tuft of hair"; Gr. *adenos,* gland; -oma) Soft, large protrusion on the mucosa of the large intestine.

Villus \'viləs\ (*pl.* villi) (L. *villus,* "tuft of hair") Small protrusions from the surface of a membrane.

Volition \vō 'lishən\ Deliberate action.

Wilson's disease \'wilsənz də'zēz\ Rare hereditary disease in which large amounts of copper are absorbed by and accumulate in the liver, brain, kidneys, and cornea. Produces degenerative changes in brain and liver tissue.

Xanthoma \zan'thōmə\ (Gr. *xanthos,* yellow) Fatty, yellowish colored plaque deposit in the skin.

Xerophthalmia \ˌzi,räf'thalmēə\ (Gr. *xeros,* dry; *ophthalmos,* eye) A disease of the eye in which the cornea and conjunctiva become dry.

Zwitterion \ˌtsvid·əˌrīən\ The term given to amino acids to describe the capacity, when ionized in a solution, to behave as either an acid or a base depending on the need of the solution in which they are present. This dual nature makes amino acids good buffer substances.

Zygote \'zī,gōt\ (Gr. *zygotos,* yoked together) Fertilized ovum; the single cell before the division process starts.

Index

Recommended Daily Dietary Allowances, cont'd

Mean Heights and Weights and Recommended Energy Intake

Category	Age (years)	Weight (kg)	Weight (lb)	Height (cm)	Height (in)	Energy Needs (with range) (kcal)		Energy Needs (with range) (MJ)
Infants	0.0-0.5	6	13	60	24	kg × 115	(95-145)	kg × 0.48
	0.5-1.0	9	20	71	28	kg × 105	(80-135)	kg × 0.44
Children	1-3	13	29	90	35	1300	(900-1800)	5.5
	4-6	20	44	112	44	1700	(1300-2300)	7.1
	7-10	28	62	132	52	2400	(1650-3300)	10.1
Males	11-14	45	99	157	62	2700	(2000-3700)	11.3
	15-18	66	145	176	69	2800	(2100-3900)	11.8
	19-22	70	154	177	70	2900	(2500-3300)	12.2
	23-50	70	154	178	70	2700	(2300-3100)	11.3
	51-75	70	154	178	70	2400	(2000-2800)	10.1
	76+	70	154	178	70	2050	(1650-2450)	8.6
Females	11-14	46	101	157	62	2200	(1500-3000)	9.2
	15-18	55	120	163	64	2100	(1200-3000)	8.8
	19-22	55	120	163	64	2100	(1700-2500)	8.8
	23-50	55	120	163	64	2000	(1600-2400)	8.4
	51-75	55	120	163	64	1800	(1400-2200)	7.6
	76+	55	120	163	64	1600	(1200-2000)	6.7
Pregnancy						+300		
Lactation						+500		

From Recommended Dietary Allowances, Revised 1979. Food and Nutrition Board National Academy of Sciences–National Research Council, Washington, D.C.

The data in this table have been assembled from the observed median heights and weights of children together with desirable weights for adults for the mean heights of men (70 in) and women (64 in) between the ages of 18 and 34 years as surveyed in the U.S. population (HEW/NCHS data).

The energy allowances for the young adults are for men and women doing light work. The allowances for the two older age-groups represent mean energy needs over these age spans, allowing for a 2% decrease in basal (resting) metabolic rate per decade and a reduction in activity of 200 kcal/day for men and women between 51 and 75 years, 500 kcal for men over 75 years, and 400 kcal for women over 75 years. The customary range of daily energy output is shown for adults in parentheses and is based on a variation in energy needs of ±400 kcal at any one age, emphasizing the wide range of energy intakes appropriate for any group of people.

Energy allowances for children through age 18 are based on median energy intakes of children these ages followed in longitudinal growth studies. The values in parentheses are 10th and 90th percentiles of energy intake and indicate the range of energy consumption among children of these ages.